Introducing The CORE

Demystifying the Body of an Athlete

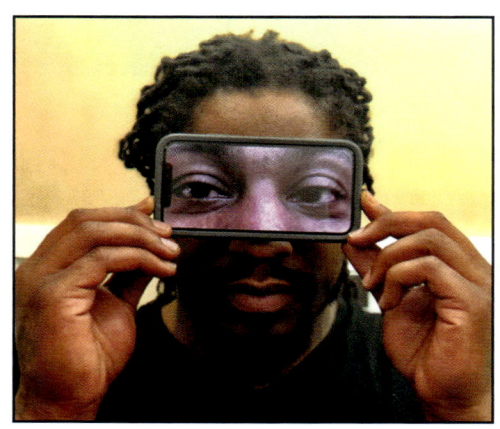

To understand the core, you must put on new eyes.
The core is like family. To go forward, your family must stay together.
—Marshawn Lynch, famous NFL running back.

Introducing The CORE
Demystifying the Body of an Athlete

Editor
William C. Meyers, MD, MBA

Co-Editors
Marc J. Philippon, MD
Adam C. Zoga, MD, MBA
Alexander E. Poor, MD
Johannes B. Roedl, MD, PhD
Jim McCrossin, MS, ATC, CSCS, PES, CES, CKTP
Alex McKechnie, PT, MCSP

Guest Writer
Michael J. Bradley, MLA

Illustrator
Rob Gordon, MFA, CMI

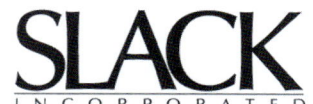

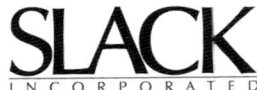

SLACK Incorporated
6900 Grove Road
Thorofare, NJ 08086 USA
856-848-1000   Fax: 856-848-6091
www.Healio.com/books
© 2019 by William C. Meyers

 Figures I-3A/1-6D, 1-5/1-6ABCDE, 1-8, 1-11, 1-12, 1-13, 1-14AB, 1-16, 1-18, 2-1, 2-2, 2-3ABCD, 2-5, 2-6, 2-7, 2-8, 2-14, 2-15, 3-1, 3-3, 3-6, 4-1, 4-6, 4-7, 4-8, 4-10AB, 4-11ABC, 4-14, 5-25, 6-1, 6-2, 6-4, 6-5, 6-9A, 7-1, 7-2, 7-3A, 7-6ABCD, 9-1, 9-2B, 11-4, 12-1AB, 13-1, 13-2C, 13-3, 13-5, 14-1, 14-2, 14-3, 14-6, 14-7A, 15-1, 15-7, 18-1, 18-2, 18-3, 19-1, 20-1, 20-4, 23-1, 26-1, 27-1, 27-3, 28A-1, 28A-5, 28A-8, 29-2, 30-1, 31-1, 32-1, 32-2, 33-1, 34-6AB, 34-7, 35-1, 40-1AB, 40-2, 40-7, 40-8 are from Shutterstock. Figures 1-7, 4-13, 5-15, 5-24, 5-26, 5-27, 13-2B, 15-8, 27-19, 29-1, 34-4, 35-3, 40-5 are from iStock. Figure 31-3 is from Colourbox. Figure 39-2 is from GoGraph.

All rights reserved. No part of this book may be reproduced, stored in a retrieval system or transmitted in any form or by any means, electronic, mechanical, photocopying, recording or otherwise, without written permission from the author, except for brief quotations embodied in critical articles and reviews.

The procedures and practices described in this publication should be implemented in a manner consistent with the professional standards set for the circumstances that apply in each specific situation. Every effort has been made to confirm the accuracy of the information presented and to correctly relate generally accepted practices. The authors, editors, and publisher cannot accept responsibility for errors or exclusions or for the outcome of the material presented herein. There is no expressed or implied warranty of this book or information imparted by it. Care has been taken to ensure that drug selection and dosages are in accordance with currently accepted/recommended practice. Off-label uses of drugs may be discussed. Due to continuing research, changes in government policy and regulations, and various effects of drug reactions and interactions, it is recommended that the reader carefully review all materials and literature provided for each drug, especially those that are new or not frequently used. Some drugs or devices in this publication have clearance for use in a restricted research setting by the Food and Drug and Administration or FDA. Each professional should determine the FDA status of any drug or device prior to use in their practice.

All opinions expressed by the authors and quoted sources are their own and do not necessarily reflect the opinions of the publisher. Any review or mention of specific companies or products is not intended as an endorsement by the author or publisher.

SLACK Incorporated uses a review process to evaluate submitted material. Prior to publication, educators or clinicians provide important feedback on the content that we publish. We welcome feedback on this work.

Library of Congress Cataloging-in-Publication Data

Names: Meyers, William C., M.D., editor. | Philippon, Marc J., 1965- editor.
Title: Introducing the core : demystifying the body of an athlete / editor, William C. Meyers, MD, MBA ; co-editors, Marc J. Philippon, MD [and five others] ; guest writer, Michael J. Bradley, MLA ; illustrator Rob Gordon, MFA, CMI.
Description: Thorofare, NJ : SLACK Incorporated, [2019] | Includes bibliographical references and index.
Identifiers: LCCN 2019002104 (print) | LCCN 2019004499 (ebook) | ISBN 9781630915162 (epub) | ISBN 9781630915179 (web) | ISBN 9781630915155 (hardcover : alk. paper)
Subjects: LCSH: Sports--Physiological aspects. | Athletes--Health and hygiene.
Classification: LCC RC1235 (ebook) | LCC RC1235 .B72 2019 (print) | DDC 612/.044--dc23
LC record available at https://lccn.loc.gov/2019002104

For permission to reprint material in another publication, contact Dr. William C. Meyers.

Printed in the United States of America.

Last digit is print number: 10 9 8 7 6 5 4 3 2 1

DEDICATION

- Our patients and the entire certified athletic training world
- All other fitness specialties
- Appreciating the history of medicine
- Leonardo da Vinci
- Brian, Erica, Riki, and Marley
- Cindy, Coleman, Remy, Corey, Jordan, and Age
- Sherry, my resident and attending colleagues, and everyone else who contributed to my well-being during the years of every other night call and then every night call
- Mom and Dad, Ann Marie, Marcia
- The North Durham Little League
- Inspiration from Steve Bandura, Mo'Ne Davis, and the rest of the Marian Anderson Monarchs
- My closest friends over the years: Joe and Annie, Ravi, R. Scott, John and Linda Nelson, the Doyk, the two Dicks, Mike Foley, Ted, Andres, Ari, Frank B., Steve Klasko, Rick Homan, Chris Wilmot, Tom Nerney, and everyone close I failed to mention
- Friends and professional colleagues
- The development of liver surgery
- Lee Hirsch, Bob Knarr, and the development of minimally invasive surgery
- The AHPBA, Tom Starzl, Bill Longmire, Marty Adson, Henri Bismuth
- Eddie Joe Reddick
- The Crowleys and Polar Beverages
- The sports world
- The sports medicine world, for accepting this outsider into it, and ISHA
- Traditional medicine and surgery
- Physicians, surgeons, and others who hold to the old principles of medicine
- Harvard University and the memories of my advisors, Bud Collins, Peter Gammons, Dr. Thomas Quigley, and Managing Editor Tom Winship
- *The Boston Globe* and *The Hasty Pudding Show*
- Botafogo and Flamengo
- David C. Sabiston
- Duke University
- Frank Bassett, Bill Garrett, and the rest of the Duke University sports medicine staff
- The Vincera Institute, Lashawn, Krista, Christy, Rita, the founding seven, our wonderful current staff, academic partners and co-owners, and the support and camaraderie you all provide

Contents

Dedication..*v*
Acknowledgments..*ix*
Editors and Illustrator..*xi*
Contributing Authors..*xiii*
Foreword by Michael William Krzyzewski..*xvii*
Foreword by James Rheuben Andrews, MD..*xix*
Foreword by Bryan Talmadge Kelly, MD..*xxi*
Introduction..*xxiii*

Section One   **The Way We Were*** **1**
*from the romantic comedy starring Barbra Streisand and Robert Redford

Chapter 1	What's the Core? It Seems Kind of Important	3
Chapter 2	New Eyes—Medicine's Inability to See the Core	13
Chapter 3	The Eureka Moment for the Core	21
Chapter 4	The Difficulty Abandoning Old Eyes—"Unseeing"	31

Section Two   **New Universe*** **41**
*from the book imprint for Marvel Comics

Chapter 5	Presenting…the Core!	43
Chapter 6	Some Concepts to Keep in Mind	59
Chapter 7	The Pubic Bone	69
Chapter 8	The "Harness"	81
Chapter 9	The Rectus Abdominis—Our "Cinderella Muscle"	93
Chapter 10	The Adductors—Demystifying Them	105
Chapter 11	The Rectus Femoris—The "Rodney Dangerfield Muscle"	119
Chapter 12	The Iliopsoas—aka the Psoas—aka the "Eminem Muscle"	129
Chapter 13	The Glutes—The "New Beauty Muscles"	141
Chapter 14	The Other Muscles—Hip and Core Stability	147
Atlas	Stargazing—Seeing the Constellation of Core Diagnoses	156
Chapter 15	So, You Want to Become a Doctor? Part One—Diagnostic Ambushes	169
Chapter 16	Fifteen Core Principles	179
Chapter 17	So, You Want to Become a Doctor? Part Two—History, Physical Examination, Imaging, and Other Tests	183
Chapter 18	Nerves in the Core—A "Fifth Dimension" *Enrique Aradillas, MD*	191
Chapter 19	The Universe of Diagnoses	203
Chapter 20	How the Core Universe Forms	207
Chapter 21	Optimizing and Fixing the Core Muscles	217

Section Three   **Hip Hop Movement*** **227**
*from the subculture that formed in the early 1970s in the South Bronx

Chapter 22	The Hip—How Far We Have Come! *J. W. Thomas Byrd, MD*	229
Chapter 23	Private Eyes on the Hip—Sometimes a Culprit in Pelvic Pain and Pelvic Floor Disorders *Struan H. Coleman, MD, PhD*	237

Chapter 24	Traps in Hip Arthroscopy...245 *John P. Salvo Jr, MD and Kevin O'Donnell, MD*	
Chapter 25	Special Considerations in Adolescents..253 *Fares S. Haddad, MD (Res), FRCS (Orth), Dip Sports Med, FFSEM;* *Feras Ya'ish, FRCS (Orth), MBBS; and Konstantinos Tsitskaris, MSc, MRCS, FRCS (Tr & Orth)*	
Chapter 26	Hip Arthroscopy—Frontiers and Limitations...269 *Anil S. Ranawat, MD; Brian J. Rebolledo, MD; and Jacqueline M. Brady, MD*	
Chapter 27	Complex Core-Hip Considerations in the Athlete— From "Lighting the Lamp" to "Getting Your Face Washed"..281 *Marc J. Philippon, MD; William R. Mook, MD; and Karen K. Briggs, MPH*	
Chapter 28	Biomechanics 　(A) Tilt and Version..295 　*Eric J. Kropf, MD; Struan H. Coleman, MD, PhD; and Alexander E. Poor, MD* 　(B) Altered Hip Biomechanics and the Muscles..303 　*Marc R. Safran, MD and Joshua Sampson, MD*	
Chapter 29	What Lies Behind the Hip—The Deep Derrière..309 *Hal David Martin, DO*	

Section Four — Shared Responsibility* 327
*from both Democratic and Republican Presidential platforms

Chapter 30	Fixing Everything—Putting the Core Universe Into Perspective 329	
Chapter 31	Managing the Ruptured Proximal Hamstring...335 *Christopher C. Dodson, MD and Daniel P. Woods, MD*	
Chapter 32	Rehabilitation and Performance—From Snake Oil Salespeople to Well-Oiled Machines.............345 *Alexander E. Poor, MD; Jim McCrossin, MS, ATC, CSCS, PES, CES, CKTP; and* *Alex McKechnie, PT, MCSP*	
Chapter 33	The Final Stage of Rehab—Getting All the Way Back...357 *Andrew Small, PT, CSCS, RSCC*D, MPhtySt, BSc (HMS-ExSci)*	
Chapter 34	Don't Forget the Thorax..365 *Tracey Vincel, PT, MPhty, CBBA and Andrew Barr, DPT, MSc Spt Sci, BSc (Hons) Physio, CSCS*	
Chapter 35	The Yin and Yang of Yoga..381 *Biz Magarity, MBA, C-IAYT, 500 E-RYT*	
Chapter 36	Perspectives of Nonoperative Sports Medicine Physicians 　(A) Nonoperative Interventions for the Management of "Hip" Pain..........................389 　*Eugene Hong, MD, CAQSM, FAAFP and Sarah C. Hoffman, DO, FAAP, CAQSM* 　(B) We Need More Studies ....394 　*David Stone, MD*	
Chapter 37	An Osteopath's View of the Core Universe—Manipulative Therapies—A Functional Approach.....399 *Jason Hartman, DO; Philip J. Koehler III, DO, MS; and Veronica Williams, DO, Illustrator*	
Chapter 38	A Chiropractor's Perspective—The Knee Bone's Connected to the Thigh Bone… ....413 *Marc Legere, DC, BS, BA*	

Section Five — Life Is a Journey* 421
*from "Life is a journey and not a destination," attributed to Transcendentalist poet
Ralph Waldo Emerson and revisited by AM O'Shea, a very smart CEO

Chapter 39	Putting It All Together—A Patient's Perspective on the Core ....423 *Esra Roan, PhD*	
Chapter 40	Final Chapter—Seeing Things a Whole New Way...429	

Quiz Answers...435
Financial Disclosures 437
Index..439

ACKNOWLEDGMENTS

- Greg Horner—book coordinator, photographer, and videographer
- Thomas Hart and Adam Miller—image consultants
- Rita Greiman—encourager and artist
- Ann Marie O'Shea, for all that she does
- Marcia Horner, for doing the rest of it
- Brooke Havens and Leigh Waters—brilliant ATCs and much more
- Struan Coleman—partner in risk
- Blake Bowden and all the other medical students who contributed
- Garrison, Connor, and Alec—proofers extraordinaire
- Nicole Curran—for taking charge
- The forbearance of my staff and their camera-friendliness

EDITORS AND ILLUSTRATOR

Michael J. Bradley, MLA
Writer
Broadcaster
Villanova University Professor

Rob Gordon, MFA, CMI
Freelance and Medical Illustrator
Charter Member of the Association of Medical Illustrators
brightinvisions.com

Jim McCrossin, MS, ATC, CSCS, PES, CES, CKTP
Director of Sports Medicine
Philadelphia Flyers
Philadelphia, Pennsylvania

Alex McKechnie, PT, MCSP
Assistant Coach/Director of Sports Science
Toronto Raptors Basketball Club
Toronto, Ontario, Canada

William C. Meyers, MD, MBA
Founder
President
Vincera Institute
Professor of Surgery
Sidney Kimmel Medical College
Thomas Jefferson University
Duke University
Drexel University

Marc J. Philippon, MD
Managing Partner
The Steadman Clinic
Director of Sports Medicine Fellowship
Co-Chairman
Steadman Philippon Research Institute
Vail, Colorado

Alexander E. Poor, MD
Partner
Vincera Institute
Philadelphia, Pennsylvania

Johannes B. Roedl, MD, PhD
Assistant Professor of Radiology
Division of Musculoskeletal Imaging and Interventions
Thomas Jefferson University
Philadelphia, Pennsylvania

Adam C. Zoga, MD, MBA
Clinical Professor of Radiology
Thomas Jefferson University
Vice Chair for Clinical Practice
Director of Musculoskeletal MRI
Department of Radiology
Thomas Jefferson University Hospitals
Philadelphia, Pennsylvania

Contributing Authors

James Rheuben Andrews, MD (Foreword)
Founder
Andrews Sports Medicine and Orthopedic Center
Clinical Professor of Orthopedic Surgery
University of Alabama Birmingham Medical School
University of Virginia School of Medicine
University of South Carolina Medical School
Adjunct Professor of Orthopedic Surgery
University of South Alabama
Clinical Professor of Orthopedics
Tulane University School of Medicine

Enrique Aradillas, MD (Chapter 18)
Philadelphia, Pennsylvania

Andrew Barr, DPT, MSc Spt Sci, BSc (Hons) Physio, CSCS (Chapter 34)
Quantum Performance Lab
Los Angeles, California

Jacqueline M. Brady, MD (Chapter 26)
Assistant Professor and Orthopedic Surgeon
Oregon Health & Science University
Portland, Oregon

Karen K. Briggs, MPH (Chapter 27)
Director of Hip Research
Center for Outcomes-Based Orthopaedic Research
Steadman Philippon Research Institute
Vail, Colorado

J. W. Thomas Byrd, MD (Chapter 22)
Nashville Hip Institute
Nashville, Tennessee

Struan H. Coleman, MD, PhD (Chapters 23 and 28A)
Associate Professor in Orthopedic Surgery
Weill Cornell Medical College
Associate Attending Orthopedic Surgery
Hospital for Special Surgery
Team Physician
New York Mets Baseball Club
New York, New York
Director of Hip Preservation
Vincera Institute
Philadelphia, Pennsylvania

Christopher C. Dodson, MD (Chapter 31)
Director of Orthopaedics
Vincera Institute
Head Team Orthopaedic Surgeon
Philadelphia Eagles
Head Team Physician
Philadelphia 76ers
Philadelphia, Pennsylvania

Fares S. Haddad, MD (Res), FRCS (Orth), Dip Sports Med, FFSEM (Chapter 25)
Divisional Director
University College London Hospitals
Director
Institute of Sport, Exercise, and Health
London, United Kingdom

Jason Hartman, DO (Chapter 37)
Miami, Florida

Sarah C. Hoffman, DO, FAAP, CAQSM (Chapter 36A)
Attending
Pediatrics and Sports Medicine
Maine Medical Partners Orthopedics & Sports Medicine
South Portland, Maine

Eugene Hong, MD, CAQSM, FAAFP (Chapter 36A)
Chief Physician Executive
MUSC Physicians
Professor
Family Medicine and Orthopedics
Medical University of South Carolina
Charleston, South Carolina

Bryan Talmadge Kelly, MD (Foreword)
Chief of Sports Medicine Service
Hospital for Special Surgery
Professor of Orthopedic Surgery
Weill Cornell Medical College
New York, New York

Philip J. Koehler III, DO, MS (Chapter 37)
Department of Physical Medicine and Rehabilitation
Thomas Jefferson University Hospital
Philadelphia, Pennsylvania

Contributing Authors

Eric J. Kropf, MD (Chapter 28A)
Associate Professor and Chair
Director of Sports Medicine
Orthopaedics and Sports Medicine
Lewis Katz School of Medicine
Temple University
Philadelphia, Pennsylvania

Michael William Krzyzewski (Foreword)
Head Men's Basketball Coach
Duke University
Head Coach
USA Basketball Senior National Team
Naismith Basketball Hall of Fame Enshrinee
Professor
Duke University Fuqua School of Business

Marc Legere, DC, BS, BA (Chapter 38)
Creator of PATCH Technique
Founder of PATCH Chiropractic
Philadelphia, Pennsylvania

Biz Magarity, MBA, C-IAYT, 500 E-RYT (Chapter 35)
Philadelphia, Pennsylvania

Hal David Martin, DO (Chapter 29)
Hip Preservation Center
Baylor University Medical Center
Dallas, Texas

William R. Mook, MD (Chapter 27)
Orthopedic Surgeon and Sports Medicine Specialist
OrthoVirginia
Reston, Virginia

Kevin O'Donnell, MD (Chapter 24)
Orthopaedic Sports Medicine Fellow
Rothman Institute
Philadelphia, Pennsylvania

Anil S. Ranawat, MD (Chapter 26)
Hospital for Special Surgery
New York, New York

Brian J. Rebolledo, MD (Chapter 26)
Orthopaedic Chief Resident
Hospital for Special Surgery
New York, New York

Esra Roan, PhD (Chapter 39)
CEO/President
SOMAVAC Medical Solutions, Inc
Memphis, Tennessee

Marc R. Safran, MD (Chapter 28B)
Professor
Orthopaedic Surgery
Chief
Division of Sports Medicine
Stanford University
Redwood City, California

John P. Salvo Jr, MD (Chapter 24)
Associate Professor
Orthopaedic Surgery
The Sydney Kimmel Medical College
Thomas Jefferson University Hospital
Director
Hip Arthroscopy Program
Rothman Institute
Philadelphia, Pennsylvania

Joshua Sampson, MD (Chapter 28B)
Clinical Research Fellow
Department of Orthopaedic Surgery
Stanford University
Redwood City, California

*Andrew Small, PT, CSCS, RSCC*D, MPhtySt, BSc (HMS-ExSci) (Chapter 33)*
Milwaukee, Wisconsin

David Stone, MD (Chapter 36B)
Department of Orthopedic Surgery
Allegheny Health Network
Pittsburgh, Pennsylvania

Konstantinos Tsitskaris, MSc, MRCS, FRCS (Tr & Orth) (Chapter 25)
SpR Trauma and Orthopaedics
North East Thames Rotation
University College London Hospitals
London, United Kingdom

Tracey Vincel, PT, MPhty, CBBA (Chapter 34)
New York, New York

Veronica Williams, DO (Chapter 37 Illustrator)
Doctor of Osteopathic Medicine Candidate
Philadelphia College of Osteopathic Medicine
Philadelphia, Pennsylvania

Daniel P. Woods, MD (Chapter 31)
Orthopaedic Sports Medicine Fellow
Rothman Institute
Philadelphia, Pennsylvania

Feras Ya'ish, FRCS (Orth), MBBS (Chapter 25)
Consultant
Trauma and Orthopaedics
Sheikh Khalifa Medical City
Abu Dhabi, United Arab Emirates

Foreword by Michael William Krzyzewski

For the past few years, we have really stressed core strength at Duke. It improves an athlete's base, and that's vital, because so much emanates from there.

Strength, power, and endurance all flow from the core. And taking care of the core is also important for increasing performance.

If an athlete is strong in the middle, his/her extremities will be helped. For years, people didn't emphasize that, and as a result there were more extremity injuries than there should have been. Nothing can eliminate those injuries entirely, but good core strength helps cut them down.

We believe in training the core and work with our players on it year-round. We do a lot of band work that helps build the core. The training methods for that area of the body have changed throughout my career at Duke. Of course, I have been coaching 41 years, so a lot of things have changed, especially since I played. Back then, we didn't even lift weights.

We've put a huge emphasis on the hips. They are vital for players to get into their defensive stance (Figure F-1), for the running we do and the explosive strength our players need. Hip strength and core strength determine whether a player has a better landing base after jumping, and we are up and down on the court a lot. If players have weak cores, they aren't landing on strong bases.

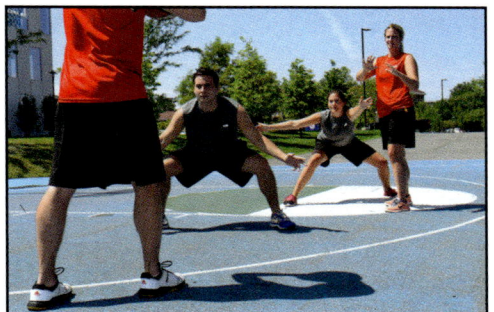

Figure F-1. The Duke University defensive stance exhibits the nitty gritty of the core's neutral engagement posture. When well executed as a team, the posture displays "attitude."

It all makes more sense. That part of the body, which has been neglected, gives the body so much. A lot of people see 6-pack abs or strong biceps or leg muscles, but that's not what we're talking about. We're talking about strength you can't see, but you see it in performance.

I think one of the reasons that people haven't done a lot with the core is that you can't see the parts of the body that make up the core. But so much emanates from that.

So, it works for us in terms of injury prevention and performance. If a player on our men's basketball team isn't physically ready to play, I don't care how much talent he has, he can't get onto the court. We're making sure he's on the court as many minutes as possible, especially our better players. When they are on the court, we want to improve their levels of performance.

Having a strong core pays huge dividends. It gives a player more confidence in his/her abilities. It provides more endurance and confidence. Any athlete has to trust his/her body. With good core strength, the athlete can have more confidence and perform to his/her top capability.

This book, and the work Bill Meyers has done in the field, will bring good core health to the forefront and help everyone—elite athletes and others—to understand the importance of a strong core for performance and confidence.

Suggested Videos

Krzyzewski M. Duke Basketball: A Clinic With Coach K [DVD]. Champaign, IL: Human Kinetics; 2003.

Open practice: defensive skill development featuring Mike Krzyzewski [video]. YouTube. https://www.youtube.com/watch?v=omg8mm6Uejs. Published November 4, 2014.

Foreword by James Rheuben Andrews, MD

The core is the latest thing in physical development and performance. Nobody ever mentioned the core until 5 or 10 years ago, and while I'm sure that some of the physical fitness gurus might have used the word, we didn't use it in sports medicine. Bill Meyers has brought the core to the forefront.

Now, even in baseball, injury patterns you see in the shoulder and elbow are related to core imbalance. If you don't have a good core, you don't have good balance, and your injury chances go up. Building the core has become a major part of the rehabilitation we do with all athletes, especially baseball players.

For example, a pitcher who is throwing from the mound and goes into the stretch position has to drive off of one leg. If he/she doesn't have a good core, he/she is going to stress his/her shoulder and elbow and create an unstable situation. We will have athletes stand on one leg and do a dip. From that, we can tell if their core is strong. If it's weak, they almost fall over.

The core is important in running, because it helps with the stability of the lower extremities. That goes for every sport. If your core is not strong, you can become either bow-legged or knock-kneed. In basketball, when you come down for a rebound, or if you are a wide receiver and land after making a catch, if you don't have good core strength, all the impact goes to the knee and ankle, and you can get injured. It's even more important for female soccer players. If they have a weak core, they have a 3 to 5 times higher incidence of tearing their ACLs as compared with men.

The work that is done to develop the core does not have the same popularity as what's done to build pecs, biceps, and quads. We can see those muscles, but we can't see the core, which is more important to overall health and performance.

This book has been needed for a long time. As much as we talk about the core, it still isn't a glamorous part of medicine. But the work Bill has done has helped the idea of core strength become more popular, and this book could be what is needed to get it more attention.

Foreword by Bryan Talmadge Kelly, MD

The timing of this book and the increased recognition of Bill Meyers' work in the area of core repair, rehabilitation, and development are perfect because progress in the field of hip and groin injuries in sports medicine has advanced considerably in the past 15 years. Treatment methods of the hip and core are moving on 2 parallel tracks.

I absolutely feel like the hip is the last frontier in sports medicine. You can compare it to the evolution of treatment of the knee and shoulder. The knee came first in the 1970s, when physicians began to treat torn ACLs differently, and the shoulder followed in the 1990s, as we developed a larger understanding of labral instability and tears. The 2000s have brought a better understanding of the hip as an athletic joint. Progress is coming, but we are learning more.

The concepts of athletic pubalgia and core muscle injuries were really invented by Dr. Meyers. Bill has done a tremendous job of figuring out the complex anatomy of the core. He noted that a lot of athletes had been suffering from groin injuries that wouldn't heal quickly and understood there was more at work than just a groin pull. Simultaneous to that, within the field of orthopedic surgery, there emerged a better understanding of mechanically derived injuries of cartilage and soft tissues in the hip joint, and our knowledge of that area grew.

The mechanical malalignment in the hip joint leads to cartilage injuries and limits motion. That can lead to injury of the joint, as well as the muscles around the joint. We have really started to understand the relationship between core injuries and femoroacetabular impingement. If the hip and socket in the hip are mismatched, there is a reduction in motion. This leads to increased mechanical injury to the cartilage and the hip joint.

Making the proper hip diagnosis can be difficult because some hip injuries can feel like groin injuries. There are also many muscles around the hip that can be affected. Things become interesting because there is so much overlap in the area. The ability to understand the pathologies is critical to providing good care for patients. This book can help in that regard.

Developing collaborative efforts like the one Bill and I have forged allows us to get athletes back to action in a timely fashion, because we know about those overlaps. Bill has done a fabulous job of figuring out where, anatomically, those overlaps are. On the orthopedic side, we have done a lot of work on the complex problems in the hip joint. It's exciting now to see the interrelationship of the 2 areas.

When someone has pain around the hip and pelvis, there are 4 layers that can be affected. There is the bony layer, which is the foundation; how does the ball fit in the socket? There is the interarticular structure that contains large, inert areas that don't have contractile components. The muscular layer is where the core comes into play. How does it respond to a hip injury? And then there is the neuro layer. How are the nerves in the area of the hip impacted by an injury to the core and the hip socket?

This is an exciting time, and we still have a long way to go. Orthopedic and general surgeons are looking at the problems and making progress in the treatments that will advance the field. Relationships like the one Bill and I have established will help us move forward. This book is another step in that direction.

INTRODUCTION

The Strike Zone

There is no more important area of the body for an athlete—okay, for anyone—than the core. It's the engine room, the place where power is generated and then distributed. Strength there makes life easier for shoulders and knees. It produces speed and explosiveness. Endurance and grit. Build the core, and you have built the house.

It extends from the chest to the thighs and includes a network of muscles, tendons, ligaments, and joints that interconnect to provide the burst necessary for optimal performance. Perhaps because this is where the body generates its power, the core just so happens to be the same as the baseball/softball strike zone (Figures I-1 and I-2), at least the way the American League umpires call strikes these days.

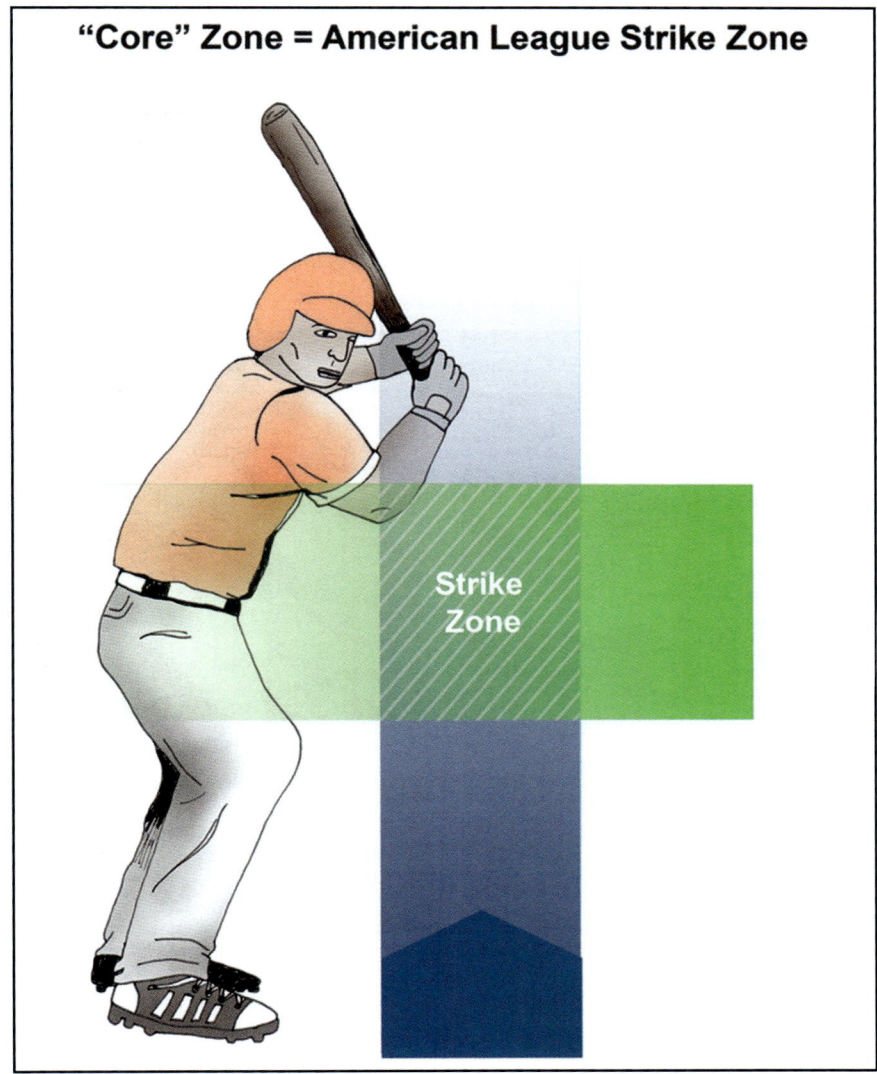

Figure I-1. It so happens that the American League baseball strike zone delineates the same area of the body we are calling the *core*. According to baseball myth, the strike zone defines the portion of the body where power and athleticism are generated. Within this area, the real battle between the pitcher and batter takes place.

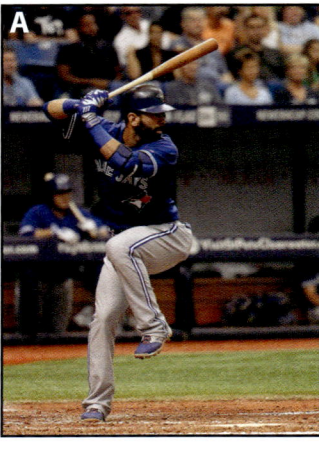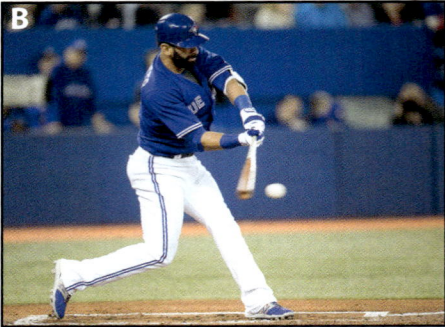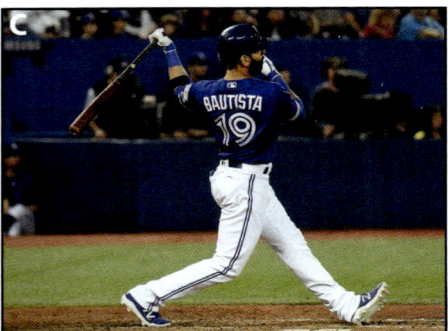

Figure I-2. José Bautista generates as much power per pound as anyone in baseball. Power, balance, and the ability to hit the ball comes from sequential movements known as 3 phases: (A) initiation, (B) acceleration, and (C) follow-through. The core governs these movements in conjunction with the brain. (Reprinted with permission from *USA Today Sports*, with permission from José Bautista.)

A set of bulging biceps or polished pecs may look great on the beach, but those who want success on the field, the court, the ice, or anywhere competition is staged need to tone their foundation.

But how does it all work? This hub is a tricky place, where the intertwining of tissue creates a series of reciprocal reactions and effects that can bring success or, in the event of a failure, agony. Understanding the relationships between the core's parts helps an athlete train more effectively and allows a physician to repair problems that arise. You may see 6-pack abs, but there is more to core strength than looking good. Much more.

The same thing happens in soccer (Figure I-3) and every other sport. The head, arms, and legs all depend on the core as their leader.

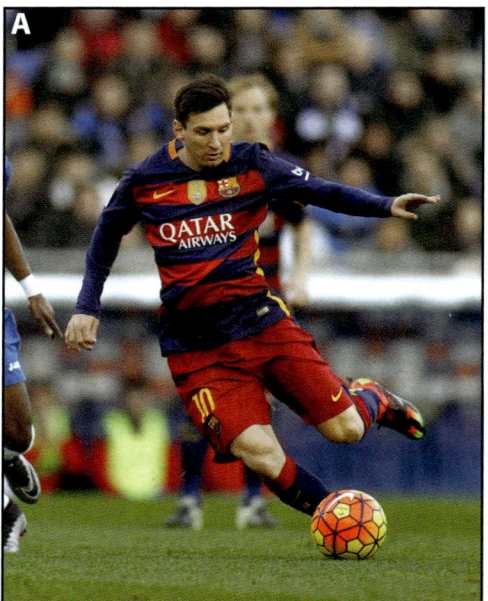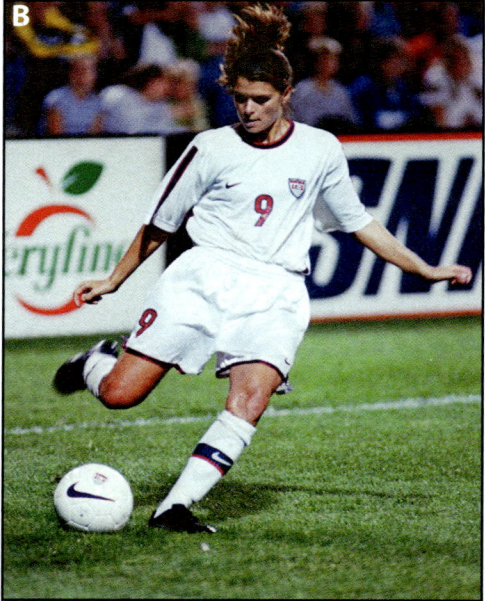

Figure I-3. Both (A) Lionel Messi and (B) Mia Hamm demonstrate the core translating into athleticism. The sturdiness of the core enables balance, accuracy, and strength. Note the harmony that both Lionel's and Mia's cores achieve with the ground. ([B] Reprinted with permission from AP Photo/Don Heupel and Mia Hamm.)

The leadership of power and athleticism belongs to the core. This last statement holds in sports and for everyday movement (Figure I-4). It also holds for both men and women. But we need to peer inside the 2 sexes and see the certain anatomical differences besides what's so outwardly noticeable. Sex differences in core anatomy seem subtle but become huge when one considers injuries that result.

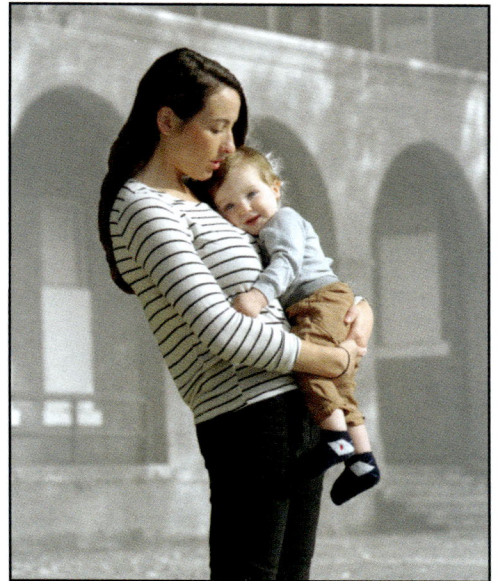

Figure I-4. The core gets involved in everyday life.

The core governs everyone's movements, not just those of athletes. This becomes more and more important as we grow older. Balance and the ability to move and not fall depend almost totally on the core and its interaction with the brain. We will talk more about that collaboration later.

The core is so important. So why has it remained such a medical mystery?

This book will explain that.

This book will provide the definitive explanation of the core. What are its parts, and how do those components work together to give an athlete the firepower he/she needs to thrive? Thanks to decades of research and experience working with the area and its machinery, Dr. William Meyers has become the nation's foremost authority on core health. He'll explain how it functions, how to build its strength, and how to repair the core when it breaks down.

Throughout his career, Dr. Meyers has seen practically every type of core injury. Through stories and anecdotes about his work with elite athletes, he will give readers a thorough understanding of the body's most important contributor to physical success and its widespread influence on the human anatomy. He will take you inside the locker room, the operating room, and onto the field to trace the arc of a performer's journey from injury to repair to return.

Calling on his relationships with athletic trainers and rehabilitation specialists, Dr. Meyers and his recognizable co-authors and co-editors will explain the secrets to a stronger core and the benefits that it will give any competitor, from the weekend warrior to the NFL star. They advise doctor and therapist colleagues on new ways to think about the core. They shall offer advice to parents of younger athletes, to help them make sure their children train in a safe, productive way that allows for maximum performance but also positive long-term outcomes. They shall explore the various treatment methods, from traditional to more unconventional, and delineate the pros and cons of each. They'll explain the state of the art and the questions that need to be answered.

No area of the body is more misunderstood than the core, what we baseball aficionados call the strike zone. *Introducing the Core: Demystifying the Body of an Athlete* will demystify the body's power plant and allow athletes of all abilities to improve their performance by strengthening and building the core to peak levels. The book will advise us all on the best way to stay in shape into our old age, to keep our balance and never unintentionally fall on our butts again.

By all measures, this book is a home run (Figure I-5).

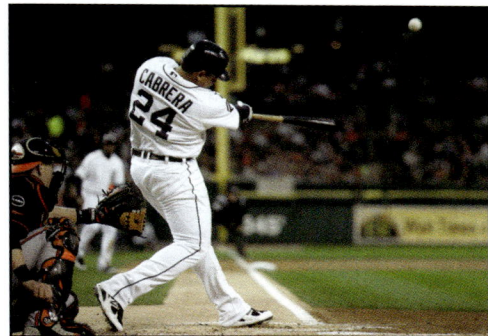

Figure I-5. Miguel Cabrera doing what he does. (Reprinted with permission from AP Photo/Duane Burleson, with permission from Miguel Cabrera.)

The Book's Outline

Like a caricaturization of the female/Venus perspective on life, the core is all about relationships. Pure transactional interactions (eg, isolated muscle strengthening) often cause harm. We shall examine the core's important relationships with the "giggle" organs, upper and lower extremities, brain, and other structures.

We intend for the entire book to bridge old and new understandings. Understand that the book focuses on a brand new field that we have helped develop. At first, the new concepts may seem unfamiliar, such as the functional anatomy of the core muscles. At first glance, some of the concepts may seem controversial. Keep in mind that these concepts should not be controversial.

To unify effectively the new with the old, we must make certain that a certain perspective prevails. With that perspective, you shall then see how the old lenses were, in fact, seeing slices of the visual fields of the new eyes. And to avoid confusion and keep that perspective, it is important that the book maintain one voice. Therefore, Dr. Meyers and his co-editors provide commentary throughout all parts of the book. Dr. Meyers has invited some world leaders to provide chapters in their areas of expertise. Their perspectives provide the knowledge base upon which some of the new paradigms are based. The commentaries chronicle how their viewpoints fit within the new understandings.

There are 5 sections of the book. The first section (The Way We Were) dissects the events that steered Dr. Meyers and his colleagues to the new appreciation of the anatomy. We promise the second section (New Universe) to be the most exciting description of anatomy you have ever read. The third section (Hip Hop Movement) brings multiple world-leading arthroscopists into the overall core picture, providing their perspectives on how the core universe works. The fourth section (Shared Responsibility) underscores the fact that a wide spectrum of folks treat the core, from traditional surgeons to alternative therapists. We must appreciate that none of us knows it all. We must respect the opinions of other specialists who work in this domain.

With some scrutiny, you will notice that some of the concepts presented in the chapters of this fourth section actually seem to conflict with other concepts in this book. Do not regard this as bad. Instead, these other perspectives may fit with our own and, in the least, make us appreciate that the core belongs to everyone. Plus, we will likely learn and get new ideas by listening to others and observing what they do.

The fifth section (Life Is a Journey) brings it all together. It shows how patients and doctors got lost within the old black-and-white world. The section starts, in a touching way, with a prominent biomedical engineering professor recounting her own personal experiences, and then providing her conclusion and advice for us all. The section ends in full Technicolor with the *Wizard of Oz* unveiling where the new world is taking us.

Throughout the book, we will let you guess whose words, among the editors, you are reading in any of the chapters or in any given section. Let us provide the following insight. This book was a group effort. The rest of us outvoted any editor who endeavored to remain humble. We needed to state things the way they are.

As a final word of introduction, let us provide a clue to the answer to a question that our world-famous medical artist Rob Gordon asked, while we were writing the book and directing him in the prospective artwork.

Rob asked us about why all the entertaining overture of the first few chapters prior to showing any of his important anatomic artwork. His question came during the long drumroll at the beginning of Chapter 5.

"This book is about anatomy. Why not start out with anatomy? Why all this other stuff?"

The answer to that question is critical to why we are writing this book. The answer shall become obvious. For now, consider a closely linked question: This anatomy has been around for a long time, before da Vinci…why the heck haven't people seen it or, at least, partially understood it?

The frustration that sprang from that question is what drove us to write this book.

The answer to that question is where the fun begins.

section one
the way we were*

*from the romantic comedy starring Barbra Streisand and Robert Redford[VID 1]

Video

1. https://www.youtube.com/watch?v=GNEcQS4tXgQ

1

what's the **core**?
it seems kind of **important**

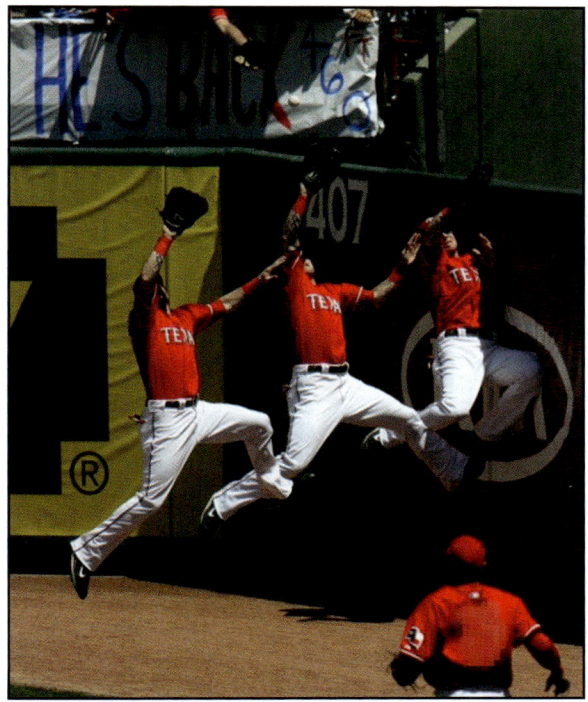

Figure 1-1. Josh Hamilton and a wall. This is the event that produced Josh's first injury. (Major League Baseball trademarks and copyrights are used with permission of Major League Baseball Properties, Inc, with permission from Josh Hamilton.)

Josh Hamilton had been given a day off, right in the middle of the 2011 World Series. Seems that "groin strain" was bothering him a lot, and Texas manager Ron Washington wanted his slugger to get a little rest. It made sense. The man who had slammed 25 homers during the regular season hadn't cleared the wall once during the playoffs (Figure 1-1).

Josh and outfield walls did not get along. He repeatedly crashed into them over the course of his career, leading to the speculation that these led to his core muscle avulsions. His first injury was definitely related to such a crash, and he set the All-Star Game Home Run Derby record the year following repair.[1] The second injury had a more occult onset and was on his opposite side.

Hamilton would go deep during the Rangers' Series loss to St. Louis. Once.

In 17 October games, Hamilton hit just .271, with that lone homer and 13 RBIs. Texas hung in for 7 games against the Cards but couldn't win the deciding game. As analysts looked back on the Series, Hamilton's performance in the Fall Classic (.241, 1 HR, 6 RBIs) was looked at as a prime reason for the loss.[2] Forget that the Rangers' pitchers gave up 42 runs. Hamilton didn't deliver, so he was branded a prime culprit.

Less than 2 weeks after the World Series ended, doctors found out exactly why Hamilton had struggled so. He had torn all 3 adductor muscles on one side of his core. It was a huge injury within the very engine room that delivered the power to his swing. This wasn't some little groin strain. It was a full tear that was in need of repair. Hamilton could have opted for surgery earlier, but there was no way he was going to miss his chance at a world title, especially since the Rangers had lost the year before to San Francisco in 5 games.

Doctors identified precisely the injury and fixed it, and Hamilton rehabbed during the winter months. The following season, Hamilton slugged 9 homers in April and went on to have one of his most productive years, slamming a career-high 43 dingers, knocking in 128 runs and hitting .285 (Figure 1-2).[3]

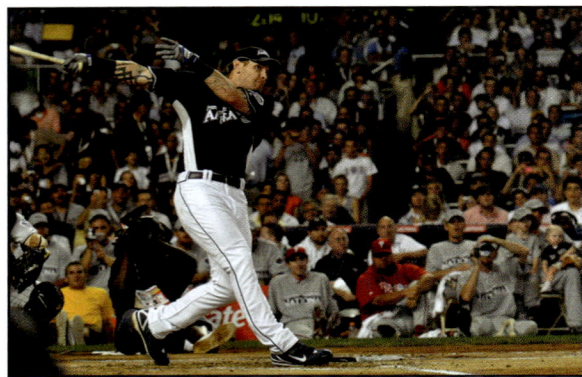

Figure 1-2. Josh setting the MLB Home Run Derby record in 2010. (Reprinted with permission from *USA Today Sports*.)

The moral of the story? The core seems kind of important.

You know Hamilton would say it is. But so would just about any athlete who needs power and energy to thrive. Football players need strong cores to generate the force necessary to overpower opponents. Basketball players need health there to attack the rim. Hockey goalies had better be able to move side to side or the net will be filled with pucks. World-class sprinters (Figure 1-3). Volleyball spikers. The list is long.

THE CORE AFFECTS US COMMON FOLK

Athletes are not the only ones. Ever bring a couple bags of groceries into the house from the trunk of your car (Figure 1-4)? If you can do that without taking a break halfway, you have built some core strength. Try carrying a teenager's book bag without a little bit of fuel in the body's engine room. If you don't have any, it's class dismissed. And don't go picking up that crying toddler without some core development, or you'll be the one throwing the tantrum.

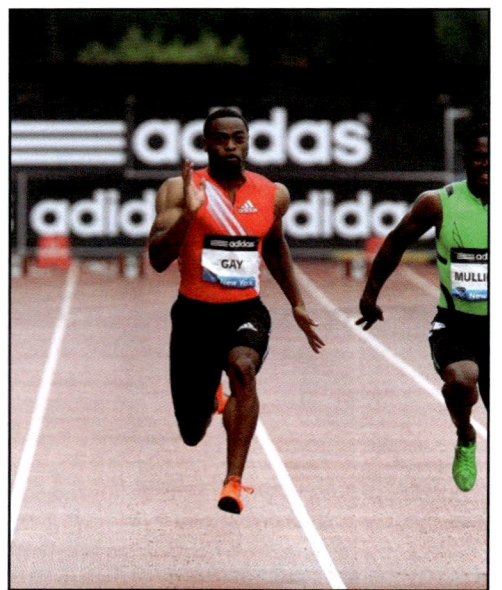

Figure 1-3. Tyson Gay fighting for first place in the 100 meters. (Reprinted with permission from Tyson Gay.)

The core serves elite athletes and everyday folks who have to carry out the tasks that get them through their days. It's the central part of the body, and it's responsible for helping everything else function at top levels. Without a sturdy foundation there, the arms, legs, and brain are vulnerable. Confidence is destroyed. Performance lags.

So, what is the core?

THE CORE IS OUR ENGINE AND TRANSMISSION ALL WRAPPED INTO ONE LARGE REGION OF THE BODY

Okay, we got that. So, it's the engine room and transmission all wrapped into one. We see that. Figures 1-5 and 1-6 show that pretty obviously. But what are we looking at? Tell us more.

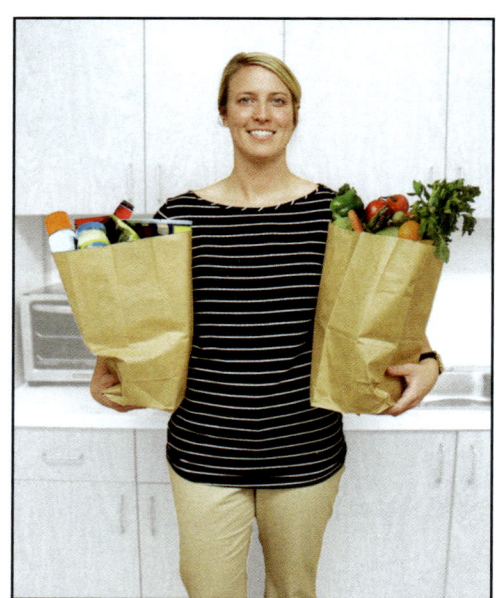

Figure 1-4. Carrying groceries requires the core.

Figure 1-5. An automobile engine/transmission.

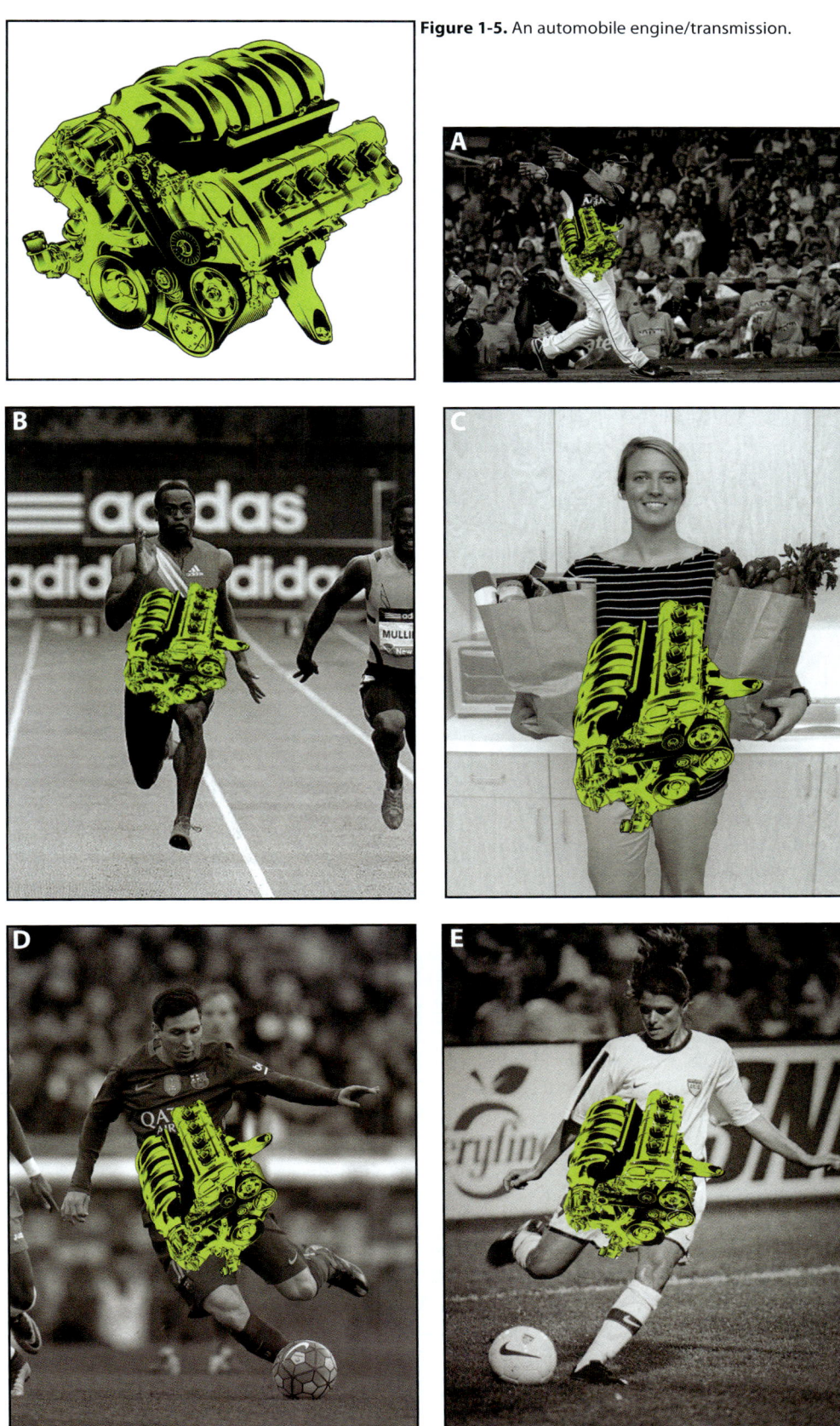

Figure 1-6. It so happens that the engine/transmission fits inside (A) Josh (Reprinted with permission from *USA Today Sports*), (B) Tyson (Reprinted with permission from Tyson Gay), (C) our grocery woman, (D) Lionel, and (E) Mia (Reprinted with permission from AP Photo/Don Heupel and Mia Hamm).

Simply put, the core is the body from the nipples to the middle of thigh, and there is an awful lot of stuff in there. Organs, nerves, muscles, and big blood vessels can all be found there. Okay, so the head is kind of important. The core is vital, too. It is amazing that nobody has really paid much attention to it until now, at least not in its complete state. Cardiologists care about the heart. Gastroenterologists worry about the digestive tract. But nobody has been concerned about the whole thing. What's in there? And, more importantly, how does it all fit together?

That's what this book is about. It discusses adductors and the rectus abdominis. The psoas and the rectus femoris. The pubic bone and the gluteus maximus. The hip joint. And the back. And then the organs and all that other stuff. The core is all of that, and believe it or not, this whole region of the body fits together. Duh! It's there. It is part of our body. Well, it is not only there, but the core actually works together and functions as a whole, just like the engine and transmission of a car, yet so much more intricately. We shall be talking about these functions; the relationships between the different parts of the core; development, repair; and rehabilitation; and much more.

THE CORE IS SPICY—SO GET OVER IT

We're going to use some spicy language here, because there are some spicy things in that core. It isn't just muscles and joints. There's sexual stuff, too. Maybe that's why everybody has been so reticent about all of this? As soon as someone mentions the pubic bone, you can almost hear the giggles, like we were in a junior high health class. Deal with it, folks (Figures 1-7 and 1-8). As you read this book, remember that giggles are okay! This region of the body is fun. Plus, a strong core can help all kinds of athletes.

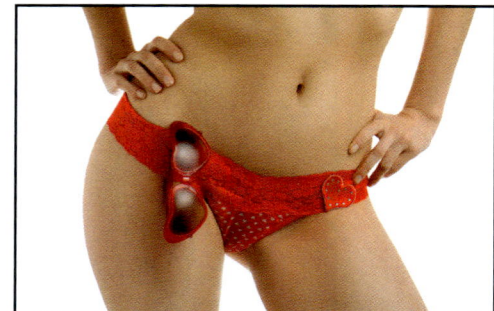

Figure 1-7. Get over it.

We said, "Get over it" (ie, get over that the core contains the "private" parts of the body). And we have to, in order to understand the core. That is not simple, and predators are out there, like Larry Nassar, the abominable family medicine guy in charge of US Women Gymnastics whose abusive and criminal actions damaged a collection of girls and young women and eventually landed him in jail, disgraced and never to practice his monstrous tactics again. Good riddance.

We all have to respect the area so much that we keep those creeps away. We need chaperoning. We need a strong, continued dialogue between physician and patient. Between physician and parent. Between everybody. This is imperative, not only to ensure the best possible care but also to ensure nothing like Nassar's atrocious behavior happens again.

But the elite athletes make the biggest news about the core. Like world-class sprinter Tyson Gay, who floundered on the track for a short while, had his muscle injury fixed, and then beat world champion Usain Bolt in the 100 meters. He later underwent hip surgery and was back winning top events at the age of 35 years.

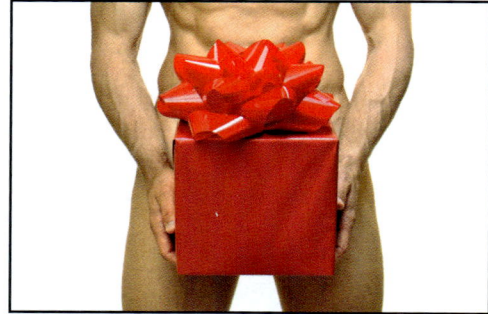

Figure 1-8. The mystery involves both sexes. This picture is shown purely for equal time. Again, get over it!

NFL cornerback Sheldon Brown saw some time as a rookie with the Eagles in 2002, but a core injury limited his effectiveness. After a doctor repaired his problem, Brown became a starter and completed his 11th year as a regular in 2013. The same story with Bills' safety Jairus Byrd. A severe core injury prevented him from playing the last couple games even though he was still named Rookie of the Year. He had to undergo both muscle and hip surgery, and 4 years later, the Bills had to franchise him in order to keep him. Tight end Jeremy Shockey knows all about what a healthy core can mean. A lot of people thought he was washed up when the Giants let him go after the 2007 campaign. And given Shockey's—let's say "enterprising"—personality and approach to the game, plenty of fans would have been happy if that had been the case. But after surgery, he became a key part of the New Orleans Saints' attack. In Super Bowl XLIV, Shockey caught a key TD pass in the Saints' victory over Indianapolis.[4-6]

It All Fits Together

One of the big things we're showing with this book is how the hip, muscles, and vital and giggle organs all work together (Figure 1-9).

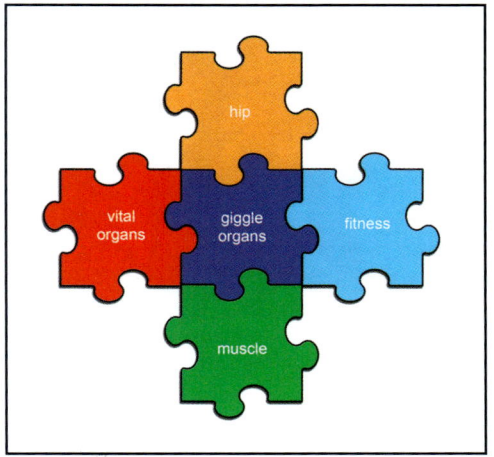

Figure 1-9.

Another big thing we expect to do by this book is to eradicate the term "sports hernia" forever from the English language. Or die trying. There is no such thing. Core injuries involve tears, pulls, and strains. They involve disruptions of big bony, muscly joints. They aren't simple protrusions or bulges. And they aren't simply hernias to be repaired by mesh. The media gets part of the blame for this. Using the "sports hernia" catch-all term is easy and doesn't require detailed explanations (Figure 1-10).

We, the medical and health care communities, deserve some responsibility here, too. A huge number of publications perpetuate that term or terms that imply that repairs of hernias will fix that one type of problem.[7-12] The anatomic region seems so complex. This complexity makes us physicians give up trying to understand the problems more, and therefore lends itself to easy-to-say, catch-all phrases—even though we all know the terms have no validity. There's an awful lot going on in the core, what with all the biomechanics and the big blood vessels and organs in there.

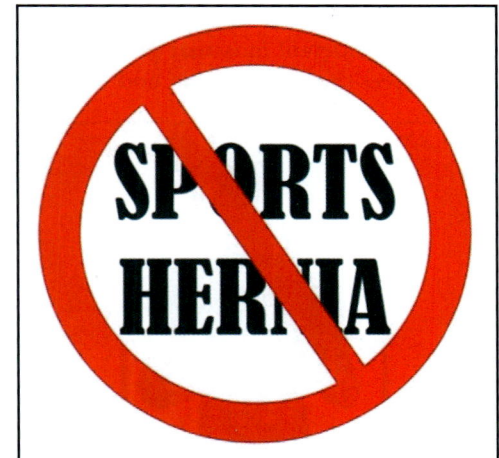

Figure 1-10.

Orthopedic surgeons tend to stay away from that stuff. Neurosurgeons will take on the spine but aren't about to go near the pubic bone. Other specialists—GI surgeons, urologists, and gynecologists, to name a few—see the core's muscles and bones simply as the black box that encloses their provinces. For too many years, we have ignored the core, and that means we haven't known what's going on. Now is the time for us all to find out.

Heath Miller found out. When he was a senior all-American tight end at Virginia, Miller sustained a core injury. On draft day in 2005, Pittsburgh was debating whether to select Miller, and the Steelers' famous team physician, James Bradley, called Dr. Meyers from Philadelphia, who had just repaired him. "Is Heath going to be 100%? I need to know now… we are on the clock." The Steelers really were. They had the 30th pick in the first round. The Colts had just taken Marlin Jackson as the 29th. Philadelphia, where Meyers lived, had the 31st. It was time.

Dr. Meyers didn't want to give any guarantees—even of his own fine work—but he did say he thought so. The response from Bradley: "That sounds like 100% to me!" Of course, there was a caveat. "And if he's not perfect," the Steelers' doctor said kiddingly, "I am going to track you down and kill you." Miller hasn't been perfect, but he's been pretty darn close, missing only 7 games during his 11-year career, playing in 2 Pro Bowls and playing on 2 Super Bowl winners. It worked out great for Pittsburgh, something with which Dr. Meyers isn't completely delighted. "I felt a little bad, because the Eagles were the next pick and needed a tight end." Things eventually worked out well for Philadelphia in that department, and you know Miller was happy with his healthy core.

It's time more people—world-class athletes and the rest of us—had that same satisfaction.

Getting the Medical Community on Board

This is the issue.

The medical community, and, for that matter, most of the established health world, sees this body region in parts and not as a whole.

This book unveils an entirely new scientific arena when we consider this area of the body as a whole, where our engine and transmission reside.

It's not always easy to get the medical community to look at things differently, but when it comes to the core, it's past time for this new perspective. This book provides that with a top-to-bottom presentation of the body's most important sector, so that mystery and confusion may vanish.

It's the vital part of the body, where just about everything that is important can be found. (Okay, so the head is kind of vital, too.) The heart, lungs, liver, kidneys. They're all there. And physicians have been trained to repair them all (Figure 1-11).

Physicians deserve trust because of centuries of study, dedication, and empiricism. But, believe it or not (sarcasm), they have weaknesses.

But do they have any idea where the core is in the body, or how the different systems all fit together (Figures 1-12 and 1-13)?

Physicians teach new physicians to practice the way they practice, to see things the way they see things. They have good reason. The reason certain procedures carry on from generation to generation is because they work. It's called *empiricism*. Aristotle understood that most knowledge derives from experience and a sense of what works. Well, the way we physician specialists see the core is through the eyes of empiricism. The

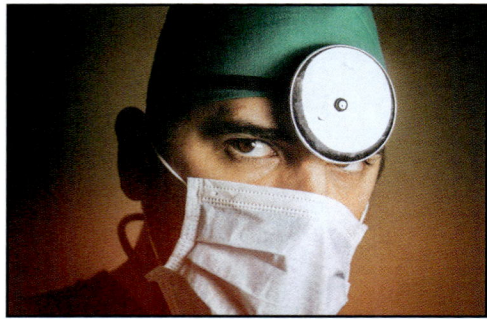

Figure 1-11. Traditional surgeons and other specialists are bound by the eyes and empiricism of their training.

urologist sees the pelvis as the genitourinary tract that resides there. General surgeons see the pelvis as the colorectum and a bunch of different muscular protrusions called "hernias." The gynecologist sees the reproductive organs, the vascular surgeon sees the blood vessels, and so on (Figure 1-14).

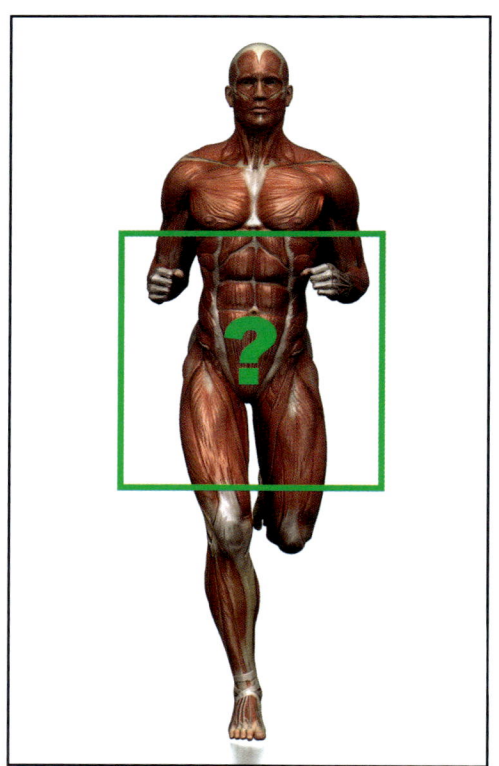

Figure 1-12. Because of the traditional methods of medical specialty training and the inherent empiricism, the core has remained mysterious.

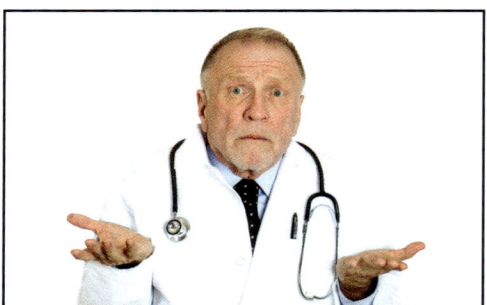

Figure 1-13. The goings-on in the core have confounded traditional physicians.

Yada, yada, yada.

Let's scrutinize the medical guys. A cardiologist is expert in matters of the heart and the circulatory system, but he/she isn't going to pay much attention to the muscles in the chest or abdomen, even though their condition is fundamental to good cardiovascular health. Nephrologists care for kidneys, but they aren't worried about the excretory system's relationship to the pubic joint. We can go on…

Back to the question, "Do traditional physicians understand what the heck the fitness people might mean by the core?"

The answer is a resounding, "Heck, no."

Well-trained surgeons should take the most blame for this failure of understanding. We can take it. We surgeons traditionally take responsibility for the anatomy. Likewise, surgeons and empiricism should also take the blame for the mistaken belief that occult hernias cause the pelvic pain of athletes (Figure 1-15).

Think in terms of the entire region that defines the core and all structures within it. The core all works together and controls the rest of the body. It's high time to pay close attention to the many relationships at work within the core and how those relationships combine to produce fitness and athleticism.

It is not just about individual organ systems. The core is a complicated collection of the body's most important components. Understanding how they all work together is the key to an integrated approach to health and performance.

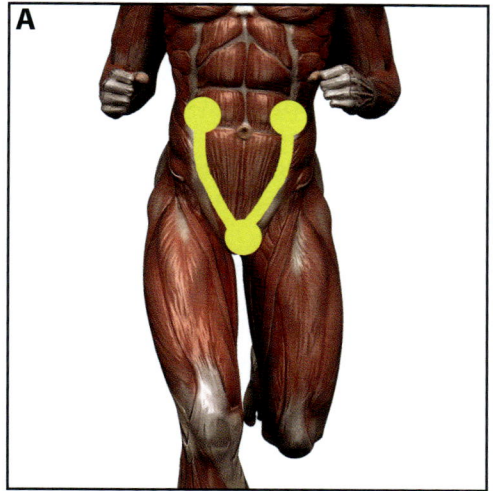 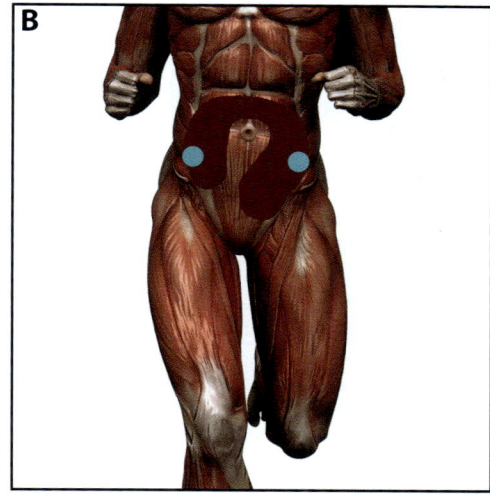

Figure 1-14. What the (A) urologist or (B) general/colorectal surgeon sees as "the core." The urologist sees the kidneys, ureters, bladder, etc. The general or colorectal surgeon sees the gastrointestinal tract and small protrusions called "hernias."

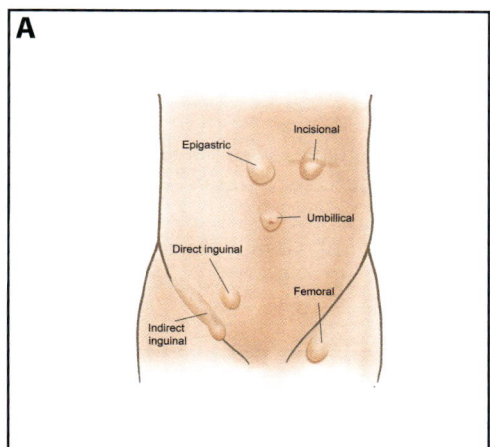 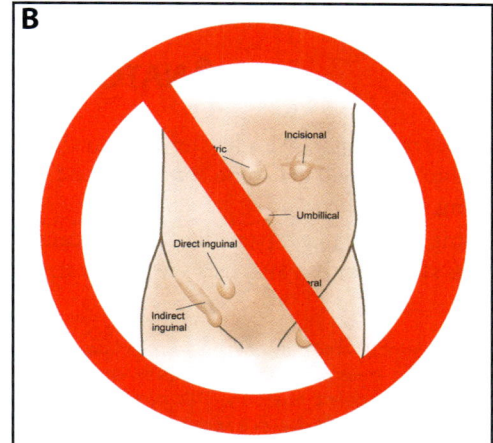

Figure 1-15. (A) Do not deny the existence of abdominal and pelvic hernias. They occur in multiple age groups, but hernias do not have a role in the mechanisms of athletic injuries to the core. (B) Thinking they do have a role leads to harm. Purge the concept of hernia from our heads!

INTEGRATION OF FITNESS AND MEDICINE

It would be hard to find someone who hasn't been told by his/her physician that it's important to exercise. Makes sense, doesn't it? Keeping the body fit and in motion is a good idea.

But once the doctor tells a patient to get moving, there is no further communication on the matter. Exercise, yes. But how? There must be a way to integrate the medical and fitness components of a person's good health.[13]

It all begins with the core. Certain exercises can hurt a person. Some people might not be healthy enough for a rigorous regimen. And building a set of bulging biceps may lead to some admiration on the beach, but it won't provide the strength necessary for performance—on and off the field. There must be a coordinated plan that allows for good core health and functional strength and flexibility. Doctors, meet the exercise physiologist. You have a lot to talk about.

We need the traditional doc spending more time with the fitness people (Figure 1-16).

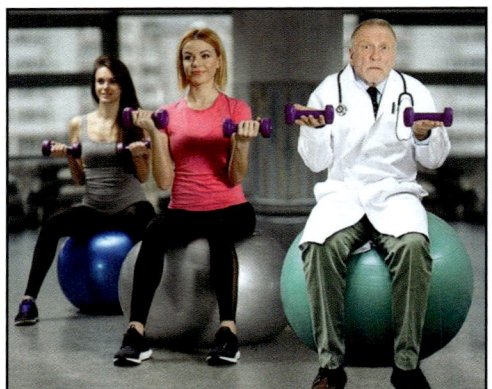

Figure 1-16. We need the traditional docs sitting on exercise balls alongside fitness experts and the rest of us.

So, as we have implied, the main impediment to the medical community's recognizing the existence of the core stems from that community's greatest strengths—the dedication of its providers and their commitment to empiricism. Physicians teach new physicians to practice the way they practice, to see things the way they see things. They have good reason. Certain procedures carry on from generation to generation because they work. Aristotle knew about this. He understood that most knowledge derives from experience and a sense of what works.

But our senses don't tell us everything. Thus, if we are purely empirical in our actions, then what happens when we encounter something totally new? Of course, we first apply again what we know has worked before, or at least the closest thing to it. In the world of empiricism, "ought" implies "can." But what if it still doesn't work? Or worse, what if there is partial success? Then we begin to "know" things with more certainty than our senses tell us. We "know" what we're thinking merely because we're thinking it. Aristotle, Hume, Peirce, Benjamin—all those philosophers/scientists—they all discussed these things. They summed it up as the failure to recognize we could be mistaken, the failure to recognize that we only have partial data.

Another way to describe our weakness as physicians is an inability to "think outside the box."

ANATOMICALLY SPEAKING

Okay, people, we're going to use a few terms hear that might make you giggle. Like "pubic bone." Let's face it, anything with the word "pubic" in it will get some chuckles. And "groin" is always good for a smile. "Pulled a groin" can get even a monastery laughing.

But you're going to have to get past all of that, because this is serious stuff—despite the relative hilarity of the vocabulary. Let's keep this stuff fun. But also let's see all the structures in there. Let's define the right terms, for example, the *hip* (Figure 1-17).

Figure 1-17. Sexual suggestion profoundly obscures appreciation of the anatomy and accurate diagnosis and treatment. This composite illustration highlights how close the hip is to other pelvic anatomy. This proximity creates enough anatomical and physiological complexity. In a sense, we have to blind ourselves to the psychological complexity built into sexual suggestion. That extra layer of complexity keeps us from seeing the problems that do occur in this region. At the same time, this part of the body cannot be taken lightly. We cannot ignore that extra layer of complexity. We need to acknowledge it. The only way to do both (ie, to focus well on the anatomy and physiology and at the same time respect the private nature of things) is to examine this part of the body in stringently proper surroundings with appropriate chaperoning. We need the anatomical/physiological understanding of the core to move forward, rather than languish in ignorance and misunderstanding. We need to eliminate the possibility of future Nassars, and to pay utmost attention to and respect for social stigmas. For example, the #MeToo movement should emphasize to us all the need for increased understanding of the pathophysiologic conditions that occur in this anatomical region. This anatomic proximity factor comes up later. We will talk more about sexual taboos that block accurate diagnosis and overall understanding of the core region. We must create an ultimate balance between medical care and personal respect.

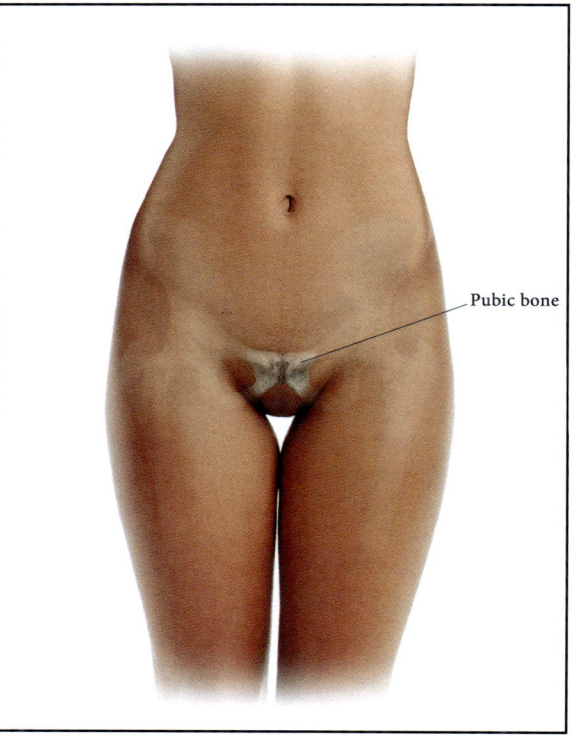

When we talk about the hip joint, we are also talking about just the ball and socket—no muscles, no nerves, or anything else. This simple definition is important. With this definition, when someone talks about the hip, we all immediately know that we are talking about the ball-and-socket hip joint and not muscles and other anatomy that surround the ball and socket. And if someone brings up "the pubic bone," we are talking about what we define as the pubic bone, and no one doubles over—unless a muscle attached to it has torn. Then, we would be in for some serious pain.

And not a bit of laughter.

A Brief Historical Perspective

It's hard to imagine that when Cro-Magnon Man suffered a core injury thousands of years ago, he was listed as day-to-day on the hunting-and-gathering injury report. But it is instructional to review the development of the human species with regard to core health, if only to chart how the change in posture over the millennia has improved strength and fitness in that area. As we have stood more and more erect, our core has changed, and that's important to understand. We also need to understand how the anatomical architecture of women fit into this postural analysis (Figure 1-18).

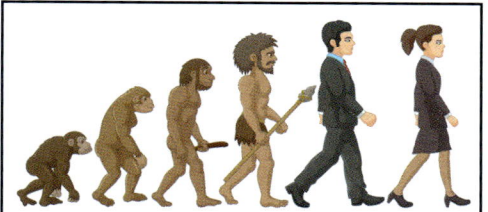

Figure 1-18. It's okay to think in evolutionary terms. Don't forget the woman in the evolution of "man" and the pelvis.

There's some personal history to be covered in this book, too, beginning with Bill Meyers' observations of a former Harvard athlete, Richie Szaro,[14] a highly recruited running back who was sidelined by a core injury that many questioned and some even considered him a malingerer. There's a story about how Meyers learned about the relationship between many of the core muscles that involves a medical student, a cadaver, and some considerable pain.

In short, good core health owes itself to thousands of years of evolution and decades of discovery, walking hand-in-hand.

See the Core Also as the Epicenter

One may also see the core as the cardinal center point. In seismology, the epicenter[15] is the point on the Earth's surface directly above the point where the fault begins to rupture, and in some cases, it is the area of greatest damage.

Anybody who has ever tried to get a group of people to do the same thing at the same time can appreciate how maddening that process can be. Well, just imagine what it's like to have joints, bones, and muscles working in concert. If everything's behaving, there are no problems. But that's not always the case.

There are 4 main components of the pelvic core (we shall get into the real 4 components later): the 2 hips, pubis, and backbone. If they are working in concert, a person can be effective. But what if the muscles don't stretch enough? Or if the hip is fine but a bone is obstructing part of the hip socket and causing muscles to tense up, mobility is limited. It is vital that everything is working in concert. For that to happen, there must be strength, flexibility, and good alignment of the area.

Communication Is the Key

Run all day. Build those beach muscles with weights all night. But when it comes to the true performance of extremities, the core is the focus. A strong, healthy core dispatches instructions to the arms and legs, allowing them to work at optimal levels. If the middle isn't sturdy, then knee ligaments can tear. If the epicenter isn't fit, shoulders blow out.

We hear all the time about how an athlete blows out an ACL while cutting, and we blame the area's instability. Often, the pressure on the ligament doesn't come from exterior forces. Weak groins destabilize legs. Lax abdominal walls stress elbows. It may not seem that way, but without a strong core, the rest of the body is compromised. It won't always result in injury, but you can bet performance will suffer. For an athlete, that's what it's all about.

Performance Anxiety

Believe it or not, there is also quite a relationship between the head and the engine room when it comes to optimal performance. The head directs those bulky muscles in the middle to drive the train. The further you move on the body from the core, the finer the movements and the more the brain matters. Fire the middle with training, nutrition, and proper care, and the machine starts to move. As it does, the extremities respond to the mind's impulses to carry out the specific chores at hand—throwing, kicking, shooting, catching.

It's a fascinating relationship, and it must all be in concert for success. If one area is too dominant, there can't be true harmony. And it all starts in the middle. You can't possibly have endurance with a flabby middle. And you can't expect the fingers and toes to do their jobs without a sharp mind sending the messages. Brains and brawn have often been at odds throughout history. When it comes to physical performance, they had better be on the same team, or nobody wins.

Read on. You will understand the anatomical bases of the above statements.

SELECTED READINGS

Zöllner F. *Leonardo da Vinci. The Complete Paintings and Drawings*. Los Angeles, CA: Taschen GmbH; 2003.
   By flipping through the pages of this enormous book, one can see da Vinci's appreciation of the importance of the core.

Meyers W, Zoga A. Core muscle injuries. In: Haddad FS, ed. *The Young Adult Hip in Sport*. London, United Kingdom: Springer-Verlag; 2014:107-119.
   This recent review emphasizes the importance of understanding core anatomy in recognizing the various injuries.

REFERENCES

1. Singer T. Hamilton's 28 sets single-round record. www.MLB.com. Published July 14, 2008. Accessed May 1, 2016.
2. Josh Hamilton: God called homer. ESPN. http://www.espn.com/dallas/mlb/story/_/id/7159892/2011-world-series-texas-rangers-josh-hamilton-says-god-called-hr. Published October 28, 2011. Accessed May 1, 2016.
3. Josh Hamilton stats, fantasy & news. www.MLB.com. Published January 20, 2016. Accessed May 1, 2016.
4. Battista J. Champs? The Saints, dat's who. *The New York Times*. https://www.nytimes.com/2010/02/08/sports/football/08super.html. Published February 8, 2010. Accessed May 1, 2016.
5. Allee-Walsh B. Dr. Meyers Makes a Difference for World Champion Saints. SportsNola. http://sportsnola.com/dr-meyers-makes-a-difference-for-world-champion-saints/. Accessed December 9, 2016.
6. Saints' Shockey will undergo hernia surgery, miss 3-6 weeks. ESPN. http://www.espn.com/nfl/news/story?id=3603003. Published September 22, 2008. Accessed October 26, 2018.
7. Swan KG, Wolcott M. The athletic hernia: a systematic review. *Clin Orthop Rel Res*. 2006;455:78-87.
8. Nam A, Brody F. Management and therapy for sports hernia. *J Am Coll Surg*. 2008;206:154-164.
9. Caudill P, Nyland J, Smith C, et al. Sports hernia: a systematic literature review. *Br J Sports Med*. 2008;42:954-964.
10. Minnich J, Hanks J, Muschaweck U, et al. Sports hernia: diagnosis and treatment highlighting a minimal repair technique. *Am J Sports Med*. 2011;39:1341-1349.
11. Muschaweck U, Berger L. Minimal repair technique of sportsmen's groin: an innovative open-suture repair to treat chronic inguinal pain. *Hernia*. 2009;14:27-33.
12. Paajanen H, Brinck T, Hermunen H, et al. Laparoscopic surgery for chronic groin pain in athletes is more effective than nonoperative treatment: a randomized clinical trial with magnetic resonance imaging of 60 patients with sportsman's hernia (athletic pubalgia). *Surgery*. 2011;150:99-107.
13. Kraus WE, Douglas PS. Where does fitness fit in? *N Engl J Med*. 2005;353:517-519.
14. High school ace Szaro lives up to publicity. *The Harvard Crimson*. http://www.thecrimson.com/article/1967/11/1/high-school-ace-szaro-lives-up/. Published November 1, 1967. Accessed October 22, 2016.
15. Earthquake glossary. United States Geological Survey. https://earthquake.usgs.gov/learn/glossary/?term=epicenter. Accessed October 22, 2016.

2

new eyes
medicine's inability to see the core

The real magic of discovery lies not in seeking new landscapes, but in having new eyes [Figure 2-1].

—French philosopher Marcel Proust (Figure 2-2).
From *La Prisonnière*, Vol V of *Remembrance of Things Past*, aka *In Search of Lost Time*.

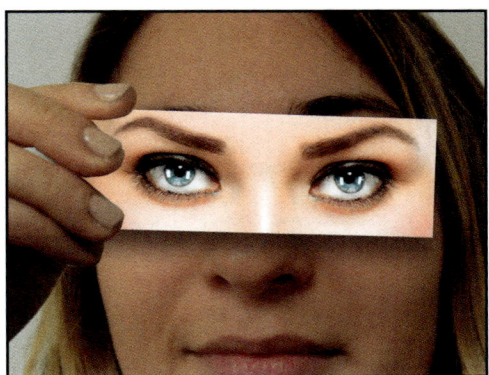

Figure 2-1.

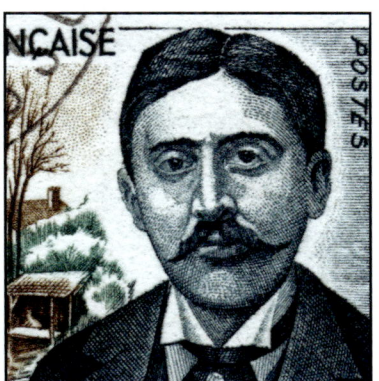

Figure 2-2. French stamp commemorating the famous French philosopher.

More About This Book

This book is about the core. What is the core? Look up the definition in the dictionary. The core is the *center*: the core of the apple, the middle of the Earth, the engine of a car, the foundation of a house. It also is the hub of activity, control central, the center of gravity. It's what makes things tick, produce, and reproduce. It's the middle of everything. Consider the different concepts about what the core represents. The core of the apple is probably most important for reproduction, and probably has something to do with growth. Our body is no different. In conjunction with our brain, our core balances, harnesses, and distributes our strength.

The house may make the best analogy. The foundation of the house is truly its balance point, when one considers the role of gravity, just like what was previously shown in the pictures of Messi and Mia (see Figures 1-6D and E). The foundation supports the walls, the insides, and everything else. And, of course, our core forms the foundation for movement and athleticism. Plus, it includes all our vital organs and interacts intimately with the brain (Figure 2-3).

The core allows us to get up from the dinner table. It generates the best athletes. A good core even makes the brain function better. One might say that the core is important. Duh! We said that before, didn't we?

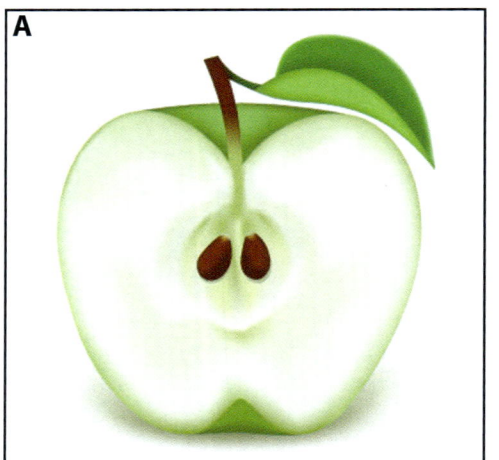
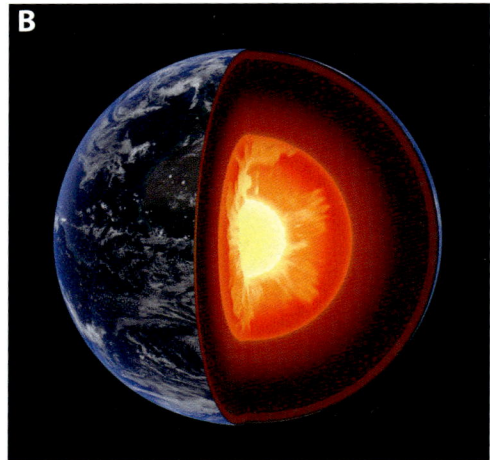
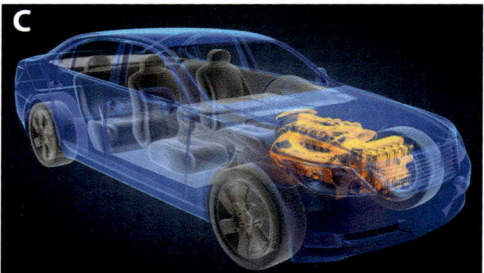
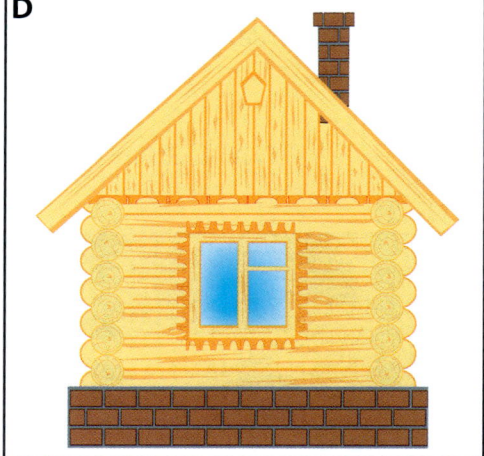

Figure 2-3. Consider all the functions of a core. The body's core does all of these and more: (A) an epicenter for regeneration/reproduction, (B) a center of gravity, (C) an engine/transmission, a hub of activity, and (D) the foundation.

THE PUBLIC SEES; MEDICINE STILL HAS BLINDERS

With respect to our body, the public knows about the existence of the core. The term *core* has come into vogue. Popular exercise programs use the term all the time. P90X, Cross-Fit, middle-of-the-night TV ads, you name it, emphasize its importance to the point of making us nauseated. They talk about the exact same body region we are talking about in this book: nipples to mid-thigh. Our point is that the public already knows this region of the body is ultra-important, yet medicine has not adopted it. The end result: Everyone purely guesses how the core works, and the knowledge gap becomes dangerous. The gap opens the door for preying entrepreneurs and snake oil salespeople. The gap leaves this essential part of our body ultra-vulnerable to injury. A good example of that danger that relates to the public's poor knowledge base about the core is the best-selling toy of a recent Christmas: the hoverboard.[VID 1]

This toy shifts the center of gravity in so precarious a way that the Las Vegas bookies would have made it the odds-on favorite to produce injury. Oh, if only we had published this book earlier, the world would be a safer place.

The public's keen recent interest in the core spawns a vigorous commercialism that takes advantage of all this ignorance. And, of course, sex plays a big role. After all, the core houses our sexual organs and is responsible for our most provocative movements. The core provides fantastic entertainment. The sex and the ignorance provide the motivation for the salespeople, not that snake oil needs more juice. Look at some of the late-night commercials. Some of them may not be dangerous. One of them certainly is.[VID 2-5]

Now look at the available information on various products and programs that are out there, such as Cross-Fit, Insanity, spin, boot camps, Ab Rail, Thighmaster, Bowflex, Chair Fitness, Total Gym, iGallop, Zumba, the 20-Minute Work-Out, and, of course, Shake Weight. See if you can tell which ones are best or where the dangers might be. Just with this exercise, you will realize the difficulty.

Now consider the paradox. Despite all this recognition and interest, docs and most of our other health care colleagues either ignore the core or deny the core's existence. Where's the disconnect? Almost no scientific efforts have been made to study this region of the body as a whole. Scientists have focused tremendously high-powered lenses on portions of the core but have not studied it as a whole. The core of the body is so obviously important…why haven't the medical scientists gotten into this field? The reason is those health professionals just don't see the core. They can't see it. They see certain parts of it, but they are essentially blind to the core itself and how it functions. They need new eyes.

NEW EYES

This book shall provide new eyes so that everyone can see the core. It reveals the basic principles of the core, the functional anatomy, and its practical aspects. It will generate far more questions than it will answer. It will point out that most popular concepts about how the core works are just plain wrong. You will also be able to deduce that most current core training methods are very bad, and that some are, to put it bluntly, dangerous.

We already talked about that "SH" term that we won't mention (intentionally) again. The point is to beware also of some of the conventional, empirical training methods.

Often, the best physical trainers unsuspectingly prescribe dangerous methods. This example may be appropriate for certain athletes but certainly not for most people: inverted, weighted sit-ups. This exercise focuses way too much in an isolated fashion on the rectus abdominis muscles and subjects them to severe "plate" injuries. The rectus abdominis muscles are part of the core "harness," which we must protect. Read further about that, and also realize that most isolated muscle exercises are really, really bad when you do too many or with too much load (Figure 2-4).

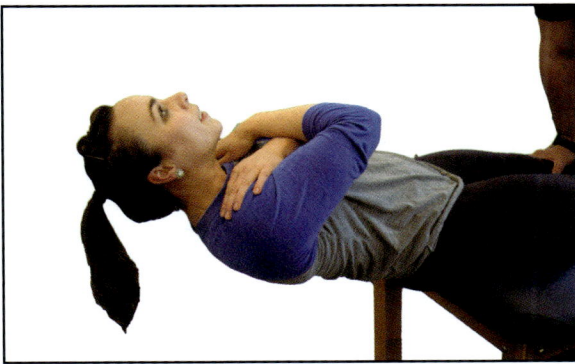

Figure 2-4. Sit-ups done in extremes of number or high load are bad (eg, the inverted sit-up in the figure should be considered dangerous). The more extreme "weighted" (weights added to the chest) sit-up is even worse.

We almost must get rid of our vision that the core is just about the upper part of our torso—the abs and above. Figure 2-5 is NOT the core. This should not be our visual.

Nor is Figure 2-6.

Our fancy should not be just the beach muscles or pure torso strength.

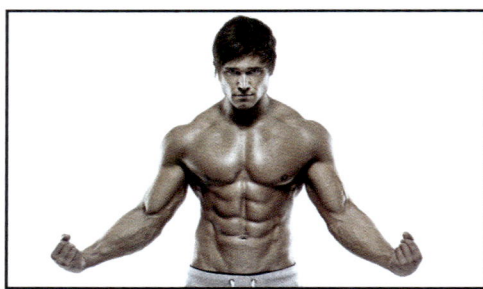

Figure 2-5. We should **not** look at just this part of the body (ie, the waist up).

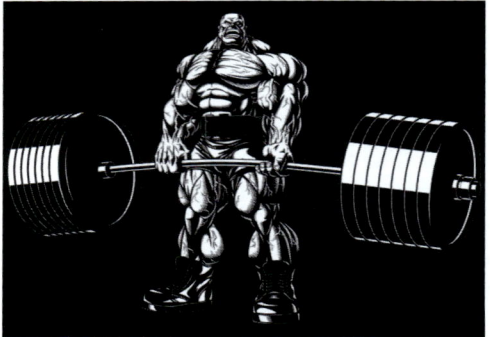

Figure 2-6. We should **not** look primarily at muscle mass.

So, if it is not about seashore muscles or pure strength, what is the core and what is it all about?

This is the core…ba dum tss!!!^{VID 6}

The core is this (Figure 2-7) and this (Figure 2-8)...

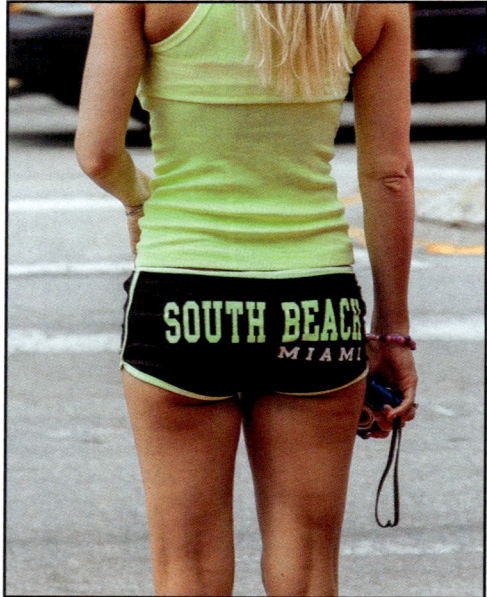

Figure 2-7. The core involves the whole region from mid-chest to mid-thigh.

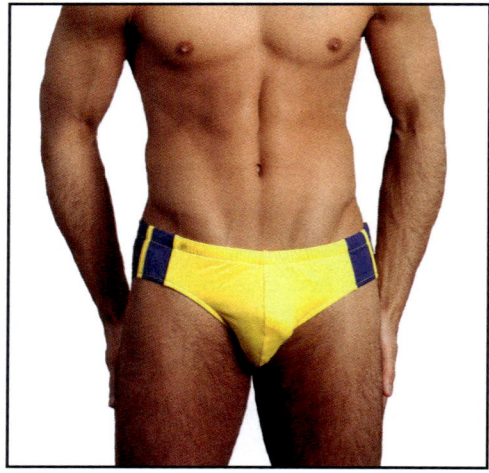

Figure 2-8. The definition does not change for the opposite sex. The core involves the whole region from mid-chest to mid-thigh. We cannot look just from the waist up, like we see in Figure 2-5. In order to understand the core, we have to look at the regions of the body equidistant above and below the core's center (ie, the pubic bone).

All we have done here is shift our view to include more of the lower body. Believe us, this should not be hard; this small shift in our visual perspective changes profoundly the way we look at our biomechanics, our real physiology. No doubt, the social taboo of looking at the body's true center has thrown off-kilter our appreciation of the anatomy. Believe us, that above-the-waist thinking has been a huge part of why we have been so blind in our medical/anatomic thinking.

WHY HAVE WE BEEN SO BLIND?

Let's first get back into why docs as a group and most medical people have not recognized the essentials of the core.

The body's core has long been staring us in the face. Yet we docs have not seen it. We have been distracted. The whole world knows it is important. So what the heck is going on? Where is the disconnect?

All we have done here is shift the view to include more of the lower body. Believe us—and this is not hard (pun not intended)—there is a lot to this shift to a lower perspective. And no doubt you are observing that "other" things have already distracted us. Precipitously, our pure medical/anatomic thinking process has been thrown off-kilter. Imagine that. That has been a huge part of why we have been so blind.

One of the reasons we have been blind to the core should now be becoming clearer. The overall answer turns out to be obvious. Docs have not seen the core for 3 distinct reasons.

First, the core is anatomically and physiologically complex. Therefore, it seems difficult to learn or understand, so we memorize the different muscles and delve deeply into the different physiologic systems within it. Of course, the core is complex. What else should we expect? It's the core, it's where everything happens. Most docs and other health care professionals will tell you they dissected the core once in their lives, over a few days in anatomy class. They memorized the many muscles and most likely passed all the necessary quizzes. That's the point. The biggest and most muscles reside in the abdomen, back, chest, pelvis, and thigh. They surround hugely important organ systems. Everything seems so detailed, so complex. That is because it is! We get lost in the core's complexity.

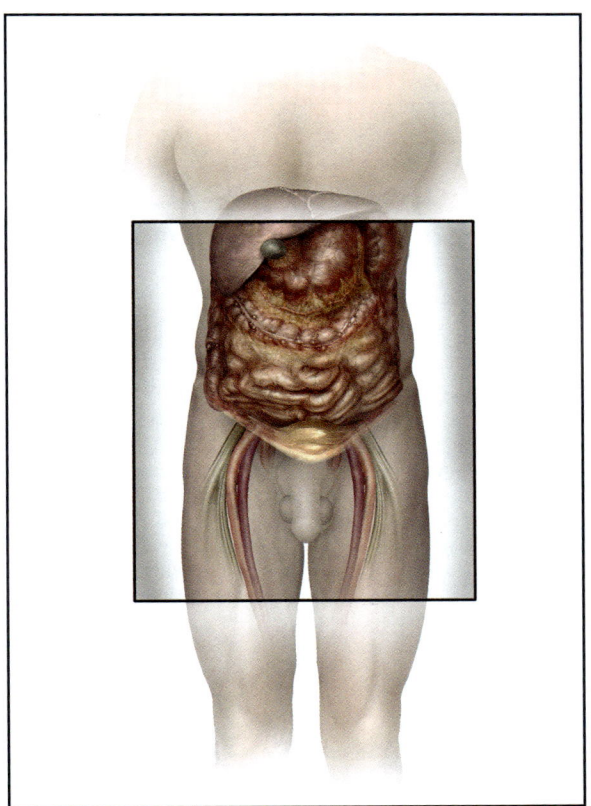

Figure 2-9. From now on, we shall call this the "fourth part" of the core. Traditional physicians work on the "systems" that reside within this nonmusculoskeletal fourth part. This is what these specialists see in this region of the body. They think primarily about the gastrointestinal, genitourinary, gynecological, nerve, blood, and other systems. Those systems are important, of course, but possible interactions with the other 3 parts are snubbed.

Second, we have only been looking at the individual parts and not the entirety of the core as a unit. It's a forest-for-the-trees thing. Docs have been studying arms and legs, the head, chest or abdomen, and sometimes the pelvis. Specialists get deep into the inner workings of the gastrointestinal system, the bladder and ureters, womb and ovaries, big blood vessels, nerves, and lymphatics. It is no wonder that they totally lose sight of the body as a whole and how the big parts are connected. (See Figure 2-9.)

Obviously, there is a lot going on both anatomically and physiologically in this region we are calling "the core." The main solid organs, the excretory system, major blood vessels, nerves, and lymphatics, they are all there alongside the hip, the pelvic muscles, the bones, and the back. Naturally, this complexity obscures our vision. As we see it, our task in writing this book is to make some of this physiology simpler.

We docs need to go up a couple of thousand feet and view the forest.

Third, it is the sex. We get lost in the sex, which is definitely distracting from the whole. And then double entendres run wild. We can't see the forest, the entirety of the unit. No matter how you describe the anatomical territory, we can't get away from double entendres. We giggle about the pubic bone and the various cavities. Yes, sex is a huge distractor. We already know that…that is not generally a very profound statement. But it is a profound statement when it comes to this region of the body. Like in the best cures for alcoholism, we have to first face up to the problem, then we can face reality.

Sex resides in the core; the core is its home. We have to accept this fact. This is not a trivial point. You will hear later more about the social taboos that affect docs in studying this area. For now, just realize that it is permissible to giggle while reading this book. Relax. Enjoy this part of the body. Read about the knees and the shoulders and be bored. You won't get bored here.

See the Body Move

Jane sees Dick. See Dick run. Dick runs after Spot. Yes, we have to go back to the Dick and Jane books to see what we are talking about with respect to the core (Figure 2-10). We even need stick diagrams.

Take the previous 3 reasons why health care professionals have been paying so little attention to the core and apply the same factors to observations about how the body moves. The same thing happens! We get lost. Complexity obscures what we see. We see the arms, legs, and head and then get lost looking at the core. We see a lot of stuff residing between the upper and lower extremities. Wow…with the heart and intestines and everything else, the area seems so complex! We see the abs and butt, and they turn into 6-packs and booties. Giggling starts. Then complexity and sensuality blinds us…again.

Stick figure diagrams work. They show what we have been missing. The core is the whole stick between the arms and legs and under the head. It is simply the connector for all the body parts. In the Dick and Jane spirit, we have fastidiously drawn a representation of the core (Figure 2-11).

Okay, back to Dick and Jane. Once we "see" the simple concept, we can walk. Once we name the different parts, we can talk and run. Then the real science begins (Figure 2-12); then we dance and frolic.

Okay, you get the point! Before we go on, here is one more crucial point. Again, it is really simple. We understand now that we need to consider the whole core, but to do that effectively we cannot ignore any single part. The region is complex, so we must simplify it. We must not forget that the core is what God or, religion aside, *something* gave us. The core is the core. It is the anatomy that we are given. We cannot change it. So we must work with it, no matter the distractions. How specialists view the core is important. But those tunneled insights should not obscure the basic concept that the core connects the other body parts. You will understand better what we mean as you read the rest of the book. As you read, keep continuously in mind the words of New England Patriots coach Bill Belichick (Figure 2-13), "It is what it is," or a Southern drawl coming from the mouth of my fellow baseball coach when we saw our youth travel team totally overmatched in Tennessee, "We shall play with what we brung." Both statements hold with respect to the core.

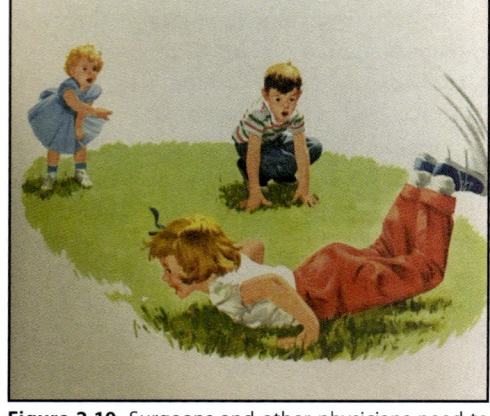

Figure 2-10. Surgeons and other physicians need to go back and read *Dick and Jane*. (Reprinted with permission from Pearson.)

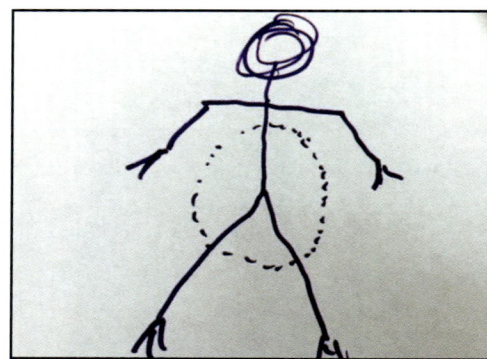

Figure 2-11. Once we see the core as a sum of its individual parts, the revelation shall liberate us. Of course, the core is a distinct region of the body. Certainly, we need to learn more about it. We need to visualize the core functioning as a whole. Without a doubt, we need to name the individual parts. The region needs intense scientific study.

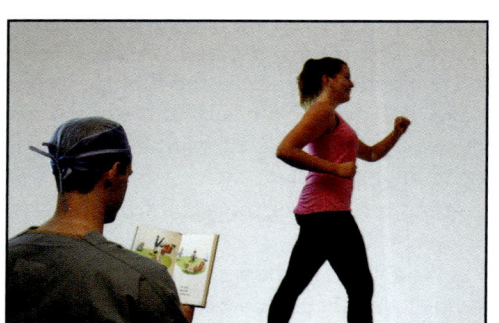

Figure 2-12. Surgeon acquiring insight into core movement.

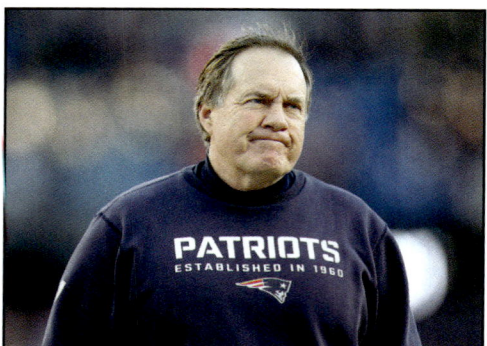

Figure 2-13. Coach Bill Belichick's "It is what it is" expression. (Reprinted with permission from *USA Today Sports*.)

So, How Do We Don New Eyes?

The main gist of this book, of course, is to learn about the body's core. We must don new eyes. As has been mentioned, many, many obstacles stand in our way. So, how do we do this? How do docs and the rest of us put on these new eyes and see the core with all this complexity, commercialism, and sex obstructing our views?

The answer is simple. Just relax and enjoy it. Remember this is a forest-for-the-trees thing. To see the forest, you just have to be willing to see things differently. As Bill Belichick also may have said, "Keep on keeping on." Continue looking. Suddenly you will don new eyes (Figure 2-14).

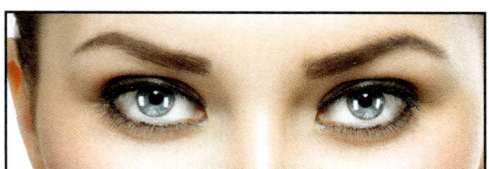

Figure 2-14. We want these eyes.

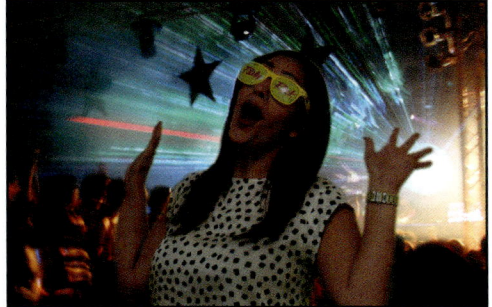

Figure 2-15. Not these eyes. No party rock frames.

Again, just relax and enjoy life and watch. Do not jump to conclusions. Do not put on sunglasses or bifocals, and certainly not LMFAO party rock frames (Figure 2-15). Put those on another time, not now.

See the core as a whole musculoskeletal system from the nipples to mid-thighs, with organs, etc, residing within it (Figure 2-16). Right now, don't think about the separate muscles and bones that reside there. Don't think about the individual physiological systems. Relax and see the forest with the various parts of the gastrointestinal and genitourinary and gynecologic systems as just a bunch of birch trees.

Think of the core as the whole region. When it comes to physical activity, it acts as a single unit. Of course, there is a lot of complexity to it; don't get lost in the trees.

Look at how the core fits together with the rest of the body—the stick diagram thing. Consider also that muscles and bones in the core sit right alongside big-time hollow and solid organs, nerves, blood vessels, and other innards. Those things do interrelate with each other. Once we have new eyes, maybe then we can listen closely to the physiologic chitchat among those anatomic neighbors. Let's find out what structures do the most communicating and with whom.

The next few chapters take a refreshing new look at anatomy and function. Be ready for it. Enjoy it. Don't just look at the diagrams and think this is "same ol', same ol'." It definitely is not that. We are telling a fun story, and this story just so happens to be true.

Once you "get" the gist, you will be amazed. You shall see that the old eyes barely saw anything. You shall discard those bifocals as well as old presumptions. Not only that, but you will want to dig the dirt to bury that ridiculous and dangerous term "sports hernia" because it causes harm, and you shall also want to throw into the same grave those outrageously treacherous sit-up regimens (Figure 2-17). We predict you will greatly appreciate the shift from abs to the butt. Check out these videos; we want you to condemn these sit-up regimens.VID 7-9

We hope you also end up laughing hysterically at "6-pack abs."

Now, let's proceed to a moment of realization.

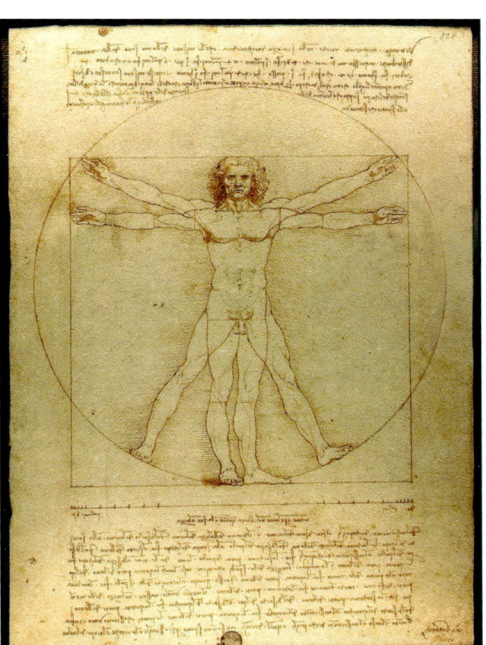

Figure 2-16. This is the core. Da Vinci saw this in the 15th century. He had new eyes back then.

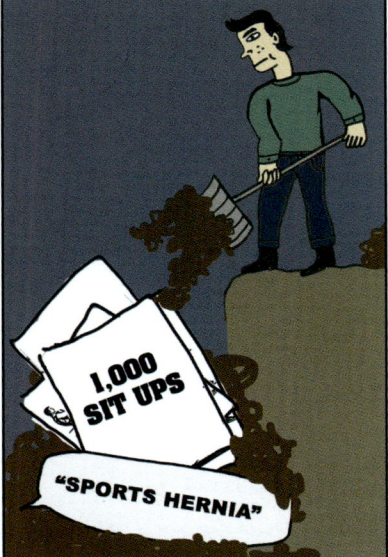

Figure 2-17. We need you to help pile on the dirt.

SELECTED READINGS

Gray WS. *Fun With Dick and Jane.* Chicago, IL: Scott Foresman & Co; 1946.
   This book is always worth a refresher, plus a reminder to keep it simple, or as the US Navy says, KISS—Keep it simple, Stupid.

Ilyas A. Local surgeon warns of hoverboard dangers. http://www.philly.com/philly/blogs/healthcare/Local-surgeon-warns-of-hoverboard-dangers.html. Published December 30, 2015.
   Read all about this popular toy. Not only does it catch on fire, it changes the center point of the core and causes a tremendous variety of injuries. And while you are reading all about this, keep in mind world champion boxer Mike Tyson on his hoverboard.[VID 1]

Holley M. *War Room: The Legacy of Bill Belichick and the Art of Building the Perfect Team.* New York, NY: Harper-Collins; 2011.
   Year after year, Coach Belichick has artfully crafted terrific football teams. One Belichick saying complements the KISS acronym: "It is what it is." Remember both KISS and the Belichick principle if the core anatomy described in this book appears complicated.

VIDEOS

1. http://www.cnn.com/videos/entertainment/2015/12/30/mike-tyson-hoverboard-fall-vo.cnn
2. https://www.youtube.com/watch?v=5xNLLk777A8
3. https://abcarverpro.com/
4. https://youtu.be/fLF8-z6ZtlA
5. https://www.ispot.tv/ad/wHw3/abdominator-unrestricted-core-enhancer
6. https://www.youtube.com/watch?v=6zXDo4dL7SU
7. https://youtu.be/B1pWxaRxEbA
8. https://www.youtube.com/watch?v=IGZOcxpRuoo
9. https://www.youtube.com/watch?v=46o0to59LIY

3

the eureka moment for the core

A Common Scenario

You are lying on your couch on Sunday afternoon, watching a pro football game on TV (Figure 3-1). And someone gets injured. Consider what you know about sports injuries.

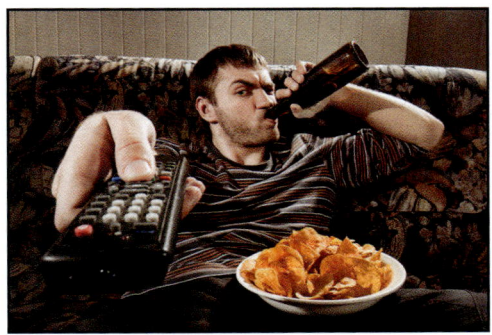

Figure 3-1. A "neutral posture" (see Chapter 32) for most of us Sunday afternoon sports critics. Not exactly what our physical therapists recommend as the best "core neutral" posture! Later chapters actually do provide insight into the best postures for watching Sunday football.

The announcer says—and you agree—that a player hurt his knee. Immediately, you start going through the possibilities. You feel confident in your knee diagnoses. Keep in mind that you are an avid football fan and not a doctor or trainer or anything else connected with health care. Whether or not you are managing an important fantasy football team, you feel pretty confident in your knowledge base. You think about the specific diagnoses and degrees of severity. It could be just a little muscle strain or bruise, and he will be back playing after just a few plays. It could be "cartilage." If so, he could possibly return, but more likely he will require quick arthroscopic surgery and be back in a few weeks. A collateral ligament is a possibility. That is worse and would take maybe 6 weeks. Hopefully, it is not the dreaded anterior cruciate tear. Then he's cooked for the season, maybe longer.

Now consider what you know if this were a core injury. You hear "groin injury," and for the zillionth time, wonder, "Where is the groin anyway?" You ask your couch-mate whether the player is tough enough to get right back and play through it. If he does not come back, you then wonder about his toughness and also the possibility of a "sports hernia." You wonder if that diagnosis is for real, and if it is, then what the heck is it? You think, why should a little tiny protrusion keep him from playing? Why can't he just play through it? You wonder about his toughness again, but admit you really don't understand these things. You bet that no matter what a "sports hernia" is, if he eventually comes back into the game, his performance will be off. He won't be what you are counting on.

Believe it or not, the above scenario reflects the exact state of medical knowledge about core injuries, until recently. For many years, docs, trainers, and physical therapists have not known more than the avid NFL or Premiership fan sitting on the couch watching the game.

Now, we should look at "the core" in a much more sophisticated way. We do know a lot more. The knowledge has just not disseminated well. A number of reasons account for the lack of dissemination, and we will get to those reasons later.

To get from the couch potato state-of-the-art to our present knowledge base, there must have been a realization moment, a "Eureka" moment. There was.

EUREKA MOMENTS IN GENERAL

A Eureka, or "aha!", moment, refers to a common human experience of suddenly understanding a previously incomprehensible concept.[1] It is named after a myth involving the ancient Greek scholar Archimedes, who realized, while sitting in a public bath, how to measure the volume of an irregular object. At that moment of realization, he leaped out of the bath and ran home naked, yelling, "Eureka!," which means "I found it." Most people who saw him running probably didn't yell "Eureka!" They probably said, "Put some clothes on." As the story goes, Archimedes had been asked by a king to determine whether a crown was pure gold or a cheaper imitation laced with silver. While climbing into the bath, he noticed that his body displaced water as he sank into it, and that the volume of water on the floor probably equaled the volume of his body immersed in the water. Since gold weighed more than silver, a crown laced with silver would be bulkier in volume than a pure gold crown if the 2 crowns weighed the same. He would tell the king in the morning! The story is probably fabricated, since the weights of crowns were never measured. But that doesn't matter. One thing for sure, Archimedes was not thinking about his core. His capable core must have facilitated his getting in and out of the bath tub effortlessly, and then his running down the street after the epiphany (Figure 3-2).

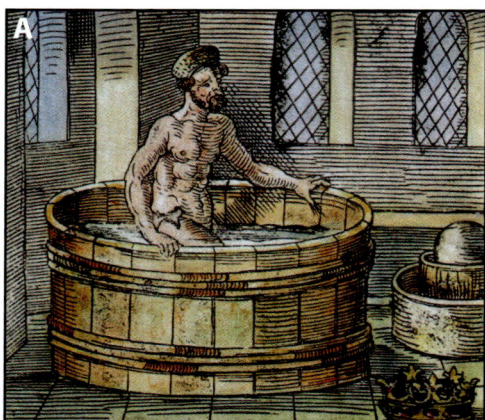 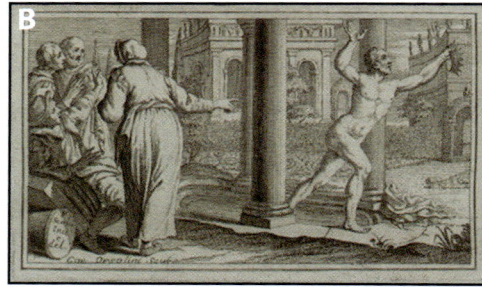

Figure 3-2. (A) Cartoon depicting Archimedes in his Eureka moment. The earliest representation of this event that we could find was in the 1st century BC, in the original German translation of the first book on architecture by Marcus Vitruvius Pollio (in the same era but not the same person as Vitruvius of the "Vitruvian Man" by da Vinci). Archimedes is at the moment of discovery and about to jump out of his bath tub. (B) Archimedes racing through streets shouting, "Eureka!" (By Giammaria Mazzuchelli [www.ssplprints.com], public domain, via Wikimedia Commons.)

Any Eureka moment of insight has a 2-stage process: (1) an impasse when no solution can be found, associated with extraordinary frustration, because all possibilities seem exhausted; and (2) a spell of heightened awareness that allows the problem-solver to identify the solution instantly despite the ordinary surroundings.

In turn, the aha! moment has 3 defining characteristics. First, it appears suddenly. Second, the moment elicits an audible exclamation of joy or satisfaction. Third, the exclaimer and people nearby also understand the solution immediately because it is so obvious and true.

THE IMPASSE WITH RESPECT TO THE CORE

Injuries to the core have always been abundant. All of us probably remember teammates, friends, or family who could not perform well because of the pain "down there." I remember my mom never being able to help to load our station wagon when we packed for vacations because of some kind of a mysterious pelvic pain. Inevitably, our loading experiences would turn into fiascos reminiscent of the Chevy Chase movie *Vacation* (Figure 3-3).

When I was a soccer goalie at Harvard, I befriended a highly recruited football player, Richie Szaro (Figure 3-4), who had been brought to the school with big expectations. But he developed a nagging injury in his groin that prohibited him from playing his position as running back. Even though Richie was in obvious pain, the coaches and *The Harvard Crimson* considered him something of a malingerer. Broken bones kept players off the field. So did torn ligaments. But a pulled groin? Suck it up!

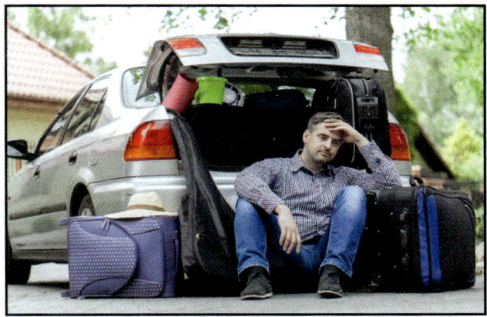

Figure 3-3. Think about the value of a good core when you get frustrated loading your vehicle.

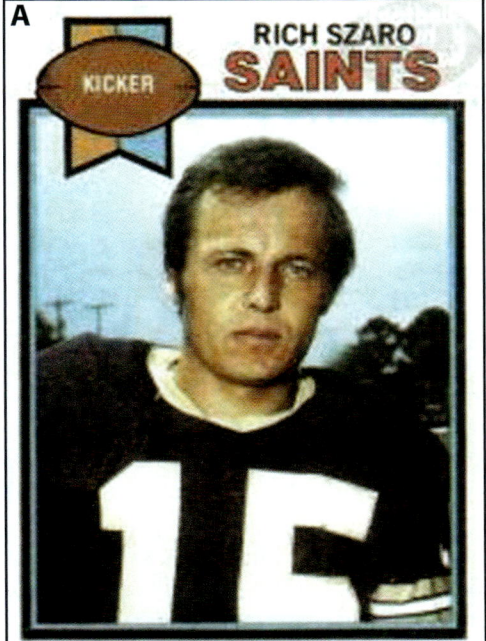

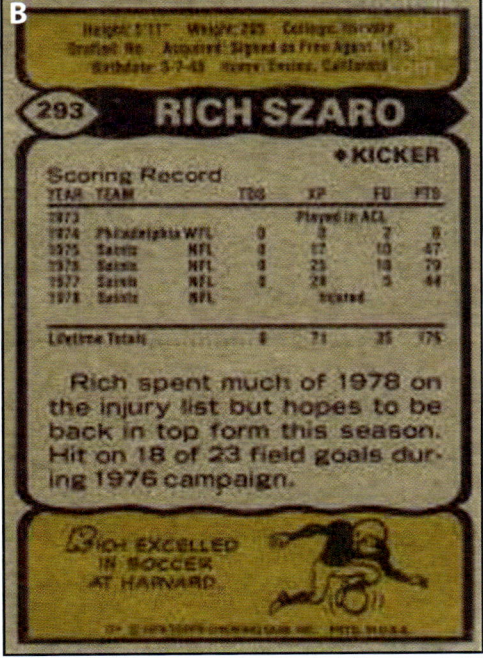

Figure 3-4. (A) Front and (B) back of my friend Richie Szaro's football card from when he played for the New Orleans Saints. He learned to channel forces and become an excellent NFL kicker until the injury wore him out. Richie won his last games by using his right, non-dominant foot for a field goal after his left side gave out. An international wholesaler stationed in Warsaw, Poland, Richie died in August 2015. (Private collection.)

I know now that this player was not faking. At the time, I knew he did not have the usual muscle strain, which, by itself, can be debilitating. Now, in retrospect, he most likely sustained a core harness muscle injury that could have been fixed, had this happened today, with surgery. Of course, that perspective comes from now and not back then. The bottom line then was that Richie had something bad. He was not faking. All his locker room mates knew that.

The old, hard-line, dictator coach of the 1960s and 1970s embodies the state of our knowledge about groin injuries until recently. Anyone who complained of them was just not tough enough. Most of us have probably had coaches like this. They weren't typically thoughtful. They did not wonder what bothered the player, show empathy, and then seek an answer. Most coaches back then were pretty powerful and just not like that (Figure 3-5).

In fairness to those coaches, the fact was that most doctors in that era had no clue about this set of injuries. The pelvis remained a mysterious, forbidden area, and without a dependable fix for the injuries, there was really no purpose for a coach to think differently. Coaches strove for team wins, and players with unfixable, disabling injuries contributed nothing to that.

Even back then, people talked about "sports hernias." Since the physicians didn't have an idea what was happening to these athletes, it made sense that the term stuck, at that time. Beginning in the late 1970s, the term received a bad name in the medical community. The outcomes from hernia repair in athletes and others with inguinal pain were so predictably

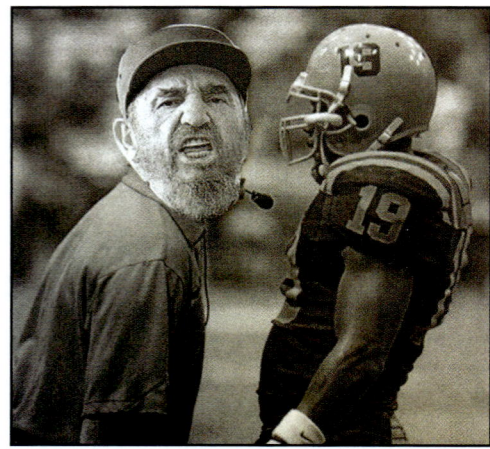

Figure 3-5. Photoshopped portrayal of the olden-days, hard-line dictator coach. The coach is saying, "Groin Schmoin! Back on the field!"

bad that it became verboten for general surgeons to perform repairs in the absence of demonstrable hernia.[2-5] Surgeons who had finished their training would flunk their oral examinations if they mentioned the term.

EXHAUSTING MEDICAL KNOWLEDGE BASES

The athlete with debilitating core pain would painstakingly go through multiple medical hoops. The rigors of medical and surgical training turn doctors' eyes into powerful microscopes that look for diagnoses that they know. We as medical

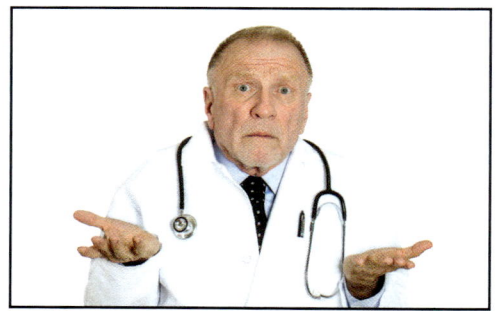

Figure 3-6. The same stumped medical person seen before.

doctors see things clearly through the lenses with which we are supplied. By its nature, training limits our supply of lenses. When people had groin pain while doing activities, they would go to multiple different specialists (Figure 3-6).

Then, the pelvis remained a mysterious anatomical region, and it remains that way for the most part. The private nature of the pelvis has something to do with this, but the main reason is that each of us (eg, physician, surgeon, physical therapist, athletic trainer) is biased by our own specific training. It is difficult to see beyond that. As mentioned, the urologist sees the pelvis as the ureters, bladder, testicles, etc. The general and colorectal surgeons think of this region as where the colon and rectum reside, as well as some protrusions called hernias. Gynecologists see what they see. You get the idea. Specialists, as the term implies, naturally hone in on what they concentrate. Orthopedists are probably best equipped to deal with the mechanics of these athletic injuries as they deal with bones and joints, but they fear misdiagnosis or injury to the genitourinary, gastrointestinal, and gynecologic structures.

The athletic trainer or doc would exhaust the use of all those specialists. Each specialist would look at the patient through his/her highly trained spectacles and rule out the various possibilities. After weeks or months without a specific diagnosis, the mystery would continue, and the frustration would grow much worse.

THE EUREKA MOMENT FOR THE CORE

One simple experiment supplied us with new lenses. It satisfied the 3 defining characteristics of an aha! moment: suddenness, joyous screams, and a simple answer. That there was also a painful scream doesn't change things. The experiment produced a simple answer that showed that the core really did exist and was not just a commercial concept. The experiment led to a whole new way to think about how the body works. It connected the signs and symptoms of many injuries to real anatomy. In this moment, we realized that the concept was really simple. Here's the story:

I became curious about this anatomy as a busy liver surgeon at Duke University in the mid-1980s. Drs. Frank Bassett[6] and William Garrett[7] had asked me to help with the school's sports teams, and I saw a number of players whose careers had been cut short by exertional pelvic pain. In medical school, the musculoskeletal anatomy had seemed overwhelming. Armed with the recent memory of physical examinations on 3 athletes who could no longer play, a medical student and I revisited this anatomy in the fresh cadaver laboratory. We were determined to think about function. We could elicit multiple sites of pain around the pubic bones of these athletes.

In the lab, it became obvious that the pubic bone was in the middle of all this activity. It was the hub (Figure 3-7).

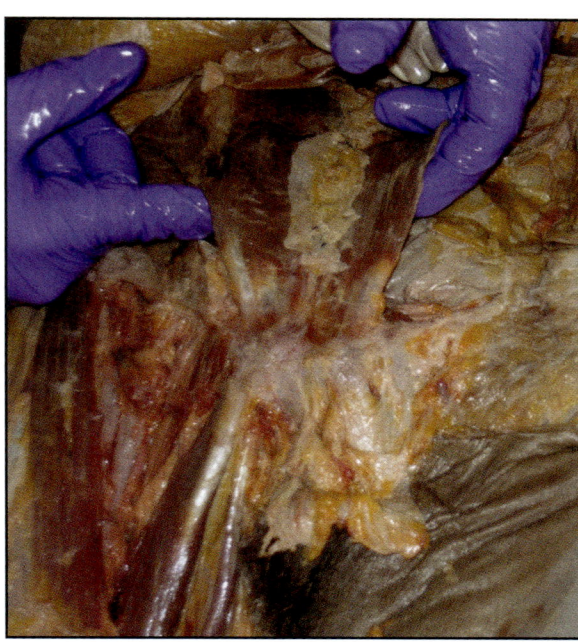

Figure 3-7. We dissected this fresh cadaver for the purposes of developing the first MRI techniques to diagnose the various core muscle injuries. The picture shows anatomy relevant to the described "Eureka" experiment. The gloved fingers hold the rectus abdominis just above where it would be cut (see Figure 3-8). The adductor muscles originate near where the rectus abdominis muscles end.

We did a stupidly simple experiment. From above the pubis, I took a Mayo scissors and cut through about 30% of the right rectus abdominis attachment while the medical student had her index finger behind the 3 adductors that attach to the pubic bone and on top of the anterior edge of the inferior pubic ramus, which has sharp, tooth-like projections. As I cut the rectus, the adductor muscles jolted posteriorly and jammed her finger into the pubic ramus teeth. She let out a scream, depicted by the tears in the figure.

She didn't know it, but that scream made medical history (Figure 3-8).

Rather than worry whether she would ever use her finger again, we immediately made the observation that forces created by the weakened rectus abdominis were being transmitted below the pubic bone. The pubic complex was acting like a joint. We had caused instability of this pubic "joint." In further dissections, it became clear the rectus abdominis, pectineus, adductor longus, and adductor brevis were the most important structures in stabilizing the joint. Other muscles passing by the joint, such as psoas, rectus femoris, and sartorius, provided additional support. A thick fibrocartilage plate lay on top of and congruent with the pubic bone, connecting the muscles above and below. There was very little real tendon.

We had discovered a new way of considering injuries in the area. More good news: the medical student's finger did recover.

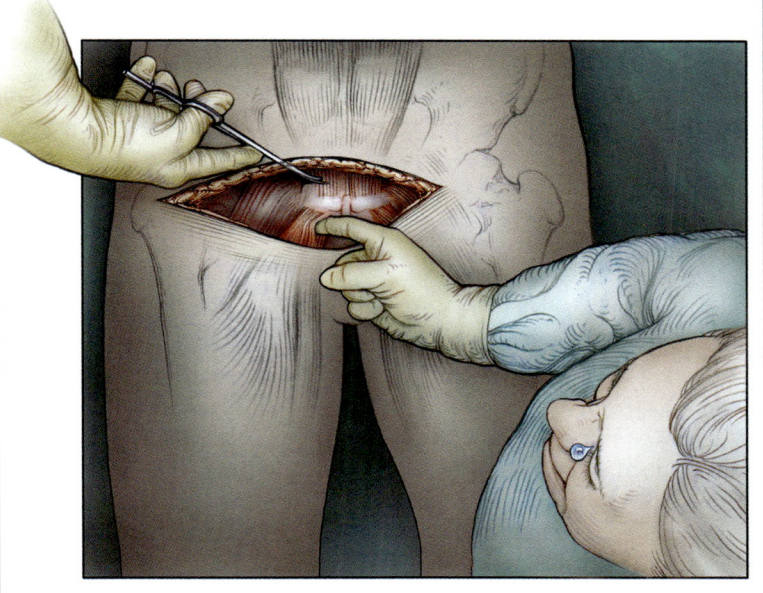

Figure 3-8. The core Eureka moment. Note the tear falling from the left eye of the medical student, due to her index finger being jammed between the adductors and the tooth-like anterior edge of the inferior pubic ramus; the pelvis had jolted forward when the rectus abdominis was cut.

Connecting the "Pubic Bone Joint" to the Hip

Further experiments on fresh cadavers reaffirmed the dynamic nature of this region. For example, dividing the same rectus abdominal muscle in the same way caused dramatic pressure changes inside the ball-and-socket hip joint. The cuts even caused our measurement needles to bend. We also found that restriction of the ball-and-socket hip joint came from not just the socket alone; it came from all the surrounding structures as well, such as the adductor muscles and even the femoral vessels. (See Figures 3-9 and 3-10.)

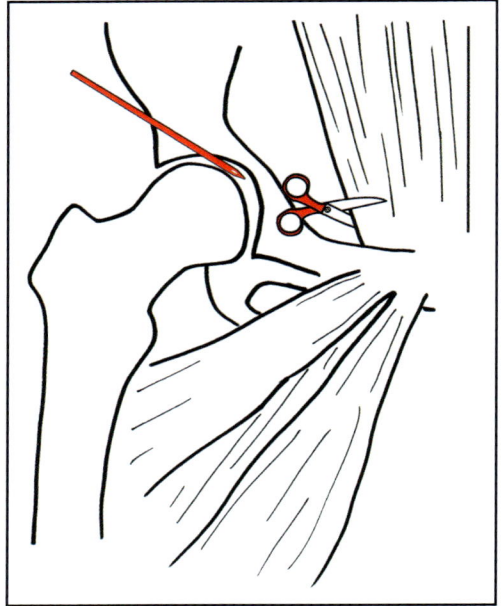

Figure 3-9. The same experiment as the core Eureka moment experiment, except with a pressure-gauge needle inside the hip joint. The pressure zoomed up as the rectus abdominis was cut.

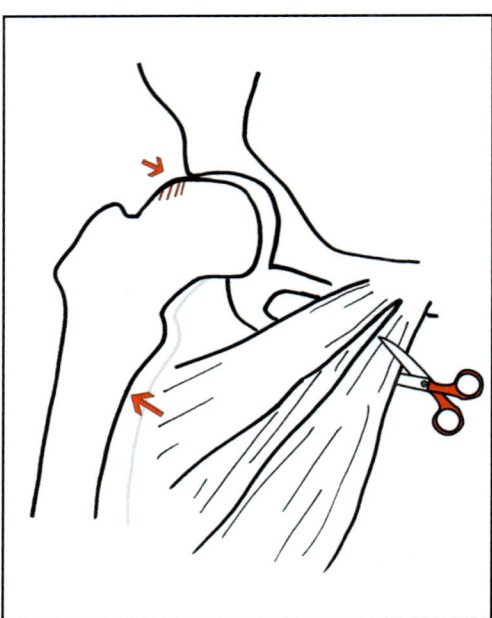

Figure 3-10. A subsequent experiment to determine the anatomical structures that restrict hip range of motion. In this case, division of adductor muscles created impingement in a cadaver with cam anatomy.

Understandably, the precise pressure values were not physiological. After all, these "patients" were dead. Nevertheless, even in the absence of life, the obvious changes meant that the entire region around and including the pubic bone had been acting together, presumptively harmoniously.

The cuts changed things. Dead people don't feel things. My live medical student did. Her finger really hurt. Imagine what an athlete, or anyone, might feel when his/her muscle or hip suddenly becomes trapped against sharp bone.

Where Next?

It turns out the whole region—chest to thighs—acts together as a unit in controlling human movement. It also turns out there is an obvious right way for the core to control this movement, and many wrong ways that lead to injury.

During the initial experiment, we felt like Archimedes. We had "found it!" The questions remained, though; how would we apply it and how were we going to convey "it" to others?

The first thing we did was to check if our anatomic findings had any clinical meaning. We operated on the 3 players we mentioned, whom we had been following in the clinic. Each had severe pain and couldn't play. Sure enough, noticeable pathology existed in the muscular areas where we predicted, and we fixed the injuries. To our delight, the operations succeeded. All 3 returned to their sports at a high level and had great subsequent seasons. That original success thrust us into a very large clinical experience with diagnosis, repair, and other methods to treat these injuries.

We published papers and presented findings at meetings.[8-10] But nobody seemed to be listening. People kept seeing the same music, playing the same old tunes. They kept misdiagnosing and performing the "same ol'" hernia repairs. Our initial findings actually stimulated some surgeons to do more hernia repairs than ever before, as if we had offered some sort of justification for them to do that. Others performed traditional hernia repairs under new names, as if the procedures were different.

We realized something was wrong when we began reoperating on so many patients.

What was going on? Why was no one listening, or at least hearing what we were saying? It was because they were not "seeing."

A Historical Perspective on the Eureka Moment

Let's summarize some of what defrocked the myth that these are hernias.

Keep in mind that the situation has grown more confusing because hernia repairs have had some success for specific injuries. Authors as far back as 1895[11-14] speculated on a dynamic musculoskeletal nature to these injuries and on changes in the pubic bone that seemed to correlate with age and soft tissue injury. A 1924 article[13] even connects changes in the inferior aspect of the pubis to prior suprapubic injury. In 1981, Nesovic suggested a muscular imbalance in footballers in Yugoslavia[14,15] and subsequently devised a number of repairs for various injuries. I may have followed in suggesting this in publication,[8] but Gilmore from the United Kingdom, and perhaps others, had been censuring the hernia theory years before that.

Seeking New "Landscapes" vs "Having New Eyes"

Remember the Marcel Proust quote from Chapter 2. Understanding the core requires new eyes.

After several early reports of successful experiences using new approaches,[15-17] an outpouring of traditional hernia surgeons and then laparoscopic surgeons sought new frontiers for their tools.[18-21] Most of the reports suggested that pain rarely improved without surgery. Most of those articles provided limited follow-up, and several reported 100% success rates—remarkable considering the wide variety of patients and absence of definitions. Consistent with those reports, in our own early experience with open and then laparoscopic hernia repair as primary treatment, pain often improved. However, we were never satisfied with the results because athletes often persisted with some degree of pain.[22,23] Thus, some success with hernia repair, as occurred years ago, plus an influx of hernia surgeons, has brought some people back to the mistaken concept of hernia as the underlying factor.

Then team physicians, physical therapists, trainers, and others with experience treating players during competition wrote about the injuries,[18] and some questioned the need for surgery. One paper narrowed the scope of patients to a certain type of adductor injury and reported good success with a specific physical therapy regimen as primary treatment.[24]

In 2008, we reported a large overall experience with these injuries characterizing the changes in the recognition and treatment over 2 decades (Table 3-1). The injuries were divided into a number of different categories based on the specific muscles involved, MRI, and operative pathology. The pubis and its attachments were undeniably important. Not all the lesions needed surgery, and when appropriate, surgery nearly always fixed the problems. Soon afterward, Muschaweck and Berger[25] reported a minimal repair technique with 100% "perfect satisfaction" at 4 weeks postoperatively. They described the ultrasonographic identification of an abdominal wall hernia as the common factor in the patients, and at least one patient also had an adductor procedure. In 2011, Paajanen et al again achieved 100% "perfect satisfaction," but this time with laparoscopic hernia surgery and at 12 months postoperatively.[26] Interestingly, Paajanen sometimes added some kind of adductor procedure to his repairs. As physicians, we are taught to challenge anything that is 100%. On the other hand, like searching for gold, zeal comes from looking for something valuable and finding something shiny. Those startling results likely represent a combination of some success and zeal.

The literature remains confusing. The numerous articles advocate many different approaches. For example, one critical review of exercise therapy as treatment for groin pain in athletes found 468 articles on the subject, and judged only 12 worthy of analysis, and determined that only 7 out of those 12 were reasonable in quality.[27]

We found 5 relatively recent prospective studies (Table 3-2).[24,26,28-30] Together, they reflect a lack of a unified theme. Hölmich's trial[24] was randomized and prospective for 2 types of physical therapy for specific adductor injuries; the authors showed that an active training protocol was better. Our 2 studies[28,30] were not randomized. This was not ethically possible

Table 3-1. Changes in Patient Profiles Over Two Decades (Data From the Third Selected Reading)

	1986-1995	2003-2008
Female	< 1%	15.2%
Age (years)	24.7 (14 to 54)	28.6 (8 to 88)
Athletes	91.1%	76.9%
Number of sports	15	32
Top sports	Soccer	Soccer, football, hockey
Number of recognized syndromes	3	19 (121 different operations)
Number of rehab/performance protocols	0	16

Adapted from Meyers WC, McKechnie A, Philippon MJ, Horner MA, Zoga AC, Devon ON. Experience with "sports hernia" spanning two decades. *Ann Surg.* 2008;248(4):656-665.

Table 3-2. Five Prospective Studies on Groin Pain in Athletes

Author	Year	Study
Hölmich et al[24]	1999	68 patients randomized to 2 types of physical therapy
Meyers et al[28]	2000	157 nonrandomized patients
Ekstrand & Ringborg[29]	2001	66 patients randomized to 4 treatments
Meyers et al[30]	2011	114 nonrandomized female patients
Paajanen et al[26]	2011	60 patients randomized to surgery vs physical therapy

Adapted from Meyers W, Zoga A. Core muscle injuries. In: Haddad FS, ed. *The Young Adult Hip in Sport.* London, United Kingdom: Springer-Verlag; 2014:107-119.

in our patient population; plus, we chose to treat a number of patients nonsurgically. In the first study, the overall 2-year self-assessed success rate was 95.4% after various types of surgery. Success was defined as at or better than preinjury levels of play. Most in the other 4.6% group were better but had concomitant hip or other problems not yet fully treated. The exact time frame for return to play was not assessed since many patients had surgery in the off-season. The second study[27] was on pelvic pain in female athletes. A variety of injuries were separated into 3 categories: hip, core muscle injuries, and "other causes," and there was considerable overlap among the 3 groups. Surgery provided markedly superior results compared to nonoperative approaches for the musculoskeletal injuries (see Table 3-2). The other 2 prospective studies[26,29] were randomized. Ekstrand and Ringborg[29] included 66 patients and randomized them to 4 different treatments, only one being surgical. The complex results are difficult to summarize, but only the surgery achieved satisfaction.

In summary, a deluge of studies now shower the medical literature on this topic. The various authors write about a variety of injuries, and it is difficult to sort out the definitions and patient selection. Stated bluntly, the befuddling literature along with a lack of a common anatomic understanding emphasized the urgency for new eyes.

One should not judge these studies too harshly. They reflect the eyes of the various authors' trainings. Many of the papers touch on important observations and contribute to our having new eyes by challenging the opacity of the pelvis and pelvic injuries.

THE NEXT PAGES

Before we get into hard-core anatomy, biomechanics, and the correct ways to identify specific injuries and prevent or treat them, let's analyze the difficulties we had in dispelling the old beliefs.

Certainly, part of the quandary came from the many pressures suddenly hurled upon surgeons by the changing health care system. Pressure mounted on physicians to justify their jobs and to refer patients internally within their corporate health care systems. Surgeons felt the pressure to do more procedures. The last thing they wanted was a whole new paradigm that threatened the way they did things.

New pressures were part of the difficulty. The main problem was that people just could not "see."

SELECTED READINGS

Taylor DC, Meyers WC, Moylan JA, et al. Abdominal musculature abnormalities as a cause of groin pain in athletes. *Am J Sports Med.* 1991;19:239-242.
The paper that resulted from our initial presentation on this subject. We introduced the term athletic pubalgia and pointed out that these injuries were not hernias.

Meyers WC, Foley DP, Garrett WE, Lohnes JH, Mandlebaum BR. Management of severe lower abdominal or inguinal pain in high-performance athletes. PAIN (Performing Athletes with Abdominal or Inguinal Neuromuscular Pain Study Group). *Am J Sports Med.* 2000;28(1):2-8.
Long-term follow-up on an early large series of core muscle injury patients who underwent surgery based on findings from early cadaveric studies.

Meyers WC, McKechnie A, Philippon MJ, Horner MA, Zoga AC, Devon ON. Experience with "sports hernia" spanning two decades. *Ann Surg.* 2008;248(4):656-665.
Overview of an extensive experience with core problems based on the anatomic principles described in this book.

REFERENCES

1. Eureka effect. Wikipedia. https://en.wikipedia.org/wiki/Eureka_effect. Updated March 28, 2016. Accessed May 3, 2016.
2. Swan KG, Wolcott M. The athletic hernia: a systematic review. *Clin Orthop Relat Res.* 2006;455:78-87.
3. Zoga A. Invited lecture. Radiological Society of North America. Chicago, IL, 2007.
4. Taylor DC, Meyers WC, Moylan JA, et al. Abdominal musculature abnormalities as a cause of groin pain in athletes. *Am J Sports Med.* 1991;19:239-242.
5. Meyers W, Zoga A. Core muscle injuries. In: Haddad FS, ed. *The Young Adult Hip in Sport.* London, United Kingdom: Springer-Verlag; 2014:107-119.
6. Frank Houston Bassett (1928-2007) was the long-revered director of sports medicine at Duke University Medical Center.
7. William E. Garrett Jr remains a leader in sports medicine and orthopedics at Duke University Medical Center.
8. Taylor DC, Garrett WE, Meyers WC. Presentation at the 15th annual meeting of the American Orthopedic Society for Sports Medicine; June 1989; Traverse City, MI.
9. Presentations at meetings of the American Association of Orthopedic Surgeons; 1997, 1999, 2007.
10. Meyers WC, McKechnie A, Philippon MJ, Horner MA, Zoga AC, Devon ON. Experience with "sports hernia" spanning two decades. *Ann Surg.* 2008;248(4):656-665.
11. Abbe R. Rupture of the tendon of the adductor longus. *Ann Surg.* 1895;2:517-519.
12. Todd TW. Age changes in the pubic bone. *Am J Phys Antropol.* 1930;14:255-271.
13. Beer E. Periostitis of symphysis and descending rami of pubic following suprapubic operations. *Int J Med Surg.* 1924;37:224-225.
14. Nesovic B. El Dolor en la Ingle de los Futbolistas. *Il Curso de la Escuela Catalana de Traumatologia del Deporte.* 1981;246-251.
15. Nesovic B. Abstract from presentation at 1988 Olympic sports medicine meeting.
16. Polyglase AL, Frydman GM, Farmer KC. Inguinal surgery for debilitating chronic groin pain in athletes. *Med J Aust.* 1991;155:674-677.
17. Gilmore OJA. Gilmore's groin: ten years' experience of groin disruption: a previously unsolved problem in sportsmen. *Sports Med Soft Tissue Trauma.* 1991;3:12-14.
18. Bisciotti GN. Athlete's pubalgia: a systematic review. http://www.kinemovecenter.it/ita/285/voce/66/athletes-pubalgia-a-systematic-review.htm
19. Nam A, Brody F. Management and therapy for sports hernia. *J Am Coll Surg.* 2008;206:154-164.
20. Caudill P, Nyland J, Smith C, et al. Sports hernia: a systematic literature review. *Br J Sports Med.* 2008;42:954-964.
21. Minnich J, Hanks J, Muschaweck U, et al. Sports hernia: diagnosis and treatment highlighting a minimal repair technique. *Am J Sports Med.* 2011;39:1341-1349.

22. Unpublished data, 1988-1993: Southern Surgeons Club clinical trials group, in conjunction with the Duke/United States Surgical Endosurgery Center, conducted a prospective analysis of open vs laparoscopic hernia repair. Performed in a similar fashion to Reference 23, data were collected on over 2000 patients and included approximately 200 patients with sports-related groin pain and no demonstrable hernia.
23. Meyers WC, Southern Surgeons Club. A prospective analysis of 1518 laparoscopic cholecystectomies. *N Engl J Med.* 1991;324:1073-1078.
24. Hölmich P, Uhrskou P, Ulnits L, et al. Effectiveness of active physical training as treatment for longstanding adductor-related groin pain in athletes: randomized trial. *Lancet.* 1999;353:439-443.
25. Muschaweck U, Berger L. Minimal repair technique of sportsmen's groin: an innovative open-suture repair to treat chronic inguinal pain. *Hernia.* 2009;14:27-33.
26. Paajanen H, Brinck T, Hermunen H, et al. Laparoscopic surgery for chronic groin pain in athletes is more effective than nonoperative treatment: a randomized clinical trial with magnetic resonance imaging of 60 patients with sportsman's hernia (athletic pubalgia). *Surgery.* 2011;150:99-107.
27. Machotka Z, Kumar S, Perraton L. A systematic review of the literature on the effectiveness of exercise therapy for groin pain in athletes. *Sports Med Arthrosc Rehabil Ther Technol.* 2009;1:5-11.
28. Meyers WC, Foley DP, Garrett WE, et al. Management of severe lower abdominal or inguinal pain in high-performance athletes. *Am J Sports Med.* 2000;28:2-8.
29. Ekstrand J, Ringborg S. Surgery versus conservative treatment in soccer players with chronic groin pain: a prospective randomized study in soccer players. *Eur J Sports Traumatol Rel Res.* 2001;23:141-145.
30. Meyers WC, Kahan DM, Joseph T, et al. Current analysis of women athletes with pelvic pain. *Med Sci Sports Exerc.* 2011;43:1387-1393.

4

the difficulty abandoning **old** eyes
"**unseeing**"

It all comes down to memory. Until you really see the light, you revert back to what your memory dictates.
—Dave McNabb, a wonderful PGA teaching pro, said this while teaching the golf swing.

Even when we must see things differently, we often do not. The following case displays some of the struggles involved in changing beliefs and attitudes.

A CORE MUSCLE INJURY THAT PERPETUATED OLD EYES

When a prominent NFL quarterback suffered a groin injury in 2005, his play suffered, his team staggered in the standings, and the fans grew restless. As time went on, the nature of the damage became public; he had a "sports hernia." The quarterback didn't describe his symptoms, other than to say that he hadn't "reached the point where I can't go. I don't see that happening" (Figure 4-1).[1-3]

It happened. Later that season, the injury got worse and the quarterback was shelved. He underwent surgery, completed an extensive rehab process, and returned the next season fully recovered. Everything went perfectly—except the diagnosis.

There is no such thing as a sports hernia. Despite repeated use of the term by athletes, coaches, the media that covers them, and even some physicians, "sports hernia" is a deceptive misnomer. There is no herniation that leads to protrusion of abdominal contents. This is not just one problem. There is not just one fix. This is a whole set of muscle injuries that involves the neighboring bones. A better name is "athletic pubalgia," but that doesn't sound like something a football player would sustain. And that can actually make some people uncomfortable because of the "pubalgia" part of it. It's kind of hard to imagine a coach dropping the word "pubalgia" into a discussion of Double-A gap blitzes and play-action passes.

Sports hernia is easy. It seems acceptable.

But it is wrong. The term has led to false assumptions and many off-target surgeries.

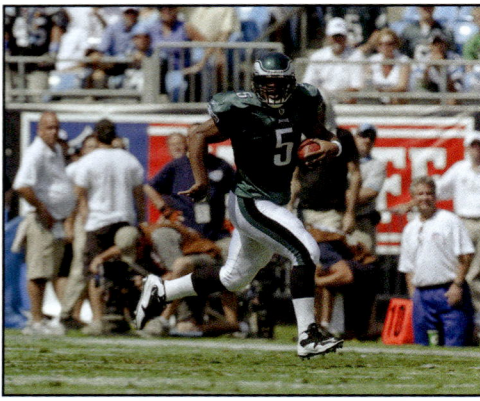

Figure 4-1. Star Philadelphia Eagle quarterback Donovan McNabb, known as a mobile, talented passer and runner. Heroically, Donovan played through nearly a whole season with a severe core muscle injury.

The injury suffered by many athletes and nonathletes is, point of fact, a set of injuries. Often, one first tears his/her rectus abdominis, then the psoas, and finally, at the same time, 3 adductor muscles on each side of the body. The name we want you to use today is *core muscle injury*. We are talking about the core—the lower back, hip joint, and skeletal muscle of the pelvis. Fortunately, he had no hip or back involvement. The core muscles get injured in sports and other activities, alone or in combination with the hip and back. These are core injuries and core muscle injuries. This quarterback's case opened many eyes with respect to the existence of these injuries.

The publicity generated also set us way back in terms of understanding these injuries. All of a sudden, the whole world "understood" these injuries were all "hernias."

This case, and Figure 4-2, illustrates the problem with old eyes looking at this quarterback's problem. His injury, in fact, was complex and required a sophisticated repair. Nevertheless, the publicity generated by his injury reinvigorated more and more surgeons to use their old eyes and treat these injuries, again, like hernias. As Proust warned, they sought the "same ol'" horizons (Figure 4-3). Inappropriate hernia repairs for these complex musculoskeletal injuries increased 10-fold.

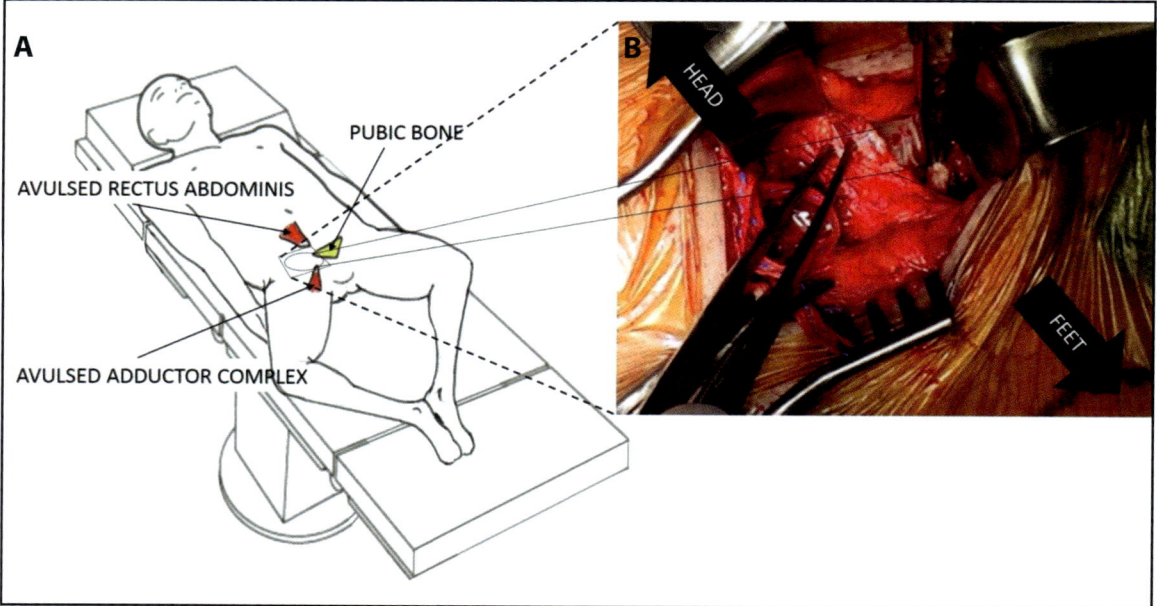

Figure 4-2. A severe core muscle "harness" injury. (A) Sketch of a severe core muscle injury in a bull rider on the operating room table with the area of incision. The parallelogram represents the frame of the intraoperative photo and the contained ellipse the skin edges in that photo. (B) Intraoperative photograph of the injury. (1) The retracted, avulsed rectus abdominis stump is above the left retractor and not shown. (2) The right forceps holds a stump of adductor. (3) The left forceps points to a subtotal avulsion of the pectineus muscle. (4) A hollowed-out right pubic body glistens behind the right forceps.

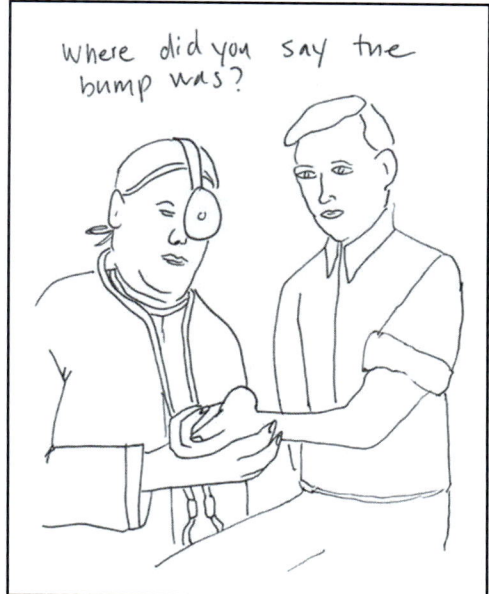

Figure 4-3. In medicine, old eyes often get obscured by our own instruments. Physicians will see the humor in this picture. A physician is looking through a device meant for reflecting light and not a telescope. The reflector should be on top of his head and not obstructing his vision.

The quarterback's injury highlighted the realization that we were not effectively conveying our findings from the Eureka moment. By 2005, we had repaired thousands of such core muscle injuries. Yet, most of medicine, and certainly the public, still knew nothing about these injuries. Obviously, despite all our presentations, the knowledge had not disseminated well. It was frustrating (Figure 4-4).

The doc in Figure 4-3 represents the same ol' docs we encountered in previous chapters, the ones with "old eyes," the eyes we had to make "unsee" what they were seeing. For years, people presumed occult hernias were the heart of the problem. And most nonsurgical health care professionals just took it for granted that hernias were the problem. Figure 4-5 shows an ultrasound that greatly aggravated the problem further.

For years, it has been known that ultrasonography can make things look like hernias by a combination of varying the locations of the probe and different types of straining. True hernias may, in fact, look like this on ultrasonography, but one can produce these findings in people who do not have any semblance of a hernia.

The unseeing problem here is sort of like the concept of group-think that led to the space shuttle Challenger disaster.[4] In that disaster, you will remember, sets of real data escalated a mistaken belief, held by multiple experts who all worked together. The final analysis was wrong, and the space shuttle crashed. In this case, a general surgeon predisposed to thinking that pelvic pains in athletes is all due to occult hernias listens to a radiologist who calls an occult hernia on an imaging study. What happened next? Of course, the surgeon, inclined to do a hernia repair, believes the ultrasound report and puts his/her instruments to work. "Another successful repair!" might be stated when the surgeon sees the patient 2 weeks after the surgery. But for how long is the patient followed? How well does the patient really do?

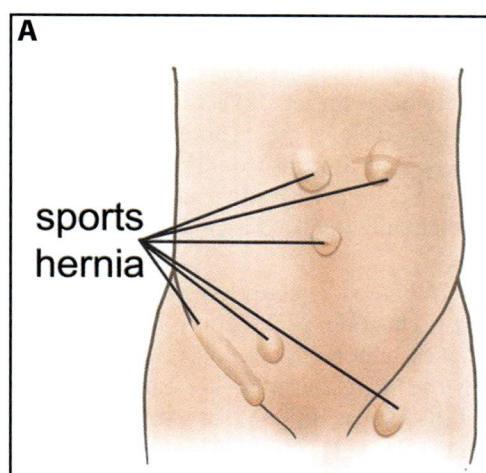 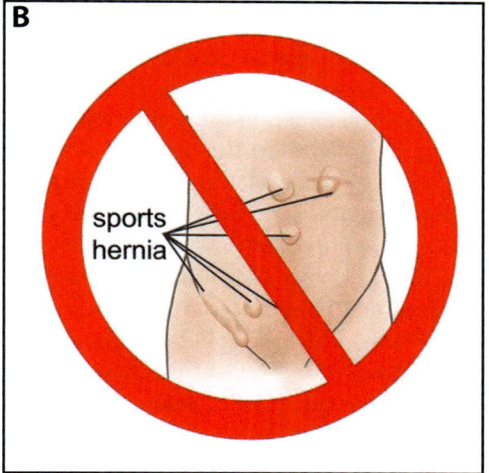

Figure 4-4. In 2005, the old concept of "sports hernia" still festered. The aforementioned quarterback's injury disseminated incorrect notions and treatments of core injuries (A and B).

Unfortunately, copious medical literature does exist that supports such diagnostic and surgical approaches. As poorly as the articles may be written, they cannot be "unwritten." The problem is a big one. It gets back to the discussion of Aristotle and Hume, etc, and the big flaw in empirical medicine (ie, "knowing" things with more certainty than our senses are telling us).

With respect to the core, physicians need to see more clearly what is really happening.

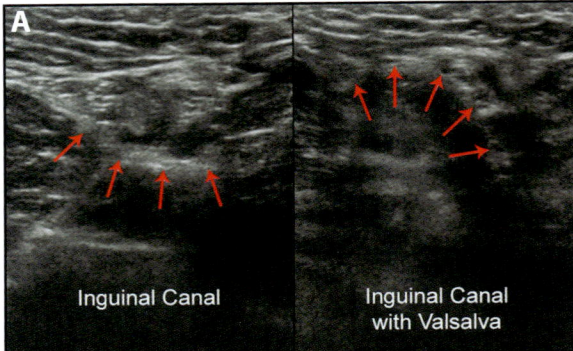 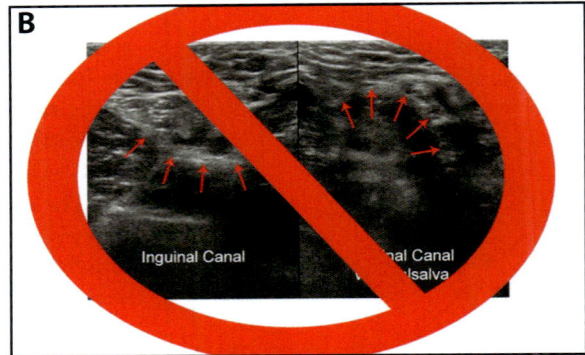

Figure 4-5. Ultrasounds exacerbate the deception of old eyes. This set of images shows how an ultrasonographer can generate what looks like an inguinal hernia during abdominal straining. The arrows point to supposed alterations in the musculature. Such alterations are normally seen with Valsalva maneuvers. The bottom line is that this sort of image can be produced in just about **any** person undergoing this dynamic examination.

Let's next address the state-of-the-art as it looks in the present literature. You will "see" that most authors still have not acquired new eyes.

WHAT HAS THE LITERATURE BEEN CALLING THESE PROBLEMS?

A year ago, I was asked by an orthopedic journal to do a review of current literature on "athletic pubalgia."[5] Even for me, having devoted 30 professional years to this topic, it was tough to even write an opening sentence for the requested literature review. "Thorny" may be a better adjective, because a quick read through the various literatures exposed so many different, often intensely competitive, biases and interests. So, any critique was likely to provoke massive grousing. My 2 goals for the review swiftly became: (1) to build some common ground, and (2) if that were not possible, to, at the very least, keep the moaning of therapists locked into old eyes at lower decibels.

Understand that the literature on this overall subject has been a mess. So, 3 colleagues and I asked 2 simple questions. The first was: What literature exactly should we review? The term *athletic pubalgia* came from a 1989 paper we presented at the 15th annual meeting of the American Orthopedic Sports Medicine Society.[6] There, we had proposed the term as an alternative to *sports hernia* because it accurately depicted, in a general way, the anatomic location of a set of pains so potentially disabling for athletes. At the time, we also knew that general surgeons would flunk their American Board of Surgery oral boards if they mentioned that other term. That latter fact emphasizes that no one in 1989 understood this pain. At that 1989 presentation, we believed athletic pubalgia potentially involved a lot of different muscles and bones intimate with some pretty important organ systems.

Keep in mind that at the time of writing this review in 2014, there were countless quasi-scientific articles on this subject. They appeared in all kinds of journals, dealing with all aspects of physical therapy, fitness health, and medicine. Some of the better articles, which we could not ignore, happened to be in popular periodicals targeting the general public. Therefore, for the purposes of this review, we chose to review only the English-written literature over the past 2 to 3 years, but not to totally ignore selected articles before that. We began with Google and PubMed web searches.

The second question we asked for this review was: What do authors call these injuries today? We simply tallied the first 100 seemingly appropriate articles, using 5 rules:

1. We searched only the time interval 2012 through 2014. Articles from other years, of course, did pop up.
2. We did not search with terms that would obviously bias the results (eg, sports hernia, athletic pubalgia).
3. We did not read articles with titles about noninjury problems (eg, inguinal hernia or gynecologic pain), unless the title suggested they might discuss injuries.
4. We excluded generally descriptive terms (eg, pelvic pain in athletes).
5. We lumped together similar terminologies (eg, sports hernia and sportsman's hernia).

Tables 4-1 and 4-2 show the results.

Table 4-1 Top Five Terms From Google	
1. Sports hernia	63%
2. Athletic pubalgia	12%
3. Core muscle injury	8%
4. Gilmore's groin	6%
5. Hockey groin	3%

Table 4-2 Top Five Terms From PubMed	
1. Sports hernia	41%
2. Sportsman's groin	24%
3. Athletic pubalgia	18%
4. Core injury	2%
5. Adductor injury	2%

Interestingly, the Top 5 from PubMed and Google were not much different. One might have expected more anatomic precision in the PubMed articles, but that did not happen. The most striking difference between PubMed and Google was the use of quotation marks around the term sports hernia. That occurred in more than 70% of the PubMed articles and just 13% of the Google article titles. From the latter observation, we surmised 2 points: (1) the authors of the articles from PubMed were indeed thinking more scientifically (ie, trying to be more accurate), and (2) the authors may have believed these injuries were not hernias.

The bottom line from this recent literature review was that people clearly no longer trusted their previous eyesight; they knew multiple injuries were operative. Plus, they knew these were not hernias. Yet they saw no consistent concept emerging. Therefore, people still labeled all these things sports hernias or pseudonyms reflecting the pathology as some kind of "inguinal disruption." Most therapists were continuing to treat all these problems by their own "trusted" methods, usually one fix for all the pathologies encountered. The "fix" always represented their training. That line of thinking also reflects the aforementioned inherent flaw of empirical medicine—"knowing" things with more certainty than what our senses are telling us (see the last section).

What the heck? Consider the frustration.

THE DIFFICULTIES

So, the literature still, mostly, reflects an impasse in understanding these injuries.

The previous chapter describes the importance of an impasse to the actuality of an aha! moment, but does not describe why a simple understandable solution to that impasse may not be immediately accepted. Logic would say that scientists would believe it. After all, this is not Christopher Columbus saying the Earth is not flat.

Perhaps we are more like Copernicus, with his *De revolutionibus orbium coelestium*, when he said the sun and not the Earth is the center of the universe. Sixteenth century religious leaders led a tempestuous charge against Copernicus, who "fortunately" died before the scorn reached full throttle.

Okay, it is not the same. This is not a religious thing. Or is it? We are saying the pubic bone is the center of the body's universe. Everybody already knows that, don't they? Maybe…but certainly not in a functional anatomic sense!

We do see reasons for the lack of acceptance of this "Copernican" understanding. The primary reason may be that this book hasn't been published yet. But we have written a great deal in peer-reviewed journals. Likely, the writings have gotten lost within the very confusing literature outlined previously.

We believe the primary reason for the lack of understanding of this concept is the "things you cannot unsee" theory about how the brain works.[7] The second reason people may choose not to accept the concept is because it conflicts with their presumptions, and sometimes their training and well-being, similar to the weakness we discussed of empiricism (Figure 4-6).

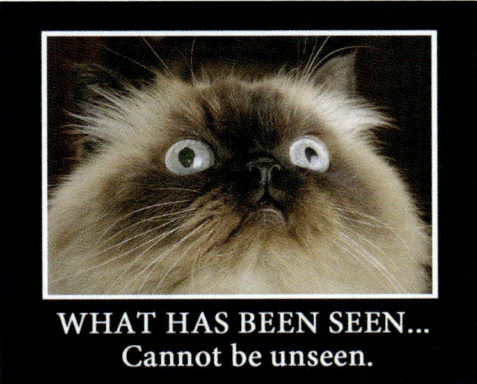

Figure 4-6. A cute photograph was the lead-in to a nice academic analysis of this phenomenon.[4]

The Primary Reason: Things We Cannot Unsee

These are like a series of aha! moments. To some degree, psychologists have been studying this phenomenon for years, when they probe patients with questions about ambiguous figures. In this theory, there are 2 or more totally plausible concepts. The perception of another way to see things is usually sudden and gratifying even if the images are not pleasant.

Here are several examples. Figure 4-7 is the international football association (FIFA) emblem for the 2014 World Cup in Brazil.

The notion behind the emblem is obvious—to promote soccer and the World Cup. This illustration of a trophy in Brazilian colors with a hand holding an abstract soccer ball served the world of soccer well.

Then Germany beat Brazil 7-1. "Out of the blue," the beautiful emblem faced tremendous criticism. Many tweeted it looked like a "face-palm." In case you don't know what that is, a face-palm is shown in Figure 4-8.

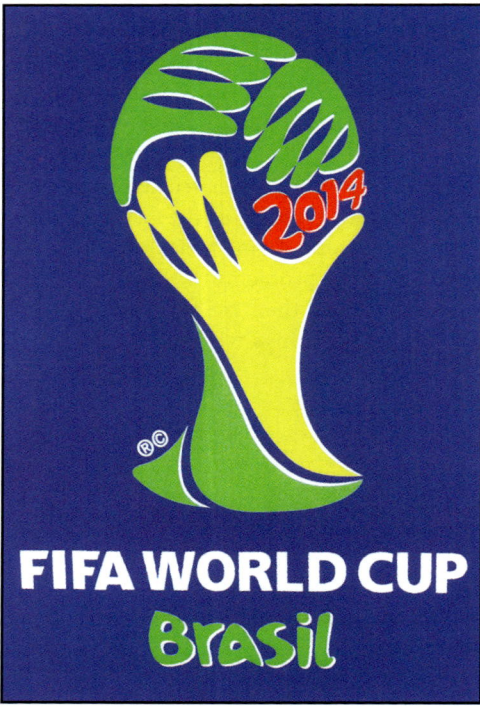

Figure 4-7. The FIFA emblem for the 2014 World Cup in Brazil.

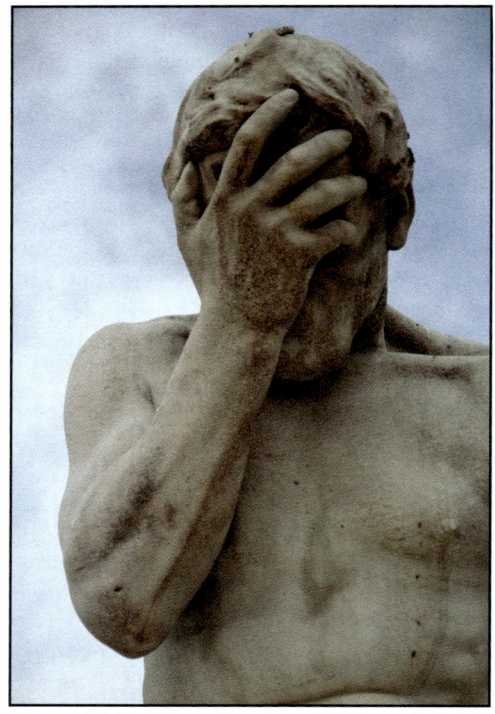

Figure 4-8. The face-palm, shown in this ancient statue, reflects frustration or incredible disappointment. The face-palm, cannot-unsee interpretation of the FIFA emblem went viral after Brazil lost to Germany 7-1 in the 2014 World Cup.

It may take a moment. Then you should suddenly see the secondary interpretation. It's like a Eureka moment without the scream. You cannot unsee what you have just seen.

Figures 4-9A and B show 2 other unsee examples. You may have seen them before. These are classic.[8]

Now consider another variation of the cannot-unsee input. Look at Figures 4-10A and B.

Now look at pictures of similar trees from 3 different perspectives (Figure 4-11). You now see different things.

You get it? Aha! The forest! It is about your lenses or introducing something totally non-tree into the picture. Look at the trees from a higher level or introduce fog or a castle and you immediately appreciate the meaning of the word forest. You need to see how the whole bunch of trees fits into the world to understand the concept.

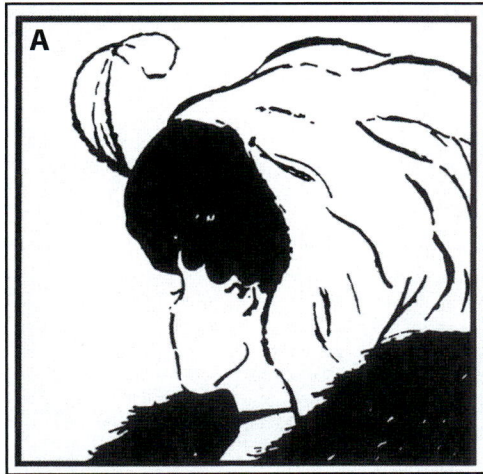
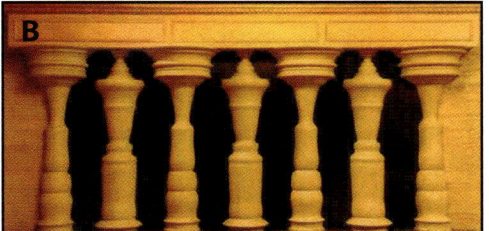

Figure 4-9. (A) The classic picture used for radiology and psychology teaching, emphasizing the point that there may be 2 drastically different ways to look at one image. Look at the picture carefully. Eventually, you should see both a beautiful young lady looking away and a depressed older woman looking down. Keep looking until you see them both… Aha! (B) Another archetypal picture that appears in multiple books and articles showing columns with shadows disclosing Charlie Chaplin–like figures.

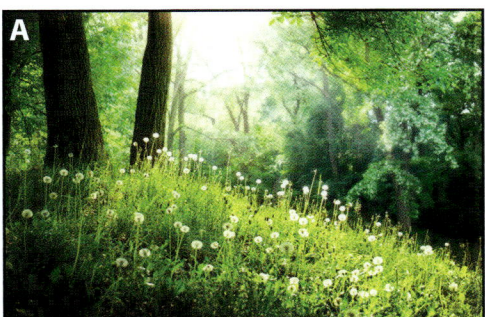
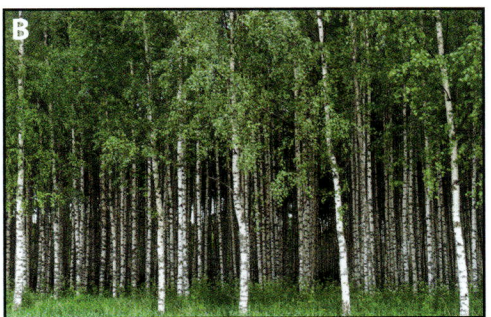

Figure 4-10. Two different views of trees. Lighting and the types of trees, etc, introduce factors that influence how you see them. Go deeper into the forest, and, no doubt, all you see is trees. Trees immerse you. This may be all you see.

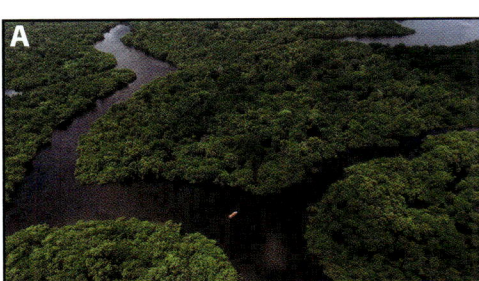

Figure 4-11. Three views of forests. (A) From a higher perspective, you see more than trees; you see water, overall tree formation, rivers, and riverlets. (B) From another perspective, you see weather effects and lighting changes. (C) With the right lighting and perspective, you might see a castle.

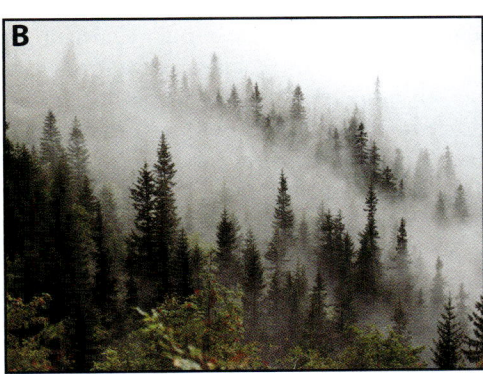
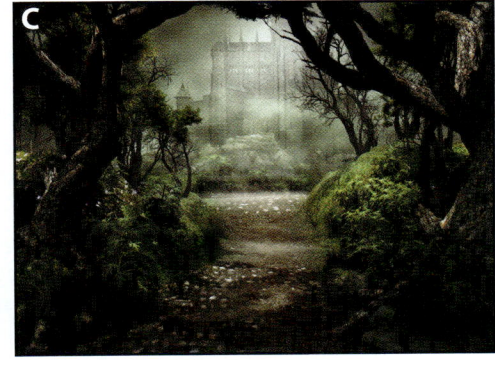

Now, one more picture that will help you understand the core cannot-unsee phenomenon (Figure 4-12). This is a taste of what's to come. What do you see here?

Don't worry. Don't dwell on the answer too much now. It's what the rest of the book is all about. Once you really see this, it becomes obvious. You will not forget it. Things get simple.

Ask yourself these questions about Figure 4-12: Do you see hernias? Or do you see lots of muscle? Do you see some areas where there may be underlying bone? Do you see symmetry? Do you see muscles that seem to connect in particular patterns?

Don't worry. You will.

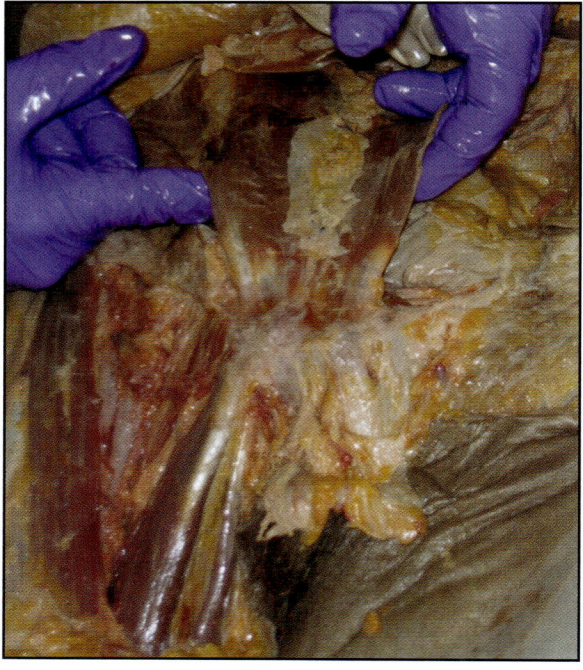

Figure 4-12. The cannot-unsee phenomenon in the core. You've seen the same picture in the previous chapter. You likely are seeing solely "trees," or muscles, or simply a forest. If you look harder, you will see superior harness muscles held by blue fingers and attaching to a firm mat of whitish tissue, and then the inferior harness muscles, and then the power muscles. You might see some sense of balance and symmetry. At this point in the book, you probably don't see these. Don't despair. Read on. You soon will see all these things.

Other Reasons the Old, Wrong Concepts Endured

Multiple factors come into play here. They include the social and professional risks involved in the paradigm-changing concept, plus commercial interests. The physician or therapist may have previously made firm observations about these matters and is convinced his/her viewpoint is accurate. Therefore, it may be hard not see that theirs may be isolated observations. The wrong notions may be bolstered by the success of certain treatments for certain patients. There may, in fact, be other plausible reasons why those specific treatments worked. Peer pressure enters into the difficulty of changing thought processes. Plus, it may take a great deal of work to understand the new concepts enough in order to develop the confidence, in fact, to employ them effectively. Generally, it is easier to go along with the old flow.

Consider the orthopedic team physician. He/She refers a pitcher for a laparoscopic hernia repair at the end of the season. The player played through abdominal and pelvic pain and, during the season, got some relief from a steroid injection by an ultrasonographer who said he/she saw a "hernia." It makes sense to order a hernia repair at the end of the season. Plus, the general surgeon, who would be doing this, is a trusted friend and colleague, and has, seemingly, "cured" a previous pitcher the same way a year earlier. Such a referral may seem an easy decision. Habit and relationships, today, still dominate these decisions. Yet, this may be the wrong decision. In fact, a number of possibilities enter into the equation as to what is the real cause of the pitcher's pain.

The main point here is that these peripheral dynamics play important roles in why simple and understandable concepts face difficulty in acceptance. They are disruptive. In Copernican lingo, this concept represents a cosmic shift. This is part of why some health care professionals have not immediately accepted the concept of core injuries. A more important reason remains. Few people, still, have not heard about the new concept.

A Final Reason Not to Accept the Concept: Distraction

Finally, look at Figures 4-13 and 4-14 for 20 seconds each. You will see another cannot-unsee theme that negatively affects acceptance of a disruptive concept.

That theme is distraction. You've got to admit that when you look at either one of these pictures, you get distracted away from the science of the core. Distraction plays out in so many ways when it comes to the core. It keeps us from concentrating on the important stuff. You smile and joke and then turn away.

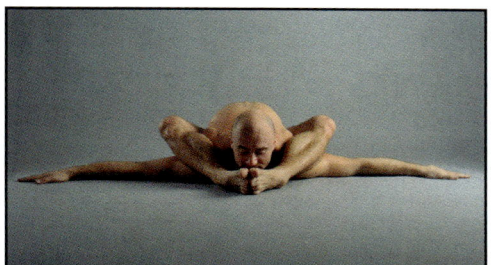

Figure 4-13.

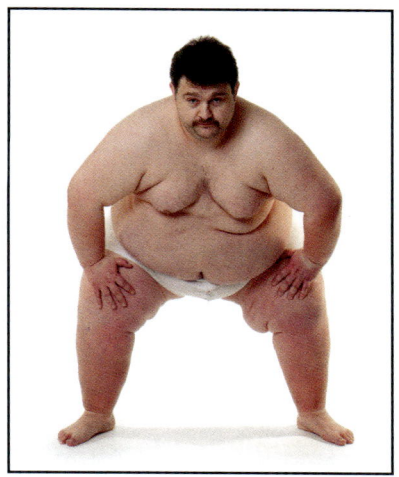

Figure 4-14.

Okay, you have stared at these 2 men long enough. You may now turn away, but do turn to the next page.

Accept the fact that you shall never get them out of your mind. No matter what you were thinking, you shall never unsee them.

We would offer our apologies, but you needed to experience these last 2 photos. Hopefully, you get it by now. But just in case you didn't, there is more to come. It's the same point we made about sex previously. It is easy to get distracted here inside the core. "Other" thoughts have blocked minds—of scientists, doctors, everyone—from a true view of the core (ie, the core concept). Sigh, giggle, do whatever you want, but then grit your teeth and hold on.

From here on in, consider sex, hunks, and funny-looking postures and adipose tissue as parts of the core. Along with that thinking, deem the pubic bone the center of the universe.

As you read more, you will see that, in actuality, it is. The pubic bone is, both anatomically and athletically, the center of the body's universe.

Let's start with a 30,000-foot anatomical overview of the core. Then we shall dive into the all-important pubic bone.

SELECTED READINGS

Meyers WC, Havens BK, Horner GJ. Core muscle injury (a better name than "athletic pubalgia" or "sports hernia"). *Curr Orthop Prac.* 2014;24(4):321-326.
   This article goes into some detail about what the world has seen and sees now with respect to the core. People are beginning to "get it."

Madrigal AC. Things you cannot unsee (and what they say about your brain). *The Atlantic.* http://www.theatlantic.com/technology/archive/2014/05/10-things-you-cant-unsee-and-what-that-says-about-your-brain/361335/.
   This is the reference and link for a wonderful discussion of the cannot-unsee phenomenon, written from a psychologist's point of view.

Weir A, Brukner P, Delahunt E, et al. Doha agreement meeting on terminology and definitions in groin pain in athletes. *Br J Sports Med*. 2015;49:768-774. doi:10.1136/bjsports-2015-094869.

This publication resulted from a consensus conference on terminology and reflects cannot-unsee difficulties cited in this chapter. Multiple surgeons, physical therapists, and other professionals interested in this region of the body met to come up with some common terms. The conclusions from this conference (ie, to divide groin pain into multiple different entities according to anatomy) fit nicely with the concept of the core and other terminology introduced in this book.

REFERENCES

1. McNabb hopes to play through pain. ESPN. http://www.espn.com/nfl/news/story?id=2174821. Published September 28, 2005. Accessed September 5, 2018.
2. McNabb to undergo surgery for sports hernia. ESPN. http://www.espn.com/nfl/news/story?id=2231967. Published November 22, 2005. Accessed September 5, 2018.
3. Doctor advises McNabb to "take it easy" in recovery. ESPN. http://www.espn.com/nfl/news/story?id=2243683. Published December 1, 2005. Accessed September 5, 2018.
4. Janis IL. *Crucial Decisions: Leadership in Policymaking and Crisis Management*. New York, NY: Free Press; 1989.
5. Taylor DC, Meyers WC, Moylan JA, et al. Abdominal musculature abnormalities as a cause of groin pain in athletes. *Am J Sports Med*. 1991;19:239-242.
6. Meyers WC, Havens BK, Horner GJ. Core muscle injury (a better name than "athletic pubalgia" or "sports hernia"). *Curr Orthop Prac*. 2014;24(4):321-326.
7. Madrigal AC. Things you cannot unsee (and what they say about your brain). *The Atlantic*. http://www.theatlantic.com/technology/archive/2014/05/10-things-you-cant-unsee-and-what-that-says-about-your-brain/361335/. Published May 5, 2014. Accessed May 3, 2018.
8. Boring EG. A new ambiguous figure. *Am J Psych*. 1930;42:444-445.

section two
new universe*

*from the book imprint for Marvel Comics

5

presenting...the **core**!

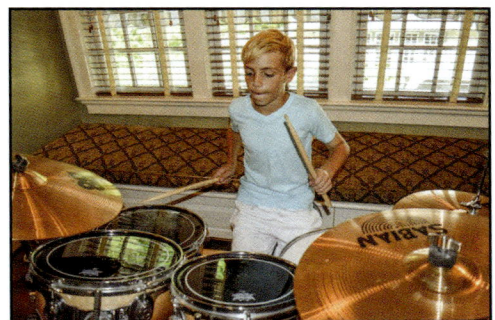

Figure 5-1.

Drum roll (Figure 5-1).^{VID 1}

It was a classic moment in Philadelphia sports—and in the world of unintentional comedy.[1] There was Eagles wide receiver Terrell Owens (nicknamed "TO"), shirtless, lying on his driveway doing sit-ups and crunches (Figure 5-2), while his agent, Drew Rosenhaus, staged one of the most curious press conferences of all time.^{VID 2,3}

While Owens worked on his beach muscles, Rosenhaus shrewdly gave one-word answers to the assembled media (Figure 5-3), who were trying to find out when Owens was going to report to training camp. He punctuated each response with a terse, "Next question," and unwittingly created a scenario that would be repeated by fans for years, often to howls of laughter.

Owens looked good knocking out rep after rep. His abs glistened in the summer heat, and he looked as if someone could hit him in the midsection with a baseball bat and he wouldn't even cringe. The witnessing world mused, "What a core on that guy, huh?"

Maybe.

Owens had a tough stomach, to be sure.

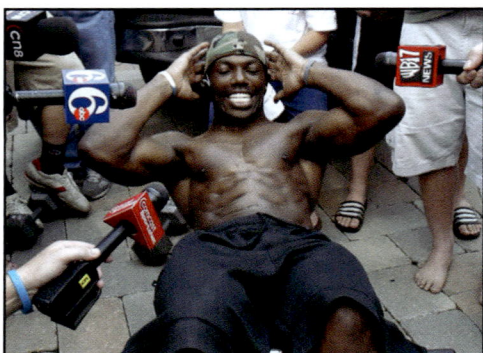

Figure 5-2. TO doing sit-ups in his driveway. (Reprinted with permission from the *Philadelphia Inquirer*.)

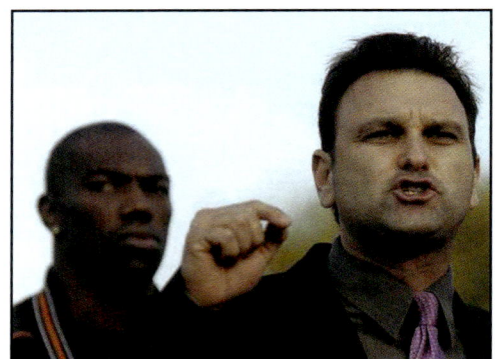

Figure 5-3. Sports agent Drew Rosenhaus at the legendary press conference. (Reprinted with permission from the *Philadelphia Inquirer*.)

THE ABS ARE BUT ONE CONSTITUENT

But the core is much more than the beach muscles found in an abdominal 6-pack. You can't blame regular folks for thinking the core is limited to the stomach area. That's what they hear whenever core strength and fitness are discussed. Strengthen the middle and everything is fine. There's nothing said about the other stuff—chest, upper thighs, rear end—and certainly nobody is talking about the genitals or pubic bone.

Ever since athletes, members of the military, or gym class students were forced to do calisthenics, there has been an interest in building a strong stomach. And as the fitness craze has boomed, trainers and other workout warriors have concocted new regimens to widen the area of attention. People are getting more powerful throughout their cores, and performance on all levels is improving.

As we mentioned earlier, the medical community has been reluctant to define and address the core. Because it incorporates so many different surgical disciplines—general, orthopedic, thoracic, neurologic, etc—no one person can handle all of it. It's unreasonable to think someone who specializes in pulmonary concerns would know the first thing about handling muscle tears in the groin area. As a result, the specialists have stuck to their areas, and instead of being considered as one entity, the core has been attacked in a piecemeal matter. Of course, that's why this book is so important and so essential to understanding the body's control.

You are going to see the anatomy of the core in its totality. Keep 2 goals in mind: (1) comprehend each part of the core and how it works with the other parts; and (2) grasp the concept of the whole core and how it controls the rest of the body. With respect to the parts, think about symbiosis. In the past, we have thought about all the different physiologic systems in this part of the body as separate species.

It turns out that these species work together effectively as one cooperative species. Again, think about symbiosis.

The chapter is a thorough study of the whole region, and not cursory explanations of parts of it. We are talking about how the whole thing fits and works.

This isn't just about sit-ups. It's about the whole core.

Next question!

THE CORE

Here is the core. The center is the same as where da Vinci placed it, at or just above the pubis (Figure 5-4).

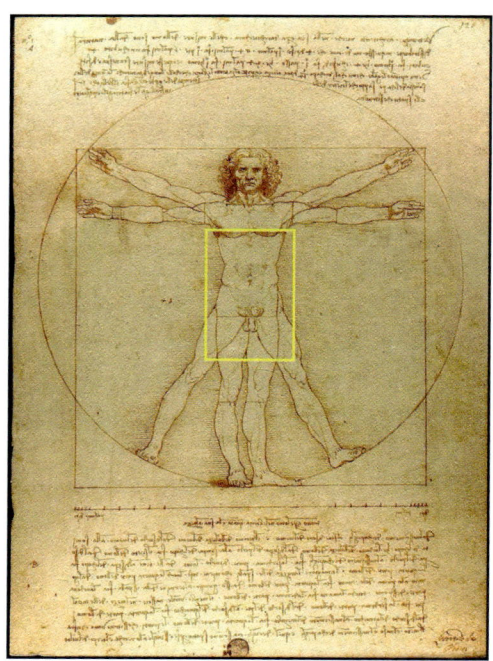

Figure 5-4. The classic da Vinci drawing with the boundaries of the core represented.

Presenting…the Core! 45

Figure 5-5 is the Vitruvian Man again and a deeper look into his core's muscles and bones.

Now consider Vitruvian Man becoming an athlete (Figure 5-6). This visualization will help you conceptualize the functional anatomy that follows.

You got it? Da Vinci "got it" with his V-Man. This part of the body is our engine, transmission, hub…

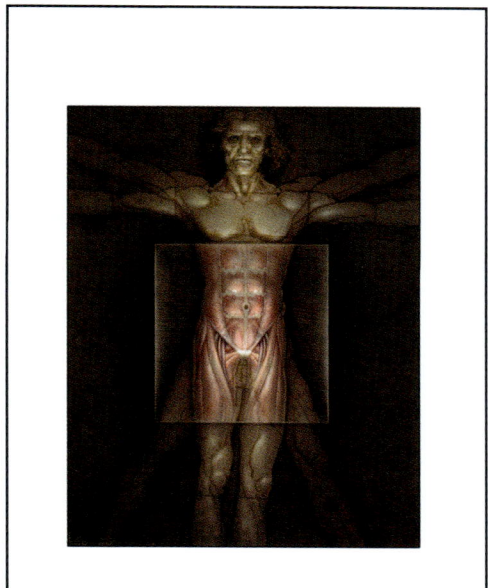

Figure 5-5.

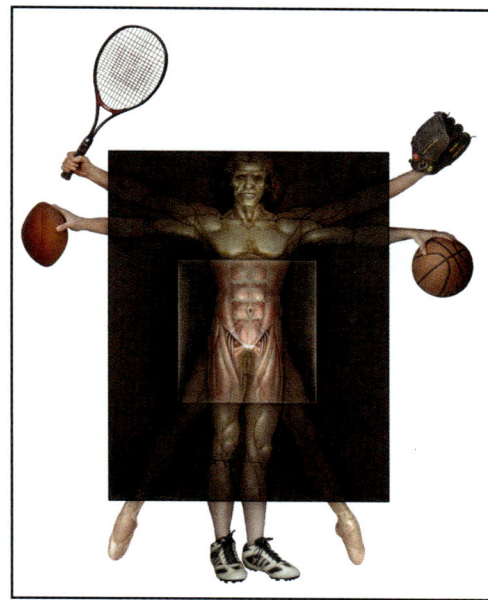

Figure 5-6.

The core has 4 parts (Figure 5-7): (A) the back, (B) the ball-and-socket hip joint with some distal femur, (C) the core muscles and the rest of the pelvic bones, and (D) all the other physiological systems and soft tissues.

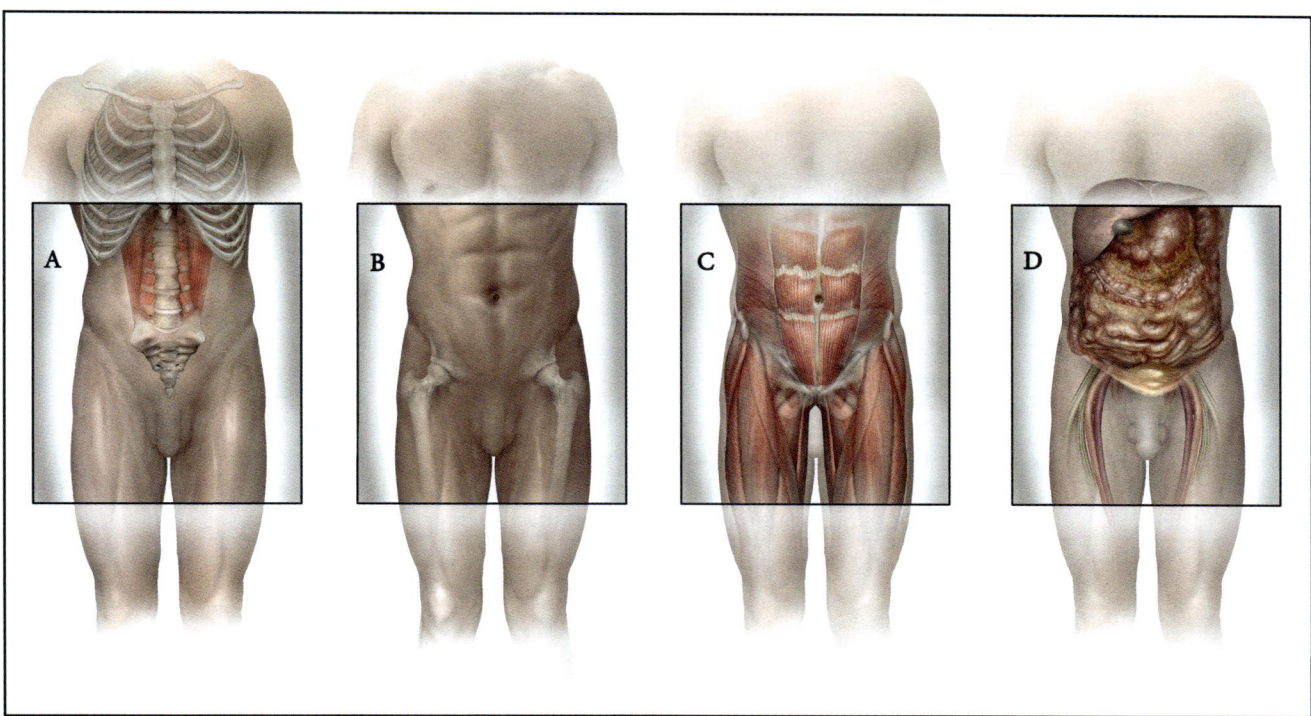

Figure 5-7.

The Four Parts of the Core

The Back (Figure 5-8)

Think of the back as still a vast unknown. Not nearly enough attention has been paid to the back. For the most part, neurosurgeons and orthopedists concentrate on the spinal cord and nerve roots and to some degree fusions and curvatures. One of the main purposes for the back is the tunnel that contains the spinal cord, which needs a lot of protection. Maybe we should call those specialists tunnel-thinkers? Okay, bad joke. Whatever the case, tunnel-thinking ignores enormous other aspects of the back. How many people in the world have undiagnosed back pain? How much of this pain is caused by pure musculoskeletal and not spinal cord problems? How much does undiagnosed back pain cost to the world? The productivity loss from that resultant absenteeism alone hurts the GDP. And think of all the emergency room and disability costs. Suffice it to say that the back is a huge and important part of the core. It deserves more attention.

In one sense—and for the purposes of this book—consider the back as a big unknown in need of much more research. Nobody has yet provided much evidence for how the muscles and bones of the back relate directly, not via nerves, to the rest of the body. Think of the back as a huge muscle mass full of important force. And think of us all as incredibly naïve for not knowing more about it.

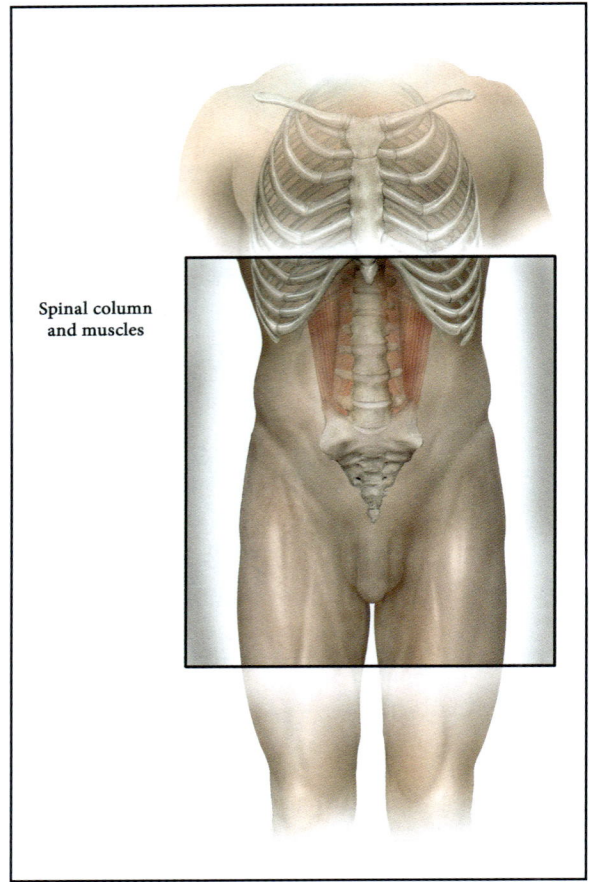

Figure 5-8. The back.

Table 5-1 Important Core Definitions	
Core	The entire region of the body from mid-chest to mid-thigh; in core parlance terms, from "nipples to knees."
Hip	Just the ball-and-socket joint and immediately adjacent bone.
Core muscles	All the skeletal muscles within the core, plus the pubic bone and all pelvic bones not considered part of the hip.
Back	The back, ribs, and all contiguous tissue within the region defined as the core.
"Everything else"	The fourth part of the core. All tissue within in the core not belonging to the other 3 parts (hip, core muscles, and back). The fourth part includes all the systems (eg, gastrointestinal, gynecological, genitourinary, vascular, lymphatic).
Core injury	Injury involving one or multiple structures within the core.
Core muscle injury	Injury involving one or multiple core muscles. Most core muscle injuries involve more than one muscle.
Harness or "harness and bridle"	The central core functional unit arising from the 2 rectus abdominis and 6 adductor muscles (3 on each side) and the pubic bone.

But the back is there, taking up a lot of space within the core. And like Coach Bill Belichick says, "It is what it is," so we have to deal with it. So, for now, think of the back in the following way. It is the whole region depicted in the following figures. In the core, the back includes the vertebral column from the mid-chest on down. We chose "the mid-chest" arbitrarily as an upper limit; this may be wrong. But as we see it now, the back unites with the chest and abdomen there in so many movements with the pelvis and thighs. This arbitrary upper limit makes sense. Of more importance is to accept that the back includes 2 main things besides the spine: (1) the massive muscle mass surrounding the vertebrae, and (2) all those anterior rings made of bone and interconnecting muscles that we call ribs.

The Hip (Figure 5-9)

This one is simple. We are talking about just the ball-and-socket hip joint. Okay, so there is a little bit of muscle in that joint…but we are not including any of the muscle outside of that joint. For the purposes of covering all the bone in the core, we accept the femur as part of "the hip" down to its mid-shaft.

The Core Muscles (Figure 5-10)

This part of the core is also easy to comprehend. The core muscles are simply all the skeletal muscles from the mid-chest to the mid-thigh, including the "internal" skeletal muscles (eg, levator ani) and the back muscles. For clarity, we usually exclude the back muscles from the discussions, because they belong to the aforementioned, still mysterious back. See Table 5-1.

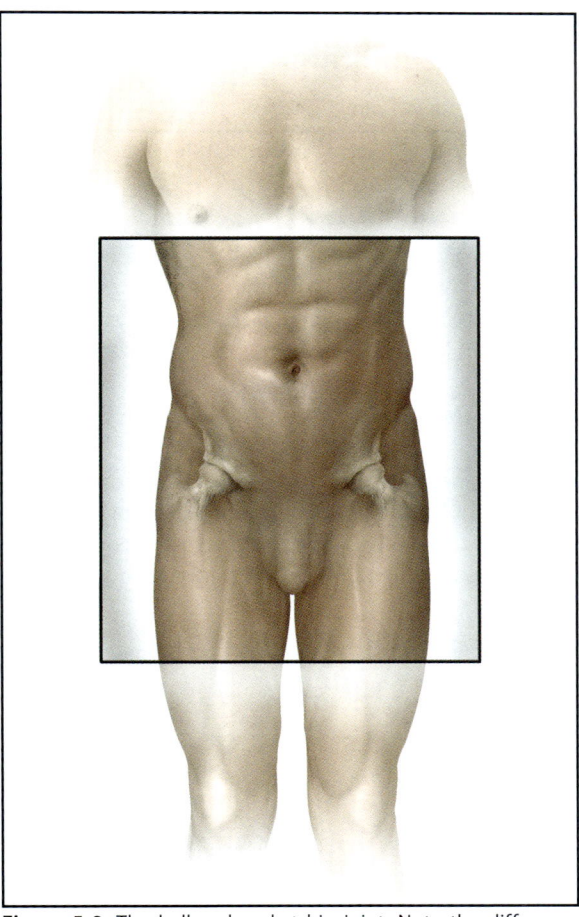

Figure 5-9. The ball-and-socket hip joint. Note the difference between what we call the hip here and Figure 5-7B, which includes the rest of the femur.

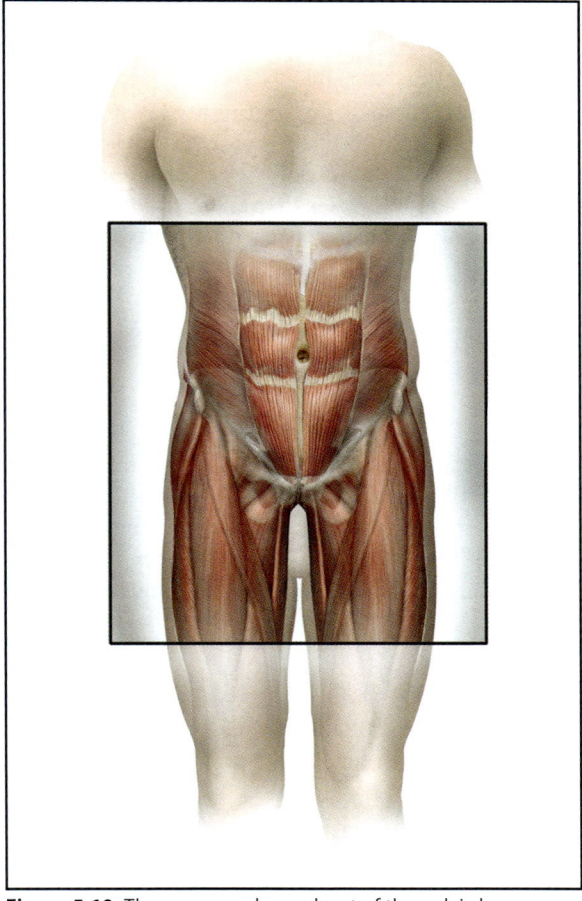

Figure 5-10. The core muscles and rest of the pelvic bones.

The "Other" Tissues (Figure 5-11)

The fourth part of the core is really, really complex yet easy to comprehend. It is a grab bag and includes everything nonmusculoskeletal that we have not yet mentioned or have forgotten to mention in this book (see Table 5-1). For the sake of comprehensiveness, this fourth part includes the gastrointestinal, genitourinary, and gynecologic systems; lymphatics; blood vessels; and nerves. Of course, we are including only those portions of these systems that reside in the core. Most of the gastrointestinal, genitourinary, and gynecologic systems do. Do not minimize the importance of these other tissues in the science of movement. You shall see numerous examples of why you should not underestimate the importance of this fourth component of the core with respect to movement and athleticism.

SEX DISTINCTIONS

Women are different than men. That's not a profound statement. Women look different than men. Again, not a profound statement.

Now let's get more profound. Think about when you watch high-level women's sports on television. They move differently, don't they? That is obvious. Men, you may attribute this to "not being as athletic." You are wrong. Women will say, "You are so wrong." They are so right.

Try out this one for profundity. Women move differently because of their core. Their core anatomy is different. The direction and strengths of forces are way different. Because of all this, they get different injuries than men, and they get different sets of injuries in different sports and other activities.

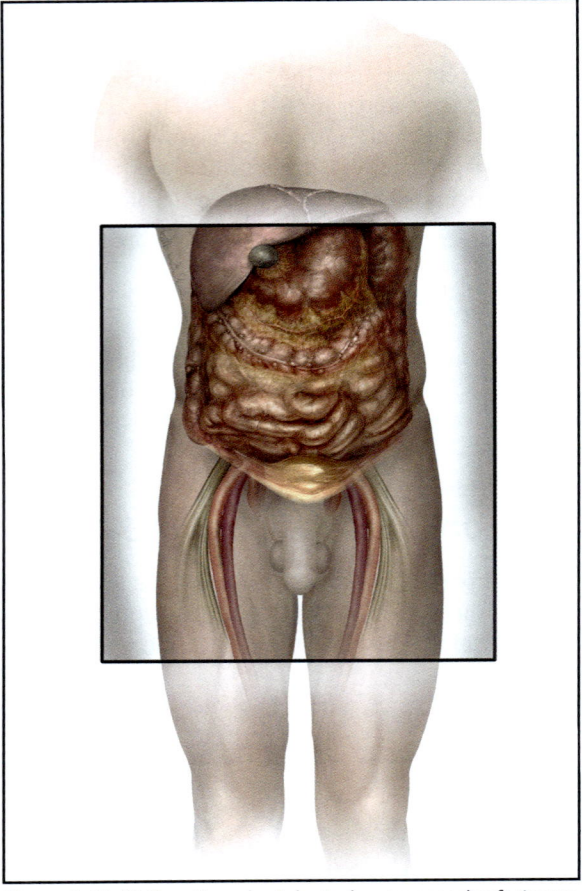

Figure 5-11. All the other physiological systems and soft tissues.

Let's get back to artwork and show women's core structure and forces and how they are different from men.

Women have wider pelves than men, particularly in comparison to their knees. Teleological teaching says this is so women may deliver babies. That may be so, but we aren't going to get into that. We are considering the forces here, etc, as they relate to movement (Figure 5-12).

Regular old radiographs show some of the principle differences between the bony pelves of women and men (Figure 5-13).

As a result of the bony structure, the forces are way different. Here is just one summary depiction of that from a previous paper. Consider the broad effects small changes in directions of forces might have. These are pretty big changes. People have already talked about the increased incidence of anterior cruciate injuries in women due to the acuteness of what is called the "Q" angle.[2] Well, it also happens that women have more stable cores in general, while their forces do shift more laterally into the hips rather than the central, pubic regions (Figure 5-14).

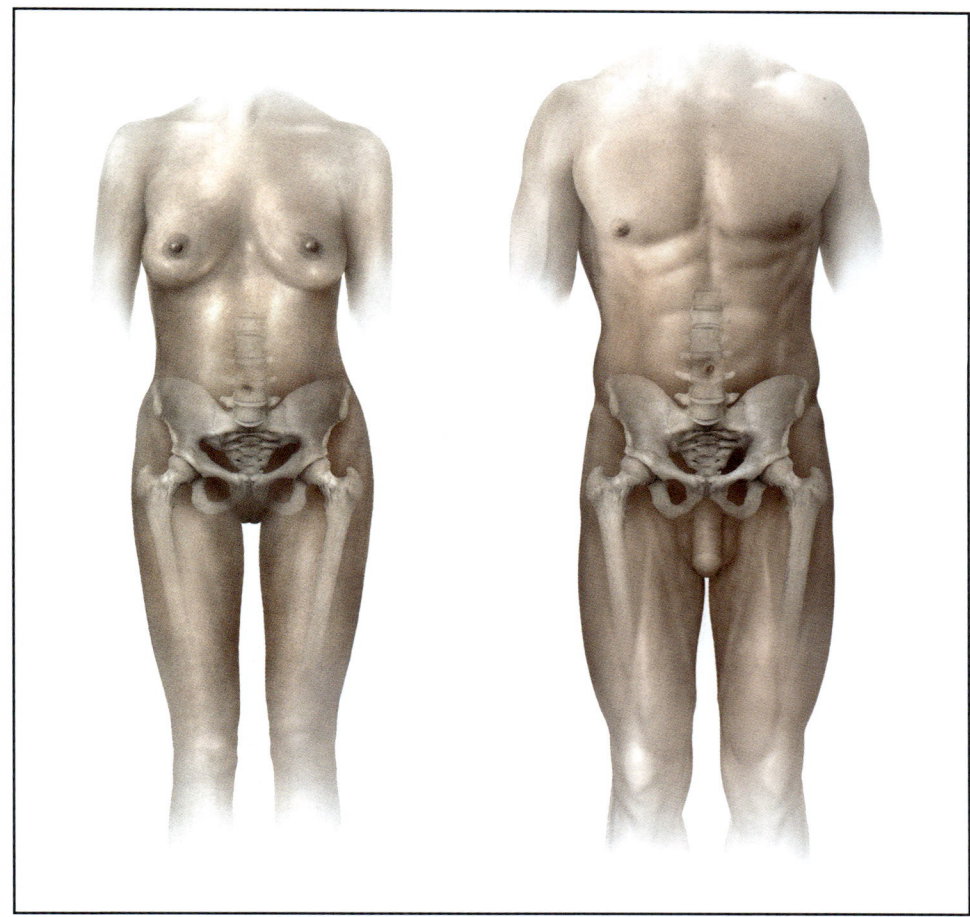

Figure 5-12. Female pelvis vs male pelvis. Subtle differences in width and alignment of the bony pelves, femurs, and knees contribute to changes in muscular forces. The man's pelvis stands a little more upright. The woman's pelvis is relatively broader.

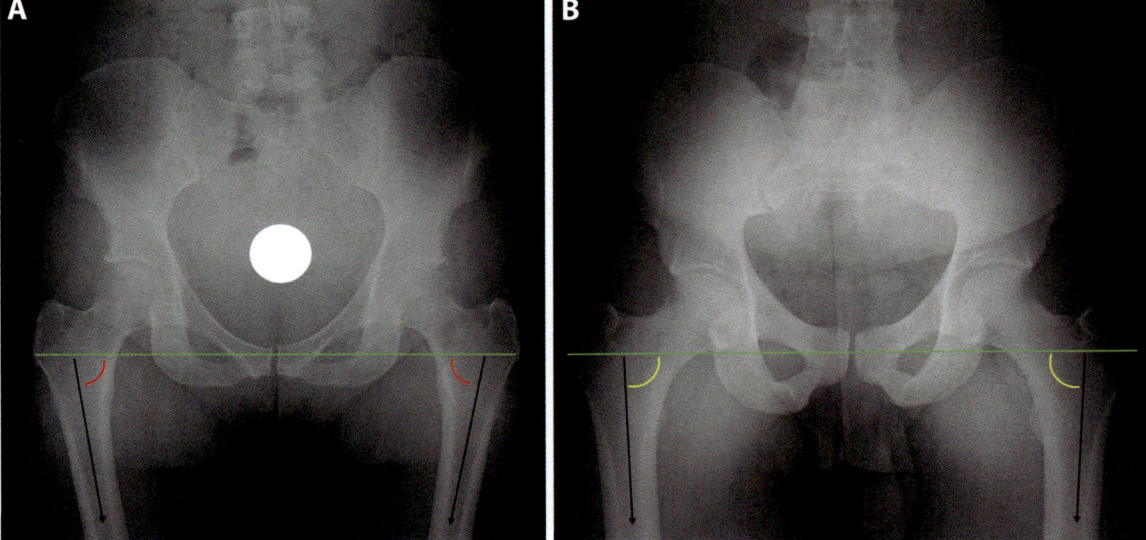

Figure 5-13. Plain X-rays of the (A) female and (B) male pelves. Interestingly, the medical and radiological literatures have focused mainly on differences in inner pelvic space (white circle) as they relate to the birth canal and delivery of babies; that space, of course, is roomier in females, even though it may not look so in these X-rays. Also, note the flatter lower bony (pubic and ischial bones) structures of women (either side of the green lines), as well as the more acute angles (red curves vs yellow curves in men) of their femurs with respect to the green lines drawn between the greater trochanters. These angle differences contribute to changes in muscular forces. Women account for only 15% of core muscle injuries, and their injuries exhibit a different spectrum of pathologies compared with men's injuries.

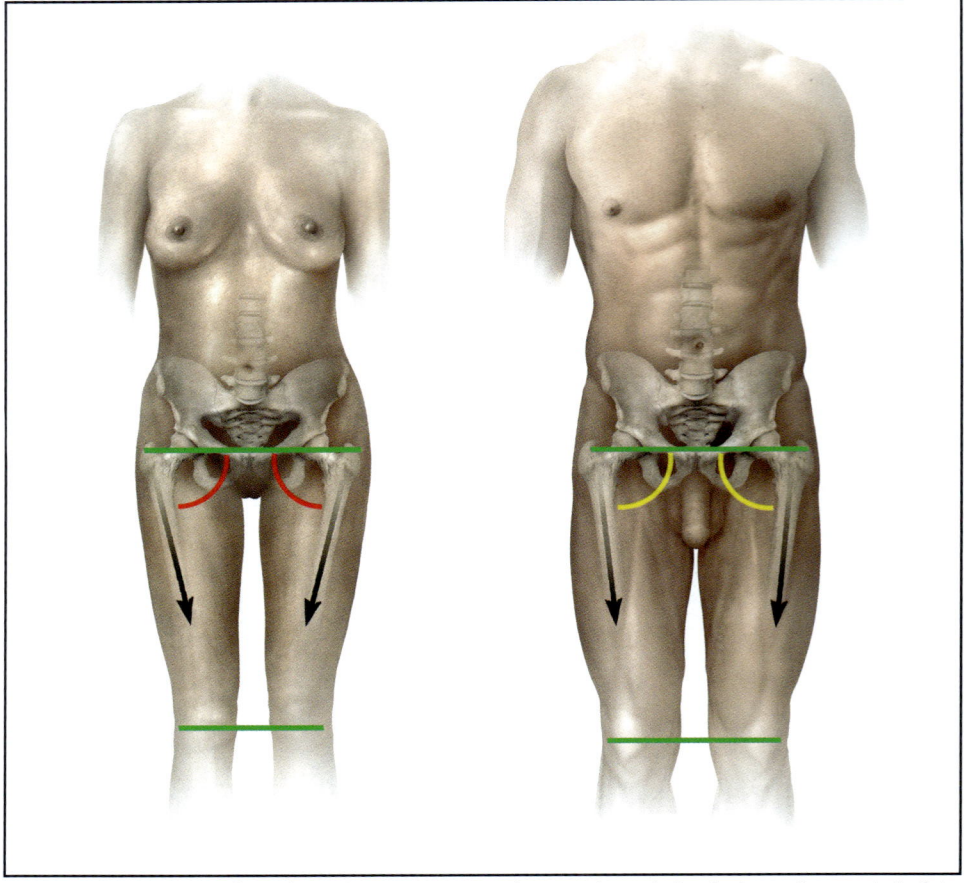

Figure 5-14. Directions of core forces in women vs men. Increased angulation (red vs yellow angles) of the femurs creates the potential for more torque in the knees of women. It is widely believed that the relative differences in widths of the pelvis and knees (green lines) respectively account for the higher incidence of anterior cruciate knee injuries in women. The same set of differences likely protects the central, pubic pelvis musculature, but not necessarily the hips.

HOW TO CONCEPTUALIZE THE BACK

The back deserves special mention here because we won't talk much about this important core part until the physical therapy chapters. We still don't know nearly enough about the back muscles' function. Our increased understanding of how the hip and pelvic muscles work exposes how little we know about the functional musculoskeletal anatomy of the back.

Currently, the best way to look at the back is as a good old-fashioned Original Slinky (Figure 5-15). Yes, the one and the same as that toy we all grew up with.

This concept is prevalent now among physical therapists dealing with the thorax.[3] It seems logical that the same concept should apply to the back.

Yes…this, of course, is quite a different way of thinking than the way most of us were taught. We will go into this reasoning more when we talk about the importance of the thorax in core physical rehabilitation. Suffice it to say here to think that the muscles around the vertebral columns work in conjunction with the ribs as a series of concentric rings (Figure 5-16).

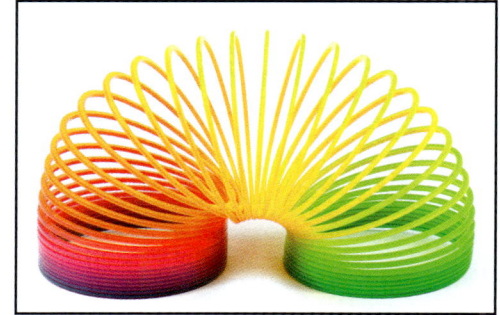

Figure 5-15. Think "retro" when you think of the back (ie, think "Slinky.")

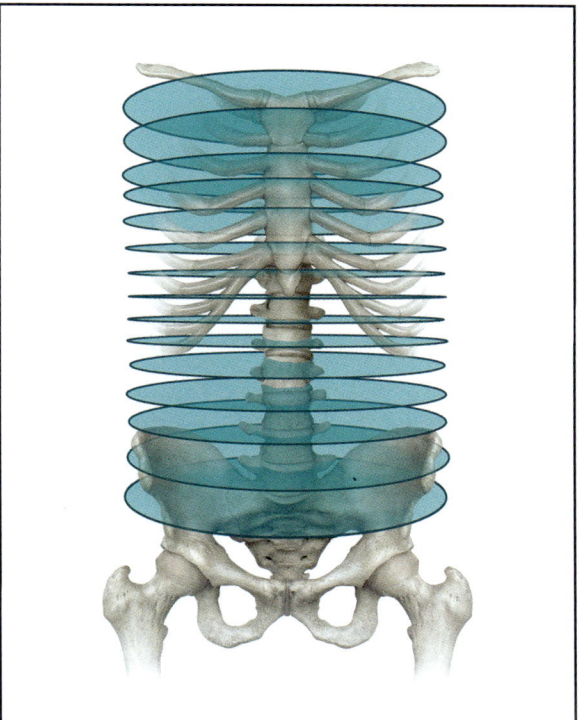

Figure 5-16.

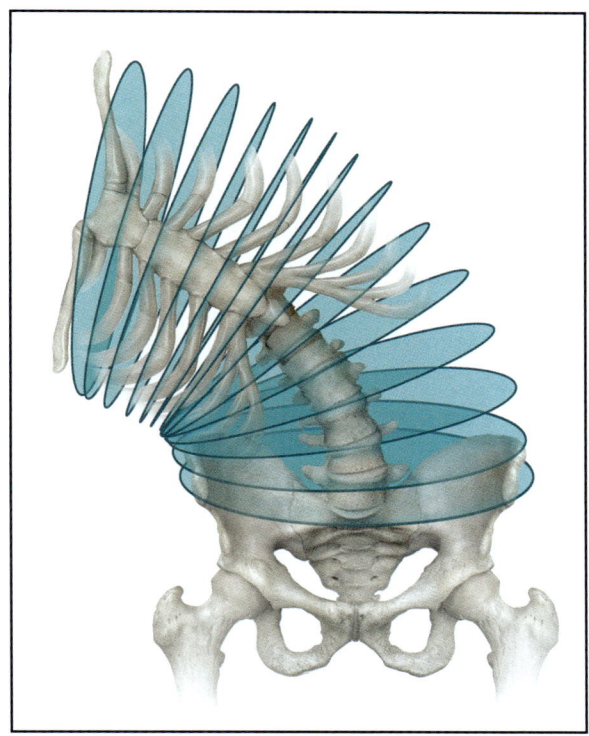

Figure 5-17. Note how the rings move like a Slinky. This model is a good functional model and in vogue in the physical therapy literature.[3] Read more about this in Chapter 34.

Simply think in terms of concentric rings extending out from the vertebrae to include 1 or 2 ribs each up top and just muscle and organs down below.

Basically, just like a Slinky, the back can bend in multiple directions and in various complex ways (Figure 5-17). The mechanics of a Slinky seem also to apply to the back and thorax. These include Hooke's law and the effects of gravitation.[4] The mechanical concepts include *simple harmonic motion* that relates to the Slinky's dangle, *equilibrium* that relates to the stationary Slinky, as well as Slinky movement such as going up and down steps that is governed by (1) the toy's mass, (2) the force of gravity, and (3) a spring constant.

What could be simpler? The back is merely the toy Slinky Dog first demonstrated by Richard T. James at Gimbel's, the Philadelphia department store, in 1943.

Okay, now that you've got this simple Slinky concept, let's put away the back and go on for now to things we know more about.

THE POWER MUSCLES AND CENTRAL HARNESS (AND BRIDLE AND REINS)

It is time to introduce how the power of the core works. This is where most of the skeletal muscles come in. Normally, the muscles connect to something sturdy—either bone or in the central areas, primarily the fibrocartilage that surrounds the pubic bone.

Think in terms of 2 sets of muscles: the "power" muscles and the "harness" muscles. The power muscles are all the muscles around the spine plus the butt muscles plus the side muscles (Figure 5-18)—in other words, everything but the harness muscles.

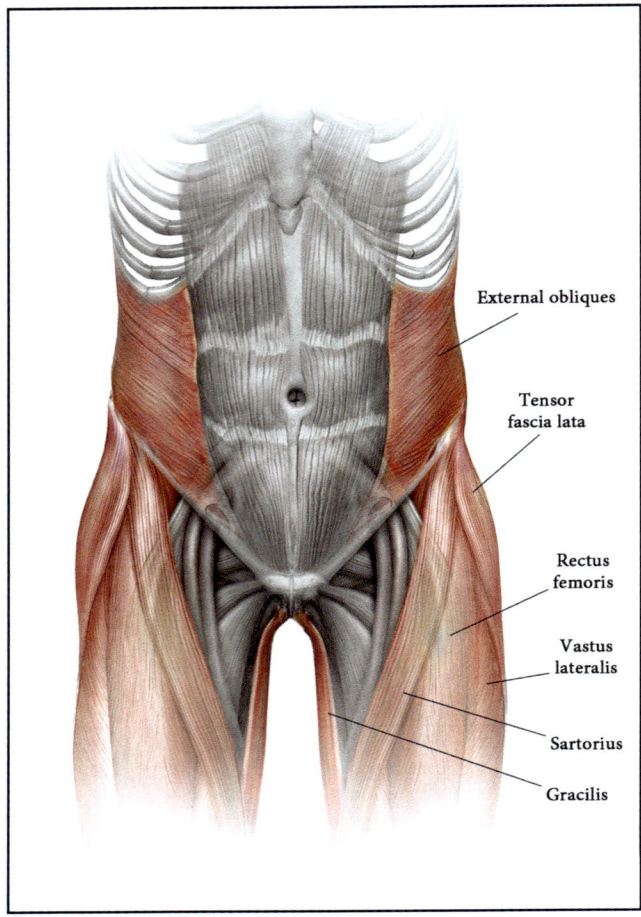

Figure 5-18. The "power" muscles.

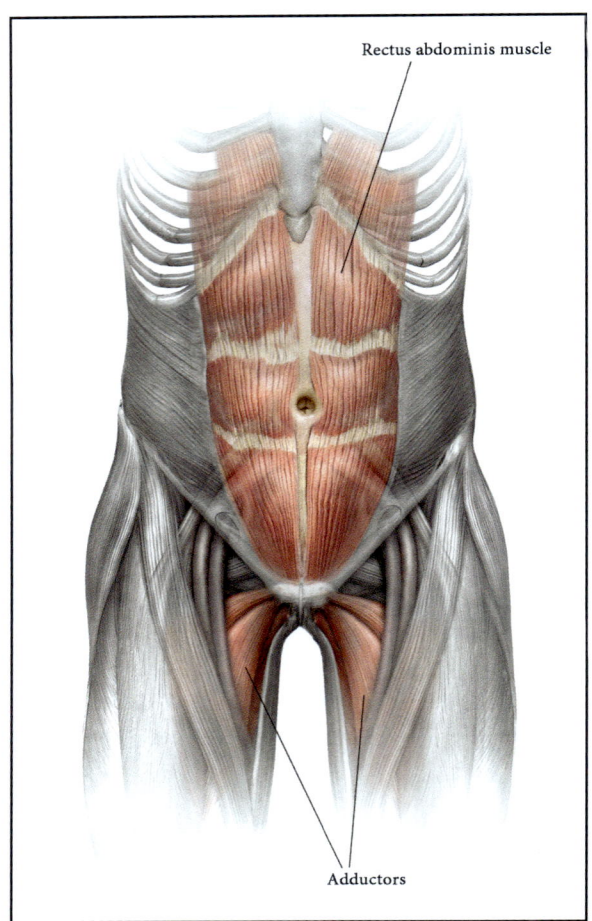

Figure 5-19. The "harness" or "bridle" muscles.

The harness muscles of the core are the central ones symmetrically arranged on either side and attaching to the pubic bone (Figure 5-19). The most important harness muscles, for an uninjured core, are the rectus abdominis muscles and 3 adductors—the pectineus, the adductor longus, and the adductor brevis on each side. The obturator externus sometimes plays an important role. The gracilis usually plays a minor role. Unquestionably, functional interchange happens between the power and the harness muscles, and other muscles (eg, the abdominal obliques) frequently contribute harnessing forces. Keep in mind that the pubic bone occupies an ultra-important central position in harnessing core power.

The harness muscles serve just like the harness, bridle, and reins of a horse. They get signals from the brain and direct the power muscles where and how to project their forces.

More About the Core's Harness

No matter the sex, the core has a harness. We shall get much more into this harness in the next chapters. Let's just introduce the concept a little more here.

The core's harness is simply those central muscles that strap to the pubic bone, superiorly and inferiorly. Think of the pubic bone as the nose and head of a horse. The harness muscles are like straps that you hold to control the horse. This harness is tremendously important for control of the core and consequently the rest of the body. The harness controls all your strength, power, and balance. In essence, it determines your maximal athleticism. With good balance and control of all those things, you develop confidence. Without it, you don't. The brain receives good or bad messages depending on that. For now, just think along the lines of: if you hop onto a horse, your goal is to become one with it, you want your brain to control it, and this requires some sort of harness (Figure 5-20).

Presenting…the Core! 53

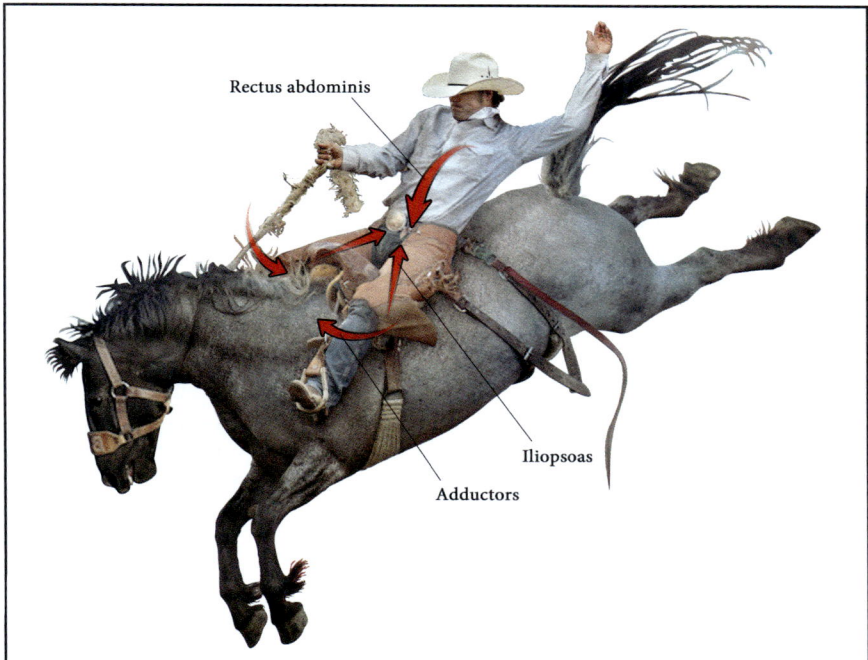

Figure 5-20. The rectus abdominis and adductor muscles control the power muscles and work directly with the brain to create our balance and athleticism. To carry this concept one step further, think about this bucking bronco rider as he attempts to join cores with the horse. Consider that he must fire maximally his harness muscles both to direct his own power muscles and also to synchronize his body with the power of the horse. With that amount of tension, slight disharmony can rip the cowboy's harness muscles right off the pubic bone. In reality, that frequently happens. Earlier, you remember, we talked about doing too many sit-ups being harmful to the same harness muscles. Think about the jeopardy bull riders experience routinely when they put those muscles into play. Not to mention their heads and necks. Are rodeo riders just plain nuts? The answer, of course, must be yes.

THE BRAIN

Let's use our brain and figure out what the brain's role is in all this harnessing of our core power. Figure 5-21 will help us think about this.

As Figure 5-21 shows, the brain sends signals to those harness muscles that balance and direct the forces of the power muscles. Think about where the horses of a stagecoach or plow get their signals (ie, from us, from our brains). The same thing happens within our own body. To prove this, all you have to do is to think about what an American football running back or a soccer player does routinely. Once the running back decides when and how much to cut in order to avoid a tackler or a soccer player decides the direction and quantity of force to use to shoot the ball, the brain sends the messages to those central core muscles where the power modulation begins.

Figure 5-21. Behind it all is the brain, directing the power of horses or our own horsepower. The brain communicates directly with the harness/bridle muscles. This picture shows the brain holding the bridle, which, in turn, sends messages to the harness.

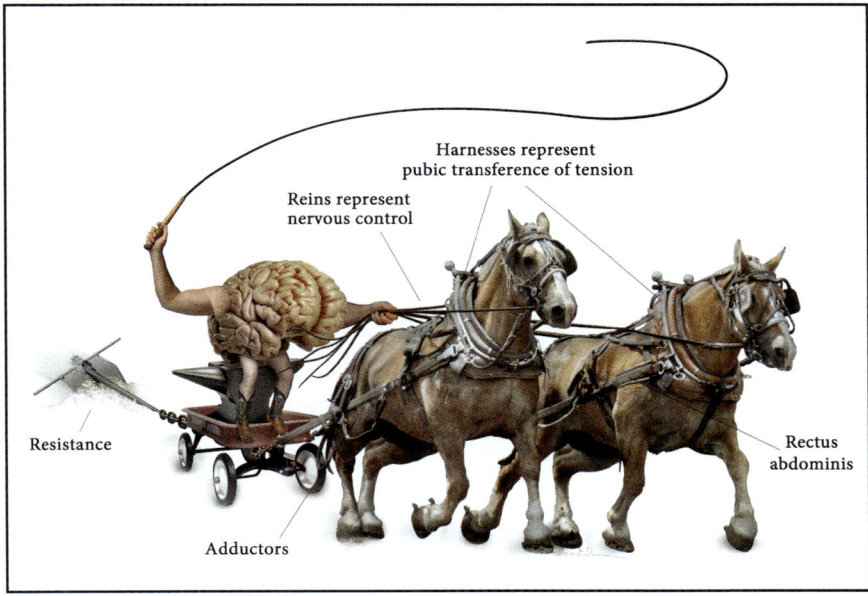

What About the Hip?

The hip is simple.

Remember, the hip, as we define it, is just the ball and socket. Yes, a tiny bit of muscle resides there (eg, the ligamentum teres). But from the standpoint of the main concept, forget the ligamentum teres for now.

While there may seem so much to consider, there is not.

Now, think anatomically. Rid your brain of all the physiology you might know. Think mechanically. Not about hormones that might be released, or remote effects, or local substances that might have direct effects on nearby tissues, or about nerves sending messages back and forth to the brain. Forget everything else you know about the body. As Rocky, our famous Philadelphia boxer might have said, "Fuhgeddaboudit." Indeed, he might have been talking about the core and forgetting all your other medical knowledge right now.

Now, with all that other stuff out of your head, answer the question: Why do so many athletes have a combination of hip and core muscle injuries?

You can answer this. Think simply, think anatomically. Think Erector Sets (Figure 5-22).

Remember the old Erector Set toy? Of course you do. It was the metal toy construction set, originally patented in 1913,[5] consisting of various metal beams with holes for using nuts and bolts and other mechanical parts, such as pulleys, gears, and wheels. What distinguished Erector Sets was the child's ability to build a model, then take it apart and build something else, over and over again. Erector quickly became the most popular construction toy in the United States. This original construction toy eventually acquired a motor, another core…perhaps the Erector Set's aha! moment! For purposes of right now, use "Erector Set reasoning."

Using Erector Set reasoning, you will discover 2 answers for why hip and muscle injuries occur together.

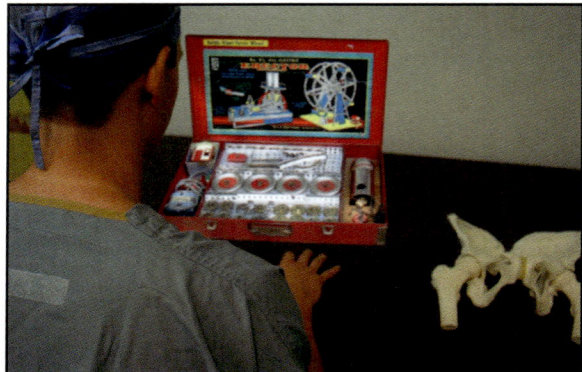

Figure 5-22. Hip surgeon studying an Erector Set.

One Solution

The problem originates in the right hip, a ball joint you made with your Erector Set.[6] Most hip problems involve bone rubbing against bone. Let's say you have already made a toy that moves along the floor, and everything relies on the free movement of the ball joint you made. Then a piece of metal bends and obstructs your ball joint from moving freely. The only way to move the toy then requires you to bend other parts of it. We shall discuss the various causes of hip impingement in later chapters. Suffice it to say right now that restriction of ball-and-socket hip movement, whether due to the ball or socket, causes limitation of movement not only of the hip but also of that whole side of the core. What then happens? Humans are usually still able to walk. Somehow the body bends to get around this new limitation. Think about all the anatomic considerations.

If the ball-and-socket joint is functionally trapped (ie, not able to move more than a certain amount), then forces must be transmitted to the other bones of the pelvis. Those bones are relatively fixed, so potential "weak" spots in the pelvis, or even the left side of the core and the opposite hip, have to come into play. Something has to happen to make up for the right-sided movement limitation. Doctors describe a Trendelenburg gait,[7] which represents an extreme of this compensatory movement, in which case the whole pelvis tilts, and the opposite hip is recruited to help make up for this problem.[VID 4]

The parallel goes on and on. The anatomic shift may cause the Trendelenburg gait and other abnormal movements of the pelvis that serve for compensation. New stresses put supra-physiologic loads on bone and muscle attachments and bones rub and muscles tear. Something eventually gives way. In cadavers, the most likely muscles to tear in these situations are the adductors, rectus abdominis, and iliopsoas. A prominent anatomic "weak spot" in the pelvic bony structure is the pubic symphysis, where the 2 halves of the core anatomically meet. Extra movement in the symphyseal joint eventually causes disruption of the fibrocartilage connections and a process called *osteitis*. We shall discuss osteitis more in later chapters.

A Second Solution

The problem originates in the muscle structure outside the hip. Let's say you have the same toy, and there is normally some limitation to the range of motion of your ball joint. And your kid sister walks by and starts stepping on the beautiful walking toy you have constructed. Besides being PO'ed, you inspect the toy. The attachments around your ball joint are disrupted and no longer can you freely move the joint. The bent parts of the Erector Set have allowed the ball joint to have more range of motion than it ordinarily would and it hangs up.

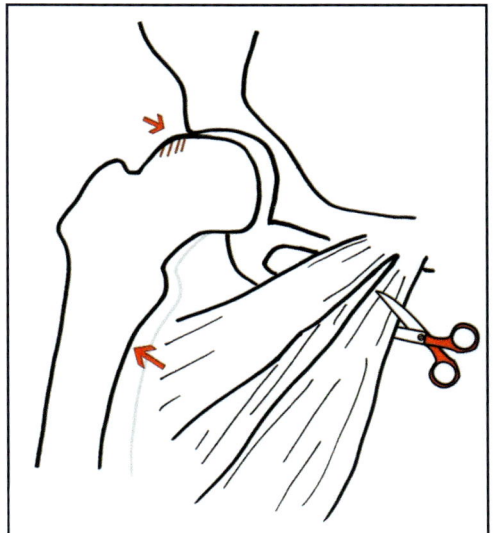

Figure 5-23. The same experiment mentioned in a historical context in Chapter 3 (see Figure 3-10). Using Erector Set reasoning, the adductor muscles can determine some of the hip's range of motion. Impingement anatomy has inherent evolutionary advantages with respect to leverage and the body's power. The adductors normally protect these advantages. When adductors disrupt, range of motion increases, and impingement anatomy can become pathologic. It is as if the bony anatomy and the adductors are conspiring. A once protective Brutus can turn traitor.

The same thing happens in the ball-and-socket hip joint.

Let's say the all the adductors in the right thigh detach from the pubic bone. This logically provides more range of motion for the right hip. Increasing range of motion leads to the ball rubbing against the socket and impingement (Figure 5-23).

One thing we know from multiple cadaveric dissections is that everyone has a predisposition to hip impingement. Hip arthroscopists talk about 2 main types of anatomy that lead to impingement: cam (a bump in the ball) and pincer (overcoverage of the ball by the socket). In the laboratory we can create restriction of hip range of motion in anyone who has both a hip and a socket by simply cutting through nearby structures (see Figure 3-10).

For example, in some cadavers, all you have to do is cut through adductors. In others, you have to add cutting the rectus abdominis, while in others you have to go to the extreme of dividing femoral artery, vein, and nerve. In some, you have to divide some of the bony pelvis. The point is that you can create hip entrapment simply by cutting through other core tissue.

Clinically, we see the same thing. Players have severe rectus abdominis and adductor tears then sometimes develop hip impingement symptoms. The core muscle injuries can also cause the same osteitis without any observable hip involvement.

Clinically, while we may see clearly the 2 possible explanations for why someone has simultaneous injuries, figuring out which came first is often difficult—the old chicken and the egg question.

See…the 2 solutions are simple when you use Erector Set reasoning.

Okay, next question!

GOOD CORE OR BAD CORE?

It is time to make judgments. Ponder the following pictures and judge whether you think the folks have good cores or bad cores. Look at the various body types and try to figure it out. Time for a quiz. For Figures 5-24 through 5-27, decide whether the person has a "good core," "bad core," or "can't tell." Answer by checking one of the 3 boxes next to each picture.

Take the quiz again, if you remember, after reading the rest of the book and compare your answers, and then check your answers.

(For the answers, turn to page 435.)

56 Chapter 5

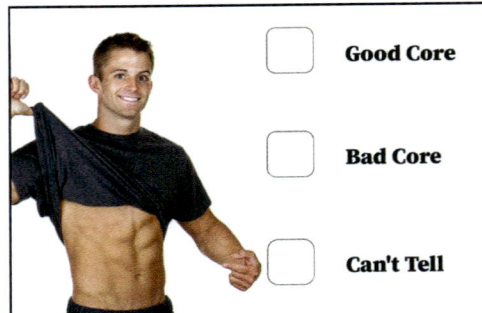

Figure 5-24.

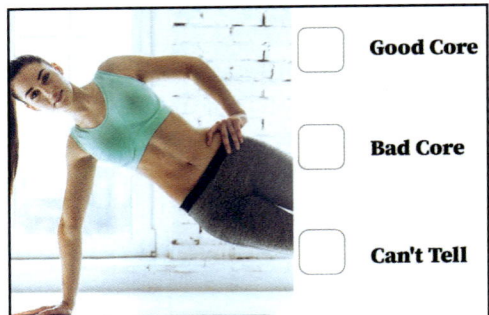

Figure 5-25.

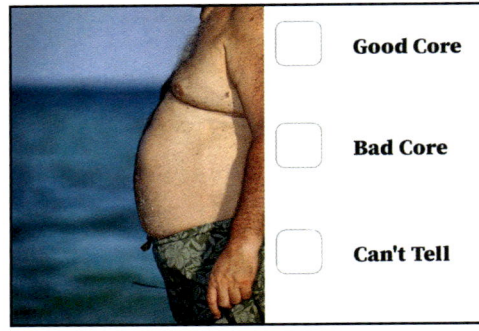

Figure 5-26.

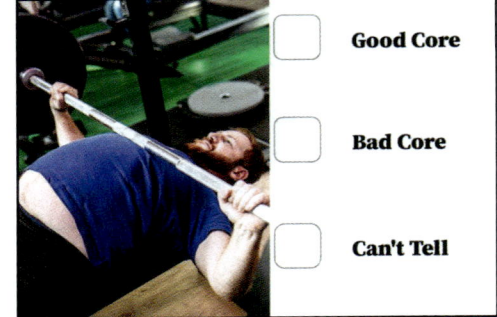

Figure 5-27.

What's Next?

We are about to dive deeper into the machinery of the core.

Selected Readings

O'Malley, CD. *Leonardo on the Human Body*. New York, NY: Dover; 1983.
   Da Vinci never published a textbook on anatomy. In fact, many of his drawings may be lost. This short review summarizes some of his contributions.

Andreas Vesalius. *De humani corporis fabrica*.
   Vesalius was the first to publish a treatise on human anatomy. In it, Vesalius endorsed the principles of da Vinci and challenged the work of 2nd century anatomist Galen. One of the few original copies, given by the founder and chairman of the first Department of Anesthesia in this country, Leroy Van Dam, to Introducing the Core *editor William C. Meyers, may be viewed at the Library of the University of Massachusetts Medical School.*

Dines JS, Altchek DW, Andrews J, ElAttrache NS, Wilk KE, Yocum LA, eds. *Sports Medicine of Baseball*. Philadelphia, PA: Wolters Kluwer, Lippincott Williams & Wilkins; 2012.
   A great sports medicine book on baseball. Although the book doesn't mention the core directly, the biomechanics discussions articulately describe some precise functions of the core.

REFERENCES

1. http://www.csnphilly.com/today-philly-sports-history-driveway-press-conference-2005.
2. Livingston LA, Mandigo JL. Bilateral within-subject Q angle asymmetry in young adult females and males. *Biomed Sci Instrum*. 1997;33:112-117.
3. Lee LJ, Lee DG. An integrated multimodal approach to the thoracic spine and ribs. In: Magee D, Zachazewski J, Quillen W, Manske R, eds. *Pathology and Intervention in Musculoskeletal Intervention*. St. Louis, MO: Elsevier; 2008.
4. Slinky. Wikipedia. https://en.wikipedia.org/wiki/Slinky. Updated January 6, 2019. Accessed January 15, 2019.
5. Erector set. Wikipedia. https://en.wikipedia.org/wiki/Erector_Set. Updated December 24, 2018. Accessed January 15, 2019.
6. Hammoud S, Bedi A, Magennis E, Meyers WC, Kelly BT. High incidence of athletic pubalgia symptoms in professional athletes with symptomatic femoroacetabular impingement. *Arthroscopy*. 2012;28(10):1388-1395.
7. Hardcastle P, Nade S. The significance of the Trendelenburg test. *J Bone Joint Surg Br*. 1985;67:741-746.

VIDEOS

1. https://www.youtube.com/watch?v=h0bArnwuhc8
2. https://www.youtube.com/watch?v=QuknFnmmWxY
3. https://www.youtube.com/watch?v=41rdU-3fiMA
4. https://www.youtube.com/watch?v=HE0lk5MVFEg

6

some **concepts** to keep in mind

Before diving into anatomical detail, let's soar up to 30,000 feet and emphasize 7 concepts you should keep in mind as you read further—about the core and how it integrates the rest of the body. You may think of real world of sports stars who illustrate the concepts. Unless a specific name is mentioned, the characters are fictional. Any resemblance to specific individuals is purely coincidental. Many of our patients do exemplify the same themes.

CONCEPT 1: THE BODY'S TRANSMISSION

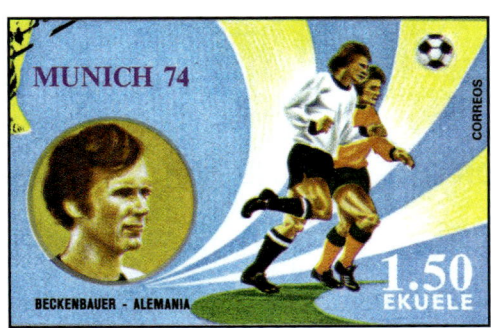

Figure 6-1. Franz Beckenbauer.

If you are going to put together a list of the toughest guys in sports history, Franz Beckenbauer (Figure 6-1) must be on the list. The soccer sweeper was the centerpiece of West Germany's teams for many years, but his performance in the 1970 World Cup semifinal against Italy might be even more impressive than leading his country to the championship 4 years later.

Early in the game, Beckenbauer suffered a broken clavicle on a hard tackle by an Italian player. Since West Germany had exhausted its 2 allotted substitutions, "Der Kaiser" stayed in the game, with a sling holding the injured arm close to his body.[1] It was unlikely the team's captain was going to leave such an important contest. Beckenbauer played his customary stout game in the middle of the West German defense for all 120 minutes, but despite his courageous efforts, Italy prevailed, 4-3, in double overtime.

Anyone who has played soccer, whether at the elite or youth levels, understands that while players aren't able to touch the ball—except on throw-ins or if they are playing goalie—the arms are extremely important for balance and in helping to ward off opponents who are trying to get the ball. To play one-armed, Beckenbauer needed more than just an iron will.

He needed a strong core.

If Beckenbauer hadn't trained his body's transmission to its peak efficiency, he never would have endured the marathon game against the Italians, much less played to his usual standard. The strength and flexibility he had built allowed him to excel at the highest level and overcome a substantial setback. No matter how strong his legs were, Beckenbauer wouldn't have been able to thrive under those circumstances without a core that was operating at its highest levels.

You can ask Mikhail Baryshnikov about that. Generally regarded as the greatest ballet dancer of all time, the Russian genius of dance brought power and athleticism to the graceful discipline, executing leaps that seemed impossible to accomplish. Though slight in frame, Baryshnikov was nonetheless a coiled spring, capable of generating great power with his jumps. (See Figure 6-2.)

His secret? Practice, of course. But more than anything, Baryshnikov had developed his engine room to the point where its output was at its apex. He displayed the results on stages throughout the world, creating a legend that will never be duplicated.

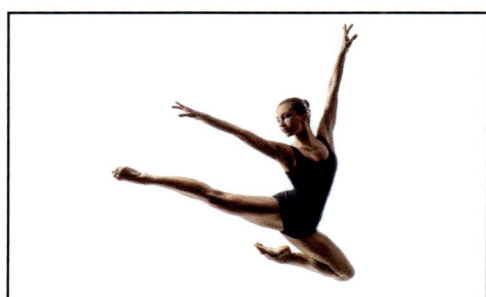

Figure 6-2. Modern ballet dancer in a move that Mikhail Baryshnikov made famous. Note the seemingly perfect form, sense of power and balance, and da Vinci/Baryshnikov focal point they call "the center."

Baryshnikov has shown that his principles of balance and power generation can be taught. He has become the master teacher. Our Chapters 2 and 7, and the pubic area at the center of the core's universe, follow unswervingly from some of his teaching.

Baryshnikov could leap, all right, but the Olympic high jumper who approached Dr. Meyers one day was able to soar. Still, he wanted to go higher and had heard about a patient of the doctor's who had gained some altitude on his jumps after some of his muscles tightened following core surgery to repair an injury. "Do the same for me," the athlete pleaded. Dr. Meyers was ready, but there was a problem.

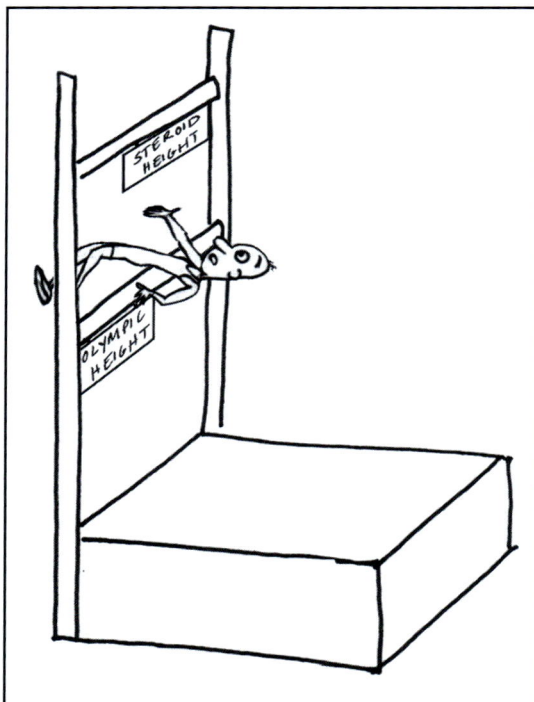

Figure 6-3.

There wasn't anything wrong with him. (See Figure 6-3.)

If surgical repair of the core could produce better results, the jumper wanted in, even if his core was without any blemish. Dr. Meyers laughed, "You have to complain of something in order for me to operate on you." The high jumper was dismayed and left the building. His knowledge of the core's importance had grown, but alas, his personal best did not improve.

The high jumper couldn't be blamed for wanting to heighten his core's performance ceiling. Repair of injuries often leads to increased results. Many of our athletes have achieved personal bests after surgery. A stronger, more efficient physical transmission will almost always aid athletes and everyday people in their duties.

In other words, if you build it, results will come.

CONCEPT 2: CONTROL OF THE EXTREMITIES

No one can say for certain if there is any direct link between the core muscle injury Chicago Bulls All-Star guard Derrick Rose (Figure 6-4) suffered during the 2012-13 NBA regular season, or the torn ACL that happened during the playoffs and his long-drawn-out return, or any of his other injuries.[2-7] There could well be a relationship between the destabilization of the core and the inability of the body to protect the legs, particularly when they are taxed so thoroughly during a basketball game. There could be a relationship between optimal core strength and ideal recovery from ACL reconstruction. Maybe there isn't.

Some Concepts to Keep in Mind 61

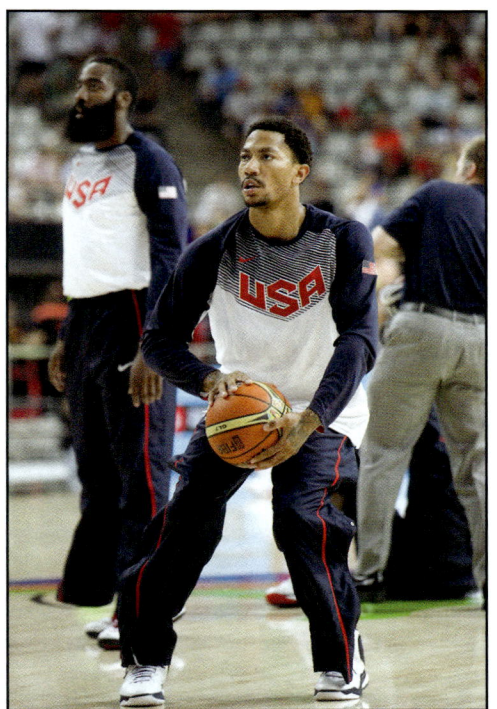

Figure 6-4. Wonderful basketball star Derrick Rose warming up with the US Olympic team.

"Something's got to give," points out BJ Armstrong, Derrick's agent and former NBA basketball great. "I weighed 175 pounds when I played; these guys nowadays are 210 and the same height. These kids are too strong. It's fun to watch lateral movement, but the body is not built to do that, at least not for long. Something's gotta give: the ankle, the hip, the knee?

"The athlete has outgrown the court. They find new ways to create space on the court. Look, for example, at Steph Curry and his 'stepback deep 3.' The court is too small. Something has to change for the safety of the kids."

BJ provided another perceptive insight, which fits precisely with the engine/transmission concept discussed in Chapters 1 and 2: "The basketball player is like a car moving at 75 mph and stopping on a dime and then changes directions beyond what it is designed to do. Other parts of the car become vulnerable."

Without having gone to medical school, some athletes and agents understand the core pretty darn well. The core is important. Core and extremity injuries are connected.

But since nobody knows for sure whether a core injury leads to an extremity injury, wouldn't it make sense to protect the extremities as much as possible by building the core and at the same time reducing isolated movement of the extremity?

Just look at what happened to Detroit Tigers pitcher Justin Verlander during the 2013 season. He had been throwing without pain, but his velocity dipped by as much as 10 miles per hour. That's a significant drop for a power pitcher. Two years after going 24-5 and winning the American League Cy Young Award, Verlander was a pedestrian 13-12 with a 3.46 ERA and 217 strikeouts.[8,9] Those last 2 stats were his worst efforts in those categories in the past 5 seasons. After the season, he was found to have torn much of his muscle mass away from the pubic bone. An inverted weighted sit-up dramatically brought the injury to light. Since repair, Justin has regained his power and command, and led the Detroit pitching staff again. In 2017, the Tigers traded him to Houston, which he helped win its first-ever World Series title. Justin's wonderful work ethic got him through all this.

Two former MLB fastball pitchers we know both suffered core injuries while covering first base on bunt plays. Both had large, protecting contracts and decided against surgery. Both struggled on the mound in the aftermath and came nowhere near approaching their previous speeds or success. Their arms were healthy, but their compromised cores didn't allow them to air it out like before.

Back in 2003, Roy Oswalt didn't want to have surgery on his core injury, either. He hurt himself in one of the strangest games in MLB history—a 6-man no-hitter. Oswalt started the game for Houston at Yankee Stadium and pitched a flawless first inning. But a "groin pull" forced him to leave the game after one frame and turn it over to the bullpen, which was remarkable. Houston relievers walked just 3 and struck out 13. Oswalt, meanwhile, didn't miss a start, despite his injury. He didn't want to take any time away from his team, and he knew he was due for a potential contract raise after the campaign, so he didn't want to take any chances. Oswalt finished 10-5 with a 2.97 ERA. After seeing his salary rise from $500,000 to $3.25 million and having his core repaired, Oswalt went 20-10 the next year and led the majors in victories.[10]

After the injury and prior to the repair, we could see slight limitation to full flexion of the left thigh. Consider Figure 6-5, and imagine Roy's left foot planted about 18 inches behind where it is. We worried that this would affect pitching mechanics. Even slight alteration in pitching mechanics can have profound injurious effects on the pitching arm. Oswalt heroically pitched with the injury, giving the Astros a chance to make the playoffs. His stride returned to normal after the off-season repair.

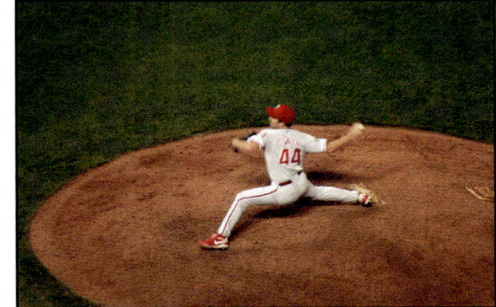

Figure 6-5. Pitcher Roy Oswalt while with the Phillies. Note his extra-long stride.

Oswalt learned that a compromised core can hamper a pitcher's ability to deliver the ball at top velocity, no matter how healthy his shoulder and elbow might be.

And if an athlete has bad feet, that can contribute to trouble with his core. That's how closely related the area is to everything on the body. Take Grant Hill.[11-13] Once considered one of the top 2 or 3 players ever to enter the NBA and heir to Michael Jordan, Hill was sabotaged by a series of foot injuries that forced him to miss sizeable parts of 4 seasons. While he tried to get healthy, he created problems for his core, demonstrating the reciprocal relationship between the extremities and the body's transmission. Fortunately, Grant underwent repair, and this wonderful player and person had a long and brilliant career.

We can't always be sure that trouble with one area leads to problems with the other, but the evidence is pretty clear that something's going on there. Physical therapists talk "kinetic chain." The key linkage is the core.

CONCEPT 3: INTERACTION WITH THE BRAIN

Star quarterbacks may find themselves on the injury report every week for many seasons, so one might say that their presence on that inventory is largely ceremonial. But, when a wide receiver finds himself on that list after suffering a severe core injury in a preseason game, the presence on that list may not be purely ceremonial.

"Groin injuries" can be substantial, and in one case a couple of seasons ago, that wide receiver chose the heroic route, opting to avoid surgery. He had missed many games the previous seasons for a variety of other injuries. He could not take the risk of missing more games if he could avoid it. It would have been too easy for management to speculate that maybe he was too delicate. Certainly, a prolonged absence would make him seem more fragile and negatively affect his career. He became sick of talking about the injury to the press and just wanted to play.

So, he returned, finally, after a number of weeks…he looked "stiff," not able to cut and weave like he once had, and he obviously wasn't able to see the defensive back right in front of him who clocked him. And he was out with a concussion for several more weeks. No doubt, the lack of mobility created a loss of certainty and self-awareness that made him more vulnerable on the field. (See Figure 6-6.)

We see this situation with core injuries time and again in many sports, not just football.

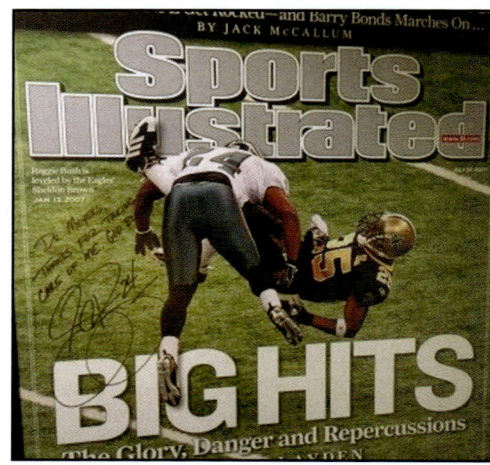

Figure 6-6. Autographed Sheldon Brown *Sports Illustrated* cover of him clocking a New Orleans Saints running back.

Profound pathways exist between the core and the brain. We already have data in the laboratory that show core injury cuts down on balance and reaction time and is a general distractor for the brain. In the previous chapter, we mentioned an "efferent" pathway (see Chapter 18) with the brain directing distribution of power via the harness/bridle muscles. The core also has afferent pathways that send messages back to the brain and interruption of that feedback pathway likely results in loss of balance, reaction time, and an awareness of surroundings. This is another potential mechanism for an injured player to aggravate the overall situation (ie, being more susceptible to other injuries such as a head injury caused by a "blind" hit and then be out to recover from his concussion). (See Figures 6-7 and 6-8.)

The decision was probably the right one for that wide receiver. The purpose of this story is not to make specific recommendations but to demonstrate the core's interaction with the neurological system. This story is not about how an injury to the area can impact nerves. It certainly can. It's more about how a finely tuned professional athlete must have the assurance from his/her engine room that it is capable of generating the necessary power, speed, and flexibility to make him/her maximally potent on the field or court. Without it, doubt creeps in, confidence suffers, and trouble looms.

By their nature, NFL games are archetypal venues for vivid hits.

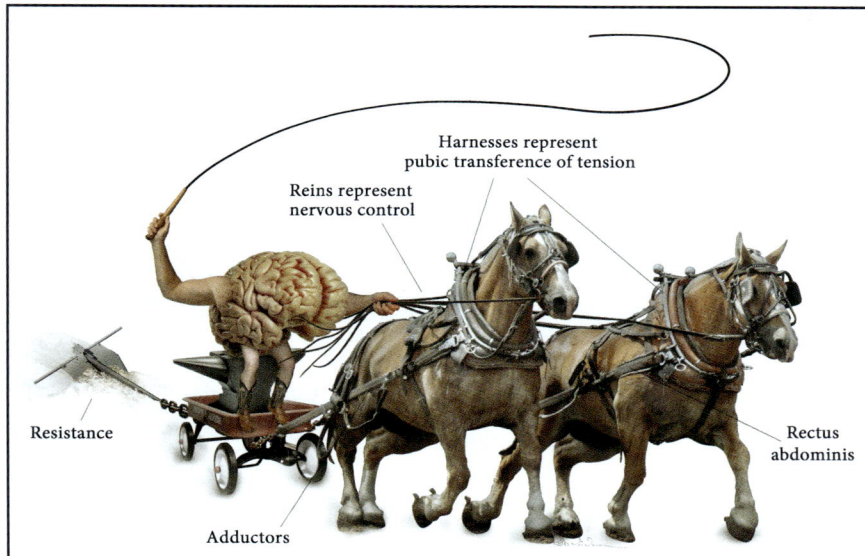

Figure 6-7. Remember this picture from the last chapter? The brain directs the horses via the reins, bridle, and harness? The brain, in fact, communicates directly with the "harness muscles." We shall go into the function of the latter muscles in the next 2 chapters.

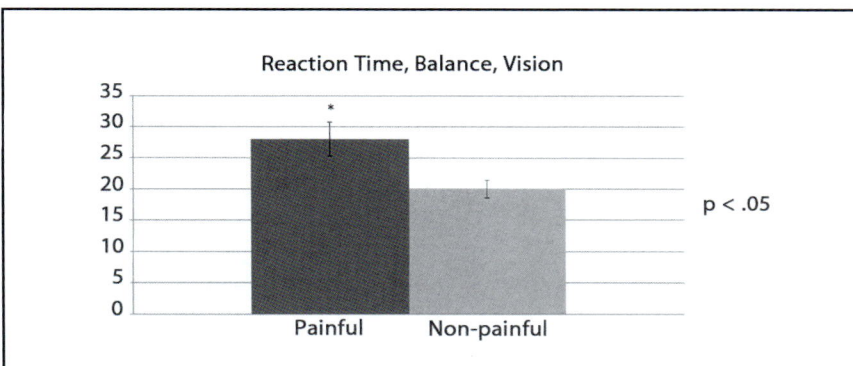

Figure 6-8. Preliminary data showing significantly decreased cognitive function after core injuries in athletes. Reaction time, balance, and vision then returned to normal after surgical correction of the injuries. No such changes occurred in normal controls.

CONCEPT 4: REMEMBER THE HIP-CORE MUSCLE INTERACTION

You know the old song: "The ankle bone's connected to the leg bone; the leg bone's connected to the hip bone…" Well, the hip bone's connected to the core muscles, and that can be an interesting relationship.

Jairus Byrd can tell you all about that. As a rookie in 2009, he intercepted a league-leading 9 passes for the Bills, including 1 in 5 straight games. His performance earned him a spot in the Pro Bowl, but in late December, he was put on the injured list with an injury to his abdomen and hip problems. Dr. Meyers repaired the muscle tear, but Byrd's hips continued to give him trouble. So, Dr. Bryan Kelly of the Hospital for Special Surgery fixed the hip problem, creating more flexibility—but tightening the adductor muscles in Byrd's thighs. Finally, after another procedure, Byrd was ready to go.

Talk about a wild cause and effect. For a while there, Byrd probably wondered whether the 2 areas were ever going to calm down at the same time.

Ask star NHL player Simon Gagne about the hip-core muscle interaction. He will tell you all about it! Left winger in the famous "Deuces Wild" line (named for the numbers he, Peter Forsberg, and Mike Knuble wore), Gagne played 10 years for the Philadelphia Flyers. Hip problems wore him out. Muscle-tightening surgical procedures finally relieved the pain and preserved his career. Gagne came back and reached the Stanley Cup finals with Tampa in 2010 and won the Stanley Cup for Los Angeles in 2011, alongside ex-Flyers Jeff Carter and Mike Richards.

Concept 5: Don't Forget the Back

The back is an important part of the core.

Anybody who has ever suffered a back injury, be it a sprain or a herniated disc, has received the same advice from physicians or those who have had to deal with the same thing: "Build your core." (See Figure 6-9.)

Figure 6-9. Back problems, of course, affect just about everyone. Spasmodic contractions (A) can reflect both pure muscular or more serious neurologic problems. By reports, a nondisplaced avulsion injury took down Neymar (B) in a recent World Cup in Brazil. (Reprinted with permission from AP Photo/Fabrizio Bensch, Pool, File.)

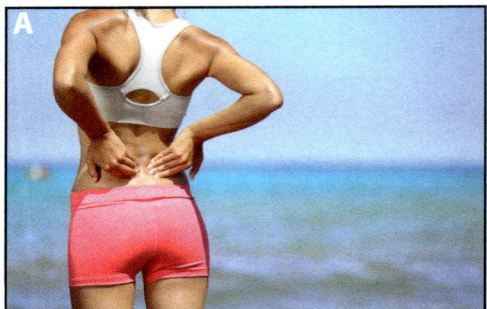
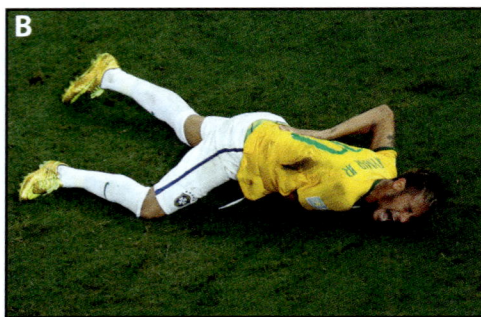

The back is the most mysterious part of the core, thanks to the elaborate network of nerves contained within it. To protect that back, it's vital to strengthen everything around it. If all you are doing is sit-ups to build strength to protect your back, you are opening yourself up to other potential issues with the adductor and rectus abdominis.

Rafael Nadal (Figure 6-10) learned all about how a back injury can sap effectiveness during the 2014 Australian Open, when he hurt his back warming up for his final match against Stanislas Wawrinka of Switzerland.[14] Instead of rolling to yet another Grand Slam title, against an opponent whom he had defeated 12 out of 12 times and to whom he had never surrendered even a set, Nadal was compromised and fell in only 2 hours.

We don't know whether Nadal's injury had anything to do with other parts of his core. Since the back is in that area, it makes sense to have everything around it working as well as possible.

A bad back can linger for a while, even after repair. Hall of Fame quarterback Joe Montana had surgery during the 1986 season to repair a ruptured disc. Though he came back to lead the 49ers to 2 more Super Bowl titles, Montana struggled with a protruding disc later in his career. He was still outstanding, but the pain did bother him and did limit his effectiveness at times.[15] Could Montana have prevented trouble by building strength throughout the rest of his core? We're not sure. It's still something of a mystery, but when you are talking about the core, you can't just focus on the front and sides. You must think about the back.

For example, a subtle groin problem can come from a slipped disc.

Of course, back injuries can be really severe and some may cause paralysis. Fortunately, most back injuries in athletes remain only mysterious, and do not cause paralysis. Certainly, though, many back injuries linger and end careers. A far greater number get better or the athletes learn how to cope with the pain. One of the biggest dangers of back injuries is the risk of causing other core injuries that result from treating the back. We shall get into this more later, but, basically, do not think of doing a zillion sit-ups as a cure for a back problem. Physical therapy must address the whole core, not just the beach muscles.

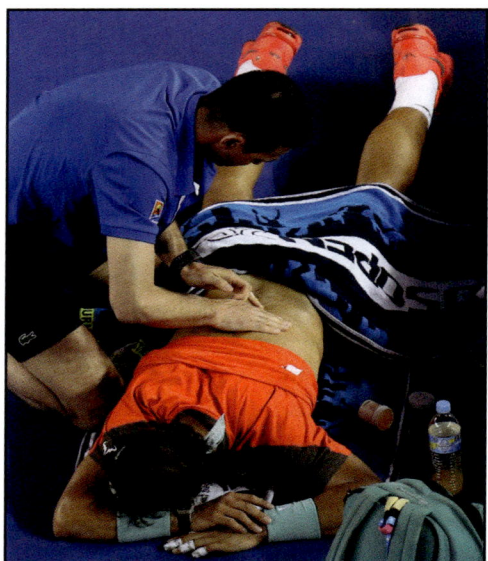

Figure 6-10. Rafael Nadal in the midst of his back problem. (Reprinted with permission from AP Photo/Eugene Hoshiko.)

CONCEPT 6: KEEP YOUR ANTENNAE UP FOR THE REALLY SERIOUS PROBLEMS

Keep your antennae up for everything else that can cause core problems!

Remember that there is a whole bunch of other stuff that resides in the core. Think about the star college basketball player who had pelvic pain whenever he went to jump or cut or shoot, and the pain was caused by a Crohn's disease fistula between his small intestine and the bladder. Or about the top marathon runner with endometriosis and terrible pain that would routinely begin at 2 miles. Or the pro ice hockey goalie with groin pain from rectal cancer. Or the young volleyball player with a synovial cell sarcoma. A long list of serious medical problems can mimic musculoskeletal injuries here. (See Figure 6-11.)

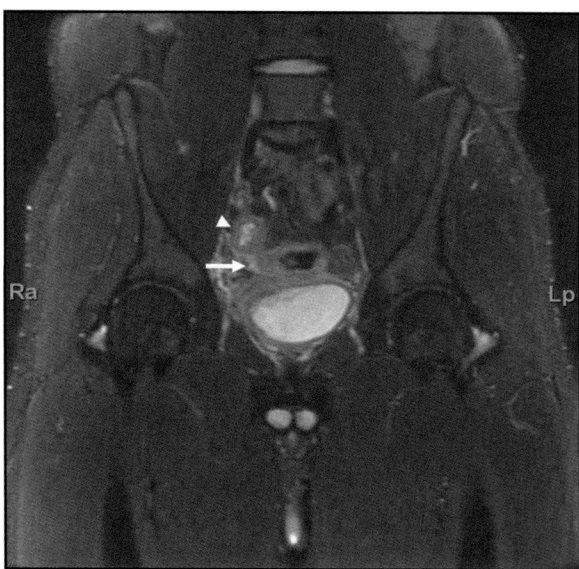

Figure 6-11. This MRI shows an inflammatory pelvic mass (arrow is in the middle of this, the entire area of white opacity is inflamed), which represents a Crohn's disease abscess and communication between the intestine and bladder (enterovesical fistula). The MRI comes from a star collegiate basketball forward with severe right-sided exertional groin pain. He had a significant core muscle injury, but the principal symptoms came from his Crohn's, which had been previously undiagnosed. The same arrow points also to a trickle of white fluid within the fistula. The arrowhead indicates the thickened, culprit bowel loop. This young man underwent a successful laparoscopically assisted bowel and fistula resection; subsequently, he had a great basketball season.

Numerous things in the core can mimic musculoskeletal injuries and impede performance. Think about the possible effects of kidney stones, constipation, appendicitis, or even reflex sympathetic dystrophy.

A whole world of possible diagnoses is out there. For obvious reasons, including that one may have to perform an abdominal, rectal, and/or pelvic examination, remember also that the training room is not the optimal place to examine an athlete with a suspected core injury. It may be necessary to perform an initial exam there. However, a physician cannot possibly do a complete examination in that setting.

CONCEPT 7: CORE INJURIES ARE MORE COMMON THAN ANY OTHER SET OF INJURIES

No one has yet elucidated the real epidemiology of core injuries. To introduce the subject, let's make an analogy with cholera in the mid-1800s.

John Snow, the father of epidemiology, scoured the streets of London for answers in 1854 with his investigatory spyglass and concluded that a water pump was spreading cholera. Nobody had the foggiest idea then that bacteria existed. At the time, most people thought the disease spread through the air.[16] "Experts" saw all kinds of manifestations of the sickness. They had a hard time linking it to a single source. Imagine the frustration of the baffled doctors as they watched scores of Londoners die.

No doubt, the epidemiologists of the mid-1800s would have classified cholera according to its clinical manifestations. They would have categorized this disease, which they found out later to have one cause, according to the signs and symptoms they saw: diarrhea, dehydration, nausea and vomiting, starvation, etc. Only later did Snow arouse suspicion that the disease had a common denominator. In fact, Snow did not link it to bacteria. He suspected contamination of the water.

That's the way it has been, and largely still is, with core injuries.[17-20] While the concept of the core creates a common denominator, most people still have difficulty seeing that. Frustration mounts from a lack of a unifying concept. The literature talks about osteitis, secondary cleft signs, "sports hernia," adductor injuries, femoroacetabular impingement,[2] etc. Like with cholera, one concept links the manifestations of core injuries.

Let's think through an excellent, relatively recent, meta-analysis of 25 articles from the literature in the *British Journal of Sports Medicine*.[18] One conclusion was that groin injuries made up 7% of all lower extremity injuries in soccer. Consider what the various authors might have meant by "groin." Next, look carefully at the meta-analysis's injury categories: hip, groin, upper leg, knee, lower leg, ankle, and foot. Then extract out conservative estimates that might fit into a category called "core." Recalculate. The number turns out to be much higher, perhaps 26%. We need a Dr. Snow to visit this region of the body.

TIME FOR GIGGLES

Okay, enough seriousness. Keep these 7 concepts in your mind, and then you can start giggling again.

It's time to pay a longer visit to the Copernican capital of the body's universe… the pubic bone. As Drew Rosenhaus might say, "Next chapter!"

SELECTED READINGS

Meyers WC, Yoo E, Devon O, et al. Understanding "sports hernia" (athletic pubalgia): the anatomic and pathophysiologic basis for abdominal and groin pain in athletes. *Oper Tech Sport Med*. 2007;15(4):165-177.
   Some of the basics for understanding core muscle injuries. The article discusses the association of hip and core muscles and several of the other concepts mentioned in this chapter.

Sommer Hammoud, S, Bedi A, Magennis E, Meyers WC, Kelly BT. High incidence of athletic pubalgia symptoms in professional athletes with symptomatic femoroacetabular impingement. *Arthroscopy*. 2012;28(10):1388-1395.
   This article establishes a profound relationship between the hip and core muscles.

Hölmich P, Thorberg K, Dehlendorff C, et al. Incidence and clinical presentation of groin injuries in sub-elite male soccer. *Br J Sports Med*. 2014;48:1245-1250.
   The guru of adductor epidemiology presents his perspective on the subject in select populations.

REFERENCES

1. Der Kaiser, the brains behind Germany. FIFA.com. Published December 18, 2008. Accessed May 6, 2016.
2. Friedell J. Timeline: Derrick Rose's injury troubles. ESPN. http://www.espn.com/blog/chicago/bulls/post/_/id/21637/timeline-derrick-roses-injury-troubles. Published February 27, 2015. Accessed May 8, 2016.
3. Chiusano S. The plight of Derrick Rose: a look at the new Knicks point guard's injury history. *NY Daily News*. https://www.nydailynews.com/sports/basketball/injuries-scarred-derrick-rose-career-article-1.2380299. Published June 23, 2016. Accessed November 1, 2016.
4. Chicago Bulls Derrick Rose knee injury torn ACL. JMRL Fitness. jmrlfitness.leadpages.co. Accessed November 1, 2016.
5. Zirm J. What's wrong with Derrick Rose? Five expert theories on the oft-injured star. Stack. https://www.stack.com/a/derrick-rose-injuries. Updated November 19, 2014. Accessed November 1, 2016.
6. An open letter to Derrick Rose's groin. *Chicago Tribune*. www.chicagonow.com. Published April 4, 2012. Accessed November 1, 2016.
7. Altergott B. Derrick Rose's epic battle with injuries: a timeline. EW Scripps Company. www.newsy.com. Published September 28, 2015. Accessed November 1, 2016.
8. Justin Verlander stats, fantasy & news. www.MLB.com. Published January 20, 2016. Accessed May 8, 2016.
9. Kepner T. Justin Verlander and the Detroit Tigers are back for more. *The New York Times*. https://www.nytimes.com/2017/03/02/sports/baseball/justin-verlander-detroit-tigers.html?_r=0. Published March 2, 2017. Accessed January 15, 2019.
10. Roy Oswalt stats, fantasy & news. www.MLB.com. Published January 20, 2016. Accessed May 8, 2016.
11. All-Star forward will be sidelined after hernia surgery. ESPN. http://www.espn.com/nba/news/story?id=2205531. Published October 28, 2005. Accessed October 24, 2018.
12. Adler M. If Grant Hill stayed healthy… Chat Sports. https://www.chatsports.com/detroit-pistons/a/If-Grant-Hill-Stayed-Healthy-9026. Published March 7, 2012. Accessed October 24, 2018.
13. Willis J. Grant Hill talks playing through pain, opioids, and the NBA's rest problem. *GQ*. https://www.gq.com/story/grant-hill-pain-management-interview. Published October 11, 2017. Accessed October 24, 2018.

14. Newman P. Australian Open 2014: Rafael Nadal's pain brings an end to Stanislas Wawrinka's long wait for a major crown. Independent. https://www.independent.co.uk/sport/tennis/australian-open-2014-rafael-nadal-s-pain-brings-an-end-to-stanislas-wawrinka-s-long-wait-for-a-major-9085994.html. Published January 26, 2014. Accessed October 24, 2018.
15. Montana gets surgery for disk. *The New York Times.* https://www.nytimes.com/1986/09/16/sports/montana-gets-surgery-for-disk.html. Published September 16, 1986. Accessed September 5, 2018.
16. Paneth N, Vinten-Johansen P, Brody H, Rip M. A rivalry of foulness: official and unofficial investigations of the London cholera epidemic of 1854. *Am J Public Health.* 1998;88(10):1545-1553.
17. Mandelbaum BR. Sports hernias, adductor injuries, and hip problems are linked. https://www.medscape.com/viewarticle/876035_2. Published February 28, 2017. Accessed May 3, 2018.
18. Wong P, Hong Y. Soccer injury in the lower extremities. *Br J Sports Med.* 2005;39:473-482.
19. Hölmich P, Thorberg K, Dehlendorff C, et al. Incidence and clinical presentation of groin injuries in sub-elite male soccer. *Br J Sports Med.* 2014;48:1245-1250.
20. Weir A, Brukner P, Delahunt E, et al. Doha agreement meeting on terminology and definitions in groin pain in athletes. *Br J Sports Med.* 2015;49:768-774.

7

the **pubic** bone

We dance round in a ring and suppose, but the secret sits in the middle and knows.
—Robert Frost, famous poet.

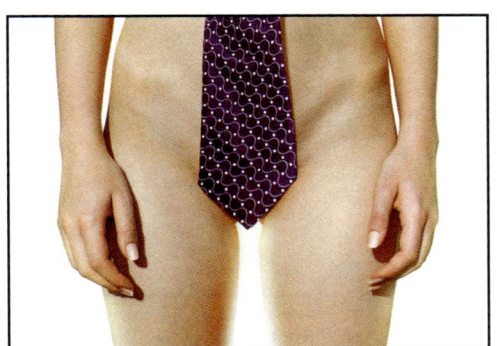

Figure 7-1. Don't giggle.

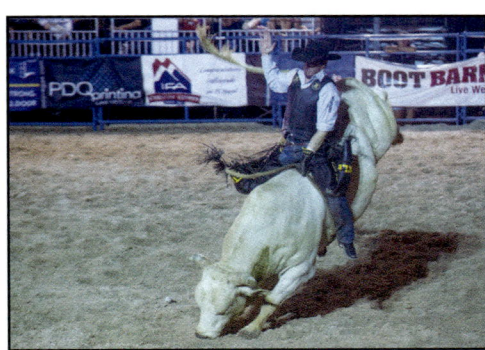

Figure 7-2.

Ask 100 people about the pubic bone, and after they stop giggling, they'll no doubt mention something about sex. Or everything about sex. And, when it comes to that, the pubic bone is definitely in play. Man or woman, it has a big role in sexual intercourse (Figure 7-1).

Bull riders look at the thing differently—for good reasons (Figure 7-2).

If you spent 8 seconds (or less) on an angry hunk of bovine nastiness, you would too. The twisting, turning, and bouncing can't be good for the body, and that pubic bone bears the brunt of the action. Imagine trying to control about 2,000 pounds of snorting cattle that doesn't want any part of you sitting on its back. It isn't easy. Even if the rider has a strong core, he/she is exposed to countless opportunities for muscles to tear and bones to break. Those who haven't built up the area might as well try the merry-go-round.

Obviously the Center

Sex, bulls…what else? What other roles does the pubic bone play? Ask a ballet dancer or a futebol jogador, or a hockey goalie, or Leonardo da Vinci for that matter…where is your "center" (Figure 7-3)? They will tell you.

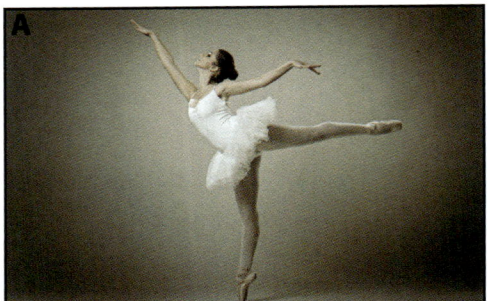 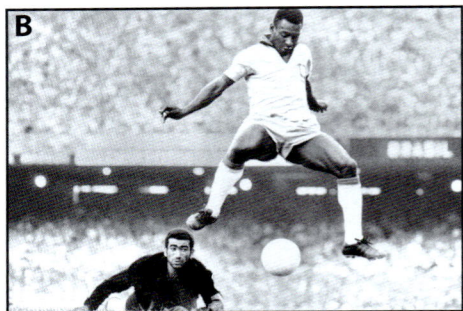

Figure 7-3. It doesn't take much thought to locate "the center" of either (A) the ballerina or (B) Pelé. ([B] Reprinted with permission from AP Photo.)

They point to the pubic bone or somewhere slightly above it. Look at what anatomists call the center of the "normal anatomic position" or what evolutionists call the bending point for human progression from a 4-legged animal to early caveperson. Consider the "set" positions of baseball or American football players. What part of the anatomy comes into play most? How does the upper body connect to the lower body? How are the muscles arranged to do this? Isn't there an obvious symmetry? What anatomic structure provides a more obvious connection point? Is it possible that the pubic bone is the center of the body's universe (Figure 7-4)?

Not that we need more convincing, but let's look at what we should already know. The following ancient observations were not simply mythical. Nobody has refuted them. Leonardo da Vinci was not out of his gourd in 1490 when he drew *Le proporzioni del corpo umano secondo Vitruvio*, the man with the supposed perfect proportions. He used complex mathematical models and a circle and a square to show that the pubic bone and perhaps an area just above it was the center of the body's universe. He even called it that. He believed literally that man embodied the universe. Da Vinci based his observations on the work of ancient Roman architect Vitruvius. Da Vinci's square, formed by arms outstretched, represented material existence, and his circle, formed by spread-eagled extremities, represented our spiritual being. It appears that the pubic center covers all the bases! Eerily, da Vinci went further and even used words for this center like "the core." His Vitruvian man became the symbol for symmetry and balance. I became queasy reading some of the da Vinci translations. I wondered if we were plagiarizing his interpretations, and was relieved when I realized it was way beyond the statute of limitations for da Vinci to sue us.

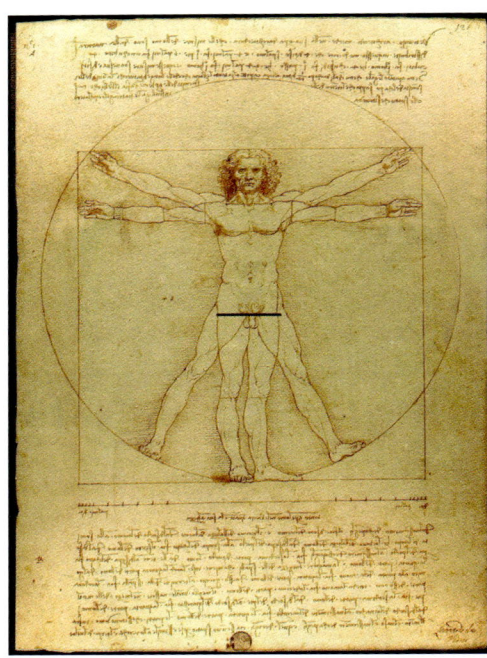

Figure 7-4. The famous Vitruvian Man by Leonardo da Vinci. You can see the horizontal line just above the base of the penis. In fact, Vitruvius, centuries earlier, had the center 1 or 2 inches higher.

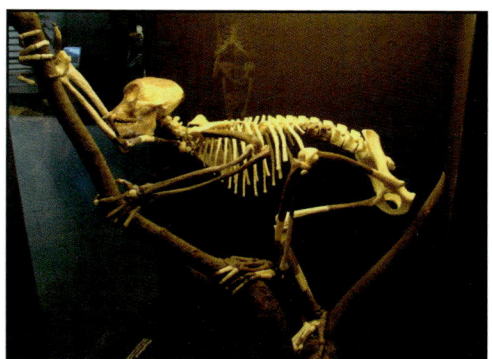

Figure 7-5. Reconstructed skeleton of the tailless *Proconsul*, a species from 13 million years ago. Note where the center-point is likely to be. (Reprinted with permission from Wikipedia. From the Museum of Anthropology at the University of Zurich. Photo taken by Guerin Nicolasn. https://en.wikipedia.org/wiki/Human_evolution#/media/File:Proconsul_skeleton_reconstitution_(University_of_Zurich).JPG.)

Now travel ahead to the 20th century. Relatively modern evolutionists reidentified the pubic bone as a crucial anatomic feature in man's progression from a 4-legged animal to the way we are now. They implied that the older evolutionists already knew this. C. Owen Lovejoy showed that a 3-million-year-old lady named Lucy[1,2] could walk and run on 2 legs, with that same bony frontal part at the center of it all, presumably in her first decades of life. Interestingly, Lovejoy and colleagues also saw that the hip sockets formed the levers providing tremendous power that would be channeled through the one and same friendly bony prominence.

So, evolutionists and ancient architects may have known far more about the pubic bone than us modern scholars (Figure 7-5).

Let's not beat ourselves up too much unnecessarily for being so innocent. How many of us serve as Little League coaches or dance instructors or commit time to teaching other activities? Certainly, we know the pubic bone area is important. We may not say it out loud, but we do. We probably don't appreciate how much we know. Baryshnikov and other ballet teachers call that anatomic area the same as da Vinci "the center point" for balance and dance. As coaches in baseball, football, soccer, basketball, you name the sport, we teach the "set position" (Figure 7-6). Think about how Coach Mike Krzyzewski teaches the defense in basketball. Bend slightly at the center, be ready for immediate power. A profile of the bony structure of the sprinter's starting position displays a "ready" position perhaps the best. Plus, we always tell athletes to "play within themselves." What do we mean by that? Aren't we advising them to stay in control of their bodies and to maintain their center points? Figure 7-6B should convince you that this starting position is natural.

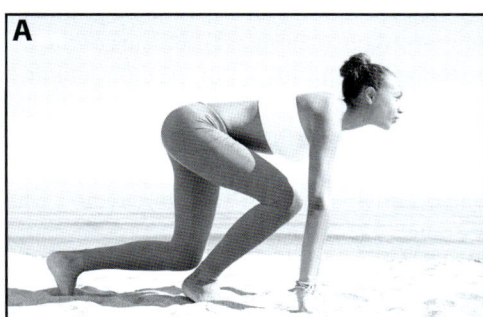
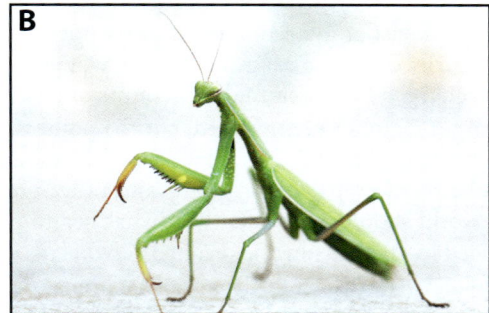
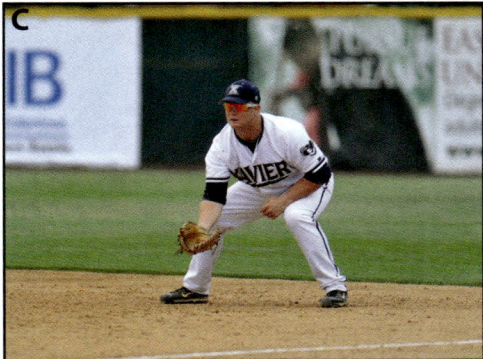
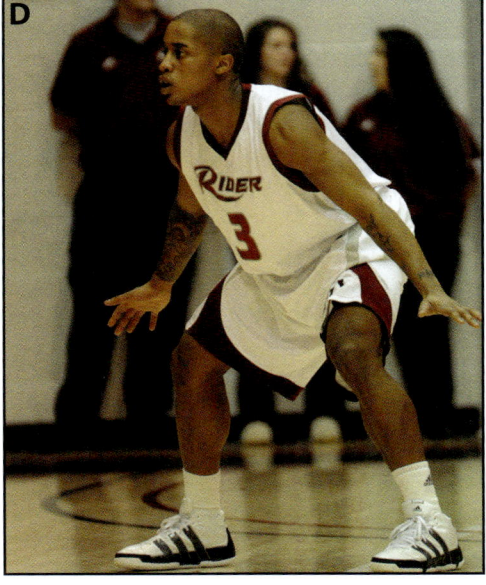

Figure 7-6. The "set" position has been with us since the beginning of man and other species. Who dares deny that the pubic bone or thereabouts is at its center? The set positions for a (A) female sprinter, (B) praying mantis, (C) baseball infielder, and (D) basketball defensive player.

Extrapolating Vitruvian Concept to Copernicus

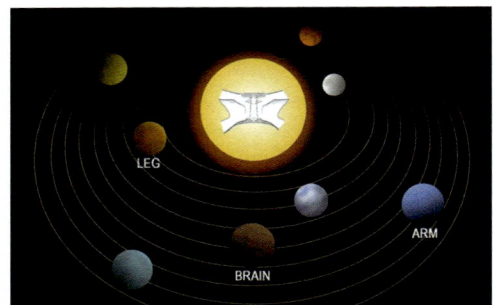

Figure 7-7. The pubic bone is the "sun" of the body's universe.

For fun, let's combine the da Vinci pubic center concept with the Copernican controversy concerning the sun at the center of the universe. Could it be that the pubic bone is the center of the body's universe, with arms, legs, neck, and head orbiting around it (Figure 7-7)? Yes. Now you've got it.

More on the Difficulty Studying This Area

This stuff seems so obvious. Then why has this anatomy remained so mysterious to us docs? Why is all this stuff not written down? To keep the mystery in sex? No, medical people don't obsess on that. The core's complexity? Maybe that's part of it. So many muscles and organ systems converge right there. Plus, medical specialists get trapped in their individual organ systems. And except for trauma and the hip, orthopedists generally fear veering into the pelvis. No medical specialty looks at the core as a whole. Could it be that? And put the sex thing on top of that. Maybe we've got something here. For whatever reason, important concepts—including the incontrovertible reality that the pubic bone is at or near the center of the core's universe—have heretofore simply not been articulated in modern times.

Before looking more closely into the anatomy and function of this important center of our body, let us render a couple more remarks about the difficulty studying this area in today's world.

Clinically, social stigmas spill over in spades to the professional side. With modern-day taboos, the whole "private area" of men and women has become almost off-limits. Detailed physical examinations are almost impossible, except when undertaken by a urologist or gynecologist, who are not ordinarily versed on anatomical problems of the hip. Yet, orthopedists do not ordinarily do pelvic examinations on women. An orthopedic hip surgeon in Vermont did do that a few years ago. Prosecutors charged him with multiple counts of rape.[3, VID 1]

No doubt, other factors were involved, but the point is that we need to redefine this specialty of the core. We need to establish principles and guidelines. Otherwise, physicians and others, with good or bad intentions, shall continue to make up their own rules. Gynecological, prostatic, and other problems occur in the same anatomic region where the hip also lies. The whole world should peer intently at what health professionals are doing when they care for patients with pelvic problems. We need to create a new field called *core medicine*.

Social stigmata carry over into the scientific arena, particularly in cadaveric dissection suites. Cadavers provide the answers to how the pubic bone works as the center of the body's universe. The dissections are not pleasant. But the smells and general disagreeableness of those travails were minor compared to the hoops of social and regulatory taboos we jumped through. It may have been easier to dissect cadavers in ancient Egypt when docs had to let dead people drift for days in the Nile so they could puncture the skin without a knife. The Egyptians would have considered themselves lucky not to have so many people standing around ready to snap cellphone photos of them.

Even educating medical students became difficult. I still dream about all the hairy eyeballs I aroused by my pointing out the pubic anatomy to our medical students at Body Worlds exhibits at the Philadelphia Museum of Art.

As you read further, imagine the difficulties we faced doing our experiments. Nevertheless, the cadaveric dissections were so important. They helped define this body region's biomechanics. With these, we also developed our MRI techniques. The logistics behind imaging these cadavers in an outpatient center were interesting (Figure 7-8).

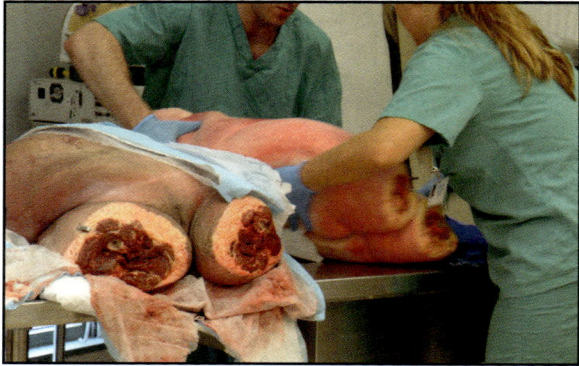

Figure 7-8. Nonembalmed ("fresh") cadavers are necessary for optimal understanding of the gross and functional anatomy of the core musculoskeleton. (Reprinted with permission from Isaac Stackell.)

What the Pubic Bone Really Looks Like

Dissecting so many "fresh" cadavers, we began to see the light shine on the real pubic and core anatomy. We saw how the 4 parts of the core fit together. One important observation was the spacious range of motion around the pubic bone. Fresh cadaver trunks rotated so readily in so many directions around that enabling bone. The region's suppleness compelled us to call it a *joint*. We referred to the whole complex as the *pubic bone joint*, distinguishing it from one of its parts—the pubic symphyseal joint. We then correlated the newly learned anatomy with the sites of pain in many athletes with clinically recognizable core injuries. On the basis of these studies over many years, we devised the many surgical techniques that generated a huge successful clinical experience diagnosing and treating such injuries.

To do those dissections, we had other limitations besides the smells and sometimes-doubtful eyes that watched us. Most of the cadavers were older and had various physical ailments. Young athletic cadavers, fortunately, did not ordinarily reach our lab; those that did often had problems, such as cerebral palsy, that limited our observations. So consider our observations subject to error. Most of our impressions seem quite well founded, but please take them for what you think they are worth. We won't be offended. All this is open to interpretation.

Think of the whole pubic bone—the hardness at the bottom of your belly—like a baseball, with a firm, compressible leather cover. The baseball turns out to be a great prop for understanding the musculoskeletal anatomy of the core (Figure 7-9).

Symmetrically, all of the core muscles cross by or attach to this baseball. Fibers of the adjoining muscles, in fact, join the cover and cross from one side to the other almost like the spiral seams of a baseball (Figure 7-10).

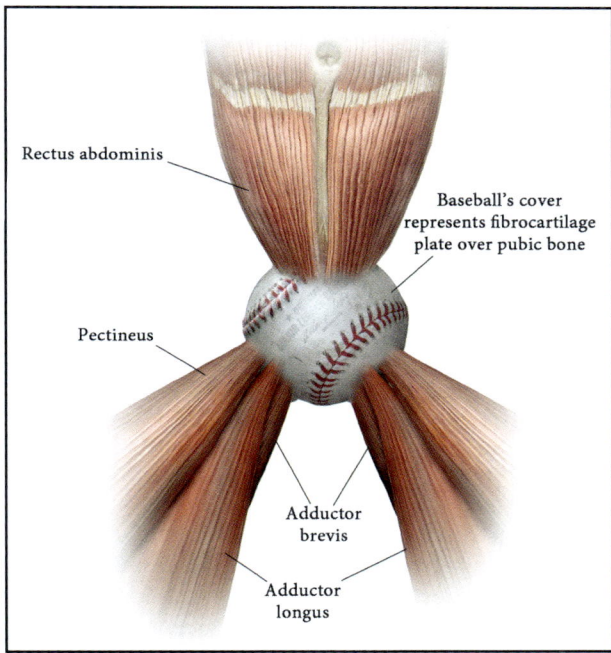

Figure 7-9. The baseball model. Think of the central core muscles as attaching directly to the cover of the baseball cover. In fact, thick fibrocartilage covers surfaces of the entire bone. The continuity of this cover establishes the basis for understanding function of the core muscles.

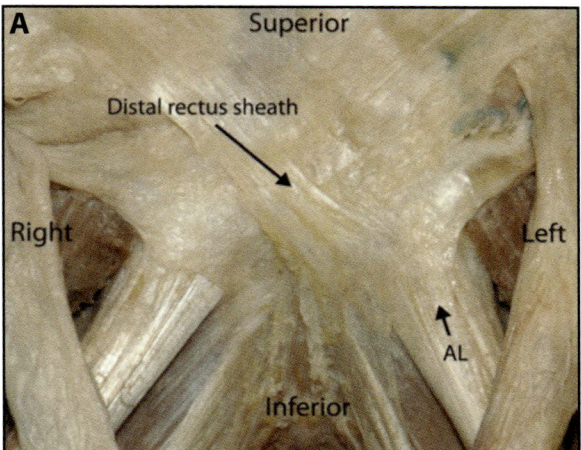
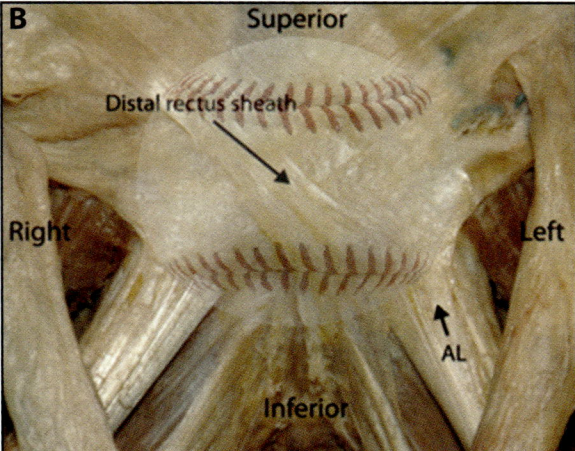

Figure 7-10. (A) This nice anatomic study illustrates the directions of fibrous extensions of muscles that blend into the fibrocartilage "baseball" pubic cover. We think of these like seams or laces. (B) Same dissection with a baseball. (Reprinted with permission from Norton-Old KJ, Schache AG, Barker PJ, Clark RA, Harrison SM, Briggs CA. Anatomical and mechanical relationship between the proximal attachment of adductor longus and the distal rectus sheath. *Clin Anat*. 2013;26:522-530.)

74　Chapter 7

That's it, the key to the core: a baseball with its cover. Of course, there is more. But if you don't get this key observation, go back to the couch and watch some more football. Actually, that's a good idea even if you do get it. Real American football puts the reality into the whole set of observations. That's how we began to understand it.

Getting back to the baseball…the pubic bone, of course, does not really look totally like that. But the concept works. There are many analogies. Think back to the Eureka experiment described in Chapter 3.

In reality, the 2 pubic bodies form a relatively round-feeling object. Thick fibrocartilage covers the whole round item. The fibrocartilage not only covers the "baseball," it extends into it and between the 2 halves as well as over the baseball and then fades along some bony extensions called the *rami* (Figure 7-11).

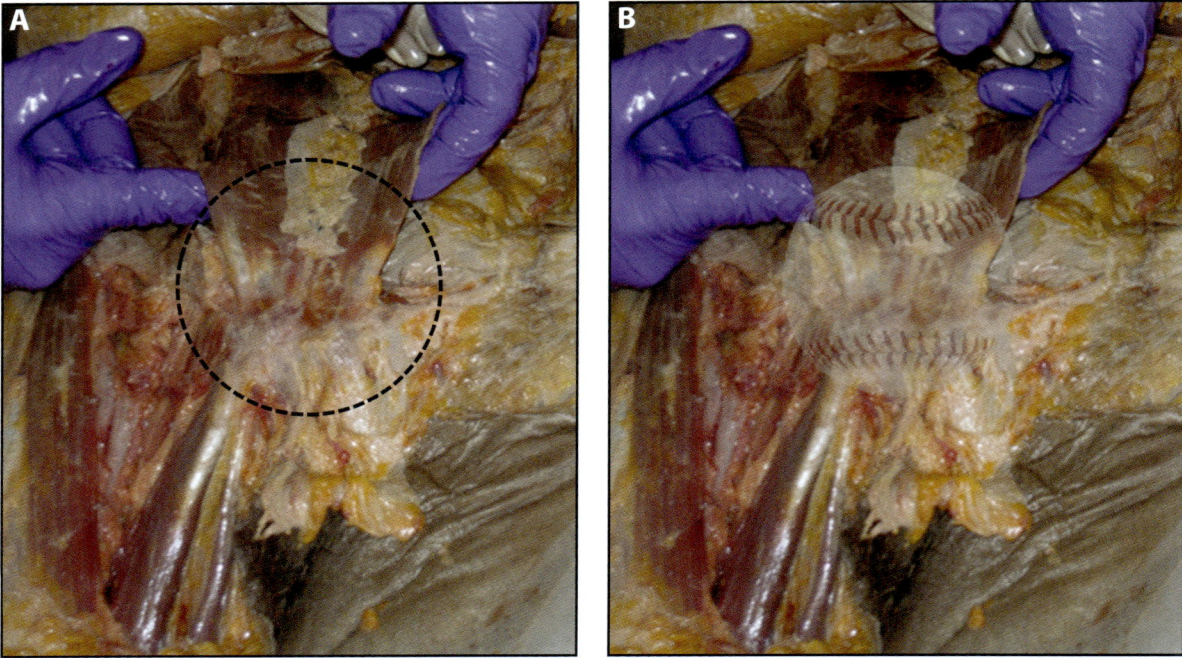

Figure 7-11. The location of the "pubic baseball" in the human. This is the same cadaver you saw before (in Chapters 3 and 4) with (A) a circle representing the location of the pubic bone baseball and (B) the baseball.

Now look back at the same cadaveric dissection picture we showed before. The yellow circle represents the baseball. Note the rectus abdominis muscle attaching from above and the adductor muscles from below. They attach to the same, hard-to-see mat of tissue. The 2 sets of muscle share the same fibrocartilage cover and therefore, from the standpoint of motor function, they connect. Also note the much larger muscle mass passing alongside the rectus abdominis/adductor complex. The fact that that muscle mass is so much larger might insinuate it provides a lot more power than the rectus abdominis/adductor complex. That has been shown to be true. Most of our power comes from our back, butt, and side muscles. We call these the *core power muscles*. We call the pubic attachment complex (ie, the rectus abdominis/adductor complex) the *harness*. We shall get into the harness more in the next chapter. For now, let's just say it serves to harness the power from the power muscles. We call the baseball cover the *fibrocartilage plate*.

For now, consider the following anatomic features of the pubic bone. These features are important to understand the subsequent chapters. Memorize them if you want, but if you don't want to, that's okay. These pages shall remain here for reference. The fibrocartilage plate connects the rectus abdominis to the pectineus, adductor longus, and adductor brevis. Other adductor muscles do not attach at the same place. The gracilis attachment is so petite and so posterior, it seems unlikely that it plays much role in pubic bone joint stability. All the harness muscles attach to the same plate so functionally they all connect to each other (Figure 7-12).

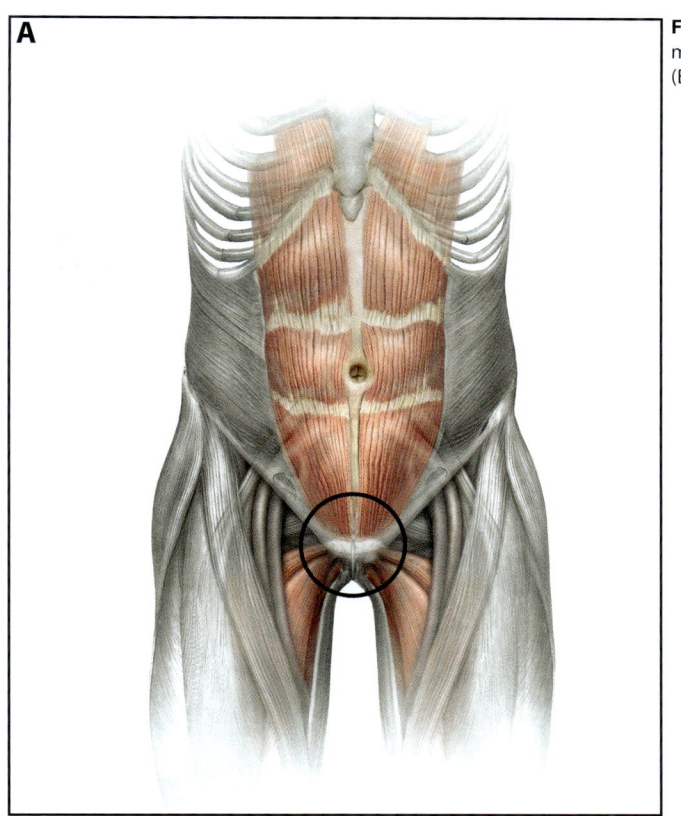
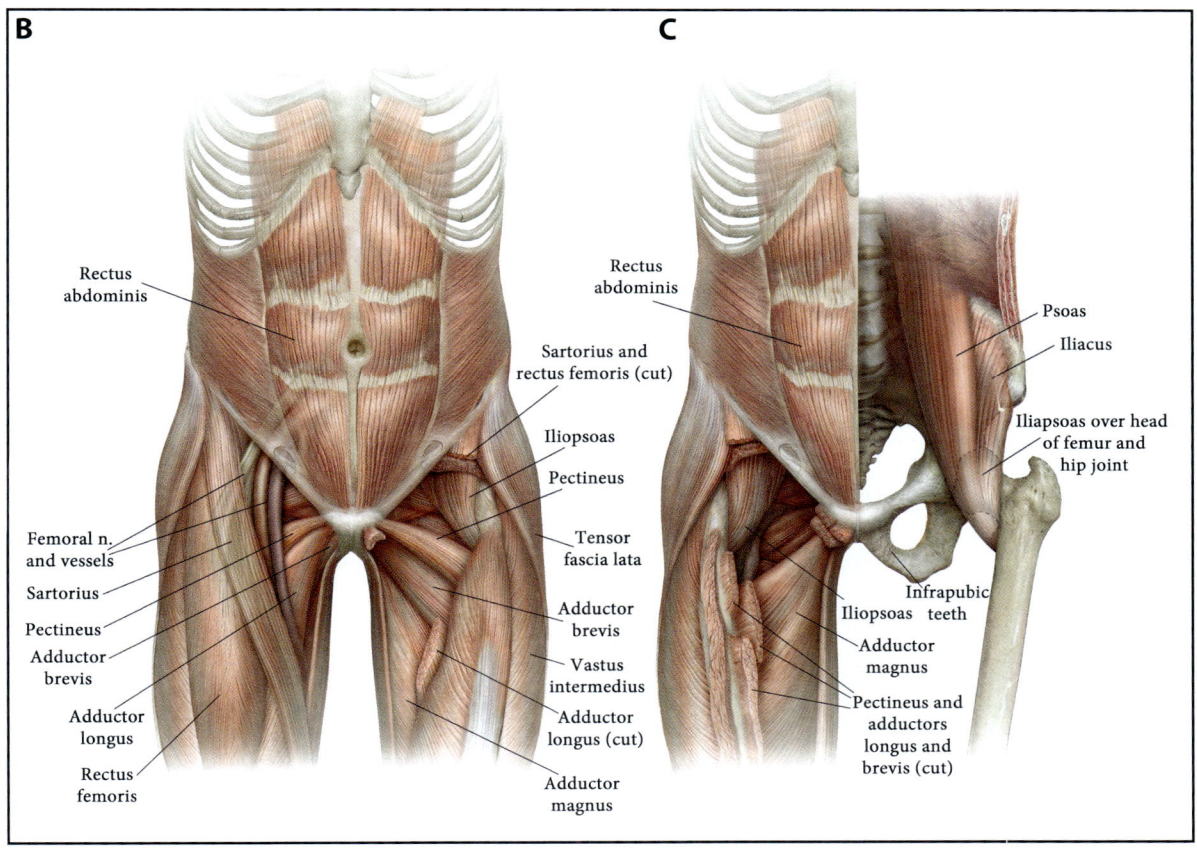

Figure 7-12. The anterior pubic bone with its surrounding muscles (A), and then with more of the muscles cut away (B, C).

Also, do not think in terms of adductor or rectus abdominis "tendons." Very little tendon, in fact, exists, and virtually all the operations were derived without consideration of any tendon residing here. We shall go into this more later. The harness muscles join with the cover of the baseball. The individual muscles and cover are all separable clinically and they dissect out easily in the fresh cadaver lab (Figure 7-13).

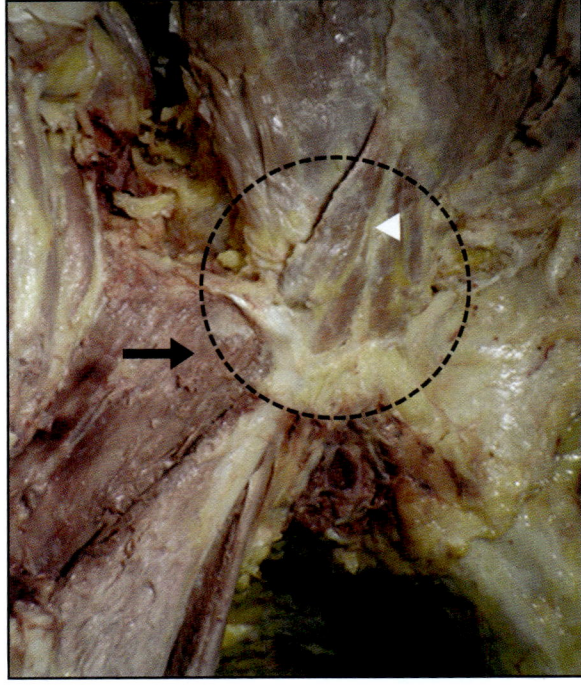

Figure 7-13. A similar photo to Figure 7-11 except of a slightly less fresh cadaver and with the same circle surrounding the location of the pubic bone. This could have been an NHL ice hockey player considering his relatively large pectineus muscles (black arrow). The cadaver also has a pyramidalis muscle (white arrowhead) overlying the rectus abdominis. A pyramidalis muscle is not present in all human bodies, and it is variable in size and shape when it exists. It lies anterior to the rectus abdominis and may connect to the adductors. In our dissections, it was invariably small. Therefore, it probably has little function.

And one final point for now with regard to gross anatomy: The pubic fibrocartilage plate (aka baseball cover) can peel off from the periosteum of the pubic bone. It is easy to separate the plate from bone in young people and more difficult in older folks. The plate becomes thinner as it travels onto the rami (Figure 7-14).

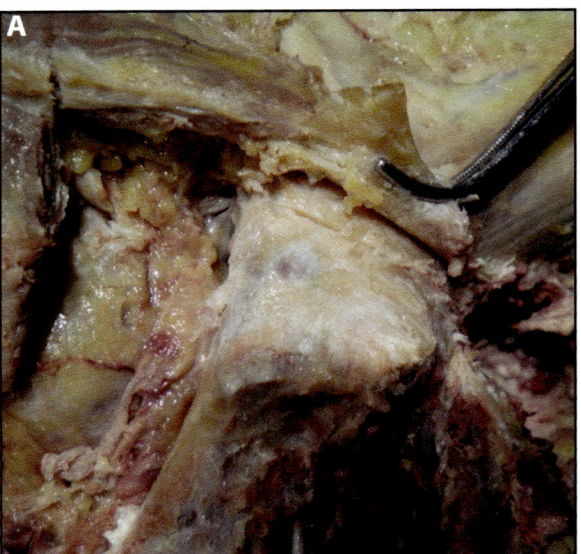 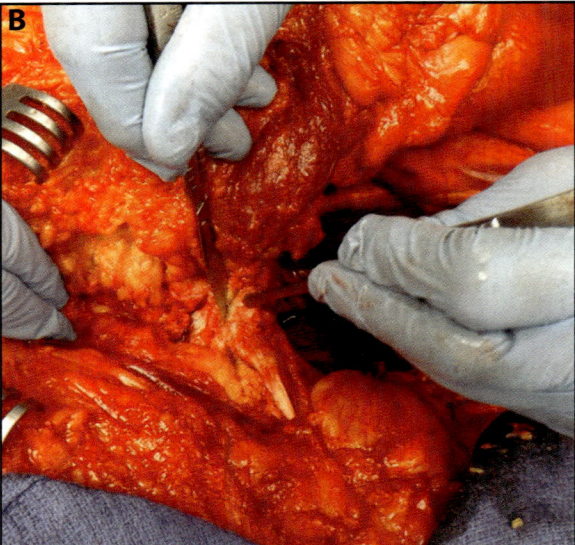

Figure 7-14. Dissecting the pubic fibrocartilage plate. (A) The central pubic bone (ie, pubic body) in a cadaver viewed from the right side. A large chunk of the right rectus abdominis muscle has been removed as well as most of the right pubic plate. We are looking at the insertion of the left rectus abdominis muscle. A clamp grabs the left anterior pubic plate at the left rectus abdominis junction. (B) The same cadaver showing posterior dissection of the plate along a ramus. The fibrocartilaginous plate becomes thinner along the rami.

MICROSCOPIC ANATOMY

So, how does the cover of the baseball connect with the periosteum and rest of the pubic bone?

The answer is that we don't really know yet, but we can peel it away in the cadaver lab. We can do that with sharp dissection, but time and again, we have to pull out heavy scissors and cut across spicules of bone. The next best observation is to cut out whole chunks of tissue and look at the whole chunk under a microscope. You can see these spicules. I like to call the technique *Schilders whole-mounts* after Ernie Schilders,[4] who exhibits these types of slides in his talks. In Figure 7-15, you can see fibrocartilage and interconnecting spicules existing together with muscle in the periphery.

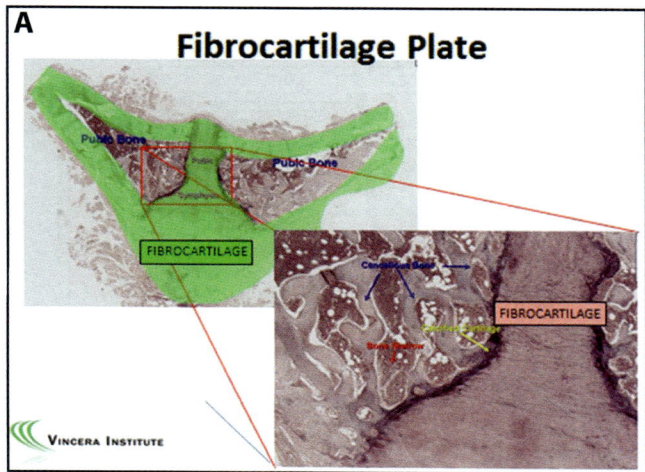
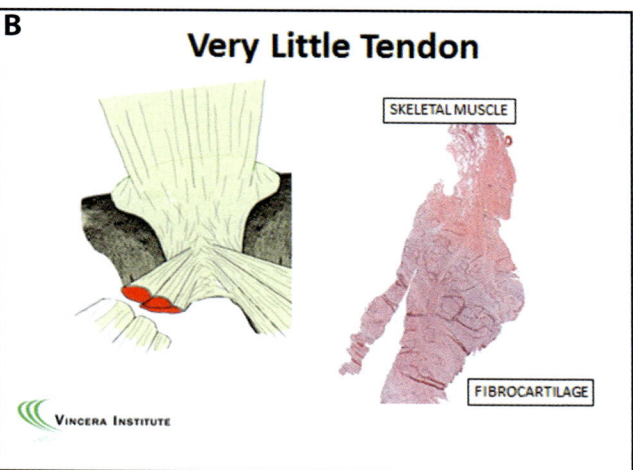

Figure 7-15. More pubic anatomy. (A) Whole-mount photomicrograph showing the fibrocartilage plate to be continuous with the pubic symphysis. (B) Gross sketch and whole-mount showing skeletal muscle blending into the pubic plate. We make the point that very few tendinous features of tendon exist in either the gross or microscopic dissections. (Reprinted with permission from Blake Bowden.)

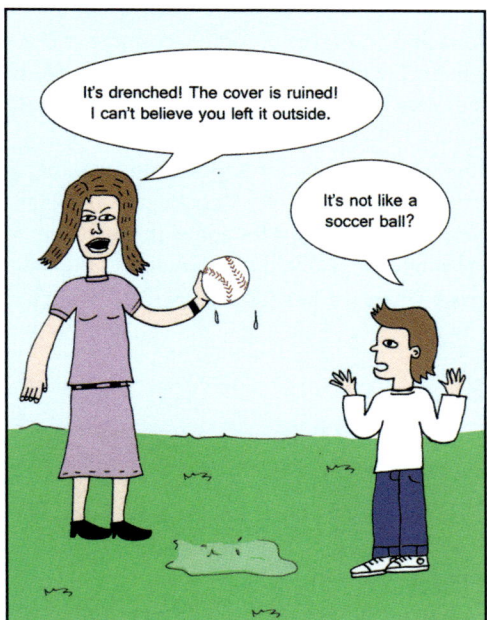

Figure 7-16.

These spicules likely rub and irritate, and fluid accumulates when there is a central core muscle injury. The injury causes an imbalance in forces and a tug of war on the cover of the baseball. The cover loosens. With movement, the process worsens. The fluid accumulation phenomenon has commonly been called *osteitis pubis*. Pain comes primarily from fluid shifts and the nerve fibers of the periosteum. With injury or any other type of force imbalance, the fibrocartilage plate can easily separate. We shall unveil more about the mysteries of this "osteitis" in the next chapter about the harness.

For now, understand this osteitis process by visualizing the baseball prop. Think in terms of an old baseball or one that has been lying outside in the moisture overnight. Your mom gets mad at you for being careless with your toy. During the night, the cover of the baseball gets wet and loosens, seams disrupt, and the cover starts to come off. You have ruined a perfectly good baseball and you pay for it with your mother's wrath. For now, that's all you need to know. Osteitis does not just "happen." There is a reason for it. (See Figure 7-16.) We shall get into this osteitis concept a lot more in the next 2 chapters.

Let's finish this chapter with the threat of providing more detail about the forces around the pubic bone than you would ever want. For this moment, simply sit back and gaze at the accompanying diagrams (Figure 7-17).

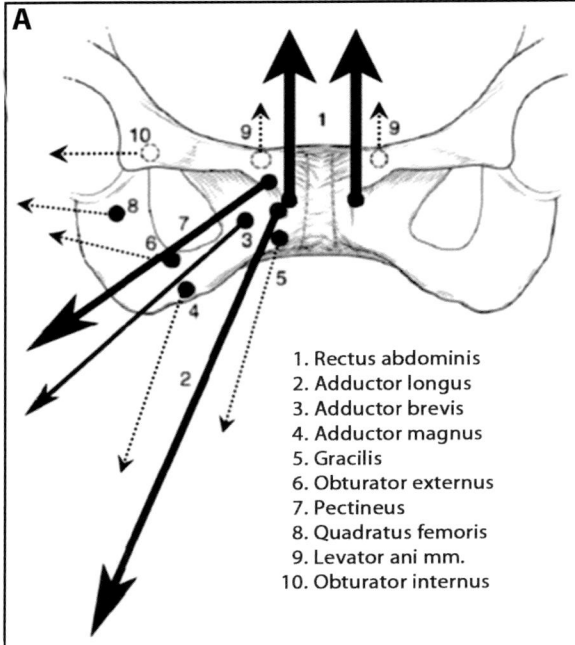
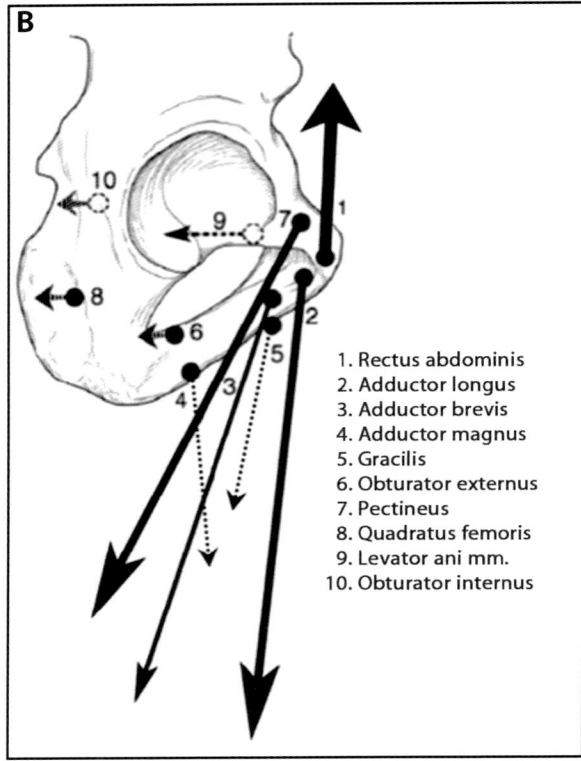

Figure 7-17. Pubic muscular attachments with approximate directions and impacts of forces with relationship to the pubic baseball.

Think about the symmetry. Welcome it. Appreciate the balance of the forces. In your head, add up the medial forces and compare them to the lateral forces. Do the same for the superior vs inferior forces, or pick any other comparison of symmetry that you might want. Jump, stand on one foot, change your body posture in various ways. Note the symmetry and how precisely your muscles compensate to achieve balance. Don't get hurt reading this book at the same time.

In fact, in the cadaver lab, we did multiple studies to determine the directions and strengths of forces around our bony friend, the pubis. Based on the origins and insertions, as well as volume, length, and width of the various core muscles, it turns out that force estimates of muscles attaching from above vs below, or medial vs lateral, or any opposite direction we chose, almost perfectly matched. A natural balance exists around this pubic bone.

Ask yourself one more question: Could detachments of muscles around the pubic bone cause important imbalances? You should be able to guess the answer.

Okay, if you've got the answer, now sigh and lean back in your chair. You now have learned a lot about the anatomy of the giggle center, the Copernican sun, pubic bone, the baseball, horse's nose, or whatever else you want to call it.

Prepare to see what happens when our body becomes dynamic like a horse, when we harness our forces, trot, run, and jump.

SELECTED READINGS

Lester T. *Da Vinci's Ghost: Genius, Obsession, and How Leonardo Created the World in His Own Image.* New York, NY: Free Press; 2012.
   An in-depth account of how da Vinci came to create his Vitruvian man and its impact.
Davis A, Stringer MD, Woodley SJ. New insights into the proximal tendons of adductor longus, adductor brevis and gracilis. *Br J Sports Med.* 2012;46:871-876. doi:10.1136/bjsports-2011-090044.
   This article points out adductor proximal anatomy to be more complex than previously described. It connects groin pathology to the fibrocartilaginous cover of the pubic bone.
Valent A, Frizziero A, Bressan S, et al. Insertional tendinopathy of the adductors and rectus abdominis in athletes: a review. *Muscles Ligaments Tendons J.* 2012;2(2):142-148.
   Using an anatomic approach, the authors focus on differences in specific sport actions and injury prevention.

Falvey ÉC, King E, Kinsella S, Franklyn-Miller A. Athletic groin pain. Part 1: a prospective anatomical diagnosis of 382 patients—clinical findings, MRI findings and patient-reported outcome measures at baseline. *Br J Sports Med.* 2016;50(7):423-430.

Data from many other studies show the same importance of the pubic bone and harness muscles. In this article, the harness was the location of pathology in nearly 80% of almost 400 consecutive patients with groin pain. The remaining 20% had pain from hip pathology.

REFERENCES

1. Lovejoy CO. The origin of man. *Science.* 1981;211(4480):341-350.
2. Lovejoy CO. Evolution of human walking. *Scientific American.* 1988;Nov:18-25.
3. Curran J. Vt doctor pleads no contest in sex case. Boston.com. http://archive.boston.com/news/local/vermont/articles/2010/01/20/vt_doctor_pleads_no_contest_in_sex_case/. Published January 20, 2010. Accessed May 10, 2016.
4. Schilders E, Dimitrakopoulou A, Cooke M, Bismil Q, Cooke C. Effectiveness of a selective partial adductor release for chronic adductor-related groin pain in professional athletes. *Am J Sports Med.* 2013;41(3):603-607. doi:10.1177/0363546513475790.

VIDEO

1. https://www.liveleak.com/view?t=739_1194041736

8

the "harness"

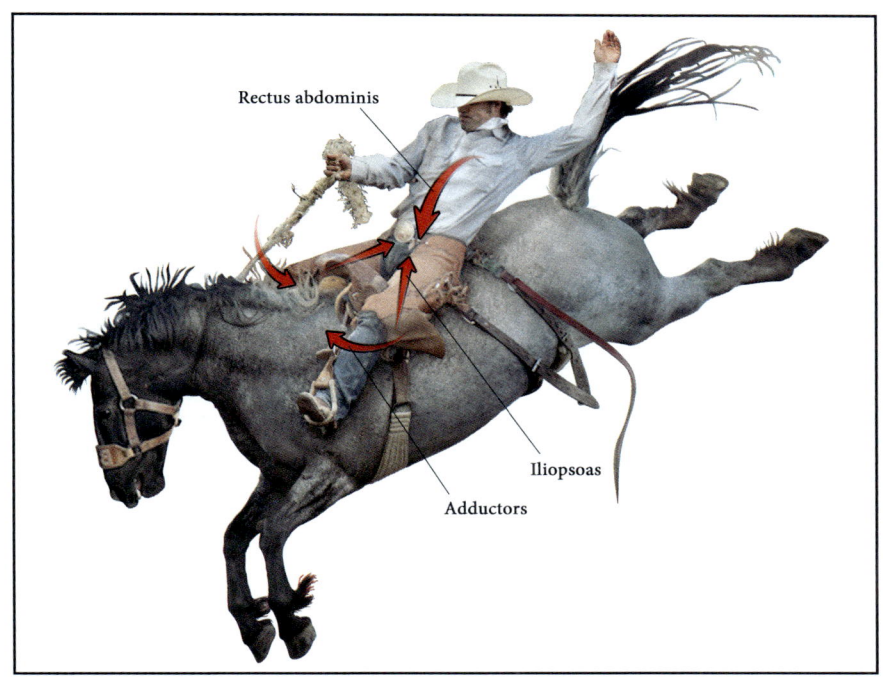

Figure 8-1.

Ready…set…Are you ready to go? This short chapter may be the most important one in the book. It introduces an essential concept for understanding the core. One might say the central concept. Dare we say the "core" concept? Sorry, we are blabbering again.

We have now established the pubic bone as the center of our body's universe. There is no doubt this is so. That's the anatomy. It is what it is. Copernicus, da Vinci, Belichick, and Krzyzewski all agree. Now we shall show how the center unites the body. We shall reveal how we control and optimally harmonize our power muscles (Figure 8-1).

The chapter is short, so no excuses… you must read it.

THE SECRET TO ATHLETICISM

To begin, think about what goes on in the core of a bucking bronco rider.

Then think about how an injury of the core may humble some of the most courageous and robust sports heroes in the world, sometimes in the biggest games of their lives (Figure 8-2).[1]

Athleticism is all about the pubic bone and the muscle harness. This part of the body, which we shall describe in detail, is the foremost dynamic area that determines the ability to stay on the horse or in the game. Of course, strength is important, too. The harness controls that strength. This harness is the main apparatus that manages the power. The harness also must communicate directly with the brain and then transmit directive messages to the torso and extremities. As you think through the analogy, keep in mind that our intact muscular harness also serves, in part, as our body's reins and bridle. Think of reins and bridles as things we also use to skillfully restrain, distribute, or liberate our power, or a horse's power, for that matter. Do not get confused about all this. Do not stick to any presupposed, strict interpretation of the word *harness*. Think of it as a controlling mechanism.

Figure 8-3 is a frontal shot of the main musculoskeletal anatomy involved.

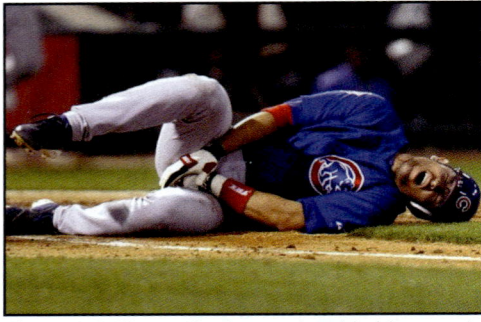

Figure 8-2. Nomar Garciaparra humbled by a groin injury that downed him taking a first step out of the batter's box. (Reprinted with permission from AP Photo/Kyle Ericson.)

HOW THE HARNESS WORKS OR MALFUNCTIONS

Remember the baseball from the last chapter. That visual illustrates the basics about how the harness works. Think of the thick fibrocartilage that surrounds both pubic symphyses and then extends more thinly onto the rami as the "cover" to a baseball. The fibrocartilage cover of the pubic bone connects with the 4 main muscular structures on each side. The spongy fibrocartilage cushions tremendous forces, as the harness directs power muscles and all the rest of the anatomy to twist, turn, and perform so many other feats. (See Figure 8-4.)

Now think about how this precious harness might malfunction. Muscles may tear. Muscles may rip right off. This injury causes a reapportionment of forces (ie, an imbalance). The remaining intact muscles "over-pull" (compensate), and a tug of war on the "baseball cover" ensues. Imagine the numerous varieties of injuries that might, and do, occur to this apparatus. Any of the muscles may tear, tears may happen proximal or distal along their lengths, or multiple muscles may sequentially tear because of changes in forces and tension. Most athletic injuries happen from "the outside." What we mean by that is illustrated by the following type of "inside" injury to the harness apparatus. Think about what happens when a big baby delivers through too narrow a birth canal. The baseball (pubic bone) splits "in half" (ie, the pubic symphyseal joint separates) from huge internal forces.

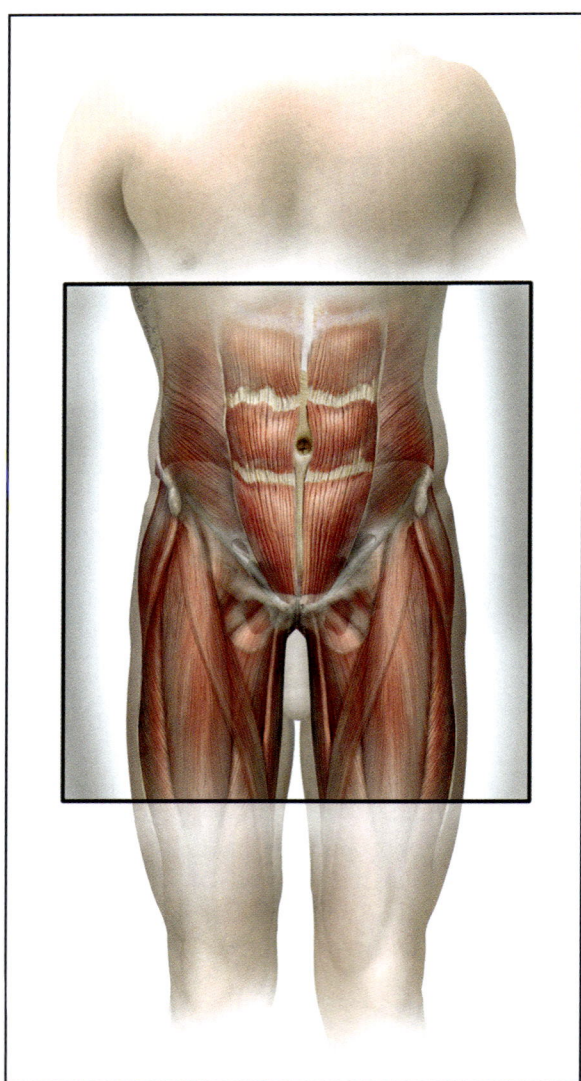

Figure 8-3. A view of the core's third part—the musculoskeletal core—from the front.

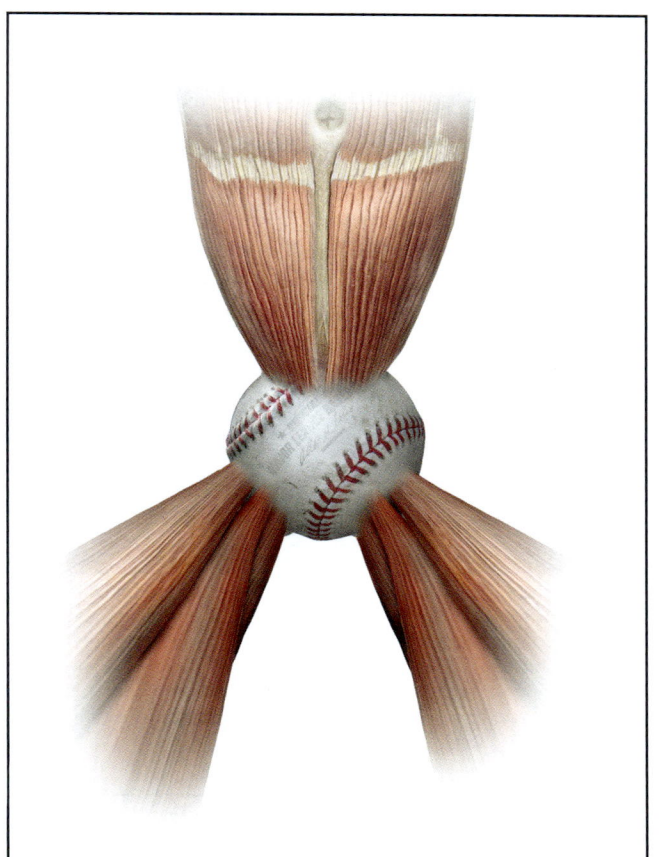

Figure 8-4.

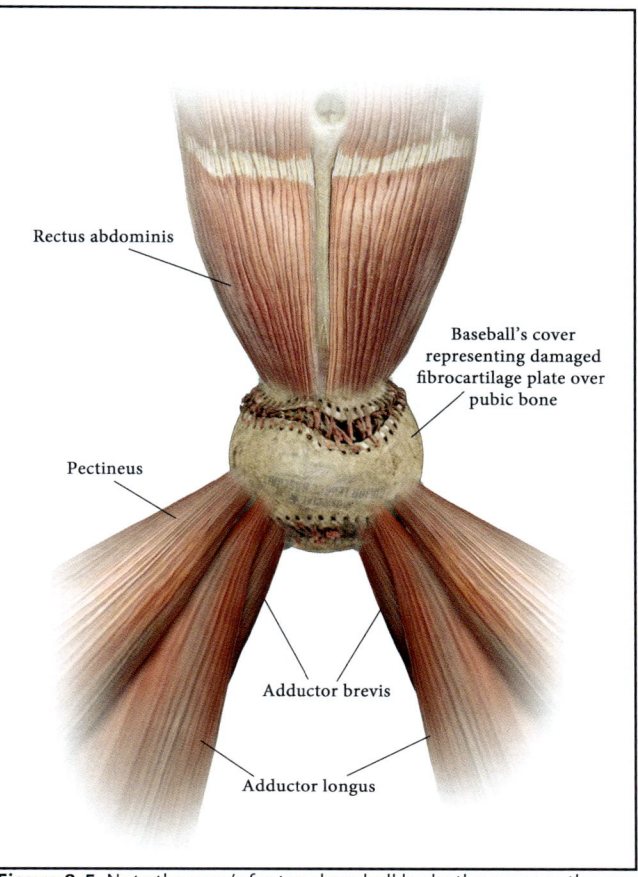

Figure 8-5. Note the core's fantasy baseball looks the same as the one above, except now the baseball's cover has become loose. The graphic does not show any muscular injury, but does illustrate vividly the main purpose of this analogy. The result of the tug of war of asymmetric forces is that seams untie and the cover loosens. This happens to the pubic bone in real life. A muscular injury initiates an imbalance of the pulls on the fibrocartilage cover. The tug of war results in separation of the cover.

Figure 8-5 portrays a fibrocartilage pubic plate separation. This is anatomically identical to the cover coming off a baseball. Okay, it is not exactly the same, but you get the picture. Fluid builds up between the pubic cover and bone, an analogous space represented by the baseball picture. For years, clinicians didn't realize what was really happening and were calling that fluid, plus the associated bone marrow edema (fluid that crosses the cortex), *osteitis*. Think of this term as vague; all the term really defines is any kind of inflammation in or around the pubic bone.

In the past, osteitis was felt to be its own process,[2,3] with its own pathophysiology solely affecting this bone. That is not accurate. That is not what happens. Osteitis is a reactive pathologic process and generally results from harness muscle injury. The injury produces weakness at one of the muscular attachment sites, and that weakness in turn causes unopposed, compensatory muscular contraction at the other 3 main muscular attachment sites. That imbalance that the forces generate results in a functional tug-of-war on the fibrocartilage plate cover, which then ends up separating from the underlying bone (Figure 8-6). Just like the baseball you left outside overnight!

A rational parallel is to the anterior cruciate of the knee. That midline structure does not heal on its own. One can build up the hamstrings and quads and make up for some of the resultant knee stability, yet the knee continues to give way during extremes of exertion.

Figure 8-7 shows the core muscular injury process that leads to "osteitis." Injury to one of the key core muscles causes other muscles of the harness to over-pull. The compensatory tugs on the fibrocartilage plate lead to the plate separation.

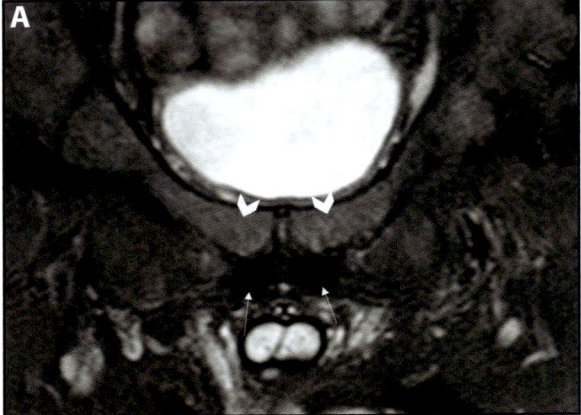
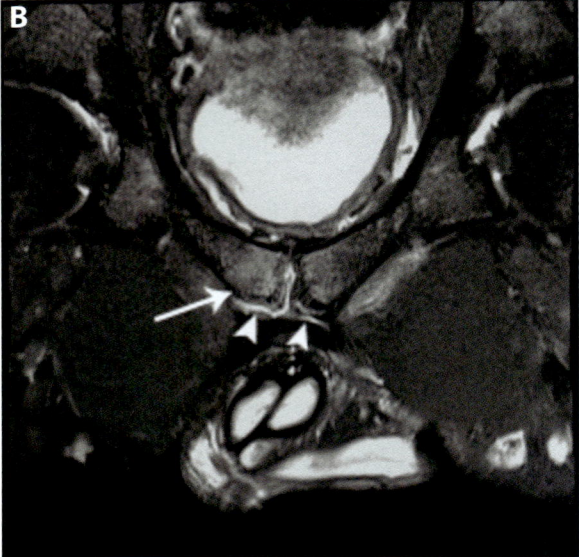

Figure 8-6. MRI of normal and injured pubic plates. (A) Normal pubic bone and plate. The arrows indicate the dark fibrocartilage pubic cover on the superior surface of the pubic bone. The arrowheads point to the pubic bone. Note the absence of whiteness between the plate and the bone. (B) Severe separation of the pubic plate. The arrowheads designate fluid in the crevices between bone and fibrocartilage. The arrow indicates bone marrow edema inside the pubic bone. The actual muscular injuries are barely seen. Intact, this harness apparatus works in concert with the brain and directs and modulates the body's power. Disrupted, the apparatus instigates problems. The loose cover slides involuntarily. Body weight forces the cover to slip. The midline becomes unstable. Building up the power muscles sometimes minimizes that instability.

Figure 8-7. This diagram shows schematically what is going on in Figure 8-6B. A right rectus abdominis injury triggers compensatory pulling by the other muscular attachments and eventual separation of the pubic plate, represented by the wider layer of whiteness on the right side (ie, between the gray fibrocartilage and the paler bone). So far, the plate separation (ie, "osteitis") process just affects the right side. With time, the left side gets involved.

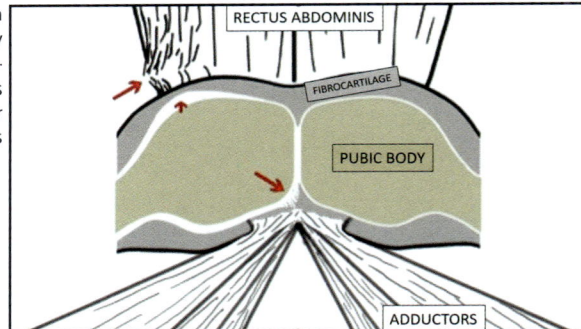

A "Crippling" Injury

The following set of MRIs shows quite graphically an example of such an injury.

Figure 8-8 shows the pubic bone losing its cover. This NFL football player had been hurting for a month. During a playoff game, he initially played in agony; then he suddenly toppled over in so much pain that he could not continue.

Now look at more of that patient's MRI images (Figure 8-9).

This NFL star had a severe plate separation injury, beginning with a right-sided harness issue. It progressed to involve the other side. He played with it, but had to compensate like mad. He remained effective until almost everything ripped off.

We described this injury as "crippling." And it was, until it was repaired. Keep in mind also that these injuries are almost always correctable surgically. This patient is now back better than he has ever been before. Even with such a severe injury, he will likely come back and remain the star he always was, or be even better.

The "Harness" 85

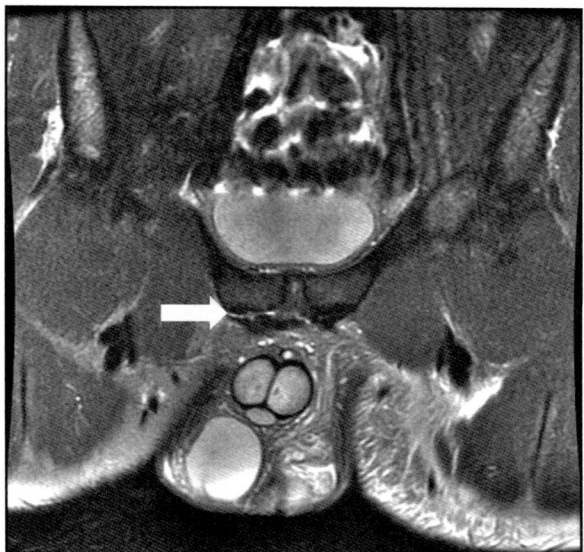

Figure 8-8. T1 axial oblique view showing a pubic plate separation (arrow) seemingly worse on the right side but with a hint of missing portion of the plate on the left side. Note the problem is on both sides. Going into the playoff game, more pain and disability emanated from the right side. During the game, something happened, and the ultimately debilitating pain suddenly arose on the left side. See how the cover of the pubic bone is coming off. Fluid, the white between the bone and dark fibrocartilage plate, spreads along the undersurface of the pubic bone. Significant edema exists in both sets of harness adductors.

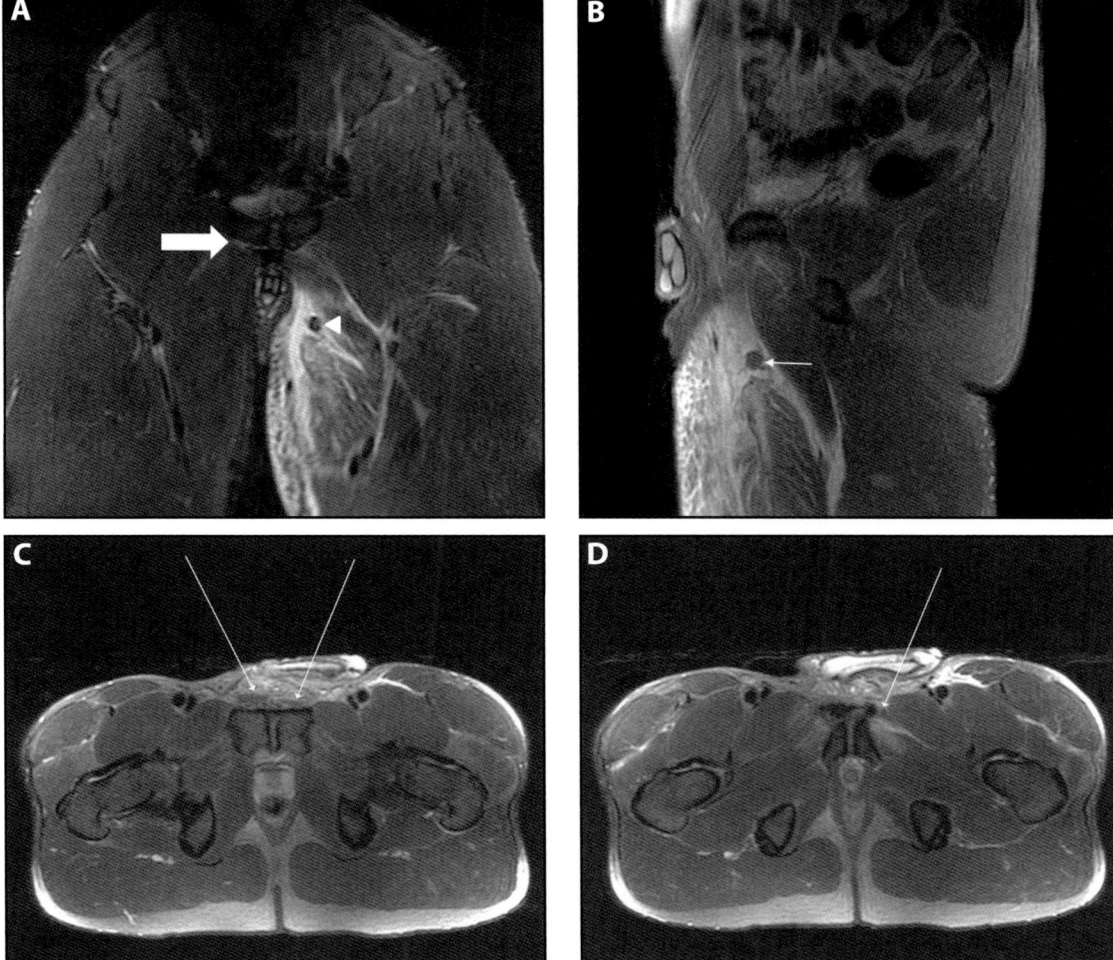

Figure 8-9. Four additional views of the same injury. Note problems on both sides. (A) Coronal stir image showing the same plate separation fluid as Figure 8-6B, some right-sided pubic plate separation (arrow), plus a big hematoma in the left adductor complex. All the white represents fluid. Note also that some plate disappears below the left pubic bone. The large adductor stump lays about 6 inches distally (arrowhead). (B) T2 sagittal image showing the same missing fibrocartilage at the left pubic bone and the same stump (arrow) shown in A. (C) T2 axial image showing an absent distal rectus abdominis muscle on the left side. (D) The same view 1 cm lower, showing missing plate on the left (arrow). Note the asymmetry compared to the right side and the adductor edema on both sides. Obviously, this is a severe injury.

86 Chapter 8

WHAT IS THE HARNESS EXACTLY?

Before we get into individual muscles (in chapters to follow), consider the harness as a whole, where it fits in the core, and its anatomical and physiological relationships with the rest of the body (Figure 8-10).

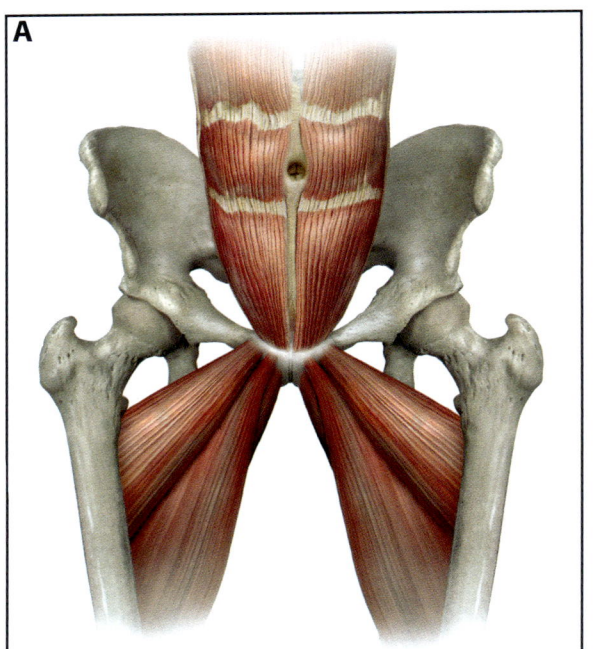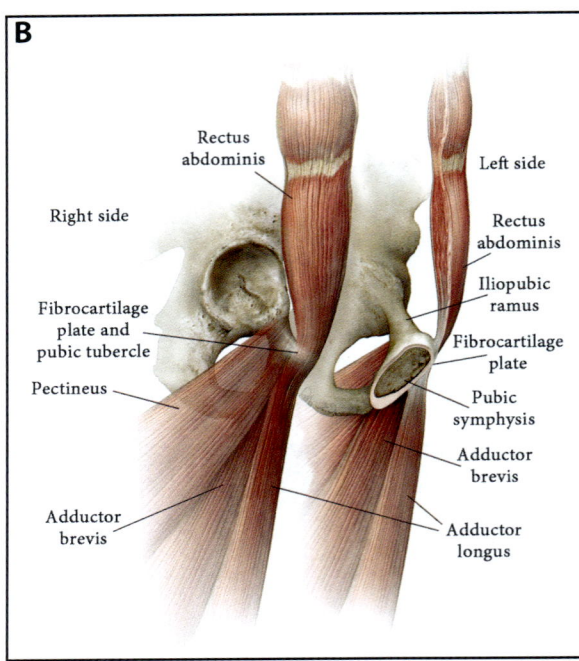

Figure 8-10. The harness is simply the apparatus that includes the rectus abdominis muscle and 3 adductors on each side connected via the pubic bodies and their fibrocartilage envelope. (A) Full frontal. (B) Oblique views.

The harness consists of the pubic bone, its fibrocartilage cover, and 4 main muscles on each side—the rectus abdominis and 3 adductors. From anterior to posterior, or, for that matter, lateral to medial, the 3 adductors are: (1) the pectineus, (2) the adductor longus, and (3) the adductor brevis. Other core muscles have some purpose in the function such as the obliques, gracilis, and obturator externus, and so do multiple internal muscles. But forget those for now. Let's keep it simple. For now, just say there are 4 muscles.

The directions of forces generated by the individual muscles of the harness (Figure 8-11) do not pay justice to the overall importance of the apparatus. The vertical and oblique natures of those forces somehow subtly tell other muscles what to do. Individually or collectively, the muscles do not compare in strength to the core's power muscles. Muscle volume measurements of the top muscles attaching of the harness match, in fresh cadavers, pretty closely the muscles attaching from below.[4] The latter fact indicates a relatively even balance of forces in normal situations.

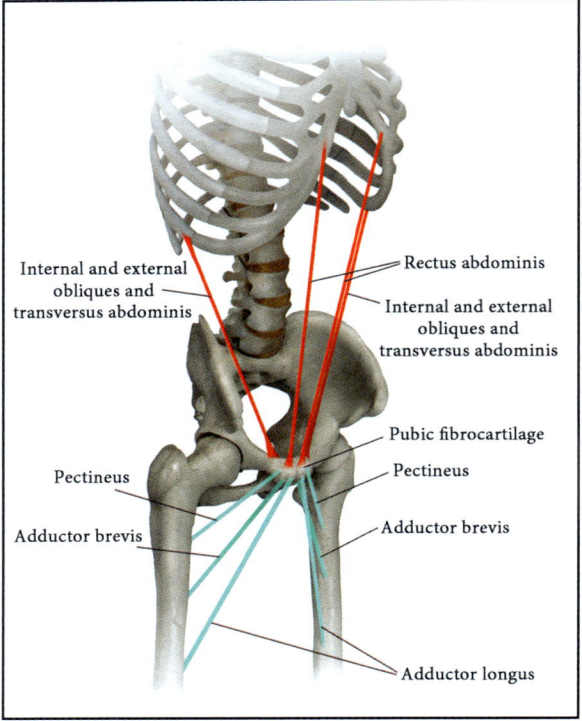

Figure 8-11. Schematic showing directions and a certain balance of forces for the "bridle" or "harness" in the normal situation.

WHERE THE HARNESS CONNECTS

As shown in the figures, the harness sits in the middle of the body. It is the most central contractile mechanism in the body. Think about the structures that lie next to the harness. Nothing is anterior or superficial to it. That direction is easy to learn. Let's consider the structures that are deep first, then the surrounding muscles and bones. Think in terms of 3 direct connections.

1. **The deep structures.** Some pretty important stuff lies inside and deep to the harness. The harness sits on top of our bladder, intestines, and other (usually) mostly hollow organs. Huge blood vessels and the ureters reside inside, while sexual organs live either inside or other places nearby. Various internal muscles work intimately with the harness. These include the coccygeal muscles (the levator ani), obturator internus, psoas, iliacus, perineal, sex muscles, and, of course, the skeletal and smooth muscles of the rectum, anus, and vagina. The harness works in profound ways with those internal organs in the delivery of babies. In other words, babies actually have to come through the harness.

2. **Adjacent muscles and bones.** Three main musculoskeletal sets of structures lay adjacent to the harness: (1) the previously described "power" muscles, (2) the ball-and-socket hip joint, and (3) the other bones, ligaments, etc, of the pelvis. The core power muscles (yes…fascia, too) lie primarily lateral to the harness: obliques, transversus, tensor fascia lata, iliotibial band, back, butt, quadriceps, and hamstrings. The harness conducts its movement symphonies through numerous fascial, bony, and ligamentous connections. It recruits the hip for melody and other pelvic bones for percussion. Using that analogy, the power muscles provide the volume.

3. **The brain.** Okay, we have covered what lies deep inside the harness and what bones and muscles surround the apparatus. One other set of connections makes this center point of the body all powerful with respect to movement. We are talking about its connection to the brain. Somehow the brain receives messages from the harness apparatus, plus, the brain sends messages back. The brain tells the apparatus how to move athletically, how to avoid a would-be tackler or how to sashay past a 7-foot center trying to block your lay-up. The brain orders the harness apparatus to do what it wants, and the apparatus falls in line and directs the power muscles and other connections what to do (Figure 8-12).

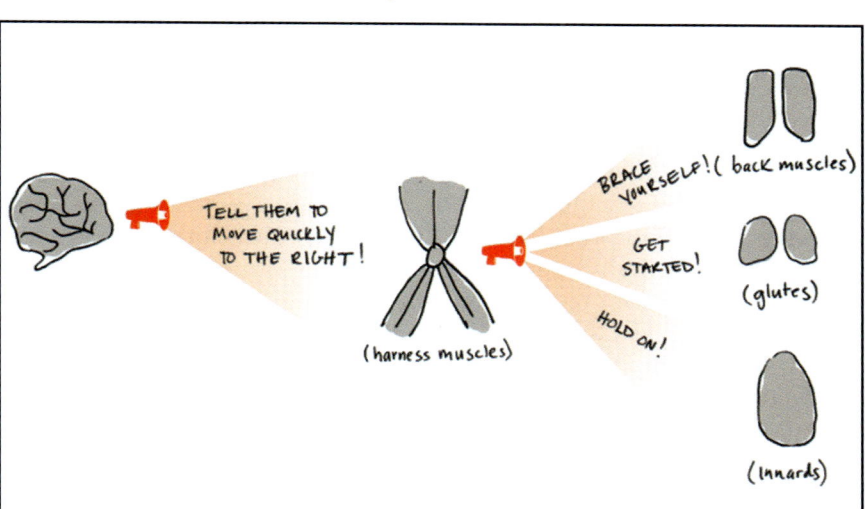

Figure 8-12. The harness as a first lieutenant, delegating responsibilities to accomplish the brain's desires.

In our clinical laboratory, injuries that caused central core pain also triggered deficits in cognitive brain function testing, such as balance, vision, and reaction time (see Figure 6-8). As mentioned in Chapter 6, correction of the injuries actually reversed those deficits. Core pain also likely affects cognitive brain function more than pain not emanating from the core.[5]

Therefore, somehow the core—and more specifically the harness—works in cahoots with the brain. Loads of peripheral nerves live in this core particularly centrally. They must receive and transmit all sorts of messages. Of course, we don't yet know the exact pathways, but that doesn't keep us from guessing. This is the primary subject of Dr. Aradillas's chapter on the nerves (Chapter 18).

So, if we go back to our horse analogy, the rectus abdominis-baseball-adductor complex about which we are talking definitely functions like a harness in a horse. It guards the insides and it gathers and conducts the core's power.

What about the connections to the brain? How do those observations fit with the horse harness analogy? Okay, perhaps the connections to the brain are less like a harness and more like reins. For an expert rider, don't reins send the messages to the horse so it does what you want it to do? Then the bridle modulates and implements those directions. Perhaps that apparatus also acts more like reins and a bridle? Okay, perhaps we are carrying the analogy too far. Hopefully by now, you already got the message.

So, How Does the Harness Cause Harm?

This harness is where we achieve our balance. This body region communicates with the brain. The brain and the harness create our athleticism. Any disruption of this area causes problems. It causes the potential for imbalance and alteration of function in the rest of the body. In short, injury to a part of the core puts not only the rest of the core at risk, it jeopardizes the function and integrity of the upper and lower extremities, neck, head, and brain. You hurt your core, you run in a distracted way. You change your pitching mechanics. You alter your gait.[6] You get clocked by a defensive back. You hurt your elbow. You tear your ACL. You retire early.

Go back to our introduction and remember the core is our engine. It is also the body's transmission. The harness is at the control center, where the captain of the body sits and presses the controls. Think about sitting at this control center, at the center of our universe.

For a moment, put on your baseball cover and become the pubic bone—at the center of the body's universe.

Be the Pubic Bone

Okay suppose you are now the pubic bone, at command central—the center of the body's universe. You are just sitting there, existing. Think about what you might experience. Use your imagination and envision the anatomy.

First, think about what's around you. We just described those things. You have the harness immediately surrounding you. Those harness muscles attach to a thick, tight, white coat that you wear proudly around you. The coat is not part of you, but it protects you and fits real snug. Next to the power muscles are a whole bunch of other muscles, powerful ones.

Deep to you are all your innards—organs, blood vessels, poop, etc. You've got your whole upper body and upper extremities, head, and neck above you; both your lower extremities below you. Yes, some external genitalia nearby. That's about it. You are not very interesting. Just like the center of the earth, that wasn't very interesting either when you first heard about it, was it? What's at the center of the earth? Just fire?

Next think about your attitude. Basically, you are just bone. You just exist there. You have 2 halves and a little bit of mobility between your 2 halves. You are connected to other bones—ischium, ilium, all that—and that really restricts you. The adjacent bone keeps you in check. There is a little wiggle room since there are numerous small, slightly mobile ligaments throughout the nearby pelvis. But basically you are an existentialist. You are Camus. Camus had one main weapon—sarcasm. You also have one main weapon—nerves. They are plentiful in your outermost thin coat that covers the cortex, in your periosteum. Anybody or anything ticks you off, you fire those nerves (Figure 8-13). You inflict horrendous pain.

So what do you experience at the center of the universe? Well, if everything is okay, things just glide along, you don't worry. But bad things can happen from all directions.

Okay, it is time to stop being the pubic bone and translate the above into clinical thoughts. Think of the pubic bone in 3 main ways.

The first way is what we have already discussed. It is the center of the core. It is the centerpiece for our balance and athleticism. That is where the baseball cover concept comes into play. Think of Bobby Mote, multiple-time world rodeo champion who has been bareback riding longer than most competitors have been alive, and the way Bobby keeps his pubic bone

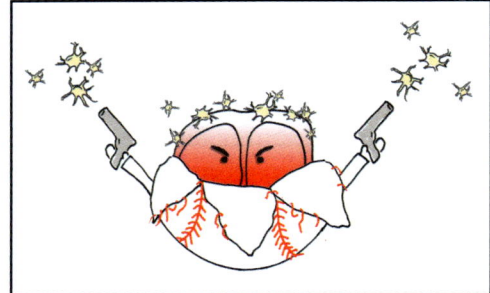

Figure 8-13. The pubic bone shooting nerve bullets at other tissues. Microscopically, the periosteum seems most loaded with neural tissue. MRI edema often corresponds to the clinical locations of pain. Most of the cover acutely ripped off the bone of star NFL center Jason Kelce. Ask him about how much pain this culprit caused!

at the center of himself and the horse. And then think of all the action that takes place around that part of the anatomy. The pubic bone does not just get affected by the surrounding muscles; one's hip causes torques on the bone that affect the central pubic bodies, the symphysis, and, alas, the other hip. See Marc Safran's chapter coming up later in the book. Marc talks in a more scientific way about this transmission of forces through the pelvic bones.

The second way to think about this centerpiece is that this location takes an immense pounding from the lower extremities and upper extremities. Think of this as the spot that gets squeezed in the process of jumping. Think of basketball players or runners. Consider all the pounding that takes place right there, the bodies landing on the court or the relentless drubbing on the pavements. Something has to give, with all that wear and tear. Again, it is usually the cover that starts to slide off. Think also of Howard Nippert, the ultra-marathoner with a tremendous blog presence.[7] Do you know what an ultra-marathoner does routinely? We are talking about hundreds of miles with all those forces continually hammering our central bone. As Howard will tell you, "I have averaged 70 to 100 miles per week for over 35 years. Something had to give." His "marathons" were each 50 miles plus.

And a third way. Think of how the pubic bone might get involved from the "inside," or even how the "insides" get affected by the pubic bone. Think about Crohn's disease, the bladder, or the prostate. Take another example, childbirth. If the baby is large enough, and the birth canal small enough, there may be such forces that the baby bangs up against the pubic bone. In the extreme, the pubic symphyseal joint disrupts, causing severe pain. Sometimes, the pain may be noticed initially after delivery, when mom returns to exercise. The disruption sometimes requires repair; fortunately, these repairs are usually successful, when one uses the principles outlined in later chapters. No longer should there be much need for the brutal and mostly antiquated orthopedic procedure of symphyseal excision, bone grafting, and insertion of a big metal vice.

Also think about the other way around. Rather than the "insides" disrupting the pubic bone, think how the bone may affect the insides. Severe inflammation in and around the pubis (osteitis) affects the bladder and nearby sexual organs. The inflammation may cause an uncomfortable feeling of a continual need to pee or outright frequent urination (polyuria) or painful sexual intercourse (dyspareunia). Think of how many people visit gynecology or urology clinics for these symptoms. Solving these underlying causes of the inflammation fixes these problems, if, of course, the diagnostician is aware of this possibility. The fact of the matter is that most specialists are not aware of this! Dyspareunia, of course, does not just have to come from just osteitis pubis; it may come from many other musculoskeletal causes of inflammation in the pelvis. Grossly underappreciated is how often the hip and acetabulum and psoas are culprits. Read about this more in Chapter 23.

NOMENCLATURE

For communication purposes, we offer the following definitions of terms. Surprisingly, anatomy books are confusing and often conflict with respect to this terminology, so we are defining these terms as we see optimal.

- **Pubic body**—This is the whole hard part of the pubis that you can feel on yourself anteriorly. You are feeling the 2 pubic bodies, right and a left, separated by the pubic symphysis. If you press down hard enough, sometimes you can appreciate a slight side-to-side shift due to a slightly pliable symphysis.
- **Pubic symphysis**—This is the space or potential space between the 2 pubic bodies. For simplicity, this is synonymous with the *pubic symphyseal joint*.
- **Pubic rami**—These are the narrow extensions of the pubic bodies. There are superior and inferior ones on each side.
- **Pubic plate**—This refers to the entire fibrocartilage that surrounds the entire pubic bone and extends into the rami, symphysis, and other pelvic bones.
- **Osteitis pubis**—Use this as a vague term for any extra fluid in and around the pubic bone. More specific terms are *pubic bone marrow edema* and *pubic plate separation*, representing the extra fluid in the bone and space between the pubic periosteum and fibrocartilage pubic plate, respectively.
- **Primary osteitis pubis**—This refers to pubic osteitis without any apparent cause. Keep in mind that almost all osteitis pubis likely has some sort of cause. For example, we know that some cases of osteitis definitely come from rheumatologic causes.
- **Secondary osteitis pubis**—Most cases have identifiable causes. The most common cause is core muscle injury. Other causes include an isolated hip impingement that causes a bony shift of the pelvis that disrupts the symphyseal joint and/or pubic plate. Likewise, the process of childbirth can cause an osteitis via direct impact and joint or plate disruption. (See Tables 8-1 and 8-2.)

Table 8-1
New Definitions

Pubic body	Each front of the pubic bone separated by the pubic symphysis
Pubic symphysis	Area between the 2 pubic bodies (aka the pubic symphyseal joint)
Pubic ramus	Each superior or inferior extension of the pubic bodies
Pubic plate	The fibrocartilage cover of the pubic bone
Osteitis pubis	Vague term for extra fluid in or around the pubic bone
Pubic bone marrow edema	Extra fluid within the pubic bone
Pubic plate separation	Pubic plate detachment from the periosteum of the pubic bone

Table 8-2
"Osteitis Pubis" Types

Primary osteitis pubis	Inflammatory process with known origination within the pubic bone itself or without apparent cause or injury
Secondary osteitis pubis	Inflammatory fluid in or around the pubic bone that can be attributed to an extra-pubic bone cause or injury (eg, core muscle injury, femoroacetabular impingement, childbirth, tumor, or Crohn's disease)

ROEDL CLASSIFICATION OF BASEBALL COVER ("PUBIC PLATE") INJURIES

Dr. Johannes Roedl has come up with a logical, radiological classification for these plate injuries. It is simple. Consider the new terminology in Figure 8-14. Call the latitudinal width of the pubic symphysis the *midline pubic plate*. All the fibrocartilage to the right then becomes the *right plate*, and, you guessed it, everything to the left gets named the *left plate*.

The nomenclature for the plate injuries (Figure 8-15) then becomes simple.

Figure 8-14. Roedl nomenclature for the anatomy of the pubic plate. (Reprinted with permission from Dr. Johannes Roedl.)

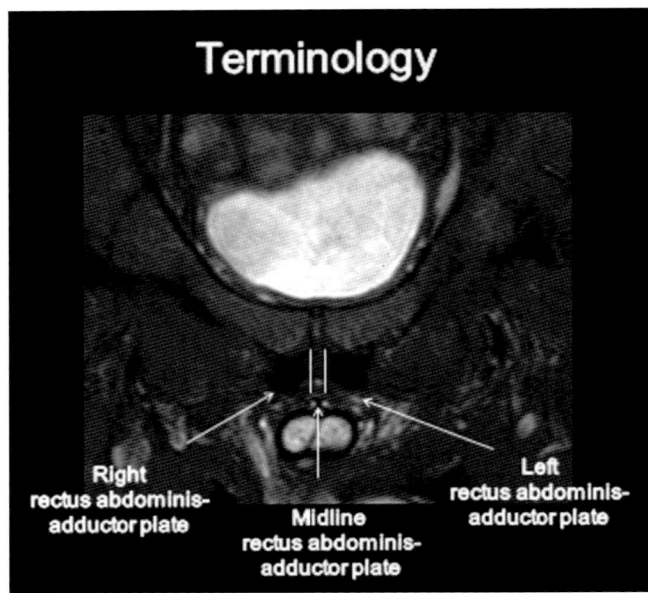

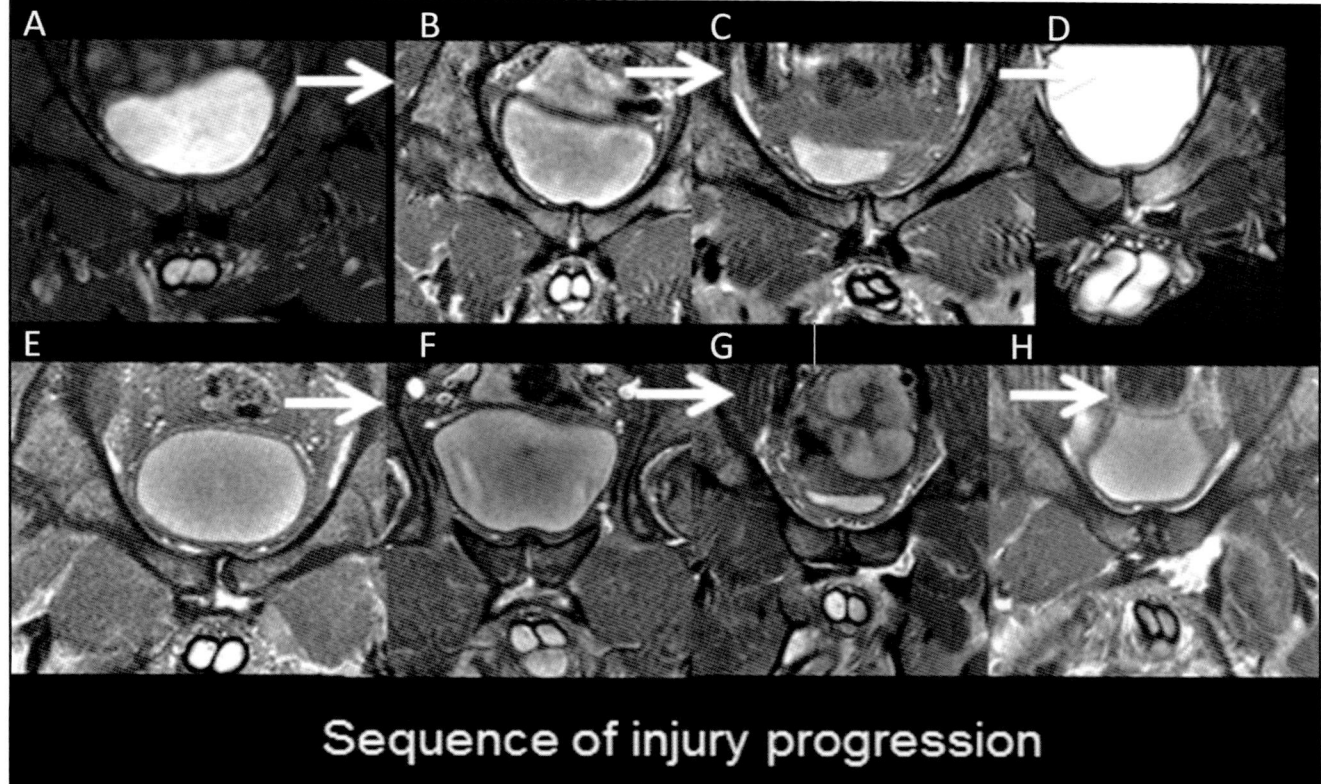

Figure 8-15. These 8 MRI images show a logical sequence of injury in an imaginary patient. In fact, the images come from different patients. (A) Normal plate. (B) Small midline injury. (C) Extension of the midline injury to involve the left plate. (D) More extensive involvement of the left plate. (E) The injury now also involves the right pubic plate. (F) The midline injury progresses to involve, rather extensively, both right and left pubic plates. (G) The left-sided injury becomes more severe. (H) Now there is a complete avulsion of the left pubic plate, which means, most likely, all 3 harness adductors and the rectus abdominis muscle are detached. (Reprinted with permission from Dr. Johannes Roedl.)

NEXT

It's time to get more familiar with individual core muscles. The nicknames assigned to each muscle spotlight our prejudices with respect to each muscle's roles or potential roles.

SELECTED READINGS

Barrey E. Biomechanics of locomotion in the athletic horse. In: Hincliff W, Kaneps AJ, Gear RJ, eds. *Equine Sports Medicine and Surgery*. Philadelphia, PA: Elsevier Health Sciences; 2013.
This chapter of equine sports medicine book goes into detail about a horse's biomechanics, its harness, and other gear. The principles are directly applicable to this chapter.

Messmer C, Kellogg RT, Zhang Y, et al. A technique to perfuse cadavers that extends the useful life of fresh tissues: the Duke experience. *Anat Sci Educ*. 2010;3:191-194.
Scott Levin, both a plastic and orthopedic surgeon and now Chairman of Orthopaedics at the University of Pennsylvania, has led the charge for using fresh cadavers in education and for studying biomechanics. He has reproduced his Duke fresh cadaver lab with added features in Philadelphia.

REFERENCES

1. Cottier A. *Steven Gerrard: Portrait of a Hero*. London, United Kingdom: John Blake; 2007.
2. Paajanen H, Hermunen H, Karonen J. Pubic magnetic resonance imaging findings in surgically and conservatively treated athletes with osteitis pubis compared to asymptomatic athletes during heavy training. *Am J Sports Med*. 2007;36(1):117-121. doi:10.1177/0363546507305454.
3. Meath forum: the war against osteitis pubis—blog. http://hoganstand.com/Meath/MessagePage.aspx?TopicID=14572. Accessed November 6, 2016.
4. Fresh cadaveric data from laboratory at Duke presented at the 6th International Society for Hip Arthroscopy Annual Scientific Meeting; 2014; Rio de Janeiro, Brazil.
5. Unpublished data.
6. Franklyn-Miller A, Richter C, King E, et al. Athletic groin pain (part 2): a prospective cohort study on the biomechanical evaluation of change of direction identifies three clusters of movement patterns. *Br J Sports Med*. 2017;51:460-468.
7. The official site of USA ultramarathoner Howard Nippert. Howardnippert.com. Published March 3, 2009. Accessed May 11, 2016.

9

the rectus abdominis
our "cinderella muscle"

I'm a girl who loves fashion. I'm such a Cinderella [Figure 9-1]—
I love to put on a great dress and heels. It's fun!
—Maria Bello, American actress and writer, from Norristown, Pennsylvania.

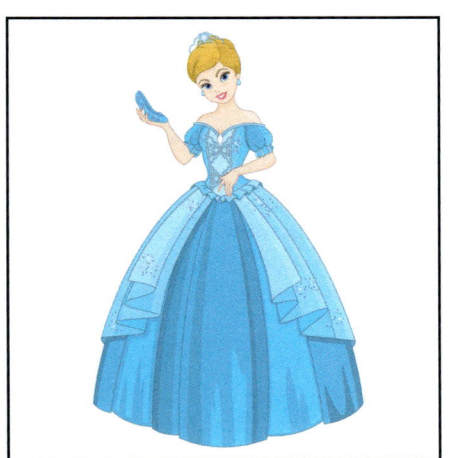

Figure 9-1. Cinderella.

NOT ALWAYS MINOR STRAINS

It was just a minor strain. Nothing serious.

The Washington Nationals' Ryan Zimmerman's rectus abdominis tweak during 2011 spring training wasn't supposed to be anything it all. Until it was.

While diving back into second base during the first week of the regular season, Zimmerman did more than just aggravate the area. He tore it up. After a month of treatment and some rest, Zimmerman was still in enough pain that in mid-May of that year, surgeons repaired the tear.[1]

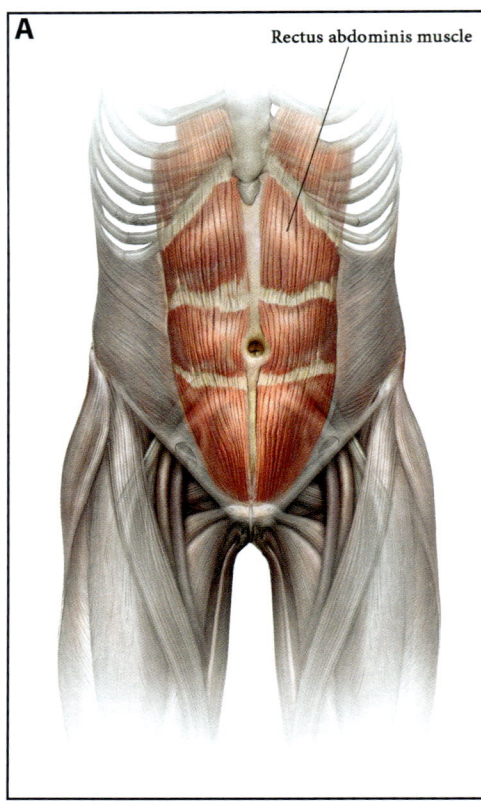

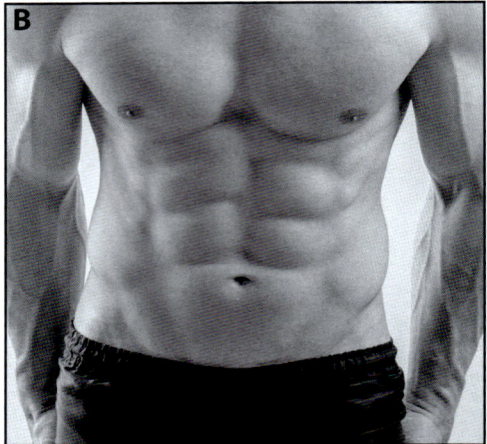

Figure 9-2. (A) Artist's depiction of the rectus abdominis muscle. (B) Prominent rectus abdominis in a male model.

Most people know the rectus abdominis as the muscle group that comprises the 6-pack (Figure 9-2). Athletes like to have nice abs, but they would rather have a collection of rectus abdominis muscles that allows them to lunge, spike, dive, pull, and perform a menu of other important functions that involve extending the body. Zimmerman returned to action and has enjoyed good health since. But there is no guarantee someone who plays baseball's hot corner and is constantly diving to stop hard-hit balls will be pain-free forever.

And he has plenty of company.

He had torn the muscle from the pubic plate (ie, the cover of the pubic baseball; see Figures 8-4 and 8-5). The muscle had twanged upward, and the bleeding end caused a big, proximal hematoma.

Yes, most rectus abdominis strains have no bad consequences. But you had better keep your eyes open for the more serious injuries. Put up your antennae for anything unusual or if pain lasts more than a few days. These injuries can be serious and debilitating. With precise diagnosis and treatment, nearly all are highly fixable (Figure 9-3).

Common Themes

From our clinical practice, we have quite a number of other illustrative cases from whom we could have chosen to lead off this chapter. Dramatic cases of the rectus abdominis ripping off the pubic bone affect various types of athletes and everyday folks, from bull riders to P90X beginners. You may have seen the famous ESPN video of the wonderful role model in baseball Nomar Garciaparra falling to his knees in pain while sprinting out of the batter's box, or know about a star for Manchester United who suddenly reeled to the ground in pain at a key time in the match. Or perhaps you heard about Jack Sock, the American tennis prodigy with the huge serve, who had such troubles with his abdomen early in his career.

You probably don't know about the young woman from Philadelphia who tore off her abdominal muscle picking up 2 cases of beer, or the 20 soldiers with badly wrenched rectus abdominis muscles after a sit-up contest at a US Army base. We have a lot of such stories. The point is that abdominal muscle injuries happen every day in athletics and routine life. Some of them get better and some of them don't.

So, what might the folks with severe injuries have in common predisposing them to such problems? One main thing: they work their abdomens out way too hard. They might do this voluntarily (eg, novice exercise enthusiasts getting back into shape, pitchers doing inverted sit-ups in off-season workouts) or they might be in situations in life where they have to work their abdomens too hard (eg, volleyball players, dancers, divers). Beyond a doubt, the same repetitive forces to the rectus abdominis muscles may have a serious toll; often, they cause enough wear-and-tear to predispose you to something bad.

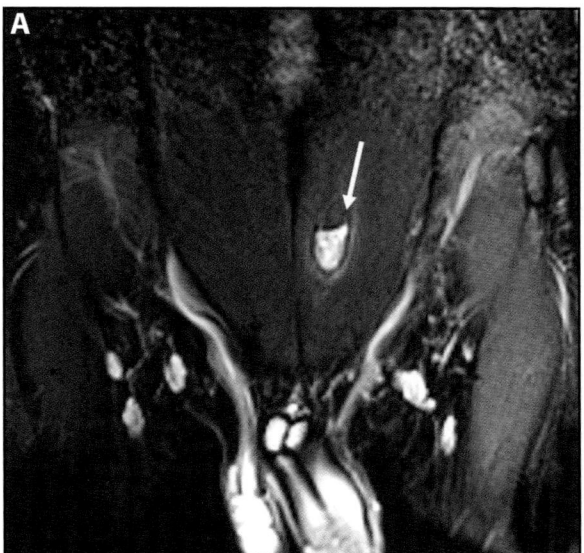 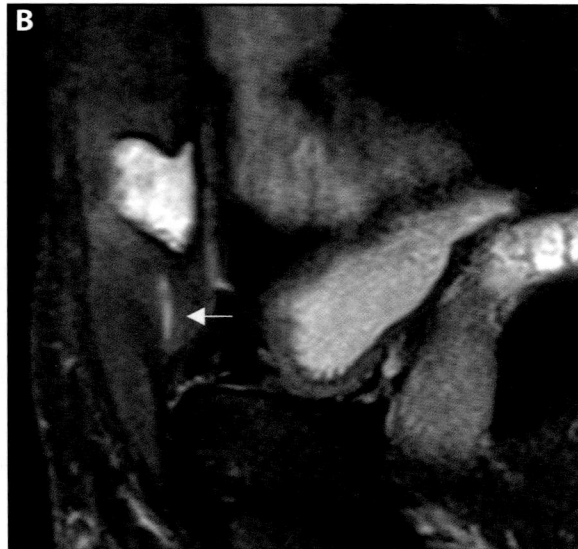

Figure 9-3. Rectus abdominis hematoma from pubic plate injury. The muscle of this major league third baseman had torn off the plate 6 weeks previously and the proximal muscle stump bled into the substance of the muscle. (A) Coronal stir image of a well-organized hematoma several inches above the plate. (B) T2 sagittal image showing the tract to the same hematoma from where the muscle ripped off the plate.

You can probably easily guess what sports or what specific positions within sports would make someone most vulnerable to isolated rectus abdominis avulsions. Think about it? The rectus abdominis primarily flexes the abdomen with the chest.

Pick sports or positions that involve a lot of flexion and extension. You've got it—tennis players with big serves, third basemen, rowers, bull-riders… The list goes on. Of course, you can get these tears in most sports. The point is that certain activities make you more susceptible to these specific injuries. And when it comes to abs, most people who try to stay in shape mistreat them. The soldiers mentioned previously are supreme examples.

We like to call the rectus abdominis the "Cinderella muscle" because it is regarded as so beautiful yet wicked stepsisters love to abuse it.

What's Obvious About This Muscle

The rectus abdominis is probably the most important of our core muscles.

It may not be the strongest. But it is so important for balance and athleticism. It connects the upper body to the lower body, it directs the mechanism that harnesses our core power and even seems to have a direct connection to the brain. It is beautiful, humble, and underappreciated. While the world may recognize its beauty, it may not appreciate its graciousness or importance. That's why the world regularly abuses the rectus abdominis muscle.

Figure 9-3 exhibits some subtle details about the rectus abdominis muscle. At the top end, it intermingles with the rib cage. On the sides, it merges with the obliques, and at the bottom, it joins with the pubic plate, which attaches to the pubic bone and rest of the harness. It forms the top part of the harness.

Think of the rectus abdominis as having 3 parts:
1. The top part where it merges with the ribs
2. The middle part, which becomes hugely important in some sports (eg, diving, tennis, gymnastics)
3. The bottom part, a key part, the connector to the thighs

In most but not all sports, the bottom part puts in the most work. Think about soccer and American football. On the other hand, rowing works more the top part.

It was upon the untimely death of this good man, however, that the stepmother's true nature was revealed: cold, cruel, and bitterly jealous of Cinderella's charm and beauty, she was grimly determined to forward the interests of her own two awkward daughters. Thus, as time went by, the chateau fell into disrepair, for the family fortunes were squandered upon the vain and selfish stepsisters while Cinderella was abused, humiliated, and finally forced to become a servant in her own house. And yet, through it all, Cinderella remained ever gentle and kind, for with each dawn she found new hope that someday her dreams of happiness would come true.

—Giambattista Basile, *Pentamerone* (1634) and *Grimms' Fairy Tales* (1812)

WHY CINDERELLA?

The word *Cinderella* has, by analogy, come to mean one whose attributes were unrecognized, and who unexpectedly achieves recognition or success after a period of neglect. So it is for the rectus abdominis muscle. It is time for that muscle to shine. Of course, Cinderella was beautiful, but we are talking about the way she was abused. If that abuse continued, she would eventually lose her beauty. Fortunately, she became recognized for her strengths—and was saved.

Of course, we all know the rectus abdominis is beautiful. "Six-pack abs" dominate the fitness culture—"30 Days to 6-Pack Abs," "The 6 Best Exercises for 6-Pack Abs," blah, blah, blah.[2] Look at Figure 9-2B. Beautiful? Yes. Subject to abuse? For sure.

Look a little closer and notice that the 6-pack doesn't really start until about the level of the belly button. Do you think that is by chance? Note the absence of folds below the belly button. There are purposes for these subtleties of our anatomy. We don't know all the reasons for the subtleties yet, but we are learning a lot of important stuff. The likely reason for the relative absence of folds below the umbilicus probably has something to do with this being the top part of the core's harness. Think about what happens in a sit-up. You use the lower half of the abdomen more the lower your upper body gets to the floor. You need that part of the abdomen to flatten out. As you reach the top of the sit-up, your head and chest bend so much more, creating an anatomic "need" for folds.

The rectus abdominis muscle has many subtleties. Few people appreciate them. For that matter, few people appreciate the muscle as a whole; we abuse it.

This story is about the Cinderella muscle of the core. It is important. It is gracious. We must treat it gently and with respect. Otherwise, we will lose it. Just like the first moral of the story *Cinderella*: think of beauty as a treasure but graciousness as priceless. Without it, nothing is possible; with it, one can do anything.

The fitness world focuses on 6-pack abs, making these sit-up muscles more beautiful. The world believes the more sit-ups one does, the more rectus abdominis exercises one does, the more beautiful these abs become. What the world does not recognize is all the wear and tear all this work causes and the injuries to which this subjects this muscle. The fitness world—personal fitness instructors, the sports world, even the military—does not come close to grasping how much damage this continual abuse causes.

The massive number of sit-ups recommended by "fitness experts," the ab exercise machines out there, fitness magazines with all the pictures, they all feed a culture of lust, greed, ignorance, and abuse of this muscle. If you come away with one theme from this book, come away with this theme: Lust may be okay, so long as you protect the rectus abdominis muscle.

We must protect our Cinderella.

THE WAY IT WAS

The rectus abdominis muscle belongs to no medical specialty. If one had to identify a medical specialist that "owns" or knows most about this muscle, it would be the general surgeon. But the general surgeon's knowledge base concerning this muscle is shallow. For years, surgeons only viewed it as part of the abdominal wall that holds in the guts. They debated such "important" things as whether it is better to cut across it transversely or vertically, and of course, that great medical mystery was never solved.

General surgeons never talked about the importance or function of this muscle in terms of fitness or health. The general surgeon considers the muscle with respect to the occurrence of certain types of hernias, defined as protrusions through the abdominal wall. They pay attention to the occasional tumors that occur here, particularly ones that need to be cut out, like desmoids and the more aggressive sarcomas. The fact remains: General surgeons, and basically all medical specialists for that matter, think of the rectus abdominis muscle merely as one of the muscles that keeps the insides of the belly from falling out. That's it.

THE WAY IT IS

So, you've already heard the Cinderella story. Think of the rectus abdominis muscle as amazing, that it does so, so much and that it is so, so beautiful. And that we still have so much more to learn about it.

Anatomically, the muscle is quite variable—sometimes having 2 heads in its distal aspect and sometimes 3, and sometimes associated distally with another muscle called the pyramidalis (see Figure 7-13). The rectus abdominis joins with the ribs in complex ways. It does such subtle things as house certain intercostal sensory nerve branches that can cause great pain. The muscle provides astonishing coil and spring that fits well for jumping, extending, and flexing. Think of its function for divers, gymnasts, and ballet dancers.

The muscle is so important in the harness mechanism. It provides some strength, but not nearly as much for which it is given credit, but directs the power from all the muscle adjacent to it, like the side and back muscles. It harnesses the strength from those muscles so that we use it efficiently. In a sense, it also provides both the bridle and the harness for control of this strength. This muscle is super important for the harness/"pubic joint" concept. It is also the great communicator for the core to the brain in matters of athletic activity. Think about it. If you are sprinting hard and want to suddenly shift to the right or left, what muscles does your brain first ask to tense up first? No doubt it is the rectus abdominis, and then the brain asks it to coordinate with the rest of the harness mechanism and the adductors. MRIs show that the rectus abdominis also quickly atrophies in response to injury or nonuse. The latter fact provides added testimony and circumstantial evidence for how much we ordinarily use this muscle and how truly important it is.

Add to this knowledge base that this muscle is easily injured from overuse or too much force, usually from abdominal hyper-extension or thigh hyper-abduction.

Because of its intimate relationship to the pubic bone and thighs, we have seen multiple problems related to the rectus abdominis muscle. Most commonly, the problems occur in association with adjacent bony and muscular structures. For now, let's consider some of the syndromes that we have identified that are just *relatively isolated* to the rectus abdominis muscle.

Rectus Abdominis Atrophy

We see this so commonly now on the side of primary injury. The presumption is that the lack of connection to the pubic plate or pain, or both, leads to avoidance of using the muscle. Atrophy is a regular finding with mesh used in hernia repairs. Somehow, the mesh fibroses and fixates the underlying or overlying muscle rendering it less mobile or functional. There is debate about whether the dominant or nondominant side houses the bigger rectus abdominis in upper extremity–dominant sports, such as baseball or tennis. One paper attests to the nondominant side being bigger in tennis players.[3] We have seen dramatic differences in rectus abdominis size in athletes, but in a much more unpredictable fashion than that paper would suggest. And in our clinical experience, the dominant side seems to be larger, except when there is an injury (Figure 9-4).

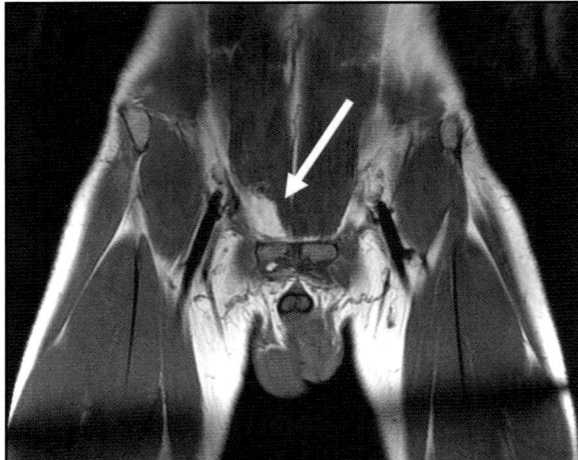

Figure 9-4. Rectus abdominis atrophy in a 24-year-old professional soccer player with right adductor pain. We speculate that abdominal detachment was the primary event leading to pubic plate separation and adductor injury. This fat-sensitive MRI image shows atrophy and fatty replacement of the right lower rectus abdominis muscle.

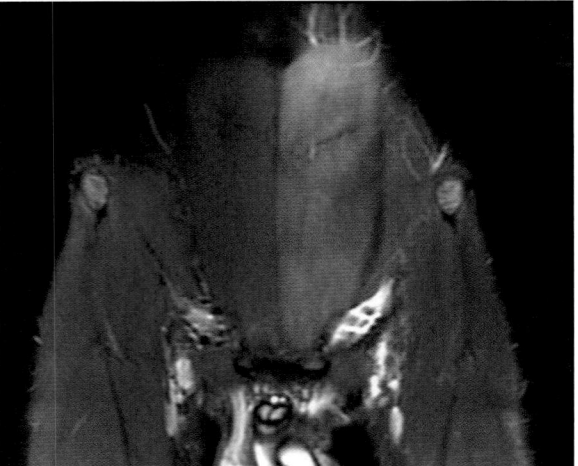

Figure 9-5. Rectus abdominis compartment syndrome. This fluid-sensitive MRI image shows a white appearance of the entire left rectus abdominis muscle in a star high school basketball player. The opacification represents swelling from nonstop muscular contraction in futile attempts to compensate for a severe hip impingement.

Rectus Abdominis Compartment Syndrome

We see this a lot. It can be a primary problem resulting usually from a muscle tear, hematoma, and fibrosis. The scarring renders the muscle less useful and results in pain with any sort of light or vigorous contraction. Or it can be a secondary problem related to compensatory response. We see it most often in patients with painful hip syndromes. The rectus abdominis muscular compartment continually contracts presumptively in response to pain and teleologically to prevent the hip from rotating too much. The continual contraction again leads to wear-and-tear injury, hematoma, and fibrosis (Figure 9-5).

Mesh Syndromes

In addition to causing atrophy, the mesh often causes pain by direct involvement of nerves or by fixating the muscle so that compensatory movement mechanisms must be invoked. Not only does the mesh often not relieve the pain of these core muscle injuries, it often adds to the pain and this then aggravates the whole situation. Pain causes more rectus abdominis nonuse and atrophy. The mesh may also migrate and impinge directly on more nerves (Figure 9-6).

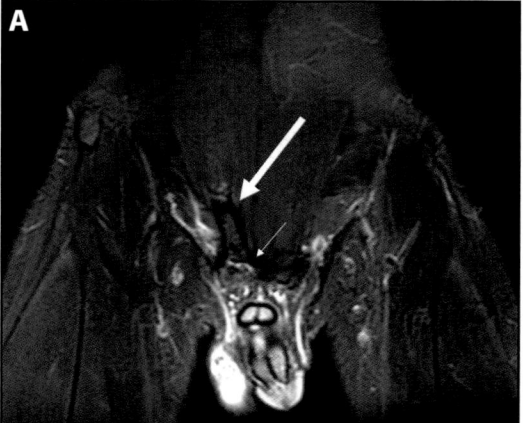
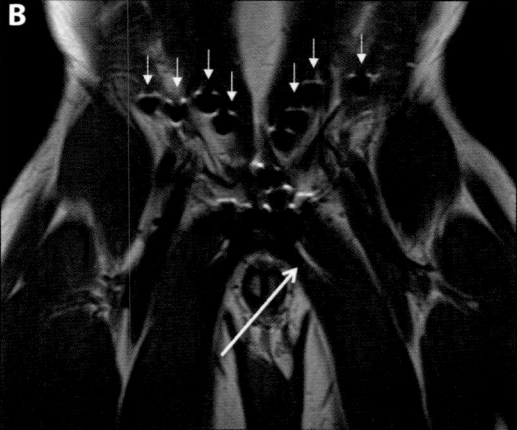

Figure 9-6. Two examples of mesh problems. (A) MRI image of an Olympic diver who could not compete for over a year after a "hernia" repair. Severe scarring and atrophy of the rectus abdominis muscle related to right-sided mesh (arrow). Note the irregular appearance of the distal muscle on the right side compared to the left. Below the mesh is a transverse white line that represents the untreated injury (small arrow). (B) Up-and-coming star professional shortstop whose hernia repair done during spring training did not work; he missed the entire regular season. Note the numerous clips from surgery creating "swiss cheese" artifacts (multiple short arrows) and the untreated left adductor injury (long arrow). The metal artifacts obscure the extent of the rectus abdominis/adductor pubic plate injury. The player also had a severe hip problem.

Rower's Rib Syndrome

This syndrome is more common than one might think. Sometimes, it requires surgery. It has become "classical" in our clinic for the sport of crew. It results from disruption of the upper rectus abdominis attachments onto the ribs and adjacent soft tissues of the chest. This is a wear-and-tear phenomenon and may totally disrupt the rib-muscle interfaces so important for rowing, tennis, throwing, and even gardening. The muscular disruption causes a painful subluxation of the ribs. At surgery, ribs will likely need to be respected and sometimes mesh required to fill the resultant muscular defect and prevent protrusion of abdominal or chest contents (Figure 9-7). (See Video 1, which brings you into the OR and shows how you can manually dislocate the rower's ribs. Rib removal and muscular repair fixed the problem.)

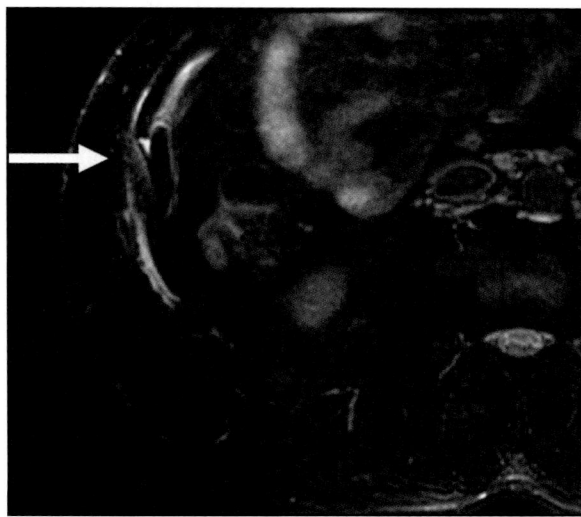

Figure 9-7. Rower's rib syndrome. Olympic rower with unrelenting, right-sided, oblique muscle pain, preventing training. MRI reveals inflammation and irregularity of ribs and adjacent muscles (arrow).

Intercostal Sensory Pain or Entrapment Syndromes

It turns out there are a number of real nerve entrapment syndromes that involve the rectus abdominis muscle. The most publicized syndrome is the anterior cutaneous nerve entrapment syndrome.[4] It is a chronic pain syndrome from terminal branches of the lower thoracic intercostal nerves "entrapped" in abdominal muscles, causing a severe localized neuropathic pain usually in ventral portions of the abdomen. It is frequently overlooked and unrecognized, but is very fixable by release of the muscle or fascia and/or excision or division of nerves.

Isolated Tears

Most often, muscle belly tears resolve without sequelae, but be aware that they may not and may lead to chronic pain, which may have to be injected or fixed directly. Large gaps, however, in high-performing athletes may be better addressed acutely since one may control the hematoma and repair the muscle directly. Be aware that these injuries may also occur in conjunction with oblique or other injuries.

Isolated Avulsions

These tend to be serious and can occur proximal to the pubic fibrocartilage plate, as well as include a portion of that plate. It is usually best to repair this acutely, and the player may be able to get back in 3 weeks. Often a muscle tear in this location would require 6 weeks to resolve nonoperatively. Keep in mind that we have seen rectus abdominis avulsions in association with oblique muscle avulsions. Several NFL seasons ago, we saw that in running backs, all of whom got back to 100% after surgical repair. One high-level college quarterback did not undergo surgery and never got back. The team's sports medicine staff had advised against it. That QB has still not gotten back. Most rectus abdominis avulsions occur in association with other injuries, the most common "other" injury being adductor avulsions (Figure 9-8).

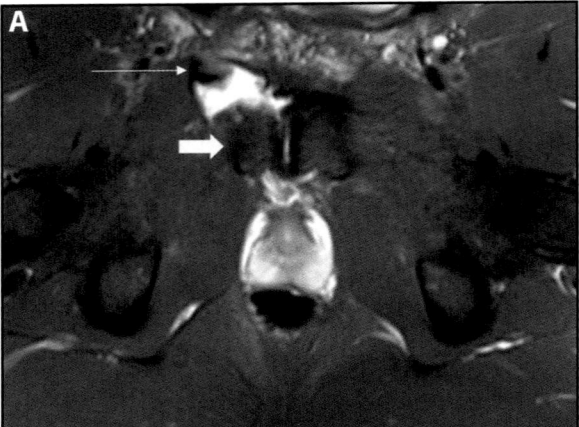
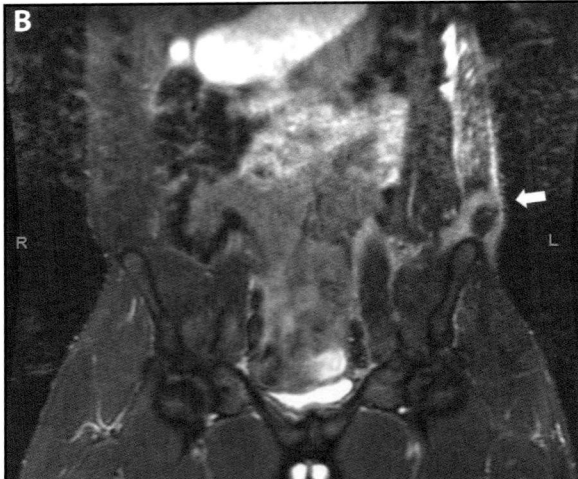
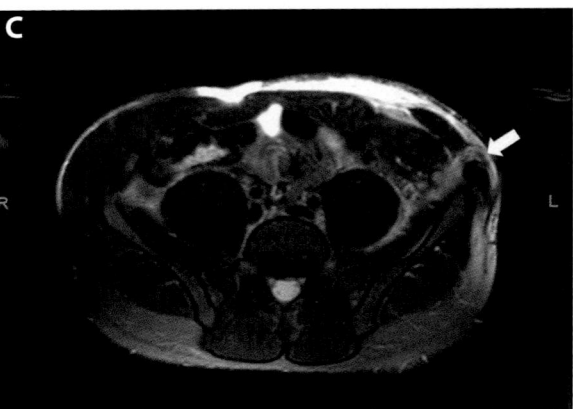

Figure 9-8. Rectus abdominis avulsions. (A) MRI image of a complete right rectus abdominis avulsion in a bronco rider. The long thin arrow indicates the rectus abdominis stump. The short thick arrow points to the pubic bone. The white in between is blood. (B) Coronal stir image and (C) T2 axial image display a complete left oblique muscle avulsion from the iliac crest, in association with a rectus abdominis avulsion (not shown) in Andre Ellington, an excellent NFL running back. The arrows in B and C point to blood and retroperitoneal contents within the avulsion gap. All the above avulsions were repaired surgically. The athletes returned to their sports in 6 to 7 weeks.

Diastasis Syndromes

Insurance companies love to say that rectus abdominis diastases do not cause pain and surgical correction of diastases is purely cosmetic, thereby avoiding payment for these procedures. The fact of the matter is that many of these are painful in athletes who regularly use their upper abdominal walls, such as rowers, gymnasts, and wrestlers. Ask Danny Briere, the famous NHL player, about core muscle injuries and diastases. Basically, this can be a shearing or attenuation injury evolving from real tears, thinning or spread of muscular tissue, and a painful separation of the rectus abdominis laterally from the midline. Often, extremes of exertion are required to demonstrate the syndrome. It is true that diastases may cause tremendous cosmetic problems, for instance, professional female wrestlers after they return after pregnancy. On the other hand, many of these women also had true rectus abdominis injuries as part of the reason they develop the enlarging diastases when they do. The problem is not entirely congenital. Consider that true hernias do often also occur in association with these rectus abdominis diastasis injuries (Figure 9-9).

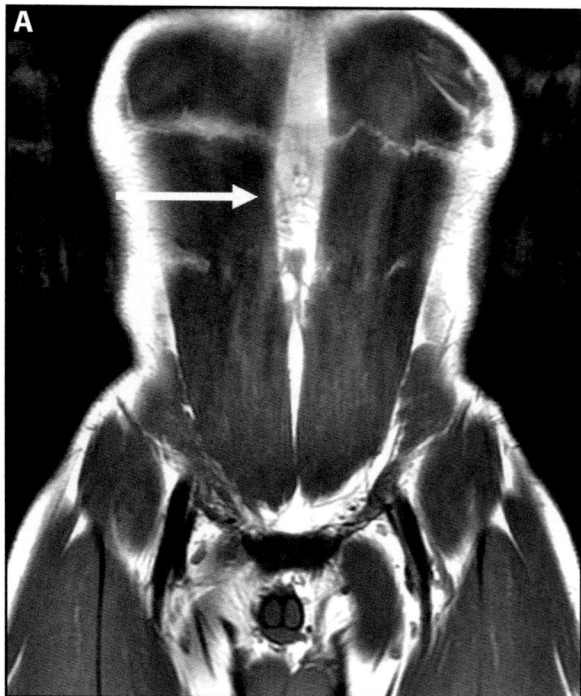 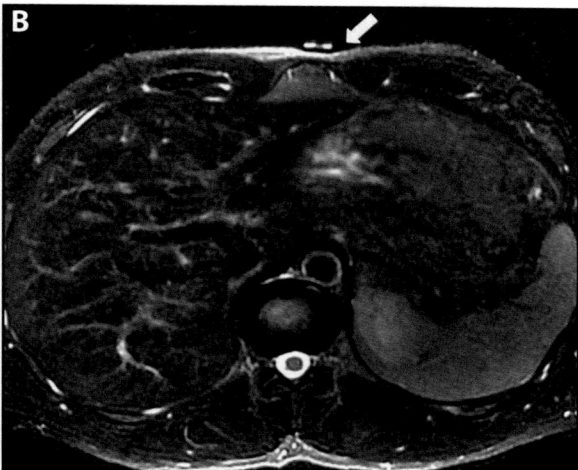

Figure 9-9. Rectus abdominis diastasis in a star NHL center. (A) T1 coronal image. The arrow indicates the diastasis, which appears white compared to the more lateral dark normal muscle. Note the small white circular structures. Those represent true hernias in evolution through the thin abdominal musculature of the diastasis. (B) T2 transaxial image showing the midline thinness (arrow) of the abdominal wall.

Weightlifter's Syndromes

Weightlifters, by the nature of what they do, develop a variety of different muscular tears and true hernias in unusual locations both within and remote to the rectus abdominis muscles. It is common for these tears and true hernias to occur through or immediately adjacent to the rectus abdominis muscles. One should not be surprised by an unusual location of abdominal wall of a demonstrable bulge in these folks. Rarely they are associated with pain. That's just what these folks get.

Spigelian Syndrome

We see a tremendous amount of pain at precisely this location, the lateral edge of the rectus abdominis sheath two-thirds of the way down (the arcus semilunaris) where the posterior sheath essentially disappears. There may or may not be an actual weakness or protrusion there. What has not been reported well is that there is routinely a large bed of nerves in this location and with trauma they often stretch or become impinged related to muscle shifting from the injury.

Epigastric Artery Syndrome

This is fortunately rare and we have seen only 2 cases of this. This was severe pain after hernia repair, each time with a staple or stitch injuring the inferior epigastric artery and causing a false aneurysm. We cured each case with aneurysmectomy.

Neurological Syndromes

Don't underplay this possibility when there is a combination of pain and weakness. Realize that our knowledge of the neural anatomy of the abdominal core muscles is rudimentary at best. Neurological derangements probably happen a lot, particularly when there has been previous surgery. A bunch of peripheral motor and sensory nerves travel transversely from the spine to the obliques and rectus abdominis muscles that we know next to nothing about. Think about how common it is for an athlete to say, "I am just weak on that side." Figure 9-10 illustrates a case of profound right-sided abdominal weakness in an athletic female caused by previous surgery.

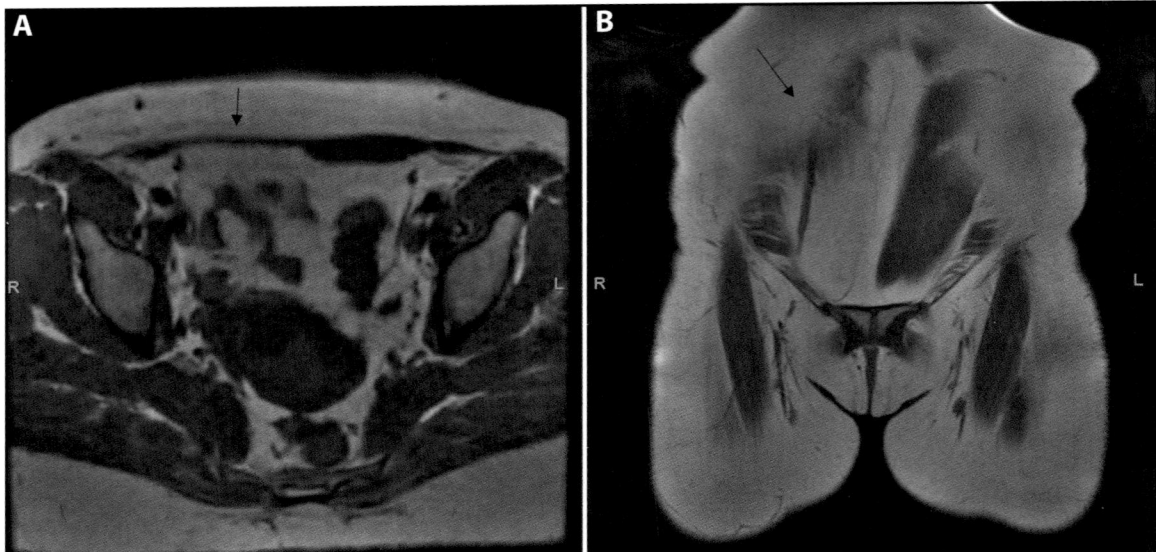

Figure 9-10. Neurological injury causing rectus abdominis atrophy. This previously athletic young lady could never get back to her fitness routine after a 6-inch right vertical flank incision that went through the muscle. Two years afterward, an MRI showed this. (A) Transverse axial view: Obvious atrophy (arrow) of the right rectus abdominis muscle that began about 2 inches below the rib cage and extended to about 1 inch about the pubic bone. (B) Coronal view: The same patient showing fat infiltration (arrow) replacing space previously occupied by muscle. A portion of the oblique muscles were also involved. These neurological syndromes are more common than one might think and pose difficult questions with regard to therapy.

Tumors

Don't forget that various benign and malignant tumors also occur here. We have seen desmoids, endometriomas, schwannoma, teratoma, sarcomas, and others.

BACK TO THE HARNESS

Realize also that there are a huge number of rectus abdominis injuries that involve the harness mechanism, as opposed to the ones listed above "isolated" to that muscle. We talk about these injuries more in later chapters. People may argue that certain portions of the obliques or transverse muscles are also involved in these injuries. Let them argue this. These critics are right. Their criticism does not make too much difference, so long as they "get" the basic concept.

Be careful, though. Those folks/critics may also be subtly arguing for the fallacious concept that there is just one type of pathology (ie, occult hernia). Remember, this is the concept that we have to wipe off the face of the earth. That argument leads to misdiagnoses, failed surgeries, and disaster stories. To become convinced of the falsity of that thinking, all one has to do is see some of these severe injuries at surgery, or simply listen to the horror stories of patients in the waiting room of our clinic. We sometimes see a dozen patients a day who had undergone unsuccessful hernia repairs.

Okay, it is time to go down a centimeter or two. Yes, just 1 or 2 cm! That's the distance it takes to get to the adductor attachments onto the same "baseball" fibrocartilage pubic cover (see Figure 7-11).

Remember that plate baseball concept? The rectus abdominis attaches more inferiorly onto the pubic bone plate than most people appreciate. Because of that, the rectus abdominis attaches right above the adductors (Figure 9-11).

In the next chapter, we take that tiny step down to the adductors.

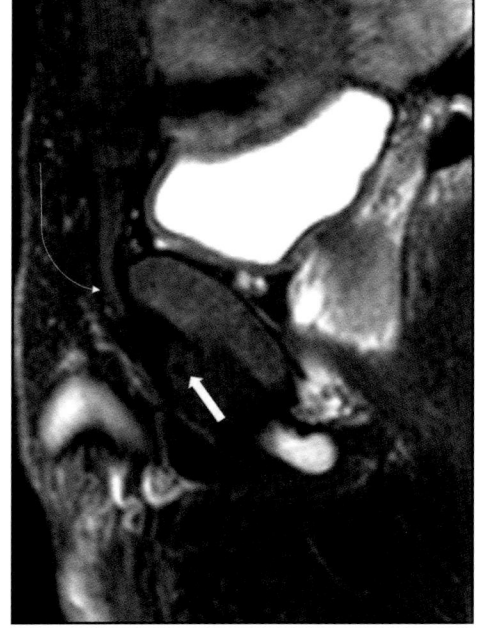

Figure 9-11. Sagittal MRI showing the close proximity of the distal end of the Cinderella muscle (long, slender arrow) to the proximal adductor attachments (thick arrow). In this picture, the 2 attachments are separated by 1 to 2 cm of pubic fibrocartilage plate.

SELECTED READINGS

Matsuda DK, Meyers WC, Larson CM, Zoga A. Athletic pubalgia: current concepts and evolving management. Round tables. *Orthopedics Today*. February 2011. http://www.healio.com/orthopedics/arthroscopy/news/print/orthopedics-today/%7B43a716b9-cc96-47aa-aa71-897fdb62866c%7D/athletic-pubalgia-current-concepts-and-evolving-management. Accessed November 6, 2016.
   Excellent discussion of state-of-the-art treatment at that time with emphasis on the rectus abdominis muscle and its relationship with adjacent anatomy. Variety and patterns of injury, including sports specificity, highlight some of the discussion.

Meyers WC. "Sports hernia" in the baseball player. PBATS Newsletter. November 2011.
   The rectus abdominis plays an important role in just about all sports, including baseball. The necessity for repetition of the same exact movements during practice makes baseball an interesting sport for study. Players at different positions tend to get different injuries.

Rectus abdominis. Kenhub. https://www.youtube.com/watch?v=Axquij1mhTo. Accessed August 1, 2016.
   A short, fun review of the classic teaching about the rectus abdominis. Don't mind the obvious error in anatomy (ie, the artwork showing too many lower abdominal folds).

Sperstad JB, Tennfjord MK, Hilde G, Ellstrom-Engh M. Diastasis recti abdominis during pregnancy and 12 months after childbirth: prevalence, risk factors and report of lumbopelvic pain. *Br J Sports Med*. 2016;50:1092-1096. doi:10.1136/bjsports-2016-096065.
   This recent article represents the new attention to rectus abdominis diastasis in sports medicine. The condition can become a real problem, particularly in female athletes.

REFERENCES

1. Kilgore A. Nationals third baseman Ryan Zimmerman to undergo surgery, will miss six weeks. *The Washington Post*. https://www.washingtonpost.com/sports/nationals/nationals-third-baseman-ryan-zimmerman-to-undergo-surgery-will-miss-six-weeks/2011/04/30/AF5cVkNF_story.html?noredirect=on&utm_term=.5b8ab976116c. Published April 30, 2011. Accessed May 18, 2016.
2. Custom core zone. www.theabscompany.com. Accessed May 18, 2016.
3. Sanchez-Moysi J, Idoate F, Dorado C, et al. Large asymmetric hypertrophy of rectus abdominis muscle in professional tennis players. *PLOS*. http://journals.plos.org/plosone/article?id=10.1371%2Fjournal.pone.0015858. Published December 31, 2010. Accessed August 1, 2016.
4. Van Assen T, de Jager-Klevit JWAJ, Scheltinga MR, Roumen MH. Chronic abdominal wall pain misdiagnosed as functional abdominal pain. *J Am Board Fam Med*. 2013;26(6):738-744.

VIDEO

1. https://youtu.be/bZXRw5f4qgQ

10

the **adductors**
demystifying them

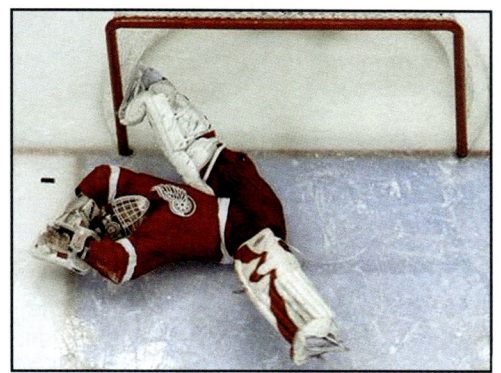

Figure 10-1. Dominik Hasek kick save. (Reprinted with permission from AP Photo/Paul Sancya.)

The puck is sailing toward the lower corner at about 100 mph, and there's little chance of its not settling into the back of the net. Goal!

Until the goalie flings his foot over his head and to the side and redirects the compressed rubber disk into the corner. Kick save—and a beauty (Figure 10-1).

Goalies have to repeat that kind of behavior several times during a game and hundreds of times throughout a season. They stretch and strengthen and do everything they can to create the flexibility necessary to play their position. But it doesn't always work.

Ask Dominik Hasek. The outstanding goalie tried to kick away a puck and suffered a big tear of the adductor.[1] He said he heard a pop and felt a burning in his groin. He wasn't kidding. That's some serious stuff.

The adductors help goalies do the splits. They allow pitchers to overstride in their wind-ups to generate maximum speed on pitches. They help defensive linemen charge forward to overpower blocks by sturdy offensive linemen or drop back into pass coverage to prevent backs from getting open. Without good strength and flexibility in the area, disaster can strike, repair might be necessary, and the puck can end up in the net.

The Top Ten Points to "Get" About the Adductors (Table 10-1)

1. Most docs do not know the subtleties of adductor function.
2. The most important function of the adductors is their role in the core's harness. The individual adductors do not usually work in isolation. And as a group of muscles, they work alongside other muscles that complement their forces.
3. Simple distal muscle belly strains are common and usually resolve spontaneously,[2,3] whereas proximal injuries at the pubic plate part of the harness are usually more serious.
4. The 3 most important adductors in the core are the pectineus, the adductor longus, and the adductor brevis. The adductor magnus is large and the gracilis long, but neither muscle is nearly as important as the other 3. The latter 2 do not attach to the more central portion of the pubic apparatus and therefore are not fundamental to the harness mechanism. In fact, the more central obturator externus has considerably more harness function than the gracilis or magnus (Figures 10-2 and 10-3).

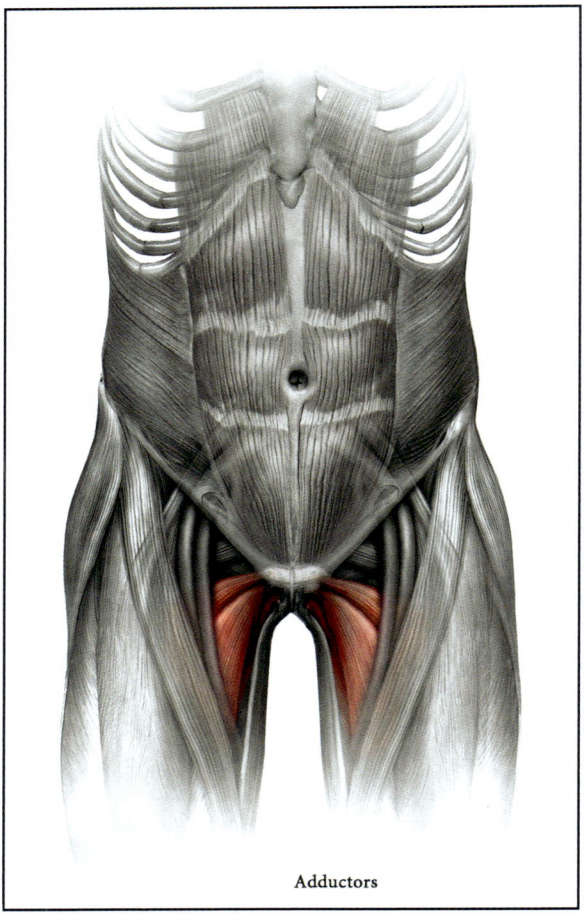

Figure 10-2.

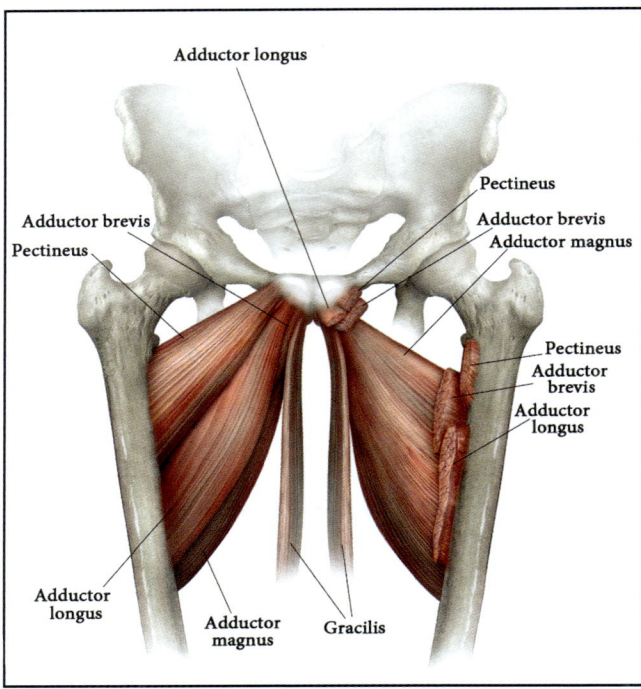

Figure 10-3. Adductors and their attachments.

5. Most proximal adductor injuries also involve the pubic plate, other adductors, and the rectus abdominis.
6. Bilateral injuries are common, via the pubic plate/harness mechanism.
7. Adductor repairs should be the primary type of surgical intervention for detached adductors, along with repairs of adjacent injured structures. Repairs usually require loosening (decompressing; eg, fasciotomies and epimysiotomies) the muscle belly compartments. Those are sometimes called *compartmental releases*, which may cause confusion. See the next point.

8. Adductor "releases"[4-6] are bad. The term commonly describes detaching the adductor muscle from its attachment on the pubic bone. Detaching any muscle from its attachment, as one should expect, causes weakness. This is particularly true of the adductors. Such detachments may relieve pain but detaching something, by its nature, creates weakness. Significant weakness in a high-performance athlete certainly usually requires reattachment. The important question looms: Why not just repair the adductors? The answer is that proper repair requires keen understandings of both the anatomy and pathophysiology of the injuries. Those understandings have not been part of surgeons' knowledge bases. The techniques for successful repairs turn out to be straightforward; there are many and one needs to choose the right one for each patient.

9. The anatomy of each adductor is readily identifiable, yet most people think in terms of old paradigms. The most important anatomical points to know are:
   - Adductor attachments onto the pubic plate are very important.
   - Very little tendon exists. One may argue that the attachments look like "tendons."[7] Forget that, that gets everybody thinking wrong when it comes to repairing them. Instead, think in terms of the muscles attaching directly into that fibrocartilaginous plate.
   - A number of anatomic subtleties exist. These relate to both various structural configurations and relative sizes of muscle, fasciae, and epimysia. There are distinct anatomical patterns for each adductor. Actually, the sport makes a difference. For example, skaters—both figure skaters and ice hockey players—have large pectinei, relative to the other 2 adductors of the harness.

10. A wide variety of adductor injuries exists varying from complete avulsions at the pubic attachments (which usually involve other structures) to more distal muscle belly injuries that do not involve the plate. The injuries may be acute or chronic and often involve a combination of acute and chronic processes. Any of the 3 main adductors may be involved, and commonly more than one adductor is involved at the same time.

Table 10-1
Top Ten Adductor Takeaways

1. Most docs do not know the subtleties of adductor function.
2. The most important function of the adductors is their role in the core's harness.
3. Simple distal muscle belly strains are common and usually resolve spontaneously, whereas proximal injuries at the pubic plate part of the harness are usually more serious.
4. The 3 most important adductors in the core are the pectineus, the adductor longus, and the adductor brevis.
5. Most proximal adductor injuries also involve the pubic plate, other adductors, and the rectus abdominis.
6. Bilateral injuries are common.
7. Adductor repairs should be the primary type of surgical intervention.
8. Adductor "releases" are bad.
9. The anatomy of each adductor is readily identifiable.
10. A wide variety of adductor injuries exists.

Old Beliefs That Are Just Plain Wrong

- Adductor injuries are all "groin strains" and an athlete can grit through these.
- Surgery is rarely necessary.
- When surgery is necessary, one should do a "release" (ie, cut the adductor from its origin). One can do this without worry. It cures the problem. There is no loss of strength, etc.
- If you really want to repair the adductors, anchor them back to the pubic bone.
- Adductors all do the same thing.
- The tendon is the important part of adductor structure.

DEBUNKING OLD DOGMA (FIGURE 10-4)

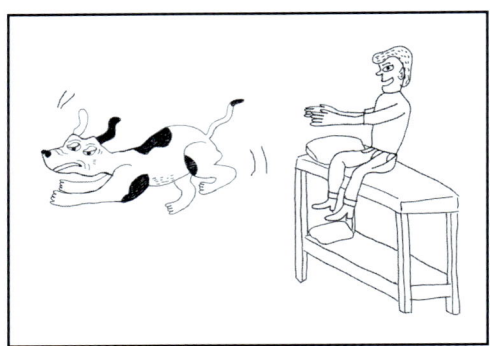

Figure 10-4. Debunking old dogma.

We are not going to spend time exhaustively explaining why each of those old beliefs just ain't true. That would only fuel controversy.

Instead, accept as reality that this area of the body has (had) remained mysterious for a long time. And accept that successful surgical experience in about 20,000 patients says that these old beliefs are wrong.

Plus, consider all the athletes that you have read about, whose careers ended or failed due to groin injuries. Logic should also enter into the debunking. For example, doesn't it make sense that... detaching a muscle would cause weakness? Or that repairing muscles so that they function normally should help? Think about other questions: Shouldn't the fact matter that the adductors don't attach directly into bone? Might not anchoring them to bone, where all the nerves are, cause pain? Shouldn't anatomical variations matter and enter into formulas for choosing the best type of repair?

The main point: Keep on reading. Ask Dick-and-Jane type questions. Continue the logic.

ANATOMICAL REALITIES

Three important anatomic points stand out.
1. The arrangement and muscular integrity of the adductors matter. Think of muscle as the functional tissue and muscular attachment as all important. Fascia and epimysium protect the muscle and provide some firmness but this tissue does not contract.
2. When muscle pulls away from its attachment, collagenous tissue may be all that is left. Function suffers and pain ensues. With time, the fibrous tissue thickens and tension increases. Our guess is that most pain comes from the pubic fibrocartilage pulling away from the periosteum, which has a rich, neural complex.
3. The harness adductors are primary protectors of the hip. As depicted in Figure 10-5, we performed multiple studies in fresh cadavers that showed this. Other structures sometimes played roles as well, such as the femoral artery and nerve. In fact, cutting the adductors sometimes produced impingement in fresh cadavers with cam or pincer anatomy. This led us to the conclusion that adductor or harness injury could cause clinical impingement signs and symptoms. Empirically, the clinical corollary rings true in many of our patients—that the harness adductors are primary protectors of the hip.

Many of our patients with manifest femoroacetabular impingement also have elicitable adductor signs. They also have adductor strictures, certainly the consequence of longstanding injury and the fibrosis related to injury and sustained compensatory contraction. From the combination of anatomic and clinical information, we could not help but conclude that the harness adductors serve as primary protectors against hip impingement.

Figure 10-5. This drawing has been shown before and reflects one of multiple sets of experiments performed in the fresh cadaver laboratory with one purpose in mind: to determine which anatomic structures, other than the ball and socket, limited the range of motion of the hip. It turned out that all 3 harness adductors played huge anatomic roles in most but not all people (er...ah...cadavers).

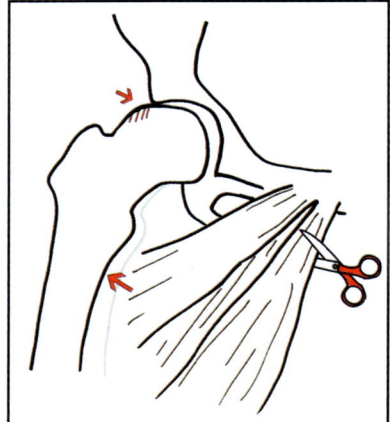

Some Adductor Disorders

Case 1. Simple Adductor Muscle Belly Strain

A 27-year-old NHL hockey player suddenly feels a "rip" in his proximal right thigh pushing off to his left during a game. He tries to continue but it hurts too much to play. See Figure 10-6.

This "strain" represents probably the most common injury that we or most athletic trainers/team docs see in most sports. It usually does not need surgery. The choices are between physical therapy alone or injecting it with something plus the same physical therapy. Empirically, some of these patients seem to get back more quickly with a steroid injection. We treated this patient without injection and just active physical therapy, massage, oral anti-inflammatories, and symptomatic progression back to full hockey. He returned at full speed in 1 week.

Note that in the above paragraph we said the injury usually does not need surgery. This player was a goalie. There is a syndrome we call baseball pitcher hockey goalie (BPHG) syndrome. This represents a scarred down version of Case 1, the consequence of repeated injuries in precisely this same region. What distinguishes the syndrome is scar and muscle entrapment leading to a compartment syndrome. We shall get to BPHG now.

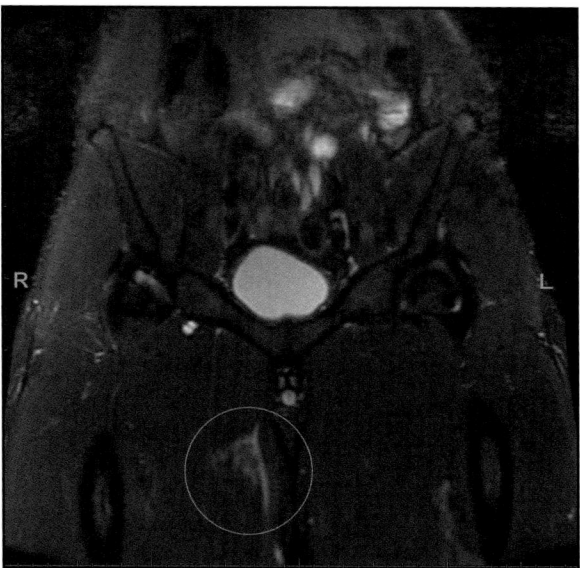

Figure 10-6. Initial imaging of an NHL center's injury. The MRI shows whiteness (within the circle; ie, likely acute hematoma with edema) in his right adductor longus muscle belly and nothing else. This is a coronal stir image. The rest of his core anatomy was intact and the injury began 2 inches away from the pubic attachment.

Case 2. Baseball Pitcher Hockey Goalie Syndrome

This is also an NHL goalkeeper with a similar story to Case 1 except repeated episodes of the same thing. He was fine each time between episodes, each of which took about 1 to 2 weeks to get over. See Figure 10-7.

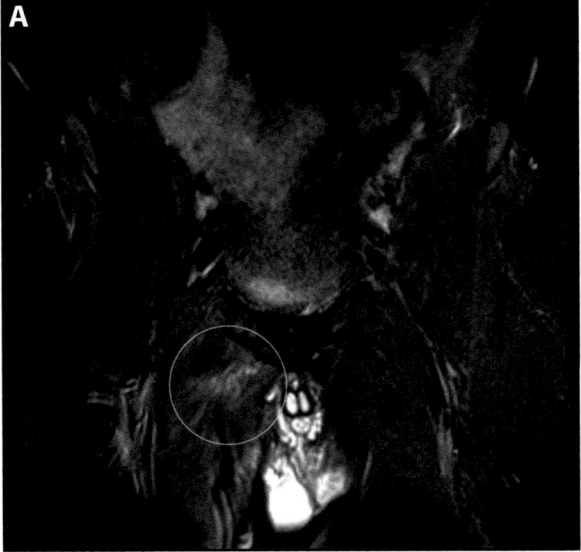
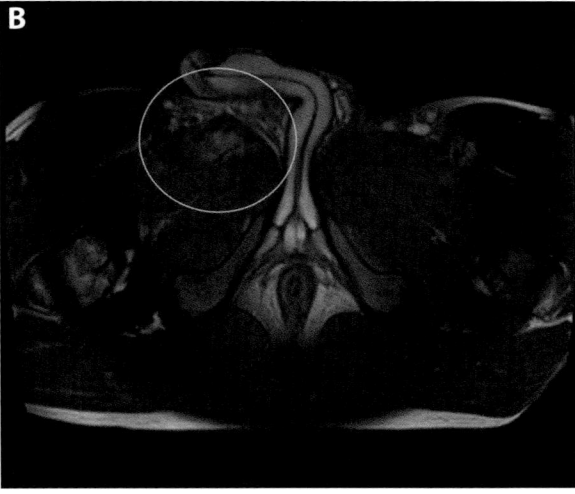

Figure 10-7. BPHG syndrome in an NHL goalie. (A) Coronal stir and (B) T2 transaxial images showing both acute edema and considerable fibrosis consistent with BPHG syndrome in an NHL goalie.

We usually let the clinical situation dictate the indication for surgery. This patient opted to have surgery at the end of the season. He underwent a compartmental decompression.

Most athletes with this syndrome get through without surgery. The decision for surgery arrives by subjective criteria, usually based upon the degree of pain, performance, and/or lost playing time. Consider the number of times in his career Roger Clemens had groin episodes and was placed on the disabled list.[8-10] Should he have had surgery? That is an open question. He had a pretty good career.

On the other hand, consider Roy Oswalt, who played heroically with pain and the same injury for the last quarter of a season when the Astros were in a fierce pennant race. And that was during Roy's contract year. Think about what Roy was risking—a severe arm injury related to a compensatory change in his pitching mechanics. Fortunately of course, he survived that and off-season surgery and had a great career. Roy's commitment to his team plus his tremendous career, despite all this, attests to his great strength of character.

If you know those 2 pitchers and are a baseball aficionado, you probably are guessing about the mechanism of this injury. Roger and Roy had something in common in addition to the "R" at the beginning of their names—their pitching mechanics. They both had extra-long strides. No doubt that type of stride helped their power and ball movement. And almost certainly, that relative biomechanical "isolation" of the thighs, certainly common in hockey goalies, plays some kind of pathophysiologic role in this injury.

Then along comes an NFL linebacker who later became a Hall-of-Famer. He had the same injury. Jokingly, he wanted us to add linebacker or defensive end to the name of the syndrome. Of course, we see the same injury in other positions and other sports—it is not exclusive to those 2 positions.

To stay in the linebacker's good favor, we told him that we officially changed the name of the syndrome to BPHG-LB!

Case 3. Adductor Heterotopic Ossification

Over the past several years, we have seen an alarming number of athletes with heterotopic ossification (HO) associated with the administration of platelet-rich plasma (PRP). Certainly it would take many cases to prove an association, but 8 patients within a year seemed a lot. We do occasionally see adductor HO in the absence of PRP but on the order of less than one case per year. Surgery after PRP can be difficult anyway, owing to the tremendous induced fibrosis, but HO can make the dissections tons more difficult. Below is the letter to pro team docs and athletic trainers that our observation prompted.

Dear Team Physician/Athletic Trainer,

I feel compelled to email to you all our recent observation that platelet-rich plasma (PRP) appears harmful in the short or long term for proximal adductor injuries. The early evidence is that it causes heterotopic ossification (HO), which can be devastating to the careers of some athletes.

Over the past year now, we have seen 8 such patients (severe HO after PRP). The HO developed within 2 weeks to 6 months after treatment(s). All required surgery and one patient developed a persistent HO problem, although he has continued to play at a high level.

As you know we see many (20 to 40 per week) new patients with various types of core muscle and/or hip injuries. And of course, the injury itself contributes to HO occurrence. Please note as well that all the cases mentioned had severe HO in the distribution of the injections.

Up until recently, PRP has been only a rare treatment for these injuries. Only 12 patients in total answered in their questionnaires that they had received any kind of PRP treatment for these type injuries over the same time period. That calculates to be a 67% incidence of HO after PRP. Plus, we have had only a total of 10 cases of severe adductor HO over the same time frame. Considering the over 1400 operative adductor cases over this time frame, that calculates to be an overall HO rate of 0.7%. At the same time we had only 10 cases of severe HO.

So, 80% (8 of 10) of the patients who had HO had received PRP. Interestingly, one of the other 2 had received another form of stem cell injection into the area. Keep in mind our questionnaire does not ask about other stem cell treatments.

Yes, questionnaires may provoke various types of bias and we cannot with certainty state that PRP is causative in any or all of these cases.

Yet, this early evidence is compelling enough for me to send out this email, prior to any publication, as a warning or a simple "heads-up" for this potential severe complication.

All my best,
Bill

The following is one example of a case of adductor-plate HO. This happened to a well-known defensive back whose college team won a national championship and he became a first-round choice. The injury and treatments occurred during his college years. This football player suffered a Grade 1 injury to his adductor and plate during his freshman season. He underwent 2 courses of PRP, which did not help. His performance suffered more as he became less able to adduct, flex, or extend his thigh. He developed a golf ball of calcium prohibiting those actions. The mass turned out to be mostly removable from surrounding tense, almost immobile tissue. His adductors still feel like "rock," but he has returned to stardom without pain at least up until this time. See Figures 10-8 and 10-9.

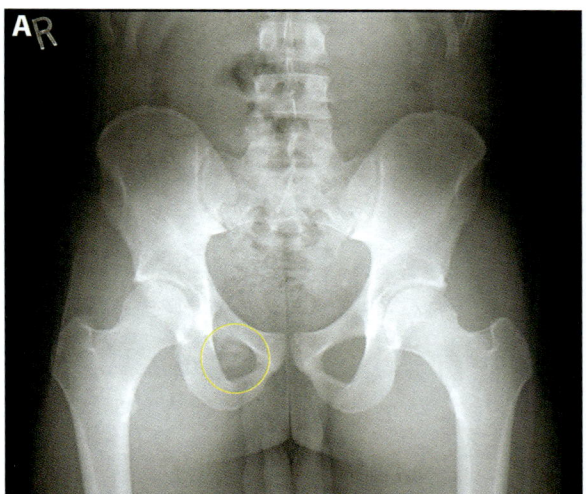
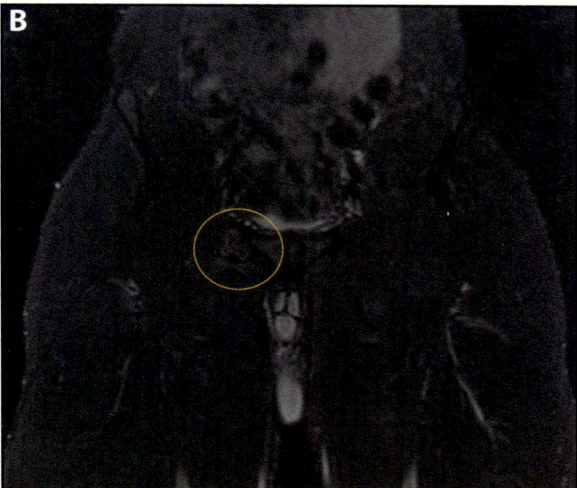

Figure 10-8. Adductor HO can occur in the absence of PRP. We have recently been seeing HO, however, primarily after PRP administration. The following images come from a college football defensive back who temporarily retired because of it. After repair excision of the HO, he was drafted in the first round and became an NFL star. (A) Plain X-ray. Note the subtle white calcification (circle) within the obturator foramen of the right pelvic bone. (B) MRI. We call this baffling display of tissue (circle) a "gnarly" appearance.

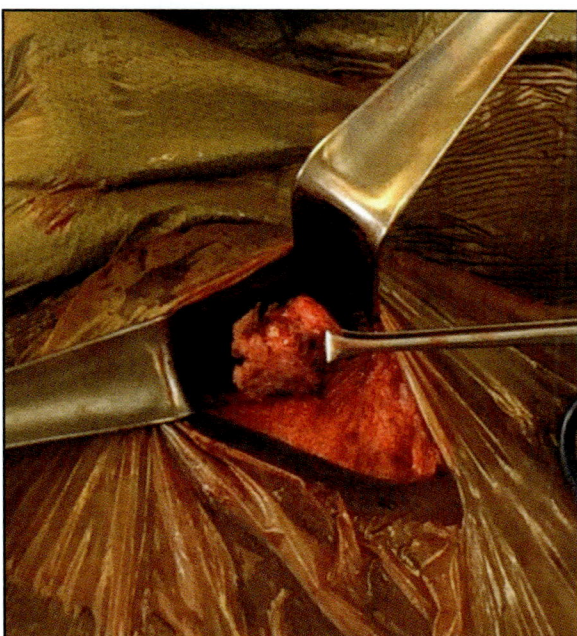

Figure 10-9. Intraoperative photos of another case of heterotopic bone related to PRP, this one in this NFL defensive back. The photo shows a chunk of bone that was removed. In this patient, multiple chunks of bone were removed from within the adductor muscle belly where the PRP was injected as well as from the skin of the scar from a failed mesh hernia repair operation. The latter finding suggests that PRP may have more than just a local effect.

Case 4. Adductor/Pubic Symphysis Disruption

It is important to realize that disruptions can occur in various ways. The symphyseal joint, in fact, is prone to disrupt if there is severe enough force and the adductor and rectus abdominis muscular attachments stay mostly intact. Interestingly, we saw this 3 times in one season, all in top professional goalies. Ask veteran NHL goalie Curtis McElhinney about this. The pain came out of the blue during a twist and described as "searing." Everything in this injury is reparable. One directly sews the muscles of the pubic plate back to where they are supposed to be after reducing the pubic body separation. Curtis remains playing well 5 years after repair.

Figure 10-10 shows a butterfly goalie with a definite plate separation at the adductor level on the left where the disruption began. Plain X-rays, Flamingo views, and MRI bring out the complete symphyseal disruption. Keep in mind that this injury was totally fixable without fixation devices and the player was back in action at 3 months. This player is now one of the top NHL goaltenders.

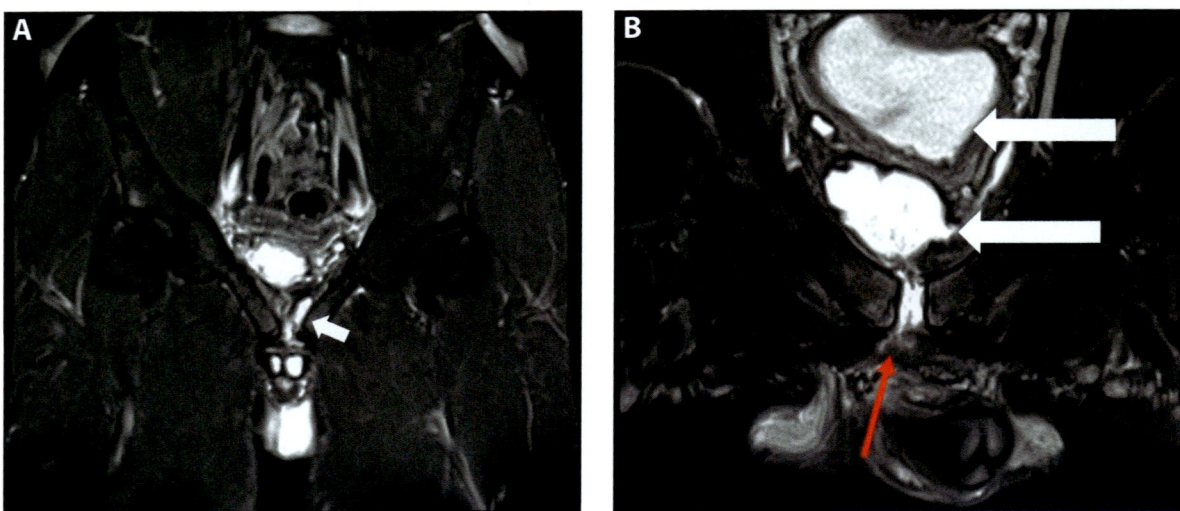

Figure 10-10. NHL goalie with symphyseal plate complete disruption. He had dislocated his entire pubic symphyseal joint. His 2 pubic bones had been plunged back into position prior to these MRI images. The dislocation came from a combination of a forceful kick-save and adductor traction. (A) T2 image showing severe widening of the joint and fluid tracking superiorly (arrow). (B) T2 image demonstrating the pubic plate disruption (arrow) and the "double bladder sign" (thick arrows) representing a big hematoma between the real bladder (top thick arrow) and the injury.

Case 5. Adductor Avulsions

Any of the adductors can be injured separately or in combination with others. Figure 10-11 shows an isolated pectineus avulsion in one of our up-and-coming young US soccer players. Most avulsions are immensely fixable. An isolated pectineus avulsion is a little less common than the adductor longus or brevis. The specific choice of repair depends on the exact pathology and individual's precise anatomy. In general, the earlier you get in there, the more technically easy it is to get a good, tension-free primary repair. This patient's repair took place 6 weeks after the injury and fortunately was still straightforward. We did this in combination with arthroscopic repair of his hip.

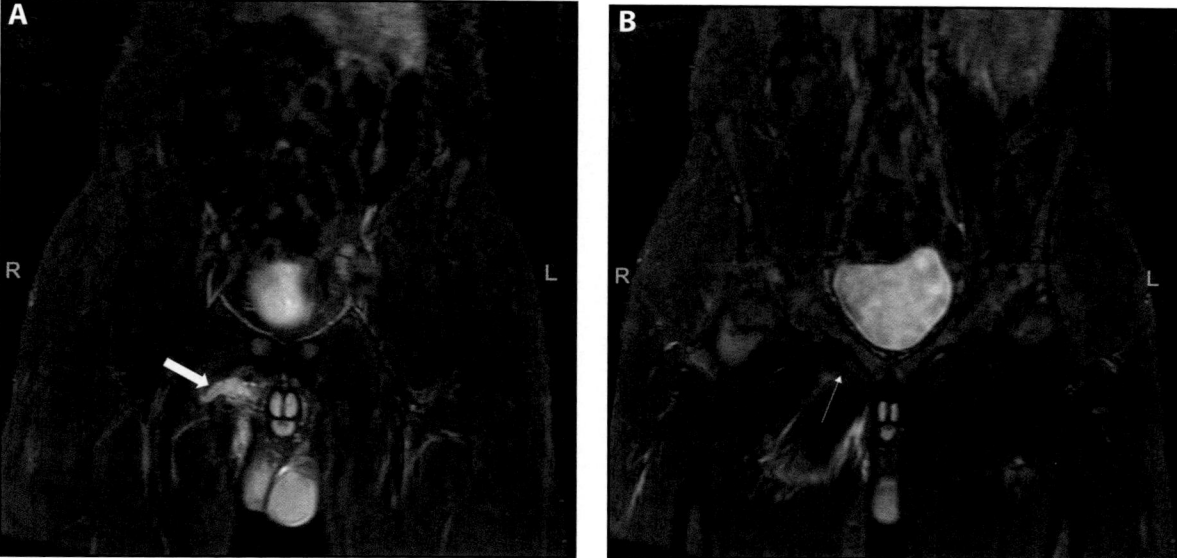

Figure 10-11. Isolated pectineus avulsion in an MLS player. The 2 MRI images are only 1 cm apart. (A) shows a complete pectineus avulsion and (B) shows that the adjacent adductor longus is completely intact. The arrow in (A) shows blood within the crevice of the avulsion. The arrow in (B) shows the adductor longus continuity.

Case 6. Adductor-Plate Disruption Natural History

We believe that most midline plate injuries as pathology that generally does not heal on its own. Think of them like anterior cruciate knee injuries (ie, a midline disruption that causes instability). Because it is midline, the disruption does not have the adjacent tissue immobility to be able to heal without treatment. Both types of injuries lead to instability and more injury of adjacent tissue. Certainly, one will accept that with most ACL injuries, one can build up enough strength in the quads and hamstrings, etc, that one may be able to perform fairly adequately many functions.[4] Yet there remains an instability that hurts performance. The same is true of these midline core muscle injuries. One can build up adjacent muscles and this can help function considerably. Yet, considerable slippage of the pubic plate remains and this leads to more compensation and progressive injury.

Take, for example, Brad Smith, the heroic NFL wide receiver and kick return specialist. He began his career in the NFL as a quarterback attesting to his athleticism. Preservation of his NFL career, as well as various other factors, entered into decisions about whether or not to operate. Brad sustained the first injury while running back a kickoff. This was an acute adductor avulsion several centimeters away from the insertion. We elected to watch this and it completely healed. A full season later, he developed severe rectus abdominis and adductor pain in the preseason and elected to have a subtle plate injury injected with steroid, but 4 games into the season, he lost his wish to treat this injury nonoperatively. He completely tore off all 3 adductors plus his rectus abdominis on the same side. Because of Brad's high pain threshold and wonderful work ethic, he was back playing at full speed 3 to 4 weeks later. See Figure 10-12.

In other words, with respect to their natural history, these injuries tend to be progressive.

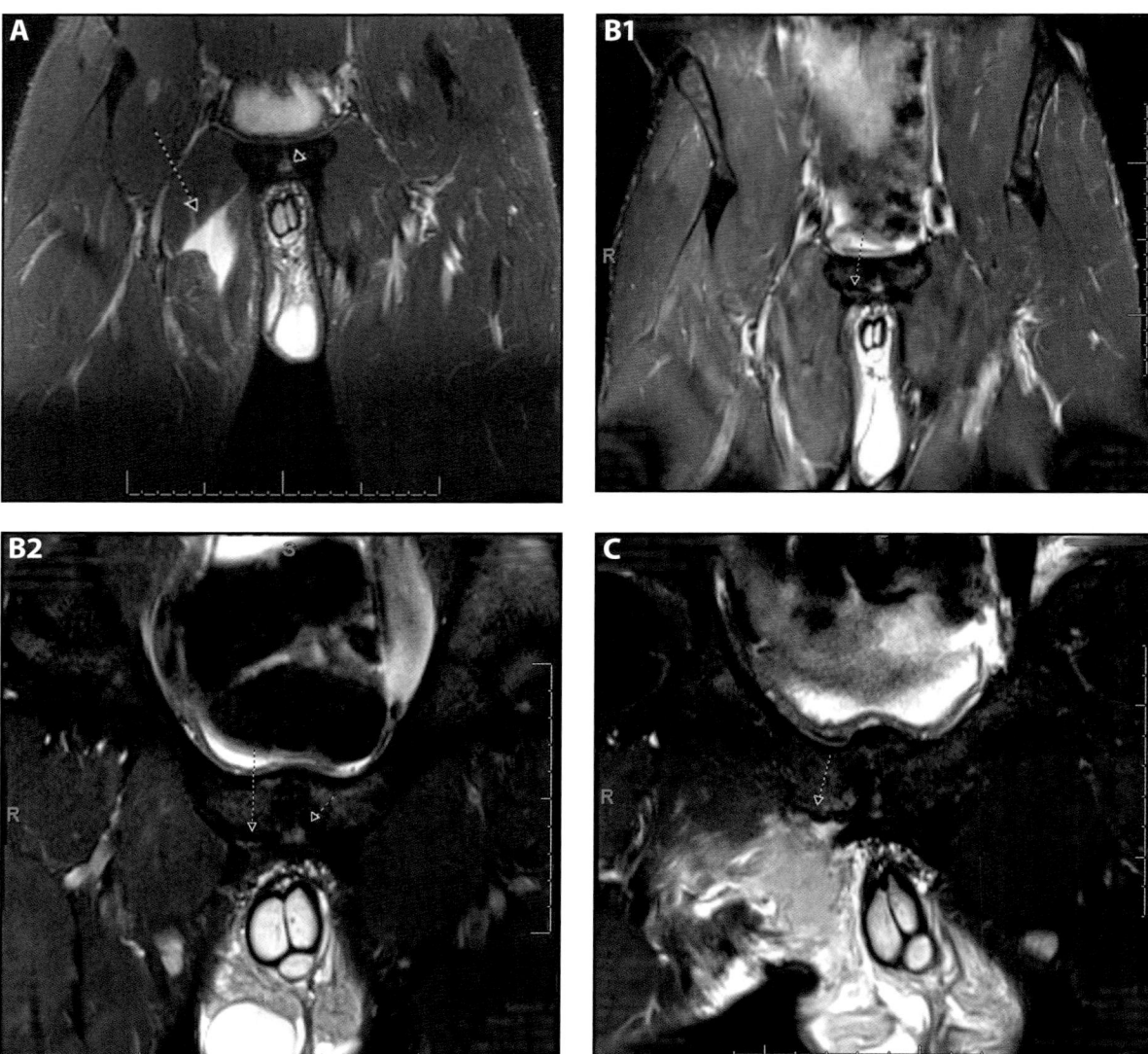

Figure 10-12. These injuries tend to be progressive. This is an NFL quarterback, who, because of his great speed and hands, was converted to a wide receiver. (A) shows a near complete adductor longus avulsion several centimeters distal to its origin on the pubic plate. The arrow points to blood. The arrowhead points to a coincidental, tiny midline pubic plate separation. (B1) and (B2) show complete healing and a subtle but new plate defect. The wide receiver continued to play and ended up with a complete disruption of all the attachments. (C) shows the absence of the entire right-sided pubic cover and replacement by a huge, white blur representing blood where muscle should be.

Case 7. Adductor Magnus Injury

This muscle is large, expansive and primarily supportive. It is important because of its size and strength. Small or isolated tears are common. Surgery is necessary only rarely. See Figure 10-13.

Case 8. Core Harness Injury

Of course, as you now know, the adductors and rectus abdominis muscles do not live in isolation. They work together via the pubic bone. When there is a severe proximal injury of any of the 3 harness adductors, the rectus abdominis almost has to be involved, considering it shares the same pubic plate (ie, baseball cover) attachment. The complementary situation holds a severe injury of the distal rectus abdominis muscle attachment (ie, at least one adductor almost has to be involved). We have many examples of these type injuries. Figure 10-14 represents one.

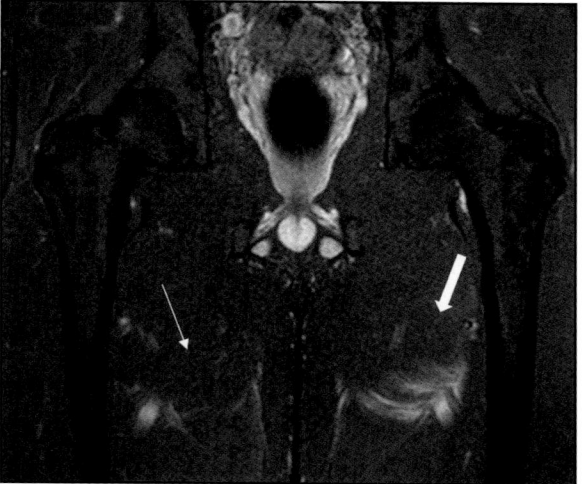

Figure 10-13. Adductor magnus muscle belly injuries ("strains") are common and rarely need surgery. This bilateral injury occurred in a bull rider.

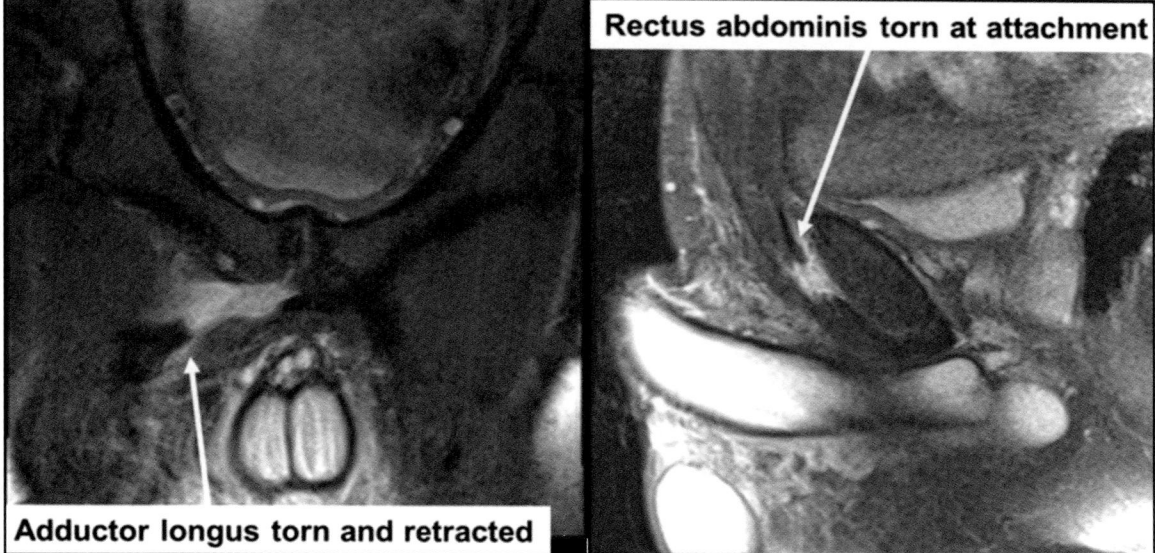

Figure 10-14. National champion figure skater with a severe rectus abdominis-adductor-pubic harness/bridle injury. This acute injury occurred during takeoff for a triple Axel (named for the famous Norwegian Axel Paulson). Functionally, the initiation of the leap "broke the bridle," immediately rendering all the power muscles useless. He fell to the ground powerless. Note the simultaneous avulsion of both the adductor longus and rectus abdominis muscles with their segments of plate. In fact, this injury was rather easy to repair since it was so demarcated. Surgery was performed on the second day after the injury.

Case 9. Combined Hip/Adductor Injuries

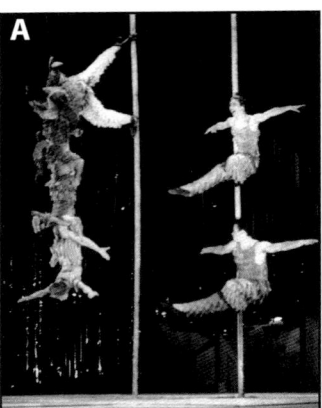

As we have mentioned, and shall continue to mention ad nauseam, the harness and other core muscles work alongside hip function. The 2 sets of structures have many biomechanical and other intimate relationships. Like men and women, the relationships are not just one-way. The adductors protect the hip, and dysfunctional adductors subject the hip to harm. Complementarily, bummer hips cause mischief with the adductors. The brain, heart, and extremities may contribute to these relationships in both good and bad ways. Figure 10-15 represents a "fun" example of these dysfunctional anatomic relationships.

Let's give this real circus performer the fictional name Rafael the Magnificent.

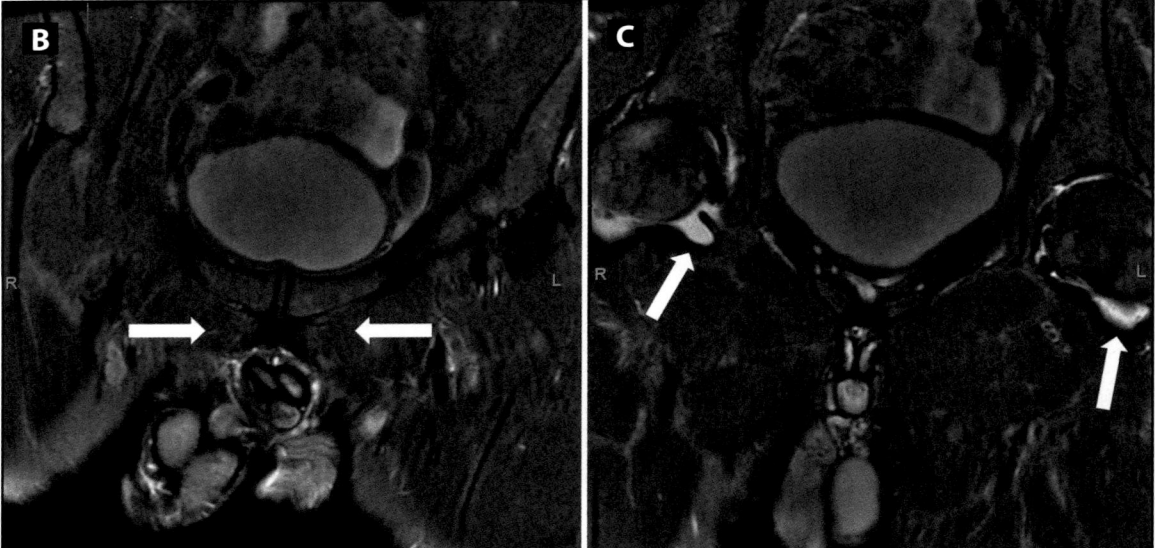

Figure 10-15. Born with the name Joe Dombrowski, Rafael, at age 10, was enthralled by the circus. He "always" knew he would become a circus acrobat and trapeze artist. His heart said this was the right thing to do. So, of course, at 16, he decided to run away from home and join the Pickle Brothers Circus. The problem was that his core anatomy did not agree with his heart and brain. He had pincer hip anatomy, which severely limited his hip rotation. He would never do the splits like he desired, nor be the Dominik Hasek (see Figure 10-1) of the circus. Those "silly" anatomic hindrances became only minor annoyances for his heart and brain. He practiced and practiced, and sure enough, he broke through the bony obstacles, gained more flexibility, and actually did pretty well in the circus. Rafael's core anatomy is now paying for what his heart and brain decided. Rafael now has continuous pain and needs total hip replacements. But remember, he did have a successful career in the circus. The MRI shows his hips and core muscles 25 years later, at age 41. (A) Pickle Family Circus. (Reprinted with permission from Aidan O'Shea.) (B) Chronic scarring, degeneration, and symmetrical partial separation and atrophy of the adductor attachments. Other views show bilateral plate detachments. This symmetrical pattern indicates overcompensation from the hips. (C) Hips with destroyed cartilage, labra, and acetabular bone.

SUMMARY

- The adductors are pretty important.
- They are complex and have multiple functions, and can suffer multiple types of injury.
- Yet, when you get right down to it, they are pretty understandable. It comes down mainly to understanding their anatomy and how they interact with the rest of the core.

SELECTED READINGS

Meyers WC, McKechnie A, Philippon MJ, Horner MA, Zoga AC, Devon ON. Experience with "sports hernia" spanning two decades. *Ann Surg.* 2008;248(4):656-665.
At the time of writing this review of our overall experience, we talked about doing both adductor "repairs" and "releases." In fact, we were not detaching the adductor muscles; we were performing fasciotomies, epimysiotomies, and other types of muscle belly decompressions.

Tips for turnout—achieving the ultimate range. The Ballet Blog. http://www.theballetblog.com/portfolio/training-turnout-part-1-achieving-your-ultimate-range/. Accessed August 2, 2016.
This article shows how dancers have really gotten into the anatomy of the core muscles. The article includes accurate anatomical diagrams and a downloadable Ebook on tips to improve your range, with special attention to advice for parents.

Hölmich P, Thorborg K, Dehlendorff C, Krogsgaard K, Gluud C. Incidence and clinical presentation of groin injuries in sub-elite male soccer. *Br J Sports Med.* 2014;48(16):1245-1250.
This excellent article asserts many inarguable facts about the adductors.

REFERENCES

1. Czech goaltender Hasek is out with groin injury. *Los Angeles Times.* http://articles.latimes.com/2006/feb/18/sports/sp-olyrep18. Published February 18, 2006. Accessed May 17, 2016.
2. Hölmich P, Thorborg K, Dehlendorff C, Krogsgaard K, Gluud C. Incidence and clinical presentation of groin injuries in sub-elite male soccer. *Br J Sports Med.* 2014;48(16):1245-1250.
3. Serner A, Tol J, Jomaah N, et al. Diagnosis of acute groin injuries: a prospective study of 110 athletes. *Am J Sports Med.* 2015;43(8):1857-1864.
4. Akermark C, Johansson C. Tenotomy of the adductor longus tendon in the treatment of chronic groin pain in athletes. *Am J Sports Med.* 1992;20(6):640-643.
5. Gill TJ, Carroll KM, Makani A, et al. Surgical technique for treatment of recalcitrant adductor longus tendinopathy. *Arthrosc Tech.* 2014;3(2):e293-e297.
6. Schilders E, Dimitrakopoulou A, Cooke M, Bismil Q, Cooke C. Effectiveness of a selective partial adductor release for chronic adductor-related groin pain in professional athletes. *Am J Sports Med.* 2013;41(3):603-607.
7. Strauss EJ, Campbell K, Bosco JA. Analysis of the cross-sectional area of the adductor longus tendon: a descriptive anatomic study. *Am J Sports Med.* 2007;35(6):996-999.
8. Boston's Clemens goes on disabled list. http://articles.latimes.com/1993-06-22/sports/sp-5645_1_disabled-list. *Los Angeles Times.* Published June 22, 1993. Accessed October 24, 2018.
9. Curry J. Clemens on disabled list after aggravating injury. *The New York Times.* https://www.nytimes.com/2002/07/14/sports/baseball-clemens-on-disabled-list-after-aggravating-injury.html. Published July 14, 2002. Accessed October 24, 2018.
10. Clemens' MRI shows he has scar tissue injury in right groin. ESPN. http://www.espn.com/mlb/news/story?id=2892971. Published June 4, 2007. Accessed October 24, 2018.

11

the rectus femoris
the "rodney dangerfield muscle"

I can't get no respect.

—The famous line from the monologues of comedian Rodney Dangerfield (Figure 11-1).

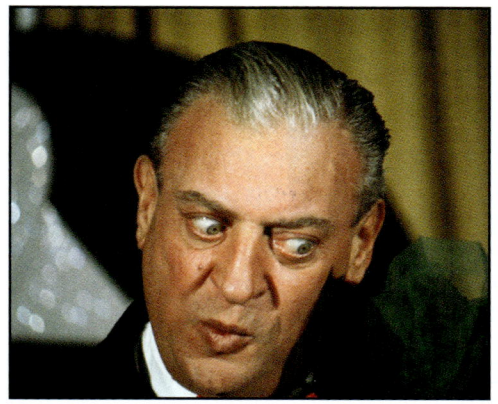

Figure 11-1. Rodney Dangerfield, the famous comedian who "gets no respect." (Reprinted with permission from AP Photo/Douglas C. Pizac.)

If you have ever watched David Lee play basketball, you might wonder how someone that big can jump that high, that quickly. Lee is a rebounding machine, and when he gets the ball close to the basket, opponents tend to get the hell out of the way, lest they show up on a poster featuring one of his monster dunks.

But all of that was in jeopardy before the 2012 playoffs, when Lee tore off his rectus femoris muscle.[1] That's the big boy in the quadriceps, the main muscle that runs from above the knee to the hip and is important for stability. The conventional wisdom was 3 to 5 months of rest and rehab to recover from the injury. So, Lee went back and played, despite the serious problem, which was repaired during the off-season. He even helped Golden State in its first playoff berth in 6 years.[1]

Injuries like this one should not have preset solutions. A savvy group of docs allowed Lee to play through his problem. Meanwhile, the athletic Sacramento Kings' Carl Landry tore his rectus femoris before the 2013-14 campaign and opted for surgery.[2,3] He missed 3 months of the season but came back healthy and worked his way back into the team's rotation. It's an individual thing.

Sometimes the prevailing belief needs be challenged, particularly when it's based on broad-spectrum data and no logic. Consider the NHL player who tore the muscle. Advised against surgery, he never got back on the ice. Finally, he went over the boards with frustration and sought new opinions. His hip had become compromised by unwelcome bone growth spurred by the torn muscle.

INTRODUCING THE RECTUS FEMORIS MUSCLE

More than any other muscle in the body, and just like Rodney Dangerfield's persona, the rectus femoris muscle needs a new or proper introduction to the sports medicine and fitness worlds at large (Figure 11-2). Those worlds have largely ignored this muscle.

For years, the muscle has gotten no respect and it still gets no respect. Come on, people…this muscle is important. Recognize that fact. That should be obvious simply from the massive position it occupies in the thigh. Not only does it command a huge presence, it also is the main muscle directly connecting the pelvis to the knee. It guards the hip. It compensates for the knee and the hip. It originates from one of the 3 pelvic bones, the ilium, and becomes the most anterior knee attachment, the patella.

Steve Martin was right: "A day without sunshine is like, you know, night." The rectus femoris muscle is so large and obvious (Figure 11-3). It's like night and day, some things are just so obvious.

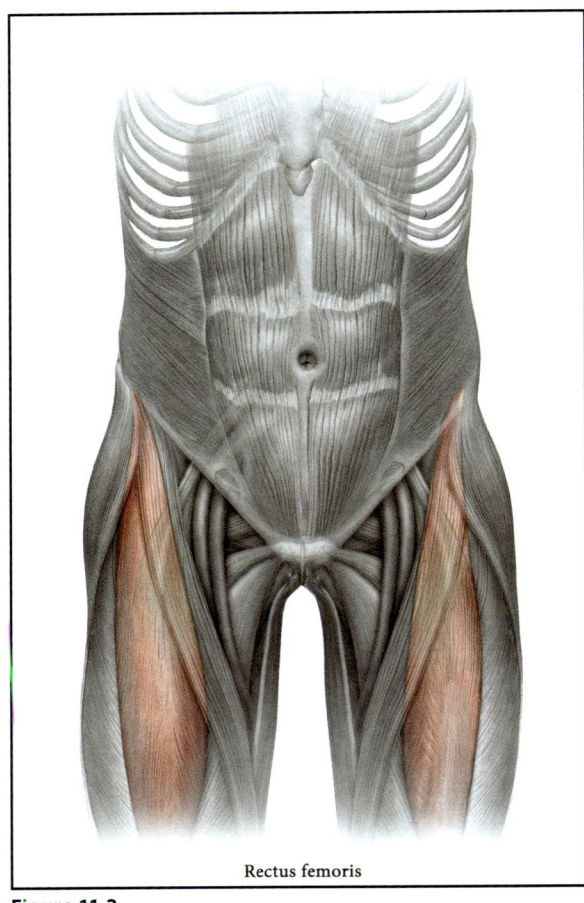

Figure 11-2.

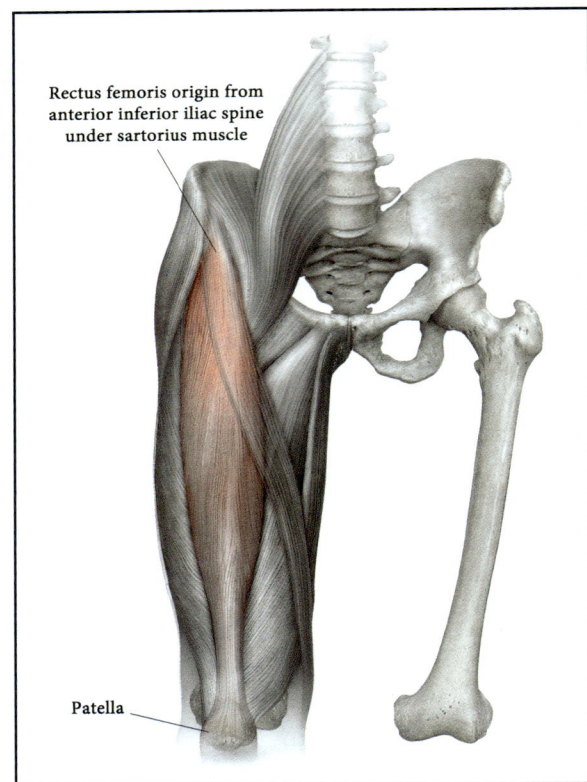

Figure 11-3. A more complete view of the rectus femoris.

And just like center/power forward David Lee or the massive players Shaquille O'Neal or Kendrick Perkins have such presence on the NBA court, we have to take notice of this big muscle. We must respect the presence in the thigh of this muscle, if only simply for the fact that it takes up so much space. It should be overstating the obvious to say that this muscle must be important for overall core or thigh stability. It's like day and night.

But that has not been the case. Its importance has been incredibly downplayed. When the rectus femoris gets ripped off, most surgeons have just said, "Oh, the rectus femoris doesn't matter, the thigh will function fine without it." Now, sit back in your chair, take a swig on your whiskey and puff of your cigar and ask the 2 obvious questions, "Where are the data for this lack of importance of the rectus femoris muscle?" And, "Who are these laissez-faire promoters kidding?" (See Figure 11-4.)

Simply said, the rectus femoris muscle gets no respect. That's why we call it the "Rodney Dangerfield muscle."

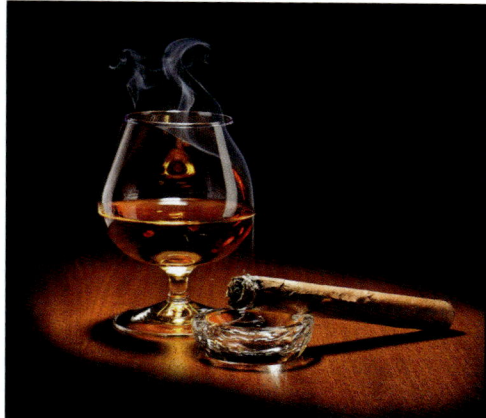

I was such an ugly kid, when I played in the sandbox the cat kept covering me up.

I remember the time I was kidnapped and they sent a piece of my finger to my father, he said he wanted more proof.

—Rodney Dangerfield.

Figure 11-4.

SO...WHY NO RESPECT?

So, where did our cheeky attitude come from with respect to the rectus femoris muscle? We're not sure. It probably came from us surgeons generally never attributing much importance to fixing muscles. For the most part, orthopedists have focused on the traditional joints and not on soft tissues; historically, orthopedists casted off soft tissue work to general surgeons. And as mentioned before, general surgeons don't generally think about biomechanics. In other words, the specialties of medicine exist as little fortresses without much communication between them. A lot of territory exists between the fortresses. The final reason for the attitude comes from the same terrain: surgeons just hadn't paid enough attention to develop the techniques for repairing the rectus femoris and other core muscles.

Whatever the case, a 2009 article in the *American Journal of Sports Medicine* certainly bolstered the same laissez-faire brashness. The conclusion in that article was: "Proximal avulsions of the rectus femoris can be treated nonoperatively with a high degree of predictability for return to full, unrestricted participation in professional American football."[4]

That oft-quoted conclusion became sports medicine dictum: Leave all ripped-off rectus femoris muscle alone.

Now consider 4 facts about that paper.

1. It reported only 11 patients.
2. This was a pure data-based study.
3. It came from the NFL.
4. The proband of that paper (ie, the player who triggered the interest for the authors to write it in the first place) reportedly ended up having hip surgery due to a complication of not having repaired the muscle in the first place. He apparently developed heterotopic ossification (HO), which led to hip impingement.[5]

Let's look even deeper into the printed observations in that paper. The careers of only 6 of the 11 injured players were available for analysis, and 2 of those 6 were place-kickers. We already mentioned the proband, who continued with symptoms. The second player interviewed was a long snapper, not exactly the most strenuous position, and he played for 2 more seasons. No mention was made about whether his avulsion was of the direct or indirect head of the rectus femoris for 9 of the 11 players. The authors recognized that most avulsions occur in the indirect head and not the direct head, the most important attachment. It turns out that avulsions of the indirect heads are relatively minor injuries and don't usually require surgery. We have subsequently found that place-kickers suffer primarily indirect head avulsions. One of the only 6 players followed up in the paper persisted with symptoms. Interestingly, in the paper's discussion, the authors mention multiple outside reports of failed attempts of nonoperative management. They also mention that these injuries are likely underreported.

So, let's summarize. The primary paper in the literature bolstering a routine nonoperative approach to complete avulsions of the rectus femoris muscle had follow-up on only 6 patients, only 2 of whom were interviewed had surgery. Two others of the 6 likely had injuries that ordinarily never require surgery (ie, indirect head tears), and the 1 remaining player was a long snapper. Plus, 1 player, likely the one with persistent symptoms, played just 1 more year in the NFL. That means, using the most favorable possible statistics, the nonoperative approach, so eloquently endorsed by this article, had a 50% or 75% failure rate in the 4 patients with injuries possibly germane to the topic.

Plus, most of the case reports and small case series in the literature at that time and including the ones cited by the authors of that paper endorsed operative management of rectus femoris avulsions, usually after a trial of nonoperative therapy.[2,3,6,7] It is difficult to find anything at all on acute operative repair of big avulsions, even though they happen frequently.

Therefore, judging from the data presented in that bolstering paper, it should be clear as day that the authors' conclusion is just plain wrong. Not only that, but it also seems obvious that rectus femoris injuries ought to be associated with significant disability. It turns out that more information on this muscle simply does not exist in the medical literature.

So... bearing in mind how much space the rectus femoris muscle occupies in the thigh and how little attention this enormous muscle gets, what's the story? Shouldn't we take this muscle much more seriously?

Talk about no respect.

Rodney, move over...

RECTUS FEMORIS INJURIES

To be fair, the above NFL database study also does not say that these players do better with surgery. The paper simply concludes, albeit wrongly, that nonoperative treatment is the way to go. We docs sometimes jump to conclusions on the basis of bias or minimal data.

It is time to discard this attitude and keep an open mind about rectus femoris injuries. Treatment likely depends on the situation. We have not yet published our full experience, yet we know that selected patients with complete rectus femoris avulsions do very well with repairs. Plus, seeing more and more such injuries in high-performance athletes, we can say, without uncertainty, that certain types of injuries left untreated lead to suboptimal performance and premature retirement from sports. Like other core muscles, quite a variety of injuries befall the rectus femoris muscle. Here are a few examples.

Keep in mind the anatomy of the rectus femoris muscle. Its main head originates from the anterior inferior iliac spine (AIIS), and its minor (indirect head) originates from a small grove posteriorly in the acetabulum. They quickly join and become a big muscle bulk that flattens and narrows as it becomes the patella. Three muscles named vastus (medialis, lateralis, and intermedius) combine with the rectus femoris to become a large fleshy mass of muscle known as the *quadriceps mechanism*. Surgeons tend to give the 3 vastus muscles too much credit. But face it. Those 3 other muscles just don't make up for loss of their leader, the Rodney Dangerfield muscle.

Case 1. Acute Complete Avulsion

A professional basketball player experiences a sudden pop in his right anterior thigh. The player still felt weak at 6 weeks after the injury. An initial MRI showed a "strain." Figure 11-5 is the MRI 6 weeks after the event.

The player still underwent repair and was back at full performance at just 3 months postoperatively. There was considerable atrophy and retraction of the muscle stump. Yet, the repair went well, and the muscle was easily mobilized. Muscle mass and function fully returned. These repairs are much easier if they are done within the first week or two of the injury.

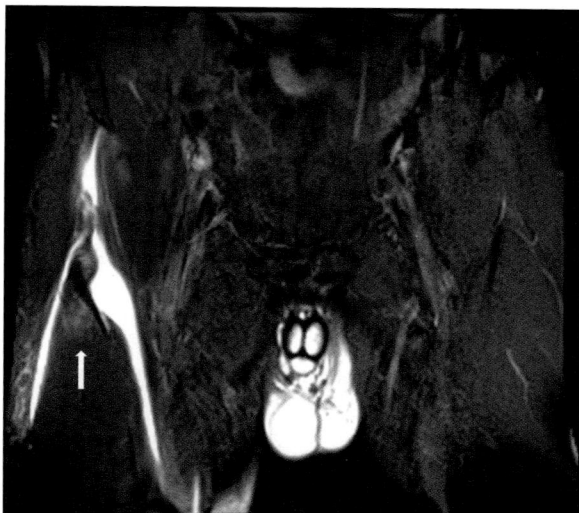

Figure 11-5. T2 coronal image of the NBA player with a complete rectus femoris avulsion. Arrow points to the main, now shredded stump of the muscle retracted 5 to 10 cm away from its origin on the pelvic bone. The white represents blood and reactive fluid. Note the shredded appearance, which represents that the muscle ripped like a telescope. Obviously, the entire rectus femoris is ripped off. It is not possible to discriminate between the direct and indirect heads, nor does that make a difference in treatment of this patient.

Comment: *Repairs of rectus femoris avulsions turn out to be very straightforward for the most part, and with good mobilization and without much tension, good primary repair can lead to early return to full performance.*

Case 2. Second Complete Avulsion on Top of an Untreated First-Time Avulsion

This patient initially ripped his entire rectus femoris muscle off at its origin near the hip. Untreated, he developed severe new bone formation as part of the healing process. When he got back to play, he ripped off the same muscle again, but in a new location (ie, below the previous bone-laden healing point). The healing process caused a new area of traction for the muscle to tear off.

An NFL linebacker had a complete avulsion of the rectus femoris that was treated nonoperatively and never got back to full play after a season and a half. Then, finally, during preseason camp after he was resigned by another team, he experienced another acute "pop" a couple of inches down from the rectus femoris insertion. It turns out that he had formed tremendous HO at the AIIS. At surgery, we (1) carved away the HO, actually relieving chronic hip impingement symptoms, and (2) did a direct muscle-to-muscle repair of the second, more distal avulsion. The player returned to full action in the NFL the following season without pain and still performs well 2 years later. (See Figure 11-6.)

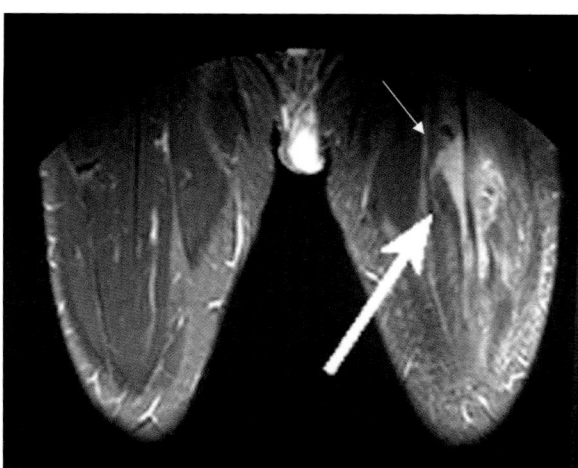

Figure 11-6. Avulsion "after an avulsion." Arrows point to the proximal (thin arrow) and distal (thick arrow) muscle stumps. This NFL linebacker had a lot of proximal HO. One can see a small, thick, dark stump of fibrosis next to the proximal stump. Interestingly, a symmetrical-looking stump appears on his other (right) side. In fact, he had also developed a similar, less severe injury on that right side.

Comment: *With so many "nonrepairs" out there, this situation of avulsion on top of an old avulsion is not rare.*

Case 3. Complete Avulsion Without Repair; Then Many Years of Adductor, Vastus, and Other Muscle, Knee, and Hip Injuries

A prominent major league shortstop rips off his left rectus femoris muscle and goes through an entire season with pain there, as well as compensatory symptoms in other regions of the core. He can still palpate his own rectus femoral stump whenever he flexes his thigh. He also developed chronic knee issues. Midway through the next season, he starts to rip off muscle after muscle. Over a 2-month time frame he tears off the adductor longus in 2 locations distal to its pubic plate attachment, the pectineus (completely) and adductor brevis. In addition, he develops 2 large adductor magnus muscle belly tears and rips his pubic plate at the origin so that it begins to involve the rectus abdominis on that side. At surgery, the rectus femoris stump is too frozen to do a repair. The other muscles turn out to be reparable and he gets placed on a rigorous core training program and does well for the next 2 years, until he has to have his hip repaired arthroscopically due to the resultant HO and impingement. He continues with problems, now more on the opposite side. He still stars for one of the MLB lead contenders. (See Figure 11-7.)

This player, as well as a number of others whom we care for, is not unique.

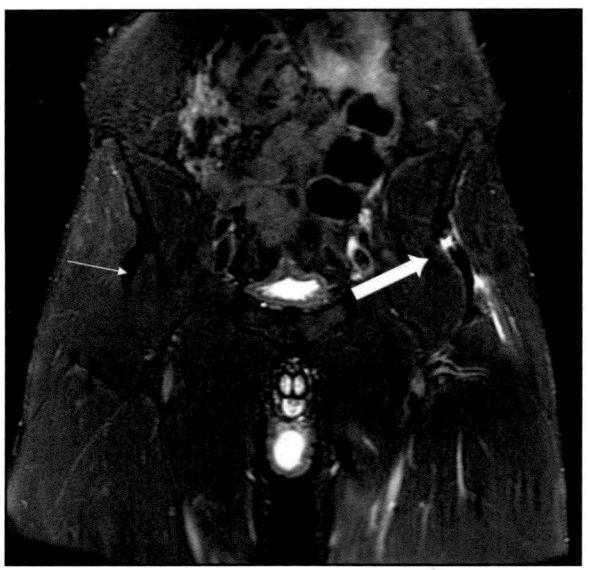

Figure 11-7. MLB shortstop with a small acute left rectus femoris avulsion (thick arrow). But, the shortstop also had a chronic right rectus femoris avulsion. Note the unrepaired stump (thin arrow). For years after the right-sided injury, the patient suffered from numerous injuries to other core muscles. The point is that, untreated, rectus femoris avulsions tip the core's balance and lead to other core injuries on either side. This shortstop also developed knee problems on the side of the untreated injury.

Comment: *Loss of the rectus femoris causes a "thigh instability" that puts the other muscles, the pubic joint, the hip, and likely the ACL of the knee at risk. We see this situation over and over.*

Case 4. Rectus Femoris Indirect Head Avulsion

One of the top NFL placekickers develops a "pop" at the right (dominant foot) rectus femoris insertion site. The MRI is clear; it shows an avulsion of *just* the indirect head. This took 2.5 months to resolve, but it did so completely. The player returned to his occupation without further difficulty.

Comment: *In our experience, indirect head rectus femoris injury does not usually require surgery, so long as good imaging shows the direct head to be intact.*

Case 5. Rectus Femoris Heterotopic Ossification Leading to Hip Impingement (Figure 11-8)

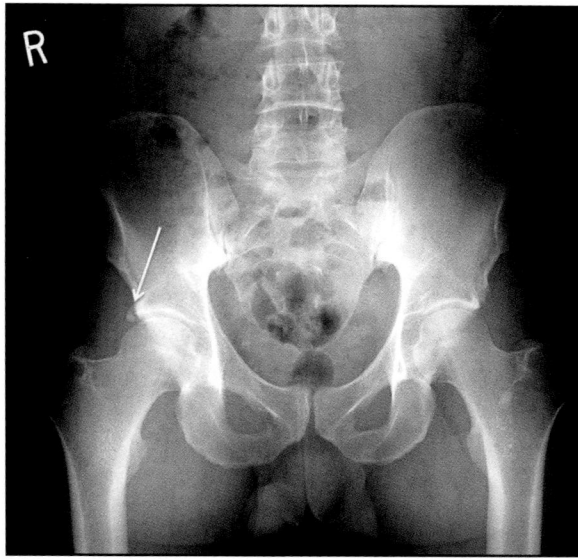

Figure 11-8. An X-ray of a soccer player with HO from an old rectus femoris injury, which led to hip arthroscopy. This HO was seen at surgery. From the image alone, one cannot tell that the new bone is not a bone chip from pincer impingement.

Comment: *We have seen many cases of HO following rectus femoris avulsion leading to hip surgery. It is difficult to say for sure that the rectus femoris avulsion alone can cause hip problems. But the coincidence occurs so frequently that it is hard not to believe a contributory mechanism.*

Case 6. Rectus Femoris Compartment Syndrome Complicating Hip Impingement Surgery

A high-level Argentinian soccer ("football") player underwent a seemingly successful arthroscopic femoroacetabular impingement (FAI) surgery. Most of the symptoms went away. Yet, he still had considerable pain with active and passive flexion and extension of the hip. It turned out that the pain was coming purely from a tight rectus femoris compartment, which, no doubt, developed as a compensatory mechanism from years of impingement. He underwent a rectus femoral compartmental (fascial/epimyseal) decompression. Pain completely resolved, and the player returned to full play and has had no pain for over 2 years after that. No doubt, the rectus femoris muscle is a key protector of the hip. (See Figure 11-9.)

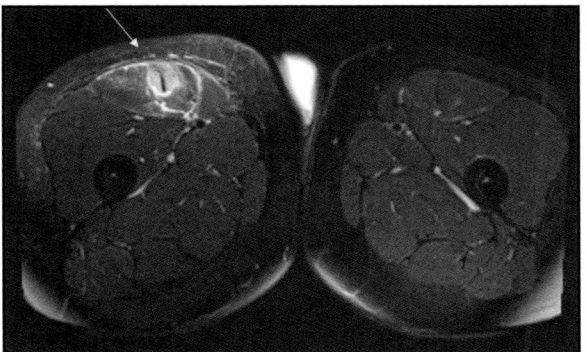

Figure 11-9. A player with severe (arrow) rectus femoris reactive compartment syndrome.

Comment: *Rectus femoris compartment syndrome occurs frequently as part of the hip impingement syndrome. We see this both before and after hip arthroscopic repair. It seems that both the rectus femoris and adductors are principle protectors of the hip and serve, in part, to prevent maximal range of motion of the hip. Of course, like with other muscles throughout the body, continual muscular spasming leads to injury and stricture.*

Case 7. NBA Player Returns to Full Play Just Four Weeks After Complete Rectus Femoris Avulsion

This veteran center's career was on the line. It was just 2 months before the start of the season and he was going into his contract year when he "popped" the direct and indirect heads of his rectus femoris muscle. He knew he was already "trade bait"; plus, he knew he was going to be on the free agent market at the end of the year. As he explained, it was "ultra-important" that he be on the court at the start of the season in order to show that he was healthy. Also, he announced that he was "deathly afraid" of general or spinal anesthesia and would not consent to that. The direct stump was just 1.5 cm away from the AIIS. The repair was performed under local anesthesia. Generous fascial/epimyseal decompression allowed the muscle to come right up and be sutured to the fibrocartilaginous plate and adjacent muscle. He had an excellent season and still plays as a back-up center in the NBA. (See Figure 11-10.)

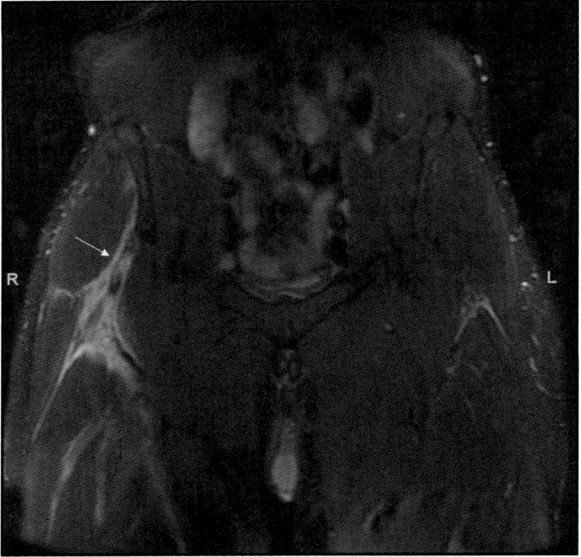

Figure 11-10. Right rectus femoris avulsion in an NBA player. The injury was repaired under local anesthesia. The arrow points to retracted rectus femoris heads.

Comment: *We are not advocating the minimally invasive approach as a routine technique. It worked in this case. The clinical situation seemed fitting for us to try something new. One might also ask if this unusual situation warranted the risk of platelet-rich plasma. We remain afraid of platelet-rich plasma here and in the adductor region because of an inherent risk of HO.*

TREATMENT ALGORITHM

As you can tell from what we just said, we do advocate a more aggressive approach with complete avulsions of the rectus femoris muscle. See the proposed general treatment algorithm (Figure 11-11).

Of course, the numbers are too few to ever have a good, randomized, prospective analysis that might prove what this algorithm represents. In recommending this algorithm, we revert back to olden days of logic, judgment, and empiricism. Hume might call that triad of cognitive function "the informal logic of scientific inquiry."[8] The triad here comes alongside an immense experience with these specific injuries. The primary 2 points of this chapter are (1) the logic stinks when it comes to a dogmatic, nonoperative approach with respect to rectus femoris injuries; and (2) we need to pay more respect to Rodney Dangerfield.

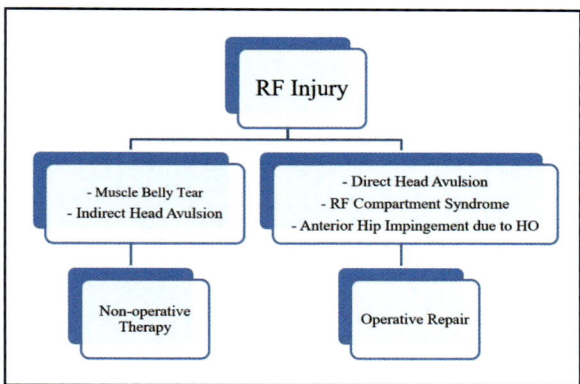

Figure 11-11. Algorithm for treating rectus femoris injuries. Certainly, most tears in the substance of the muscle or of the indirect head should initially be treated nonoperatively. We strongly advocate early operative repair of direct head avulsions in most athletes or other patients. Severe rectus femoris compartment syndrome is an indication for operative decompression; the same can be said for rectus femoris HO leading to hip impingement.

NEXT MUSCLE

So much for the rectus femoris muscle. There is so much more to say, but we shall end the discussion now.

In the spirit of Drew Rosenhaus's Terrell Owens "next-question" press conference (see Figure 5-3), it is time to declare: "Next muscle!"

SELECTED READINGS

Meyers WC, Havens BK, Horner GJ. Core muscle injury (a better name than "athletic pubalgia" or "sports hernia"). *Curr Orthop Prac.* 2014;25(4):321-326.
This relatively recently published review of core muscle injuries mentions the importance of the rectus femoris muscle and its treatment in the context of other core muscle injuries.

Gamradt SC, Brophy RH, Barnes R, Warren RF, Byrd JWT, Kelly BT. Nonoperative treatment for proximal avulsion of the rectus femoris in professional American football. *Am J Sports Med.* 2009;37(7):1370-1374.
This paper is what we are up against. The authors of the paper might give you updated scoop.

Ueblacker P, Muller-Wohlfahrt H, Hinterwimmer S, Imhoff AB, Feucht MJ. Suture anchor repair of proximal rectus femoris avulsions in elite football players. *Knee Surg Sports Traumatol Arthrosc.* 2015;23:2590-2594.
A nice case series documenting repairs in 4 soccer players. Prepare to see more papers demonstrating successful operative results.

REFERENCES

1. Thompson M. Warriors' David Lee: hip injury was worse than expected. *The Mercury News.* https://www.mercurynews.com/2013/09/04/warriors-david-lee-hip-injury-was-worse-than-expected/. Published September 4, 2013. Accessed May 22, 2016.
2. Straw R, Colclough K, Geutjens G. Surgical repair of a chronic rupture of the rectus femoris muscle at the proximal musculotendinous junction in a soccer player. *Br J Sports Med.* 2003;37:182-184.
3. Rajasekhar C, Kumar KS, Bhamra MS. Avulsion fractures of the anterior inferior iliac spine: the case for surgical intervention. *Int Orthop.* 2001;24:364-365.
4. Gamradt SC, Brophy RH, Barnes R, Warren RF, Byrd JWT, Kelly BT. Nonoperative treatment for proximal avulsion of the rectus femoris in professional American football. *Am J Sports Med.* 2009;37(7):1370-1374.
5. Personal communication with the senior author of Reference 4.
6. Irmola T, Heikkilä JT, Orava S, Sarimo J. Total proximal tendon avulsion of the rectus femoris muscle. *Scand J Med Sci Sports.* 2007;17:378-382.
7. Saluan PM, Weiker GG. Avulsion of the anterior inferior iliac spine. *Orthopedics.* 1997;20:558-559.
8. Finocchiaro MA. Empiricism, judgment, and argument: toward an informal logic of science. *Argumentation.* 1988;2:313. doi:10.1007/BF00176970.

12

the iliopsoas
aka the psoas
aka the "eminem muscle"

I am sort of hip to the younger stuff...Eminem...although he curses sometimes.
—President Barack Obama.

    As the 2005 season wore on, the 2 most used words by Philadelphia Eagles fans were "sports hernia." Even though the thing doesn't exist, there was definitely something wrong with quarterback Donovan McNabb. In quarterbacks, core problems can begin in the preseason, in the psoas muscle, with all the repetitive rotational forces incurred in throwing to their receivers. Sometimes, a steroid injection—not that kind of steroid—relieves the problem. Sometimes not.

I say what I want to say and do what I want to do. There's no in-between. People will either love you for it or hate you for it.
—Eminem.

THE SLIM SHADY MUSCLE

People either love the iliopsoas muscle or hate it. No matter the case, everybody agrees the "Eminem muscle" is important (Figures 12-1 and 12-2).

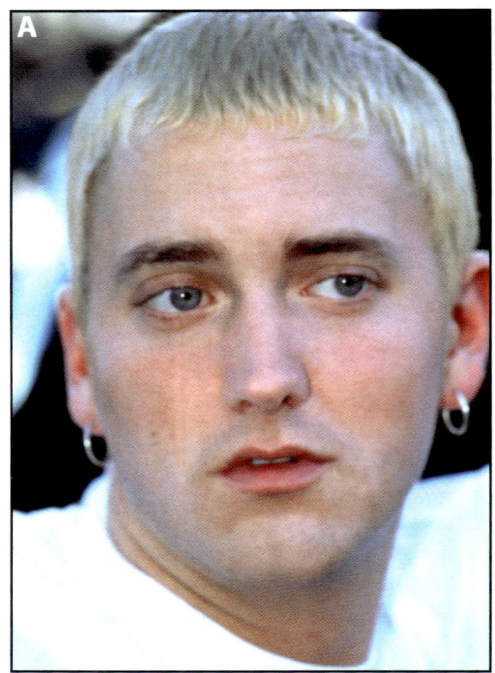 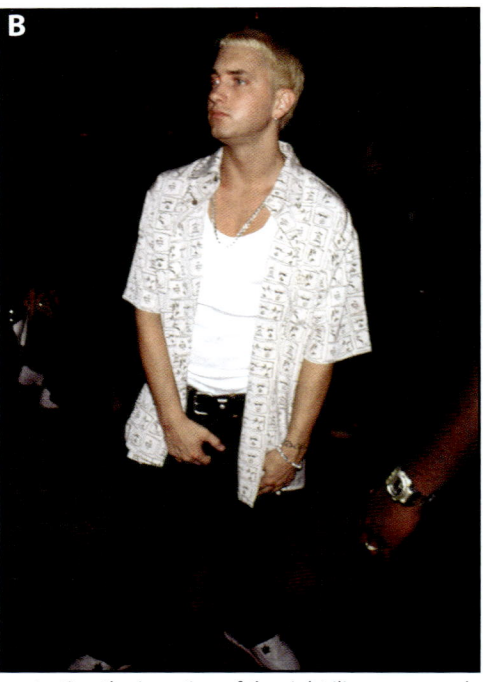

Figure 12-1. The rapper Eminem. (A) Head shot. (B) Demonstrating the insertion of the right iliopsoas muscle onto the lesser trochanter of the hip bone.

Like Eminem, the iliopsoas is big and mysterious. It somehow links the core muscles and the hip. We know that function is vital, especially for a passer, who must twist and contort his body to deliver the ball. As McNabb's core became more of a problem, it became obvious that for McNabb the psoas was calling the signals. Finally, a different set of pains became too much, and he had to have season-ending surgery.

Because of its relatively deep location, the psoas can lead some physicians to think a person's pain is due to a hip problem. Take 6-time All-Star slugger José Bautista, who struggled with pain in the area until it was found that his trouble wasn't bone but muscle related. A simple injection returned José to knocking the ball out of the park.

The psoas is a mysterious muscle (Figure 12-3). It is superficial and deep, and in part thick and in part thin. Its strong nature stabilizes things. At the same time, it may stiffen, rap, and rub you the wrong way—and generally be a pain. It's its own thing; it imitates, it mimics the adjacent troublesome environment. It also triggers headaches. Yes, it is one and the same. It's Eminem. We would write this chapter like the theatrical production *Hamilton* (ie, in rap), but we are not smart enough.

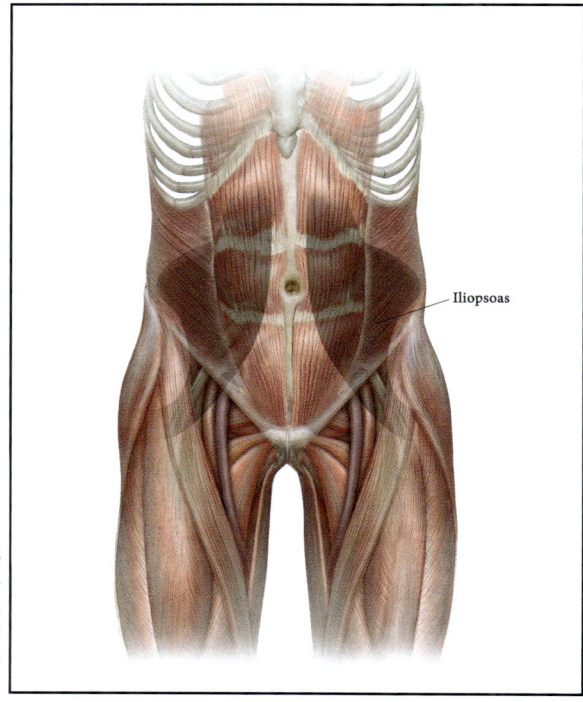

Figure 12-2. Shadowed in gray behind the anterior core musculature, the psoas and iliacus muscles join forces and form a unit. The functions may mimic actions of the harness muscles or the power muscles. The psoas protects the hip, but, when inflamed, may mimic signs of hip dysfunction. Note the shadowy "Slim Shady muscle" in this illustration. This muscular unit lurks back there. The large muscle is both mysterious and important.

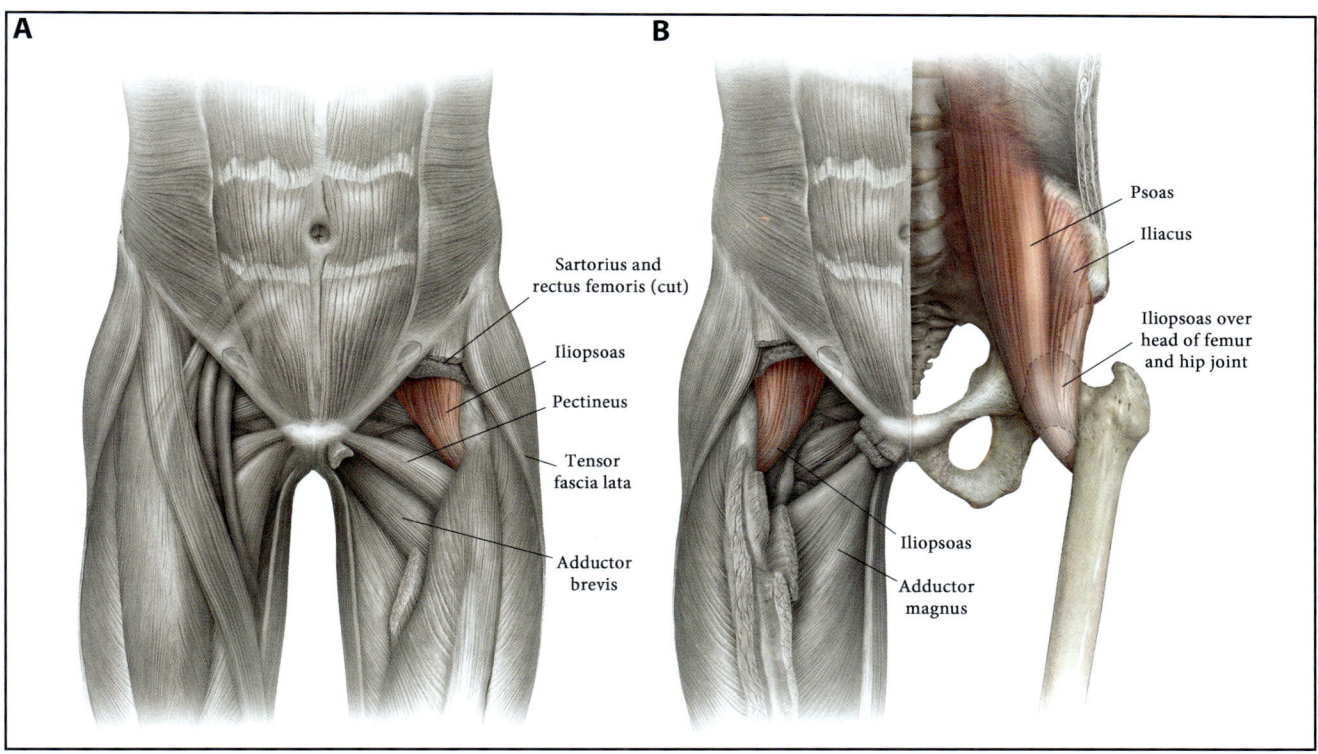

Figure 12-3. Our artist Rob now reveals Slim Shady in more realistic red, lurking behind the more superficial muscles. Various anterior muscles have been cut away in order to expose it. Figures 12-3 and 12-4 underscore some of the relationships with adjacent muscles. (A) Compare the 2 sides. The right medial thigh is intact, and the left side has 2 muscles divided. Both sides accentuate the space that may exist between Slim Shady and the other muscles. Inflammation within this space may travel in various directions and mimic hip and various muscles syndromes. (B) Two more perspectives of Slim Shady. Note the ghost of the head and neck of the femur on the left side.

The psoas is meant to be loved, not necessarily understood.

—An arthroscopic hip surgeon.

WHY ALL THE MYSTERY ABOUT THE EMINEM MUSCLE?

The answer is easy…because physicians and scientists just have not studied it enough. Failure to recognize the core as an important part of the body accounts for this lack of study. Who would have the interest to study the psoas? Orthopedists? Certainly not…the muscle is way too close to so many "dangerous" blood vessels and organs. General surgeons? No way… wouldn't that mean the general surgeon would have to know some biomechanics?

One instance in my past drives home why this muscle remains so mysterious. As a junior attending at Duke, I became the go-to general surgeon for J. Leonard Goldner, our famous Chairman of Orthopedics. One of the things J. Leonard was famous for was "anterior lumbar fusions." In his hands, and with his careful selection of patients, the procedure involved bone grafting the spine and was highly successful. It often cured long-standing, disabling back pain. Dr. Goldner operated on several such patients per week.

J. Leonard chose me to help him because I was quick and efficient and because he did not understand most of the anatomy surrounding the lumbar spine (eg, the bowel, the aorta, the inferior vena cava, all those big things that might cause him trouble). By the same token, I knew nothing about the lumbar spine. I would dissect all the organs and big blood vessels away from the psoas muscle and lower vertebrae in a lickety-split fashion. Of course, I initially felt proud to have been chosen to do this for this wonderful, great orthopedic surgeon. But the number of cases kept mounting; they took way too much time, and kept me from doing many other things I had to do. From my perspective then, I was doing all the surgical dissection, J. Leonard came in for a few minutes, sprinkled in a few bone chips, and took away all the glory! Don't get me wrong. I was never bitter. I am just exaggerating my feelings just to get the point across. I loved Dr. Goldner; he was absolutely wonderful and treated me like a son.

Thinking back on those years, I can now see what was going on. J. Leonard knew a lot about the back. He was an orthopedist who had been trained in orthopedics. He knew all about the bones and nerves. But Dr. Goldner would have gotten into big trouble dissecting away the aorta, the ureter, and everything else in this anatomic region that was so important. He might have caused sudden massive hemorrhage or poop to spill all over the spine. On the flip side, I knew all about most of those other organs back there. Because of our differences in training, I could perform all these dissections well. I had those skill sets even though I knew nothing about biomechanics. When I think about it now, neither one of us then knew much about that massive muscle staring at us in the face during those dissections—the psoas.

Bingo. In a nutshell, the above story solves the mystery. We don't know more about the iliopsoas for 2 reasons: (1) the biomechanics experts are afraid to go into this region, and (2) the people who are not afraid to enter into this region know nothing about biomechanics. Of course, the region is also deep and hard to get to. That might have had something to do with it, too.

That is why surgeons say, "Obviously, the psoas is important but…" At that point in their sentence, their voices trail off.

What We Know About the Iliopsoas

What we do know about it takes just a couple of paragraphs. Make that a couple of sentences. We can describe where the muscle sits, that it is big and strong, and that it must have important roles in the function of the hip and pelvis. We also know that its function must vary according to alterations in the pelvis's bony structure or nearby muscles. Yes, that's all we know. Two sentences, that's what it takes.

Most of the time, we can't even decide whether to call it the "psoas" or the "iliopsoas" muscle.

Where It Sits

The Eminem muscle's location is actually tricky. One can think of there being 2 muscles—the psoas and the iliacus—in the abdomen, and then 2 muscles merge as they go deeper into the pelvis and thigh. Usually as it travels down, another smaller muscle sits on top of the psoas—the psoas minor. This muscle is likely not too important except as an augmenter to the overall function of the psoas. Now that we have mentioned the latter muscle, forget about it, we shall not mention it again. Plus, we shall not use the term *psoas major*. In the spirit of keeping things simple, forget "major" and "minor." Use the term *psoas* without a modifier. We shall use of that term in this chapter both strictly to portray the specific abdominal muscle and lazily as a nickname for the whole iliopsoas. When we use "Eminem muscle," sometime we are trying to get across both the muscle's mystery and importance (Figures 12-4 through 12-7).

The psoas comes from the lateral aspects of the lowermost thoracic and most of the lumbar vertebral bodies and discs. One usually thinks in terms of it arising from T12 to L4 or L5. The iliacus comes from the anterior surface of the iliac bone, the so-called iliac fossa. For the most part, these origins don't make much difference because both fitness experts and surgeons rarely work back there. The muscles quickly become big and fleshy as they travel south and then narrow near the lesser trochanter. Clinically, we deal both with fleshy and tendinous parts after they merge. The combined muscle has a variety of different looks as it goes more distally and ends on the lesser trochanter of the femur. It can be one or multiple thick tendons or mostly fleshy muscle or both tendinous and fleshy.[1]

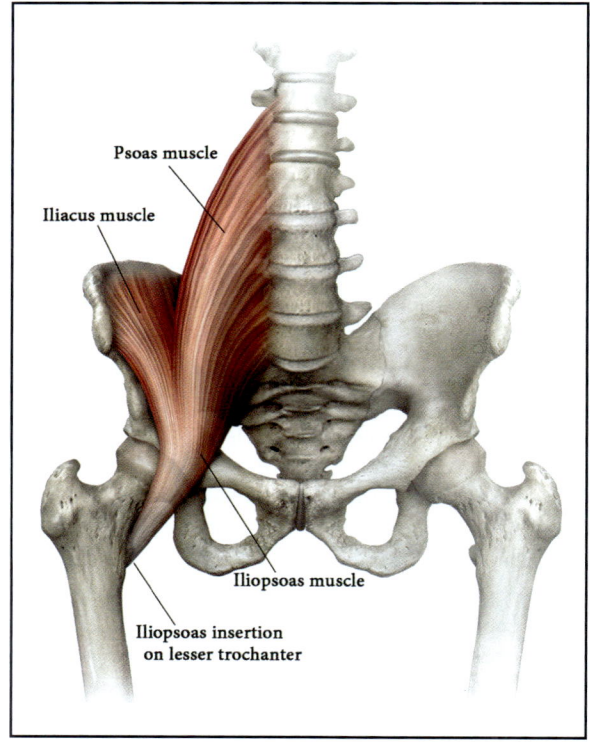

Figure 12-4. The iliopsoas forms from 2 muscles, the psoas and the iliacus, and its union is quite variable in terms of the sites of union and relative contributions of muscle bulk and tendon.

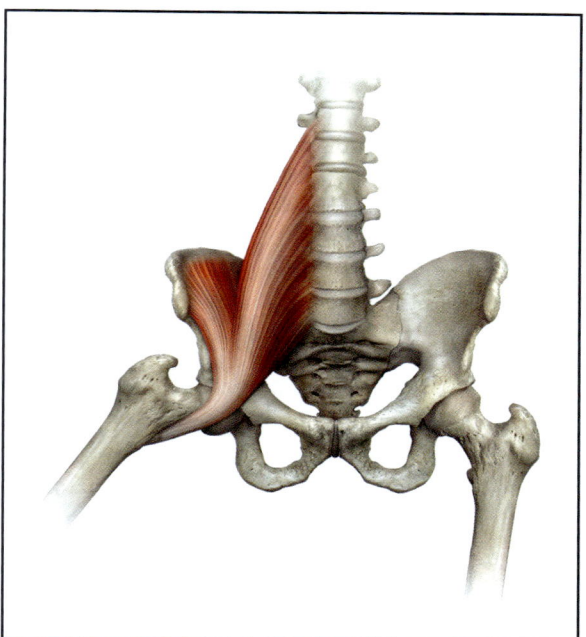

Figure 12-5. Abduction or extension highlights the muscle's intimacy with the hip. The closest areas of contact with the hip remain somewhat controversial.

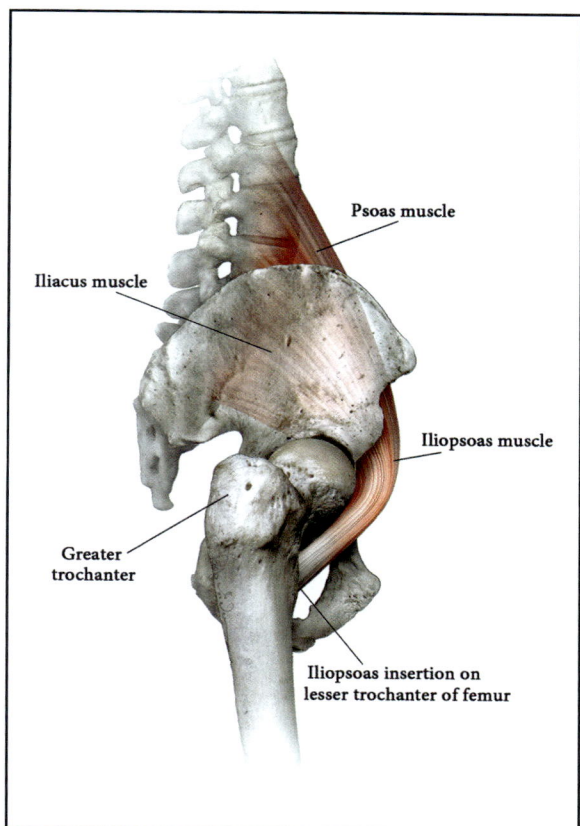

Figure 12-6. A sagittal view exhibits how the combined muscle hugs the contour of the head of the femur before it inserts onto the lesser trochanter.

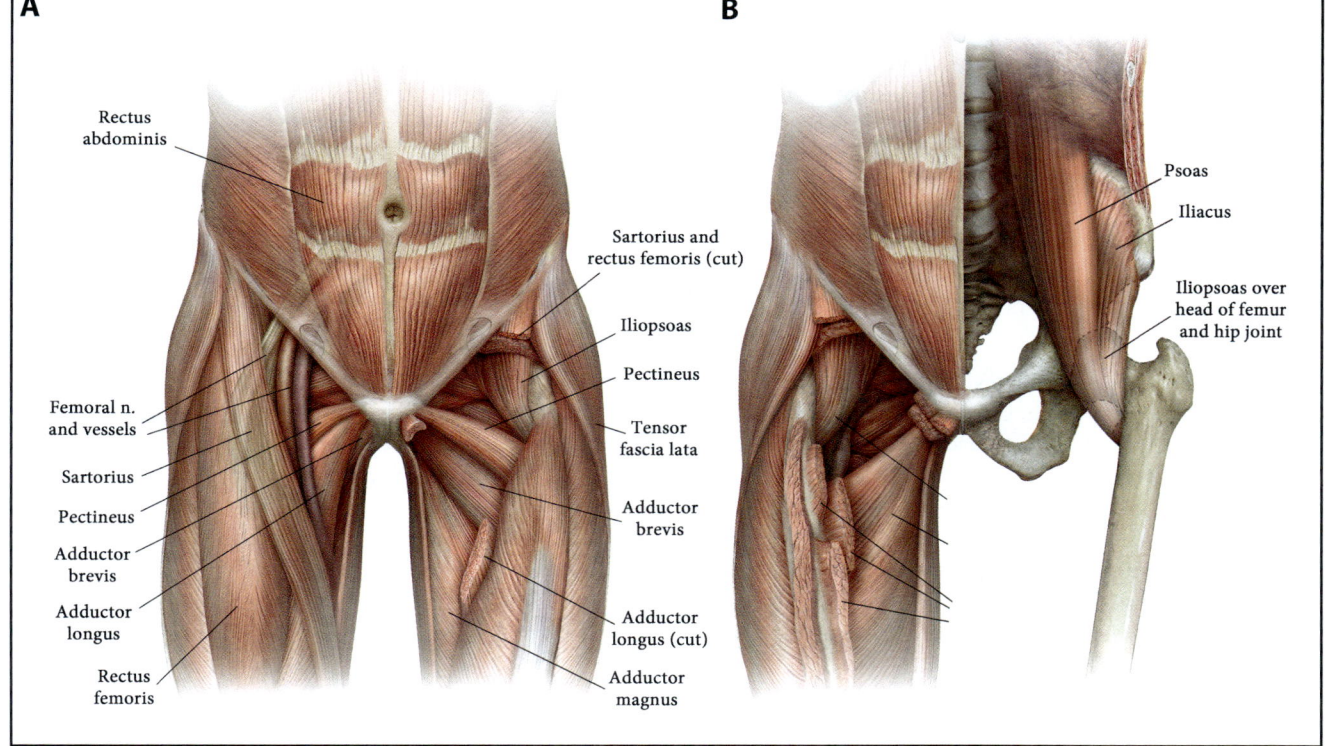

Figure 12-7. Two more perspectives on the mysterious muscle. Don't forget other nearby muscles. The rectus femoris and iliopsoas share intimate anatomic relationships in helping with the muscular component of hip stability. Note the proximity to the adductors.

Several subtle anatomic points turn out important with respect to surgery on the iliopsoas muscle and/or hip. Many of the connections of the psoas to the iliacus muscles and to other nearby soft tissues occur at or distal to the ball-and-socket hip joint. The tendon-muscle complex lies intimately anterior to the hip capsule and anterior labrum. Debate exists whether the bony "iliopectineal eminence" of the hip socket or the ball of the femur is a principal culprit in some of the severe inflammatory "hip-snapping" conditions that occur in this region. Arthroscopic hip surgeons claim that adherence to the labrum accounts for certain ("3 o'clock") labral tears.[2] The small iliocapsularis muscle might also play a role in that type of tear. It seems best to think much more broadly and in terms of a variety of anatomic factors contributing to the numerous pains that occur in this area.

An underappreciated fact is how many more connections exist between the iliacus and psoas and other soft tissues distal to the ball-and-socket hip joint and proximal to the iliopsoas's insertion on the lesser trochanter, compared to the number of connections superior to the hip joint. Our artist Rob's picture of the iliopsoas displays this observation quite vividly (see Figures 12-4 and 12-5). One simply sees more muscle connectivity the more distal you go. That anatomic fact may account for why partial lengthening procedures of the muscle's most distal aspect (ie, near the lesser trochanter) seems to carry so much less morbidity than "lengthenings" or "partial releases" at the level of the joint, where they are done during hip arthroscopy.[3] From what we have seen, the latter approach carries with it the risk of dramatic total or subtotal proximal retraction of the psoas muscle. That event can be innocuous or associated with profound weakness or pain.

Function, Strength, and Stability

Function

Functionally, think of the psoas in primarily flexion and extension and secondarily external and internal rotation. One can debate the more important function, but the more important distinction to define better is what particular part of the body the muscle is flexing or rotating. One usually thinks in terms of the psoas flexing only the hip and thigh. When one considers its long length of origin, it also serves importantly to flex and straighten the vertebral column.

Look at Rob's pictures (see Figures 12-5 through 12-7) and appreciate that rotational direction is largely determined by the body's orientation at the time of contraction. Usually, the psoas externally rotates the hip. Look at how we can barely see the lesser trochanter in the straight-on views; thereby, contraction would make the greater trochanter go posteriorly (ie, externally rotate). Geometrically though, if one is already maximally externally rotated, the iliopsoas then internally rotates.

Considering its main functions, guess which sports or positions within sports would place the psoas at most risk for injury. You are right—sports or positions with a lot of up-and-down action or ones that involve a lot of rotational action while the person remains relatively upright. Think further: basketball players, runners, quarterbacks, tennis players, divers…the list goes on. Also think of players with their own unique ways of doing things, such as José Bautista, who generates so much power with a stance with the front leg flexed and in the air and then steps down strongly at the initiation of his swing.

Strength

Muscular volume estimates of strength place the iliopsoas first as the strongest flexor of the trunk or core, with the pubic bone the center point. Certainly, the psoas is stronger than either the tensor fascia lata or sartorius. One may have a harder time arguing that in all cases with respect to the rectus femoris. The rectus femoris is usually but not always smaller than the psoas. Then one must add in location and leverage arguments. The rectus femoris is more purely anterior and takes no turns or bends at all. Its deep central location and the pulley/leverage dynamic resulting from its various turns and bends augment psoas strength enough for it to remain in first place in the core flexor category. Other arguments come into play when some of the back muscles get included in the discussion.

Okay, enough of that discussion. Let's leave this subject with one of the "central" themes of the book (pun intended). The more central the location of the muscle in the core, the more critical its function is likely to be. The psoas is strong and central. It must be pretty important.

Stability

The argument about strength and central location plays well for a key role for the psoas in overall core stability. One would guess, for example, that the psoas's strength in flexion would take some of the load away from the harness muscles (see Chapters 8 through 10) during sit-ups and protect them.

Now let's get back the psoas's anatomic location. Note how close it is to the hip. We just discussed that some surgeons speculate that it plays a direct role in the pathophysiology of some labral tears. Note in Rob's diagrams also how the strong Eminem muscle bends anteriorly around the hip joint, as if to protect it. Is it possible that the psoas plays a huge role in overall hip stability? You're darn tootin' it does. We ought to be able to draw that conclusion just on the basis of size, strength, shape, and location of the muscle. The burden of proof lies on nay-sayers who say that this is not true. One recent paper strongly implicates arthroscopic psoas lengthening including hip instability in poor clinical outcomes in patients with a certain type of anatomical orientation of their hips called *femoral anteversion*.[4]

We need to get smarter about all this. Of course, the psoas must be important for hip stability. We see patients almost every day who have done badly after arthroscopic hip surgery and psoas lengthening. Some of those patients developed real hip instability. On the other hand, the procedure has helped some patients magnificently. For several years now, arthroscopic hip surgeons have had a rather cavalier attitude about doing psoas releases at femoroacetabular impingement surgery. I am not saying we should stop doing this altogether. We just have to get smarter.

Now also consider that we see many cases of severe psoas pain after total hip replacement. These patients usually get dramatically better after psoas release.

To release or not to release the psoas, that is a real question. Certainly, there are appropriate times to do either. And the other side of the coin is that there are many patients out there with severe psoas pain and who need something aggressive done. Are there are other surgical choices? I think there have to be. Why not shave the iliopectineal eminence or other bony or soft tissue and free up the psoas in other ways?[5] That way, the psoas would stay intact. It takes 2 to tango. It takes 2 anatomical parts to impinge. If the psoas is the snapping against bone or other soft tissue, couldn't getting rid of the "snappee" be as good a potential solution as getting rid of the "snapper"?

We have to get smarter. We need more thoughtful studies. We can make some patients so much better sometimes by loosening the muscle. We can also create unstable hips and make them miserable. We've got to understand better more of the basic biomechanics and underlying pathophysiology.

PSOAS RAPS

Get it? Rap, to hit hard, the Eminem muscle, iliopsoas problems... Okay, we are stretching the analogy a bit.

Here are several case examples of psoas injuries/problems. Keep in mind 2 really important thoughts with respect to diagnosis and treatment:

1. Psoas problems can be subtle; they mimic a lot of other core injuries including those of the hip or muscles. They even mimic sobering internal problems. When considering the psoas as a cause, you must keep in mind infections of the gastrointestinal tract, tuberculosis, appendicitis, or other serious trouble. Many of the archetypal medical traps reside in the region of the psoas. For example, abscesses classically sit on the psoas muscle, psoas symptoms and signs arise, and one gets fooled thinking about benign musculoskeletal issues. Plus, even with severe, benign psoas issues, "typical" pain with flexion/extension does not have to be manifest.

2. A real psoas problem may occur as either a primary, isolated issue without any other cause or in conjunction with another core problem, such as a significant hip or other core muscle concern. When the underlying problem cannot be identified, one can guess that Slim Shady will return and would say: "Guess who's back!"

Case 1. Seemingly Straightforward Psoas Bursitis

A 17-year-old multisport high school football/ice hockey player picks up tennis and enters a top state tennis tournament and gets to the championship round. He had this intense psoas bursitis without any hip or core muscle injury. This was treated by steroid injection and oral anti-inflammatories and he returned to win the championship. He remains without symptoms 6 months later but has not returned to tennis. See Figure 12-8.

The principal message that the athlete of Case 1 sends is that psoas problems can occur in isolation. In his case, tennis seemed the precipitating factor. On his own, he chose to win the tournament but to give up tennis. Other sports were too important for him to risk recurrence of this injury.

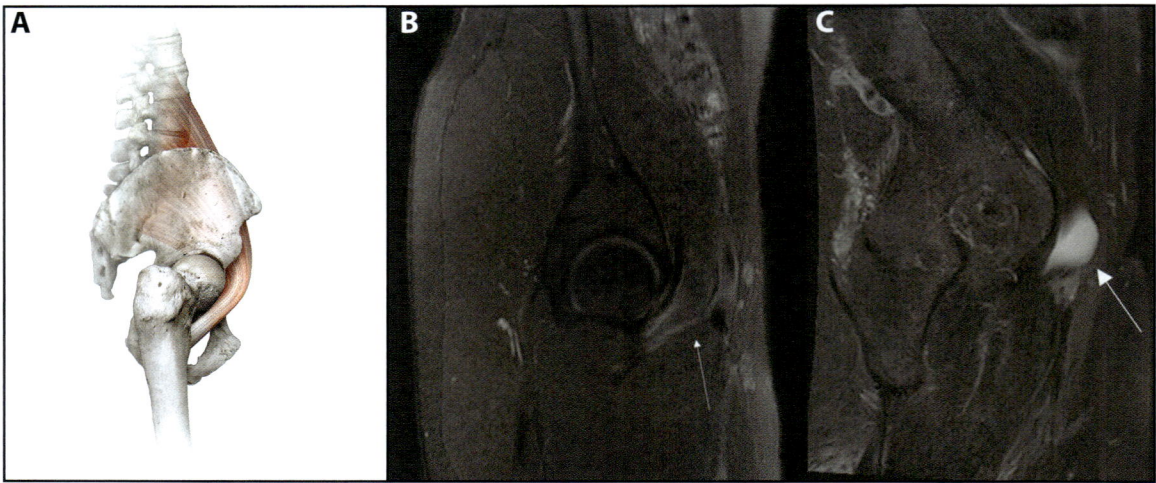

Figure 12-8. Using Rob's earlier drawing (see Figure 12-6) (A), one can easily see (B) the anatomy of this young football/hockey/tennis player's psoas strain (arrow) and subsequent bursitis in on MRI. Note the proximity of the psoas and the hip. (C) The bursitis can get so bad that it looks cystic (arrow).

Case 2. Psoas Bursitis With Core Muscle Injury

An 18-year-old highly recruited high school soccer player develops a right-sided severe pubic plate injury plus severe psoas signs and symptoms. He did not play for 3 months, and each time he got back on the field the problem returned. The MRI shows both a subtle but severe right-sided plate separation and severe psoas bursitis. Hips were normal. He underwent pubic plate repair as well as partial psoas lengthening and was back at full performance 6 weeks after surgery. See Figure 12-9.

The big question here was whether to address his obvious psoas problem at the same time since he already required pubic plate surgery. We have had numerous other patients whose psoas problems went away after repair of just the pubic plate injury. We chose to do concomitant surgeries based on the severity of his symptoms.

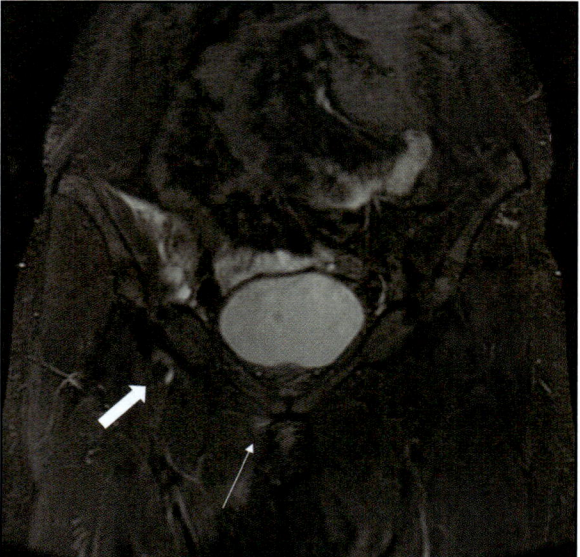

Figure 12-9. Psoas bursitis (thick arrow) in a high school soccer player with a pubic plate separation (not shown well) and acute adductor injury (thin arrow).

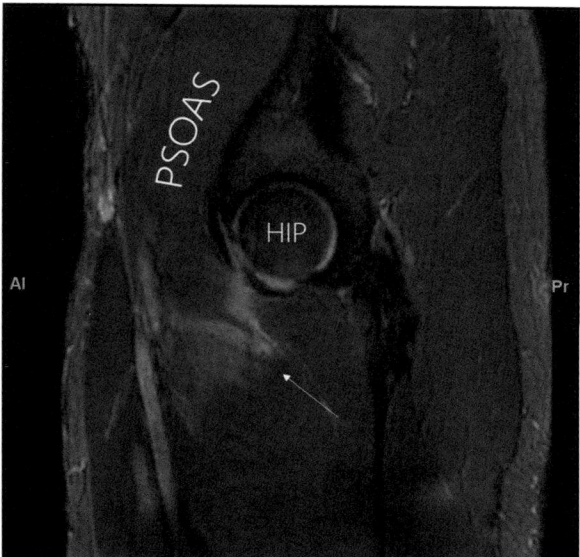

Case 3. Psoas Bursitis With Hip Impingement

A top NFL defensive end develops severe psoas bursitis 2 years after successful core muscle surgery. He underwent hip impingement surgery without psoas lengthening procedure and returned to full performance, but his team lost in the NFC Championship round. See Figure 12-10.

This patient did well after core muscle surgery, and his psoas symptoms and signs turned out to signal a severe hip problem with some arthritis. Fortunately, he has done well so far.

Figure 12-10. This NFL star had a lot of articular cartilage damage at hip arthroscopy and continued to play with minimal symptoms despite this impressive psoas bursitis. Note all the fluid (white), likely representing free communication with the postoperative hip joint.

Case 4. Psoas Retraction After Femoroacetabular Impingement Surgery

A 38-year-old government employee in DC does poorly after hip surgery. The impingement turns out to be persistent, and the psoas is totally retracted after a "partial psoas lengthening" procedure. See Figure 12-11. She underwent redo hip arthroscopy with combined open decompression and partial repair of her retracted psoas muscle. So far, she is doing much better, but she still is not perfect.

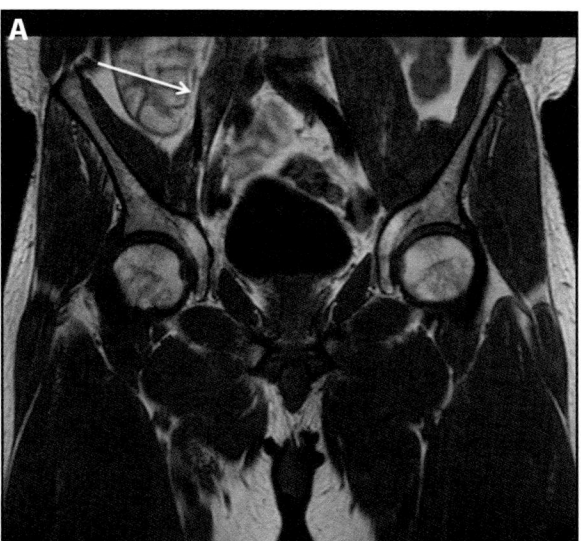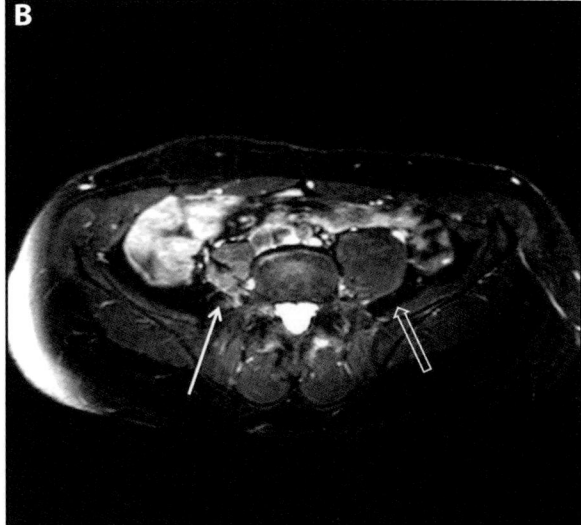

Figure 12-11. High-level governmental employee with shrunken psoas and severe pain after psoas "release" at hip arthroscopy. (A) T1 coronal image. Compare the size of the right (arrow) psoas compared to the left. (B) T2 axial image of the same. The right psoas (closed arrow) is much smaller and whiter (more swollen) compared to the left (open arrow).

Case 5. Psoas Stricture After Total Hip Replacement

This 54-year-old woman had a total hip replacement 7 years previously and developed disabling psoas symptoms escalating over 6 months. She had obvious psoas signs on examination. The hip seemed a good fit. The MRI showed psoas atrophy and stricture despite being apparently intact. She underwent trans-total hip arthroscopy and division of the stricture and has had no symptoms for the past 3 years. See Figure 12-12.

This case is just one of many cases of severe psoas problems we have seen after total hip replacement. She was unusual in that she developed problems after many years. Usually, we see this much earlier, when there are fewer imaging changes. This case shows, again, that we have a lot to learn. The hip surgery seemed to be perfect.

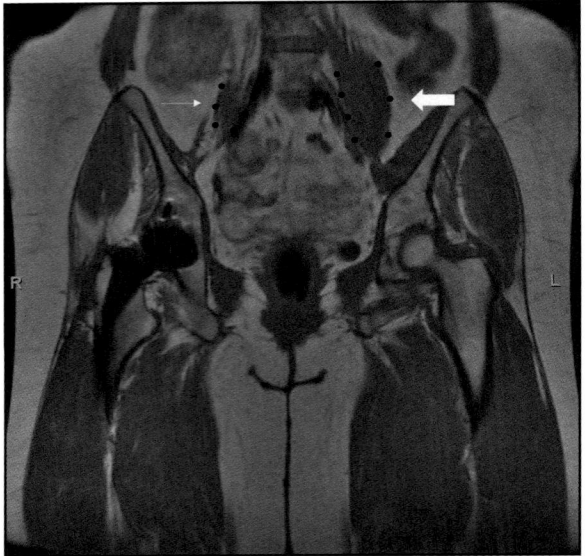

Figure 12-12. Withered psoas in a retired basketball player after total hip replacement. Distal to that was a stricture. At this level, note the difference in psoas size (dots) between the right side (thin arrow) and left side (thick arrow). The artificial hip makes imaging tricky. The artificial right hip is dark. Metal distorts the imaging.

ALGORITHM FOR MANAGEMENT AND TREATMENT OF PSOAS ISSUES

The psoas causes problems in a number of ways. We divide them into primary and secondary psoas issues, and it is usually difficult to differentiate between the two. Primary means the problem originates within the psoas or iliopsoas itself, and secondary means the culprit problem originates elsewhere. For example, a psoas bursitis in a basketball player might originate in the psoas from trauma from all the jumping up and down. But the bursitis might also come from an inflammatory response from femoroacetabular impingement or be compensatory from a big tear in one of the harness muscles.

Figure 12-13 is a proposed treatment algorithm. The point here is that no matter whether it is a primary or secondary problem, the pain may have to addressed, depending on how bad it is. There are multiple options (eg, physical therapy, steroid injection, partial lengthening procedures). The problem here is that division of psoas muscle may result in shortening, weakness, pain, and sometimes hip instability. One has to be careful, certainly. No one has perfected the right decision-making criteria. We put in "psoas repair" because we recently developed some techniques to do that, but are just trying these out, so there are no long-term efficacy results as yet.

One also must consider that it takes 2 anatomic structures to cause impingement. You know, it takes 2 to tango. Or change one word slightly: it takes 2 to tangle. Let's get even looser in our analogies: Eminem, the tango... let's stick to music. Take the guitar. Make it easier, the primitive guitar, the Diddley Bow (Figure 12-14).[6,7]

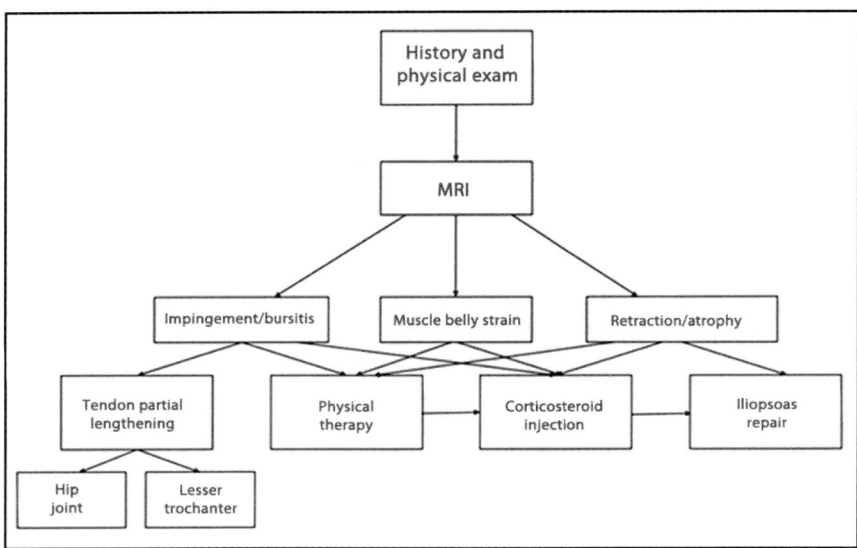

Figure 12-13.

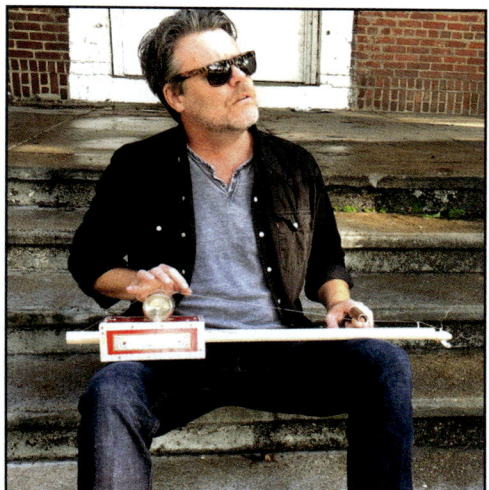

Figure 12-14. Think of the psoas as the wire of a Diddley Bow.

You make this primitive guitar with simply a board, 2 nails, a jar, and wire. Sound gets determined by the tautness of the wire and the substance around it (eg, wood, glass, or other hard substance). The psoas is the same thing; it's just a wire, okay, a little thicker and more complicated. The hip socket, of course, is the jar. The nails? The lesser trochanter and…er…ah…all those vertebral bodies and the ilium…okay, the analogy only goes so far! And yes, there is a lot more substance to the psoas than just wood or glass or whatever. But you get it. The psoas is the wire, and the hip is the jar of the Diddley Bow.

To change the sound, you somehow change the wire's tension. To do that, you have 2 choices. You either (1) work on the wire or (2) you change the size of the jar. In the case of the psoas wire, the problem is usually that it is too tight. Think of the patient making high-pitched screaming noises because the wire is too tight. There are 2 ways to loosen the wire. Either you unravel it a bit from 1 of the 2 nails or you change the tensile strength of the psoas wire.

So…jumping back to real anatomy…think of a tight psoas as too tight a Diddley bowstring! You want to lower the pitch. The conventional way to do that is either to work at the level of the hip or lesser trochanter and either divide it or "lengthen it" (ie, change its tensile strength). Why not simply change, if you can, the size of the jar? That is likely where the problem comes from in the first place. The cause of psoas impingement does not have to be the muscle itself. It could be the adjacent femoral bone, which, if shaved down, might relieve the impingement. Therefore, functionally, all we have to do is modify our techniques of femoroacetabular impingement surgery. That would serve as another kind of psoas "lengthening."

Of course, just changing the size of the jar may not be all that simple. It can get tricky. If you replace it with too small a jar, the wire gets unstable and so does the whole Diddley thing.

EMINEM ENIGMAS

Consider some of the many questions that the iliopsoas muscle leaves us with:
- Why does the psoas get so tight? Is it direct trauma? Is it compensating for other loose muscles? Is it a mechanical issue with too tight a Diddley jar?
- Why would a Diddley jar push so hard into the bowstring? Is it a ball-and-socket issue? Is it the orientation of the whole pelvis?
- What does the psoas actually do? It is so big and tensile; it must do a lot, doesn't it? Why can we usually function so well, even after it has been damaged?
- What about those few patients who do so poorly after psoas "release"? Does the problem stem from reducing the tensile strength too much? How identifiable preoperatively are the patients who do poorly? Can we tailor the amount of psoas lengthening (ie, tension reduction) based on acetabular coverage or other factors?
- Certainly, someone with severe dysplasia is at risk for hip instability no matter what you do: loosen the iliopsoas, shave bone, or change the dynamics in any way. How do you quantify how much to do, whatever you do? How much does the psoas contribute to hip stability anyway?

Okay, enough "deep" questions… for now.

WHAT'S NEXT

Enough rap. We love Eminem, but it is time to change the station.
Let's go on to the power muscles—the butt, back, and sides, and perhaps other music.
And, of course, we shall begin with the "new beauty muscles," the glutes.

Selected Readings

Fabricant PD, Bedi A, De La Torre K, Kelly BT. Clinical outcomes after arthroscopic psoas lengthening: the effect of femoral version. *Arthroscopy*. 2012;28(7):965-971.

This study highlights the complexity of the core Eminem muscle. Many patients who undergo hip arthroscopy have an element of psoas pain, and doing some degree of loosening of the psoas at the time of surgery can relieve that pain. In other people, however, releasing the psoas can lead to gross hip instability and life-long problems. This article attempts to shed some light on this subject.

El-shaar R, Stanton M, Biehl S, Giordano B. Effect of subspine decompression on rectus femoris integrity and iliopsoas excursion: a cadaveric study. *Arthroscopy*. 2015;31(10):1903-1908.

An interesting anatomic study of possible ways that shaving bone, rather than loosening muscle, might relieve psoas pain.

Brandenburg JB, Kapron AL, Wylie JD, et al. The functional and structural outcomes of arthroscopic iliopsoas release. *Am J Sports Med*. 2016;44(5):1286-1291.

This compelling case series demonstrates a high incidence of psoas weakness reduction in size after psoas release done at the time of hip arthroscopy. It appropriately warns surgeons to have a high threshold to employ this technique.

Lomax A, Bishop J, Long W. *The Land Where the Blues Began*. Independently distributed film. Amazon.com.

Think about the biomechanics of the iliopsoas muscle while watching a beautiful movie.

References

1. Philippon MJ, Devitt BM, Campbell KJ, et al. Anatomic variance of the iliopsoas tendon. *Am J Sports Med*. 2014;42(4):807-811.
2. Kopydlowski NJ, Tannenbaum EP, Smith MV, Sekiya JK. Characterization of human anterosuperior acetabular depression in correlation with labral tears. *Orthop J Sports Med*. 2014;2(10):1-5.
3. Brandenburg JB, Kapron AL, Wylie JD, et al. The functional and structural outcomes of arthroscopic iliopsoas release. *Am J Sports Med*. 2016;44(5):1286-1291.
4. Fabricant PD, Bedi A, De La Torre K, Kelly BT. Clinical outcomes after arthroscopic psoas lengthening: the effect of femoral version. *Arthroscopy*. 2012;28(7):965-971.
5. El-shaar R, Stanton M, Biehl S, Giordano B. Effect of subspine decompression on rectus femoris integrity and iliopsoas excursion: a cadaveric study. *Arthroscopy*. 2015;31(10):1903-1908.
6. Lomax A. *The Land Where the Blues Began*. Delta; 1994. Originally printed in 1970.
7. Williams DL Jr. The Diddley bow. Make. http://makezine.com/projects/make-22/the-diddley-bow/. Accessed April 18, 2018.

13

the glutes
the "new beauty muscles"

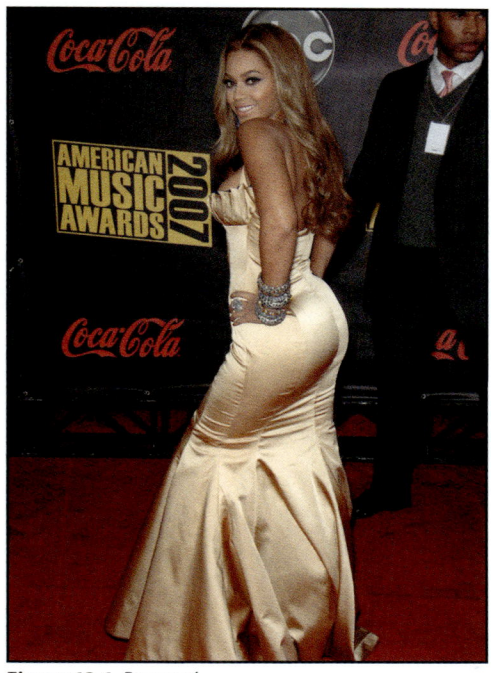
Figure 13-1. Beyoncé.

America has always had something of an infatuation with the rear end, but the last few years have signaled an unprecedented boost in attention to that area (Figure 13-1).

Perhaps the newfound fascination with the bottom is due to America's growing knowledge of core health. There's an awful lot that emanates from the gluteus region—and much of it actually has to do with athletic performance.

Check out a sprinter's glutes some time. No wonder he/she can blast out of the starting blocks and tear down the track. Golfers' first movements involve the area. Football linemen must have strength there to drive off the line and overpower their foes. It's a key to so much activity (Figure 13-2).

Build your "glute-mede" and "glute-max" and perhaps find yourself on the road to the Olympics. Keep in mind, people are still guessing here, but the glutes do seem to have a leadership role in triggering optimal core function (Figures 13-3 and 13-4).[1]

So, get off your gluteus maximus and build that core.

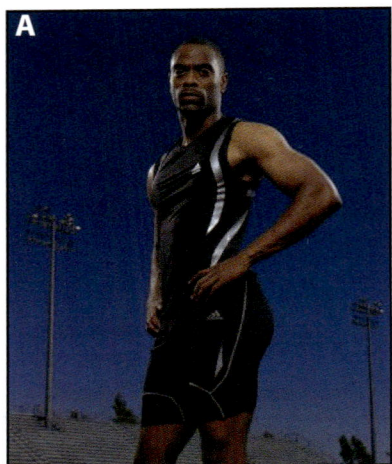
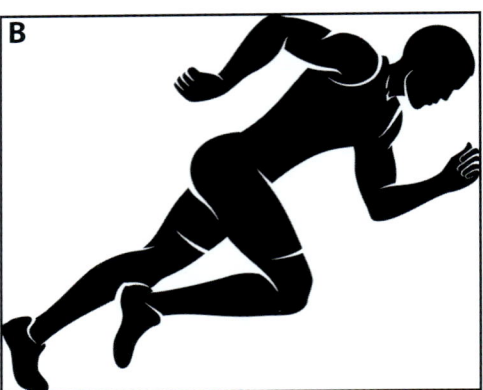
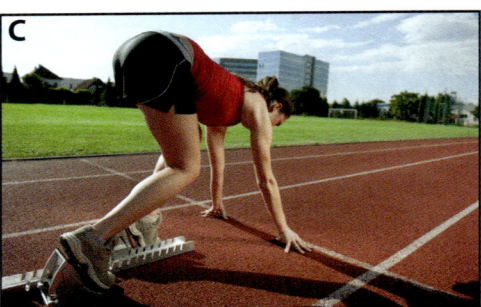

Figure 13-2. Big glutes are common in sprinters. (A) Olympic champion Tyson Gay. (Reprinted with permission from Getty Images Sport.) (B) Usual depiction of a sprinter. (C) Female sprinter.

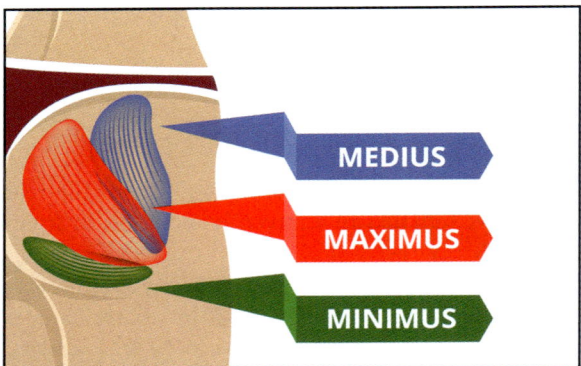

Figure 13-3. A simple way to remember the 3 gluteus muscles. The most superficial gluteus maximus is the broadest.

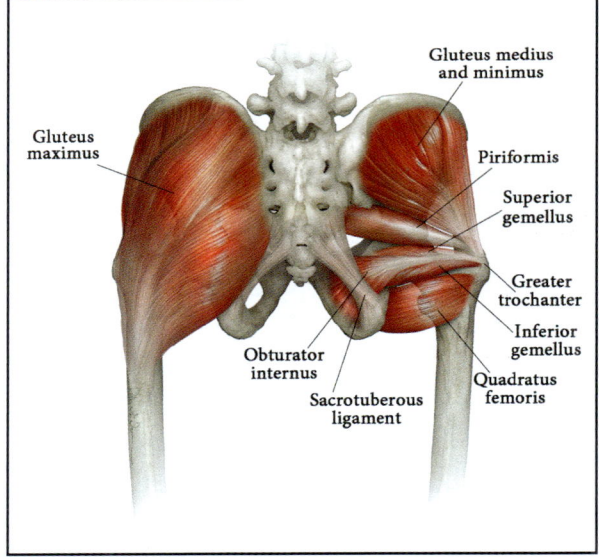

Figure 13-4. Our artist Rob Gordon exhibits the glutes. The muscular anatomy of the left "cheek" is intact. He has eliminated the gluteus maximus on the right.

Have enough electricity in your booty to jump-start the whole of New York City.

Adapted from Irish novelist Colum McCann, *Let the Great World Spin.*

GLUTEUS MAXIMUS

Of course, we must begin with this one—the largest and thereby strongest muscle in the body. Like most other anatomy of the human body, the muscle names derive from early anatomic dissections in the 15th and 16th centuries. Leonardo da Vinci (15th century) and Andreas Vesalius (16th century) get most of the glory. Let's go quickly through the anatomy, function, and a few other features of the gluteus maximus.

Implications of the Appellation

First of all, the muscle's name probably comes originally from Vesalius's *On the Fabric of the Human Body* published in 1543.[2] Vesalius highlights the muscle in his book owing to its "classic beauty" and large size, 2 things that meant one and the same thing back then, particularly when it came to the Romanesque big butts. It was all about Rome back then. Vesalius, from Brussels, which was then part of the Netherlands, ditched his given name, Andries van Wesel. No doubt, this sounded more Roman, and thus he named many of the muscles.

Gluteus maximus certainly rings of aristocracy and dictatorship. While this muscle is large and strong and beautiful, fitness experts nowadays tend to trash it—relatively speaking—with respect to its functional importance standpoint. They downplay its role in the body's initiating mechanisms and even in strength, in favor of the glute-mede and other muscles. One thing is for sure, the gluteus maximus is superficial, and as we just mentioned again in the last chapter, the more central the muscle the more important its function in the core. But it is so big, it has to be important.

Our bottom line: Respect the gluteus maximus, the largest of the 3 glutes, for more than just its size and beauty. It definitely has huge roles. Do not discard it.

Anatomy

The gluteus maximus muscle has a thick fleshy bulk that forms much of the shape and appearance of the butt. Its quadrilateral outline comes from its attachments to the inner upper ilium, lower sacrum, base of the spine, and side of the coccyx (the tailbone). It also connects with the back muscles and other fasciae. It inserts on the iliotibial band and fascia lata, as well as what we call the *gluteal tuberosity* between the vastus lateralis and adductor magnus. It is a "tough" muscle in that it has a lot of thick parallel fascicles separated by thick fibrous tissue.

Functions

In short, the gluteus maximus is big and covers a lot of space. Therefore, it should not be unexpected that it has a number of functions. One of the most important functions is to maintain the trunk in an erect posture. In other words, it is the main extensor muscle of the hip. No doubt it plays a huge role in supporting the pelvis on top of the head of the femur. The latter function becomes obvious when one stands on one leg. It also tenses the fascia lata and steadies the femur on the tibia. Different parts of this grand old muscle also participate in adduction, abduction, and external rotation.

Other Features

Basically, the gluteus maximus is a multifaceted and very forgiving muscle. Owing to its large size, one can strengthen it in many ways and most injuries involving it heal on their own. Even with massive injuries, the muscle can be sewn up easily and it heals.

The most common operation involving this muscle is implant surgery, for purely cosmetic reasons. We won't go into that. The largest literature on those procedures sits in the criminal sections of newspapers. But interestingly, the muscle can be legitimately transferred (ie, "swung around") as flaps to serve other purposes such as for preservation or augmentation of glute-mede function.[3]

In other words, one might consider the gluteus maximus another Rodney Dangerfield muscle. We should learn to love it just like the next muscle we shall talk about. Therefore, we propose to nickname this the king glute or glute-max.

Glute-Mede

Mostly because of its anatomically definable nature and importance in initiating power in proper core movements, the gluteus medius has recently become of the darling of many fitness experts and hip surgeons. Perhaps love spawned its nickname, glute-mede. If not love, then the muscle has, at least, become a best-friend-forever of most therapists.

Our physical therapists go overboard in their love for this muscle. Their passion outstrips reason. Recently, they saw the top running back in the NFL and delighted in his not having great glute-mede function. They were sure they could help improve his yardage for the next year.

Let's go over some of the same things we did for the aforementioned gluteus maximus.

Anatomy

The glute-mede anatomy is much more definable than the gluteus maximus. This thick muscle radiates broadly from the external ilium to the lateral greater trochanter of the hip. It narrows, thickens even more and flattens as its tendon inserts into an oblique fascia-bony ridge that runs antero-inferiorly, deep to the maximus.

Function

The glute-mede's function is obvious since it connects the lateral ilium to the greater trochanter of the femur. It abducts the hip and thigh. It does this along with the other glute, the minimus. The 2 muscles also internally rotate the thigh with the hip flexed and externally rotate it with the hip extended. Dysfunction of the glute-mede or paralysis by injury to its innervation, the superior gluteal nerve, leads to a positive Trendelenburg sign.[4]

Other Features

The recent interest that this muscle has sparked has led to various strengthening techniques and new surgical techniques to repair big tears when they are recognized. In our identification of the importance of this muscle, we must guard against at least 2 dangers. One, we may find ourselves focusing too much on isolated strengthening of the muscle. As we have seen with the harness muscles, too much attention to wear-and-tear injuries leads to serious injury. The other caution is to be aware that we are finding ourselves having to solve new paradoxes. For example, MRI is identifying many older nonathletic patients with severe-looking glute-mede tears. How do these rather sedate people with "hip" pain get these tears? And how do we determine which ones to repair?[5,6]

Gluteus Minimus

This muscle deserves a minimal discussion. This is basically a "mini" glute-mede in terms of anatomy and function. The minimus tends to be a little more intimate than the medius with the piriformis muscle and other deep posterior muscles. We don't know the significance of that. Obviously, the minimus is not as big as the glute-mede, but the same functional considerations hold as for the glute-mede, only a little less so. (See Figure 13-5.)

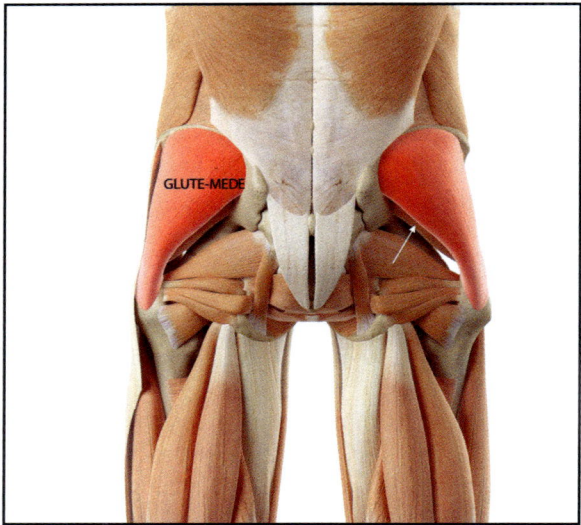

Figure 13-5. The anatomical relationship between the gluteus medius, gluteus minimus (arrow), and "deep derrière" (see Chapter 29). The minimus (arrow) lies deep, almost shadowing "the mede."

GLUTE-MEDE INJURY

Glute-mede and glute-min tendinous tears turn out to be tremendously common. Often misdiagnosed as trochanteric bursitis, the tears occur primarily at their distal attachments onto the femur. These tears produce lateral thigh pain and are a more common cause of pain there than previously realized. Technically savvy hip arthrosocopic surgeons now frequently debride, decompress, and/or reattach the damaged tendons.

Recommendations conflict with respect to what to do about gluteus medius and/or minimus injury or tendinopathy. Most everyone agrees that this is a real clinical constellation of diagnoses. Key findings on physical examination include direct tenderness, the Trendelenburg sign, abduction weakness, and pain with resisted external rotation. Imaging is useful but lacks sensitivity and accuracy.[6,7] Nonoperative treatment options remain the usual: nonsteroidal anti-inflammatories, massage, physical therapy, steroid injection, or platelet-rich plasma injection. As stated before, plenty of controversy shrouds the surgical care of these problems (eg, optimal surgical indications or best surgical techniques).

All About That Bass.

The debut single by American singer/songwriter Meghan Trainor. Lyrically, it discusses positive body image. The lyrics earned *Vogue Magazine* distinction for bringing in the "the era of the big booty."[VID 1]

IT'S ALL ABOUT THAT BASS

No matter the degree of physical fitness, it pays to develop your glutes. Nobody now disputes that stylish fact of life. The rear end has become a big part of today's beauty; it also initiates most sequential movement patterns of optimal human performance. So much so that the absence of gluteal strength has become a parlor trick for physical therapists. They love to demonstrate how one can overpower the balance of 200-pound athletes. They push the weak glute-mede athletes over with just one finger. Physical therapists love this trick because it highlights important flaws in the way people generally train. We learn more about these exercise principles in Chapter 32 on rehabilitation and performance. (See also Video 2 for a glute-mede exercise.)

SELECTED READINGS

Vesalius A. De humani corporis fabrica libri septem [Title page: Andreae Vesalii Bruxellensis, scholae medicorum Patauinae professoris De humani corporis fabrica libri septem]. Basileae [Basel]: Ex officina Joannis Oporini, 1543.
   Place yourself in a lecture hall in 14th century Padua and appreciate the beauty of the human form.
Voos JE, Rudzki JR, Shindle MK, Martin H, Kelly BT. Arthroscopic anatomy and surgical techniques for peritrochanteric space disorders in the hip. *Arthroscopy.* 2007;23(11):1246.e1-1246.e5.
   Beautiful descriptions of minimally invasive techniques for repairing gluteus medius and minimus tears. A decade later, we are still figuring out who warrants these repairs.
In the Renaissance period being fat meant to show the "value" of the human body and pureness. Blog. https://mountiangirl.wordpress.com/2012/05/12/in-the-renaissance-period-being-fat-meant-to-show-the-value-of-the-human-body-and-pureness-4/. Published May 12, 2012. Accessed November 13, 2016.
   In the Renaissance, women were considered beautiful if they were overweight or Rubenesque. This post, from just 6 years ago, says "today being emaciated means wealth and beauty." The post goes on and provides an insightful analysis of our appreciation of beauty as it relates to butts.

REFERENCES

1. Plummer HA, Oliver GD. The relationship between gluteal muscle activation and throwing kinematics in baseball and softball catchers. *J Strength Cond Res*. 2014;28(1):87-96.
2. Vesalius A. De humani corporis fabrica libri septem [Title page: Andreae Vesalii Bruxellensis, scholae medicorum Patauinae professoris De humani corporis fabrica libri septem]. Basileae [Basel]: Ex officina Joannis Oporini; 1543.
3. Whiteside LA, Nayfeh TA, Katerberg BJ. Gluteus maximus flap transfer for greater trochanter reconstruction in revision THA. *Clin Orthop Relat Res*. 2006;(453):203-210.
4. Golub BS. The Duchenne-Trendelenburg sign. *Bull Hosp Joint Dis*. 1947;8(2):127-136.
5. Domb BG, Nasser RM, Botser IB. Partial-thickness tears of the gluteus medius: rationale and technique for trans-tendinous endoscopic repair. *Arthroscopy*. 2010;26(12):1697-1705.
6. Voos JE, Rudzki JR, Shindle MK, Martin H, Kelly BT. Arthroscopic anatomy and surgical techniques for peritrochanteric space disorders in the hip. *Arthroscopy*. 2007;23(11):1246.e1-1246.e5.
7. Nho SJ, Grzybowski JS, Bogunovic L, et al. Diagnosis, evaluation, and endoscopic repair of partial articular gluteus tendon avulsion. *Arthrosc Tech*. 2016;5(3):e425-e431.

VIDEOS

1. https://www.youtube.com/watch?v=7PCkvCPvDXk
2. https://youtu.be/vuZZDAPOYUc

14

the **other** muscles
hip and core **stability**

How do we go through all the rest of the core muscles and keep things from getting incredibly boring? Don't fret. The task turns out to be simple. The rest of the muscles have a common bond; the linkage is stability. Everyone knows, or has seen, people who walk around with incredible pain that seems to reside in the core. Most of the time, the problem does stem from the core.

First, let's begin with a Freddy Krueger story.[VID 1]

Then, let us introduce you to Emma.

A Long Road to Happiness—The Saga of Hip Instability

In New Zealand, she had been an elite athlete, capable of competing for her country in international competitions in 3 different sports.

And then, she could barely walk.

The car crash was bad enough, although it wasn't so catastrophic that the police were summoned. The aftermath caused the most trouble. Well, that and the doctors.

Emma had played netball (like basketball without backboards or dribbling) and volleyball and had rowed on age group national teams for her native New Zealand. She wasn't competing at as high a level in 2013 when the car she was driving was slammed into from behind, but she was active and still training to stay in shape.

"It felt immediately like something had come right through my pelvis from the backseat," she says of the crash. "It happened so very quickly."

She wasn't immobilized. In fact, she exited the car and went about the business of collecting drivers' licenses and insurance information. Later, the pain started in her hips and throughout other areas of her core (Figure 14-1). And nobody was able to give a definitive diagnosis of what exactly was wrong.

Not that doctors didn't think they could solve the issue with surgery. Make that surgeries. Emma withstood 3 different procedures, none of which removed the pain and instability that had come to haunt her.

"Some of the doctors were honest and said they didn't know what the problem was, and others performed surgery and then told me there wasn't anything else they could do," Emma says. "A lot of them wouldn't admit they didn't know what to do.

"I felt like I was outside the scope of normal treatment. I didn't fit into any of the traditional boxes that they knew about."

She had her first hip surgery in May 2014 in Australia and hasn't been able to work—as a physical therapist and Pilates instructor—since. Things became so difficult for Emma that although she considers herself someone who won't ever give up, it seemed like the answer would never come. "My hip did not belong to me."

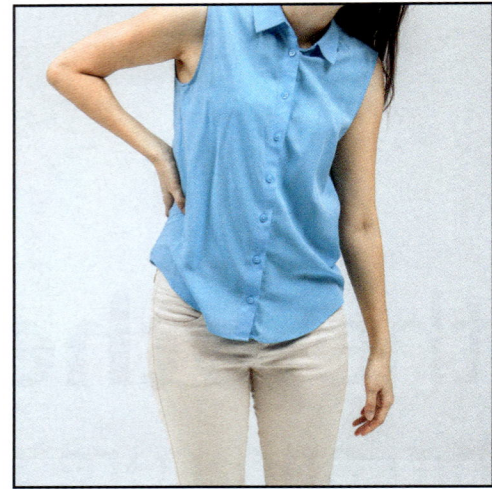

Figure 14-1.

She says, "I was absolutely distraught. I got to the stage where I could do just one outing a day, and that was it." She could barely walk. Every step felt like her her pubic bone was falling out.

Soon after Emma discovered a team of health professionals, she began the process of getting better. "They immediately picked up on what the injury was, it was a breath of fresh air," she says. The key was an overall understanding of the hip and its need for stability and full mobility. It took a combination of several months of intensive physical therapy and surgery. The team eliminated the instability Emma was feeling in her hip. They sewed some muscles together, tightened the ligaments immediately surrounding the hip, and shaved off the residual impingement in the joint so that it would be able to move freely and she would be pain-free and sturdy through her core. She felt some relief immediately after the surgery.

As she moved through the recovery phases, Emma was able to recognize a difference from the previous procedures. This time, she knew the right work had been done.

"My hip feels like it belongs to me again," she says. "It's fantastic. Before, it felt like my hip wasn't part of my body."

Emma's story exhibits the saga of hip instability. Patients often have a feeling of complete "loss" of pelvic control. The feeling goes from nipples to knees. No doubt, Emma's mild hip dysplasia played a role in this.

Her situation became complicated after a core-jolting, rear-end collision and then the hip surgery, which produced even more laxity in her ball and socket. The hip's ligamentous capsule was involved. Then came problems with more and more other muscles, then the back, and finally gastrointestinal, genitourinary, and gynecologic systems and many other visceral functions. Hip or pelvic instability is often hard for the patient to describe. The instability eventually embroils all 4 parts of the core.

Core instability ignites boundless misery.

YIKES…SEEMS LIKE LOTS OF MUSCLES

Remember that we defined the core as the entire region of the body, from mid-chest to mid-thigh, all inclusive?

That means we have still a lot of other muscles to discuss. Don't worry. The rest is easy…easy for 2 reasons: (1) because we really don't know all that much about them, and (2) because in order to understand them, all one has to do is appreciate one basic concept. The basic concept is a fresh look at what we instinctually have understood for a long time, the concept is stability. Stability is probably best understood by grasping whatever it is that we mean to communicate when we say instability. The definition of stability then becomes expressed by this simple Dick and Jane–type formula: Stability = Absence of Instability.

At this point, let us summarize what muscles and other soft tissues we have gone through thus far, and then go over the ones left to cover. So far, we have gone through:

- The harness muscles: The rectus abdominis and 3 adductors. This unit harnesses and directs the huge forces generated by the power muscles. How can you forget the pubic bone, with its baseball-like cover at the center of all this, and the coordination and stabilization it provides for the pelvis and rest of the core?
- The Rodney Dangerfield (rectus femoris) muscle: The lead muscle within the quadriceps mechanism. The under-appreciated rectus femoris probably directs and stabilizes the other muscles of the anterior thigh.
- The Eminem (psoas) muscle: This important muscle performs so many functions, many of which remain unstudied and mysterious, such as its role in central core or hip stability. The Slim Shady muscle lies so intimately with the hip and harness muscles.
- The new beauty (gluteal) muscles: These are powerful initiators of core movement as well as important spine/pelvis/hip stabilizers. Judging from their size and power, they likely play crucial roles in proper core function.

In this chapter, we shall chat about most of the rest of the muscles of the core: the tensor fasciae latae (TFL), the deeper posterior pelvic muscles, our back and side muscles, and the "pelvic floor" muscles as defined by the "uro-gynecologists." At this point, you might be thinking like Elaine from *Seinfeld*: "Yada, yada, yada."

We shall also gab about fascia, ligaments, and other "orthopedic-type" soft tissues that reside there. We shall cover the hamstring and some remaining parts of the anatomy in upcoming chapters.

Are you still worried? Do the above seem way too much to cover in one chapter? Don't worry. This chapter shall be astoundingly concise.

DEFINING STABILITY

Note that in each of the 4 bullet points describing our nicknamed core muscles, we mentioned the word "stability," yet without definition. If you look carefully within the orthopedic or fitness literature, the same thing happens all the time. Nobody defines the word *stability*. Rarely, does anybody attempt to define the term. Just about everybody in the fitness world—maybe everyone in the whole world—believes that they understand the concept of stability. Well, we don't. At least, no accepted definition appears consistently in the literature. The definition of stability remains elusive.

Well, no more. The added bonus: This chapter shall be inordinately brief.

Let's begin. And try out a definition or two. Let's start with the term *hip instability*, and from there, figure out the term *stability*. Then slog out a definition that applies to the entire core (Table 14-1).

We choose the hip first because this seems anatomically the most simple of all the 4 parts of the core (see Chapter 5). The other 3 parts have zillions of muscles or physiological systems to consider. We have defined the hip, of course, as just the ball and socket—no muscle or other organ systems involved. For simplicity, let's ignore that little tiny bit of muscle (the ligamentum teres, etc) that resides there.

Okay, got it? Let's toss up and bat around a fresh definition.

Hip instability: The femoral head ball dislodging enough from its normal position to cause disabling pain during routine activities.

Think about this definition. The femoral head is really what we are talking about it, isn't it? The "ball" of the ball-and-socket joint is what really matters, not the socket. The acetabulum may be stunted in growth or have other features that contribute to instability, but instability has to be defined by the femoral head and not the acetabulum. Pain also has to be a part of the definition, doesn't it? Pain can take on various forms. It can be a mild discomfort, pudendal in nature, affecting the compensating other side, etc. Most often, pain takes on a constellation of patterns. Whatever forms it takes, pain must help define instability.

Now let's examine the third part of the definition—"routine activities." These cover the daily activities for most of us slouches (eg, walking or sitting, getting up from the couch and going to the refrigerator). The term *routine* also covers the strenuous activities of an athlete. The bottom line here is that pain with routine activities has to cover all individuals—both us slouches and high-performing athletes. This definition says that with hip instability, the ball of the hip slips abnormally enough out of its normal position to ruin the quality of routine life of any human being, and perhaps other animals.

If we accept that definition, then the corollary definition for hip stability flows easily to mean: "the ball and socket functioning normally."

How can one argue with such profound logic? If you disagree, then please massage our ego and be courteous enough to read on, anyway!

Now consider how the term *instability* might apply to the rest of the core. Let's try out the term instability to mean: dysfunction enough to cause disabling pain during routine activities. Take the pubic bone joint as a test example; dysfunction would apply to the slippage of the fibrocartilaginous "loose baseball" cover during cutting or jumping. For the pubic symphyseal joint, it might mean the 2 sides of the pubic symphysis rubbing against each other. For the back, it might mean 2 vertebral bodies moving as a disc dislodges.

One can go on and on describing different types of core instability (eg, the rectus femoris causing instability of the anterior thigh). No doubt, many types of pelvic instability exist, yet have never been described. Consider all the different mini-joints in the pelvis and the many small parts of bones that reside there connected by large and small ligamentous structures. Also, think about the enormous number of patients in the world with undiagnosed and disabling pelvic pain who sit, over and over again, in the waiting rooms of gynecologic, urologic, and primary care offices.

Let's end this discussion by defining core instability. Let's use this extrapolation from what we have just discussed:

Core instability: Any biomechanical dislodgment within the core that causes enough pain during routine activities to interfere with one's quality of life.

Most subsequent instability discussion in this chapter shall focus on hip or pubic bone instability since we know the most about those problems.

TABLE 14-1 NEW DEFINITIONS OF CORE INSTABILITY	
Instability	Any biomechanical dislodgement of a core joint that produces unrelenting and disabling pain during routine activities
Hip instability	The femoral head dislodging enough from its normal position to cause predictable, unrelenting, and disabling pain during routine activities
Core instability	Any biomechanical dysfunction of a joint within the core that causes enough predictable pain during routine activities to interfere with one's quality of life

As mentioned, pain generation has to be part of whatever definition of instability one chooses. Therefore, in this chapter we shall succinctly list the muscles and what we do know about their anatomy and function. In so doing, keep in mind what structures lie next to what and where the nerves reside (eg, the periosteum of bones). Then one may speculate where pinching of nerves or other structures occurs.

Likewise, remember that this new look at the core is just that—new. Therefore, it is fair game for debate. It is also entirely fair game for discovery. As you read further, keep alive these concepts of stability and instability. Those concepts help keep us from too much debate. The concepts shall also help us recognize new methods of treatment (eg, new physical therapy methods, new places to inject, new surgical procedures). As treaters, one way to think about our primary goal is to transform unstable cores into stable ones.

As you read on, also think about the specific location of each muscle or muscle group and what portion of the core the muscles likely help stabilize, plus the likely importance of that contribution to overall core stability.

TENSOR FASCIAE LATAE AND THE ILIOTIBIAL BAND AND "THE LAYER CONCEPT" OF HIP STABILITY

The TFL and iliotibial band (ITB) seem like simple anatomic structures (Figure 14-2). We shall describe them simply. In reality, these seemingly simple structures are not so simple after all. They represent much more importance than a description of their location, attachments, and thick appearance. Together, they represent, potentially, a hugely important layer for hip stability.

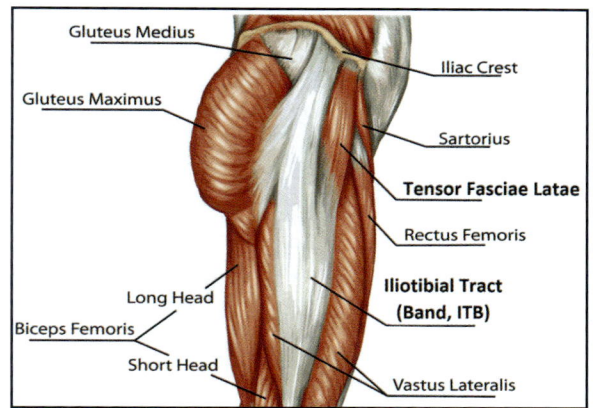

Figure 14-2. TFL and ITB, and their relationships with other structures.

Tensor Fasciae Latae and Iliotibial Band Anatomy

Here they are. The TFL sits between the gluteus medius and sartorius and goes from the iliac crest to the iliotibial tract (or "band" or ITB). Think of the ITB as a thick, sturdy fascia on the lateral aspect of the thigh, which in turn extends to below the knee. The complex helps stabilize both the hip and knee during action. The TFL tightens the ITB, and in the erect posture or during walking or horseback riding, it steadies the head of the femur outside the greater trochanter. Functionally, the muscle can be deemed an abductor like the glutes. Overall, the complex of muscles and fasciae should also be considered an external stabilizer. The latter consideration makes us contemplate about how hip stability really works. Think of hip stability as having 3 components.

A Nutshell

Okay, now the important discussion. The simple TLF-ITB anatomical apparatus just described above represents one part of a hugely important model about how the body keeps the hip and other things in the core stable. Think about a nutshell (Figure 14-3).

We use the phrase "…in a nutshell." What do we mean? We are talking about keeping something compact (eg, trying to say things in just a few words). Well, in the body, for proper functioning of the core, we also need to keep things compact. We need some type of cover or set of covers to keep things together and functioning inside. Without the covers, things get loose, they fall apart. Think of an orange. The peel does this for the orange.

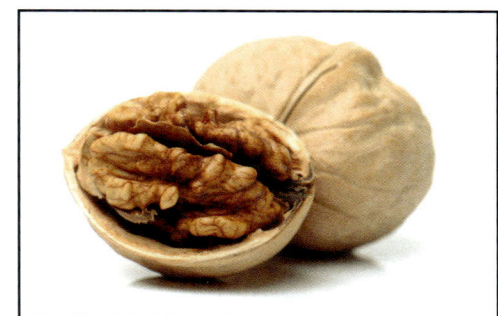

Figure 14-3. A nutshell keeps nuts compact and stable.

Well, the TFL and ITB help do this for the hip and pubic bone joints and perhaps the numerous other small joints within the pelvis. The hip, again, is the easiest core joint to conceptualize in terms of stability. Other anatomic structures, such as the pubic bone and skin, also contribute to this nutshell protection of the hip. Think of the intrinsic stability mechanisms of the hip as well as a series of protective layers outside the hip, the outermost of which include the TFL and ITB.

Intrinsic Anatomical Stabilization

Ask how does the hip ball function within the socket? What does this require? Well, it requires several things. Among these are that it needs to stay isolated, to a large degree, within its own environment without interruption by the outside world. Think about the natural anatomic factors that preserve that anatomic environment when the body is relatively still. (Body movement introduces several other factors.) First, it requires some vacuum or suction to steady the ball. Then, the shape and size of both the bony socket and head of the femur become important. Too small a socket would cause the ball to slip out. Too deep a socket and the ball would likely rub against at least one of the edges, not even considering cam bumps or pincer ledges. Finally, the ligamentum teres must supply some degree of stability, albeit minor.

Tissue Layer Components

What, then, does the hip need once you introduce movement? Preservation of the environment then requires a series of layers of sturdy tissues that protect the vacuum and keep movement inside insulated from injury. Let's now simply look at the anatomy and see what surrounds the hip. This is not rocket science, this is basic gross anatomy.

The surrounding protection of the hip has 4 tough tissue layers.[1,2] The innermost layer consists of the thick—iliofemoral, ischiofemoral, and pubofemoral[3]—ligaments on top of a delicate synovium.[4,5] The second deepest layer includes the iliopsoas and rectus femoris anteriorly, the obturator externus medially and to some degree laterally, and the whole set of deep posterior pelvic muscles that we shall describe in the following section. The third layer becomes the harness muscles—rectus abdominis, adductor longus, pectineus, and adductor brevis—femoral vessels, and sartorius anteriorly and to some degree the vasti, and the glutes posteriorly. The fourth and final layer—the nutshell—is everything else that contributes to the outermost relative inflexibility (eg, the TFL and ITB, skin, back, and pubic bone). You can put portions of the glutes in the final layer if you want; everything is arguable. (See Figure 14-4 and Table 14-2.)

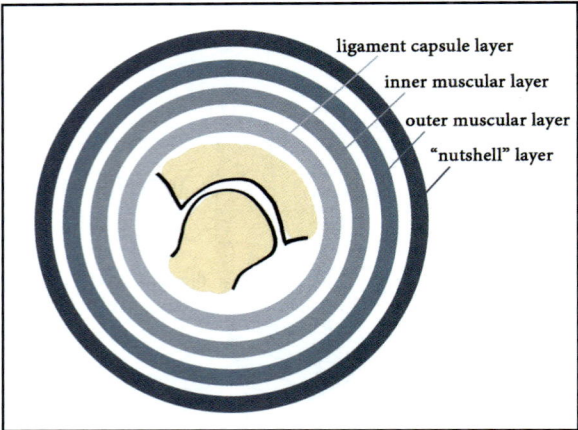

Figure 14-4. The layer concept of hip stability. Think of 4 layers plus the intrinsic stability provided by the ball and socket.

Table 14-2 ANATOMICAL COMPONENTS OF HIP INSTABILITY		
Intrinsic components	• Size and position of femoral head and acetabulum • Suction	• Ligamentum teres • Orientation of the pelvis • Other
The 4 layers: The capsule	• Synovium • Iliofemoral ligament	• Pubofemoral ligament • Ischiofemoral ligament
The deep (inner muscular) layer	• Iliacus • Psoas • Rectus femoris • Obturator externus	• Obturator internus • Piriformis • Superior and inferior gemelli • Quadratus femoris
The superficial (outer muscular) layer	• Rectus abdominis • Pectineus • Adductor longus • Adductor brevis • Sartorius • Vasti medialis and lateralis	• Glute-mede and glute-min • Gluteus maximus • Hamstrings • Sacrotuberous ligament • Sciatic nerve
The nutshell layer	• TFL • ITB • Skin	• Back • Other superficial structures (eg, fasciae, fat, femoral vessels, other vessels)

THE DEEP POSTERIOR PELVIC MUSCLES

Intricate anatomical details about the deep posterior pelvic muscles boggle minds (Figure 14-5). We don't need to delve deeply into those details right here, but see Chapter 29. Dr. Hal Martin goes into it there in fun detail. Plus, the exact routes and attachments vary as do the pathways of nearby nerves and blood vessels, rendering both learning and surgery treacherous in this area.

The Other Muscles—Hip and Core Stability   153

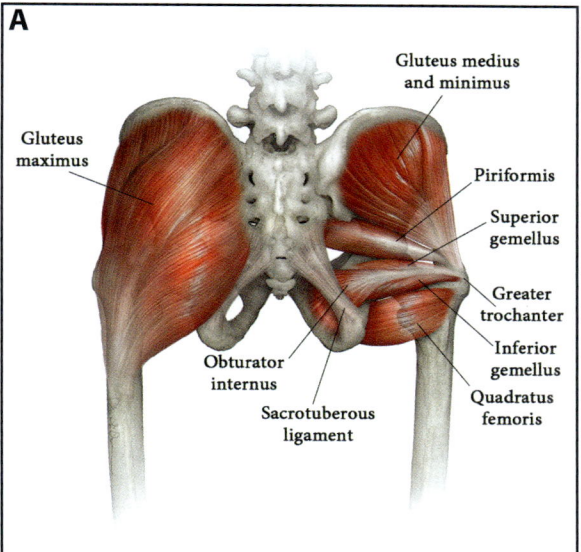
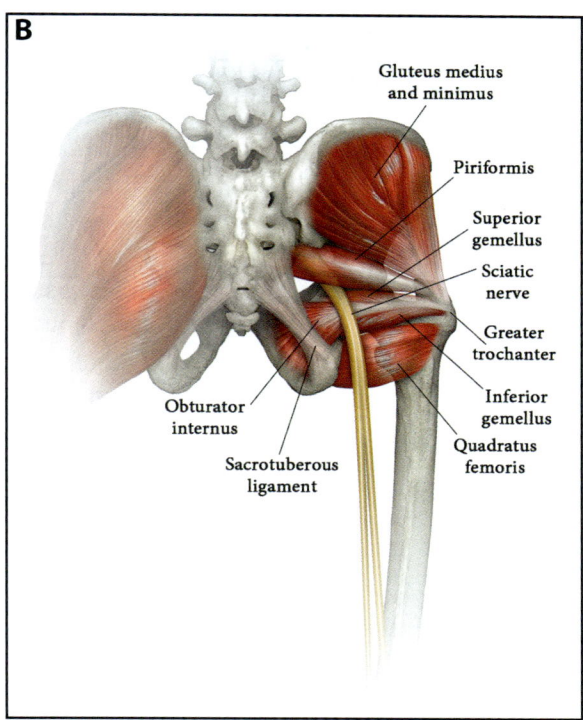

Figure 14-5. Deep posterior muscles (A) without and (B) with the sciatic nerve.

As mentioned, this group of posterior muscles does serve a stabilizing and protective role for the hip. It is probably most known for externally (or laterally) rotating the hip and their intimate relationships to the sciatic nerve. It is also often implicated as possible causes for mysterious "pelvic floor" pain. For example, usually the sciatic nerve passes between the piriformis and superior gemellus as it goes through the greater sciatic foramen and exits the pelvis, but sometimes it actually penetrates the piriformis. That anatomic variability is just one example of why diagnosis and treatment of "piriformis" or "sciatic" pain can sometimes be so difficult. A developing field is the endoscopic identification and treatment of mysterious pains that reside in this region.

As a group, the muscles may capably perform other functions, such as abduction.

THE BACK AND SIDE MUSCLES

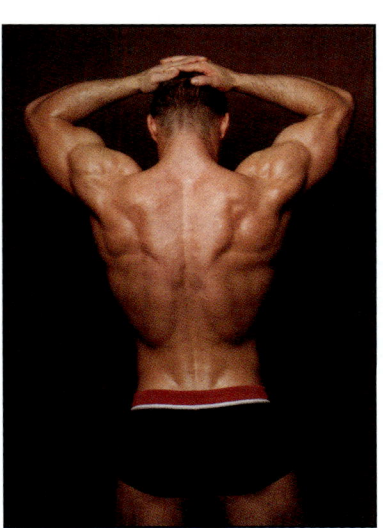

Here they are (Figure 14-6).

We shall not go into the back and side muscles in detail except in the rehabilitation chapters. We cannot do these muscles justice in this book. Suffice it to say here that, as a group, these muscles are important for power and various types of core stability. We still have much to learn about all these muscles.

Think how many of us have undiagnosed back pain.

At this point, let's play Drew Rosenhaus again (see Chapter 5): "Next muscle group!"

Figure 14-6.

TABLE 14-3 OTHER MUSCLE GROUPS		
Deep posterior pelvic muscles (the "deep derrière")	• Piriformis • Superior gemellus • Obturator internus	• Obturator externus • Inferior gemellus • Quadratus femoris
Back and side muscles	• Internal oblique • External oblique • Transversus abdominis • Latissimus dorsi	• Erector spinae • Serratus anterior • Serratus posterior inferior • Intercostals
"Pelvic floor" muscles	• Levator ani (pubococcygeus, iliococcygeus, ischiococcygeus) • Puborectalis • Transversus perinei superficialis • Transverse perinei profundus	• Bulbocavernosus • Ischiocavernosus • Vaginal • Obturator internus • Piriformis

THE "PELVIC FLOOR" MUSCLES

The domain of the pelvic floor claimed by uro-gynecologists and other specialists seems governed by 3 perspectives: (1) what you can see on looking directly down into the pelvis through a 180-degree laparoscope placed through the umbilicus, (2) what you can see externally on a standard anal or pelvic physical examination, and (3) what you can palpate through any of the perineal orifices (Figure 14-7).

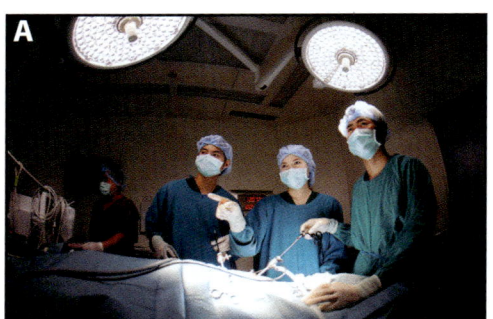
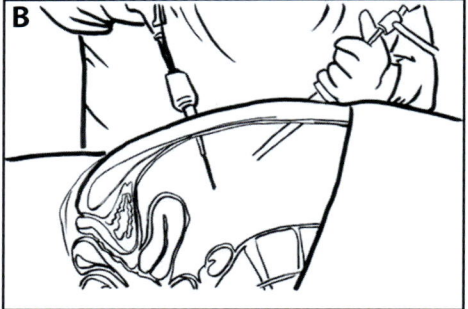
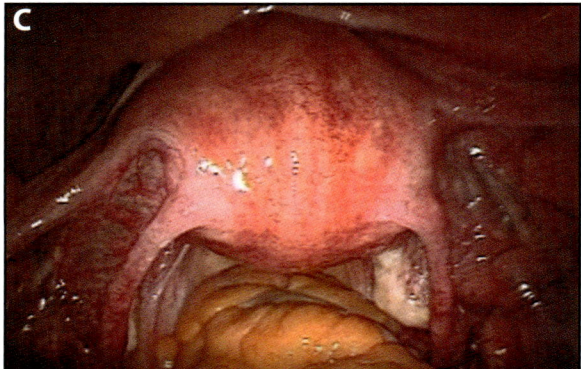

Figure 14-7. (A) Surgeons looking at TV monitor. (B) Drawing of surgeon, scope, instruments, and anterior pelvis. (C) Laparoscopic view of the pelvic floor. Note the intimacy of organs with muscles. ([C] Reprinted with permission from Jeffrey Levy.)

This obviously covers a wide region, including sometimes the acetabulum and muscles immediately surrounding the hip. It should be no wonder that alert health care personnel may find musculoskeletal pathology as the root of some of the chronic pelvic pain in their long-followed, frustrated patients. (See Chapter 23.)

In the evaluation of our patients, we constantly must remind ourselves that the gynecologic, urologic, anal, and colorectal anatomy in this region remains pertinent, both for athletes and nonathletes. One should never totally discount the potential impact of the identified uro-gynecologic diagnoses. One must proceed with caution here. Beware of the many diagnostic, social, and ethical traps.

We shall discuss more of these diagnostic and other issues in Chapter 15.

But before moving on to that chapter, let's take an MRI voyage and see what other diagnoses dwell within this core universe (Atlas).

SELECTED READINGS

Byrd JWT. Gross anatomy and portal anatomy. In: Byrd JWT, ed. *Operative Hip Arthroscopy*. 2nd ed. New York, NY: Springer; 2005.
  A definitive atlas for the fundamentals and techniques of hip arthroscopy. In these 2 chapters, the editor of this definitive atlas on the fundamentals of hip arthroscopy describes beautifully the deep anatomy involved in hip stability.

Barbera OF, Navarro IS. Gross anatomy and portal anatomy. In: Byrd JWT, ed. *Operative Hip Arthroscopy*. 3rd ed. New York, NY: Springer; 2013.
  From a very different perspective, 2 other experts describe the same hip stability anatomy as in the next Selected Reading.

Kaminoff L, Matthews A. *Yoga Anatomy*. 2nd ed. Champaign, IL: Human Kinetics; 2012.
  The same anatomy from the perspective of teaching yogini.

REFERENCES

1. Byrd JWT. Gross anatomy. In: Byrd JWT, ed: *Operative Hip Arthroscopy*. 2nd ed. New York, NY: Springer; 2005.
2. Personal communication between William C. Meyers, MD, MBA and Bryan Kelly, MD, during the development of the Vincera Institute, Philadelphia, PA.
3. Martin HD, Khoury AN, Schröder R, et al. Contribution of the pubofemoral ligament to hip stability: a biomechanical study. *Arthroscopy*. 2017;33(2):305-313.
4. Martin HD, Savage A, Braly BA, et al. The function of the hip capsular ligaments: a quantitative report. *Arthroscopy*. 2008;24(2):188-195.
5. Myers CA, Register BC, Lertwanich P, et al. Role of the acetabular labrum and the iliofemoral ligament in hip stability: an in vitro biplane fluoroscopy study. *Am J Sports Med*. 2011;39(suppl):85S-91S.

VIDEO

1. https://www.youtube.com/watch?v=lpqtLlzCA3M

atlas
stargazing
seeing the **constellation** of core diagnoses

Ground control to Major Tom/take your protein pills and put your helmet on.
—David Bowie, lyrics from the song *Space Oddity*.

For a few moments, let's drift away from "hard-core" teaching points and gaze dreamily at the many diagnostic stars in this core universe. Many stars roam across the skies. Johannes Roedl, a co-editor, has revved up the spaceship and buffed the windows for this mini-voyage. The purpose of the trip is to appreciate the enormity of this universe that we need to explore more.

Keep in mind, as you stare out the windows, that all the patients with these diagnoses had groin pain as their main complaint. In each case, a combination of history, physical examination, and imaging studies clarified the diagnosis.

This time-out shall prepare you for the chapters to come.

REGISTER OF STARS

Consider this "register" a small sampling of the stars in this space. Many more diagnoses exist in the core universe. Johannes's selection emphasizes knowing all 4 parts of the core.

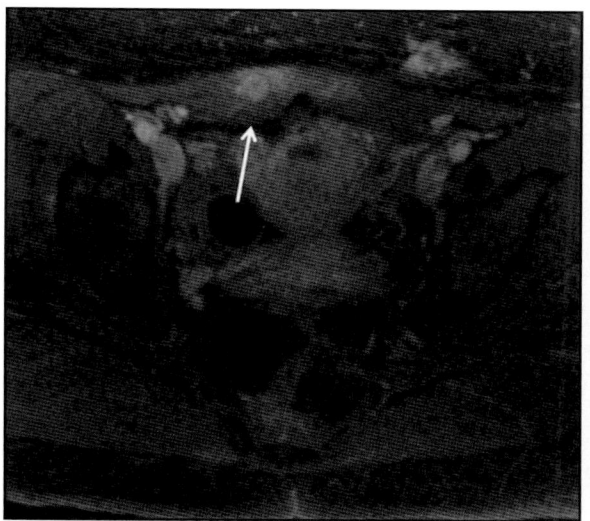

Figure A-1A. Endometrioma of the rectus abdominis.

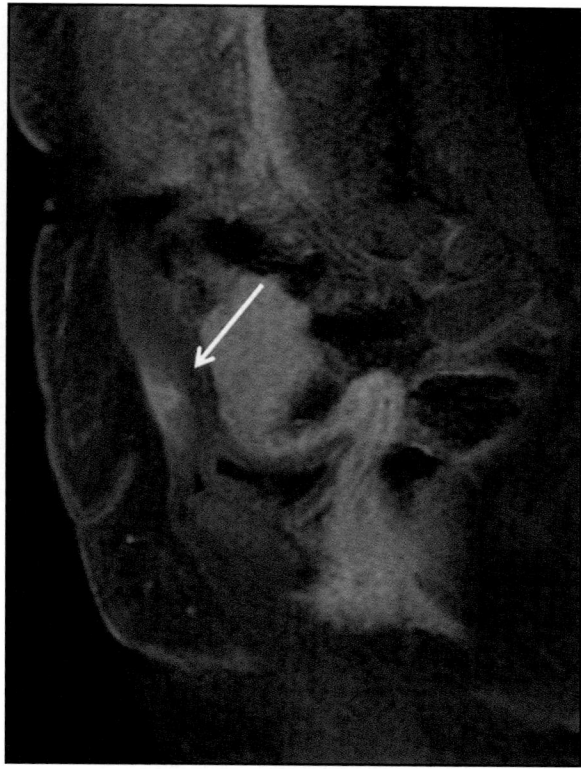

Figure A-1B. Endometrioma of the rectus abdominis.

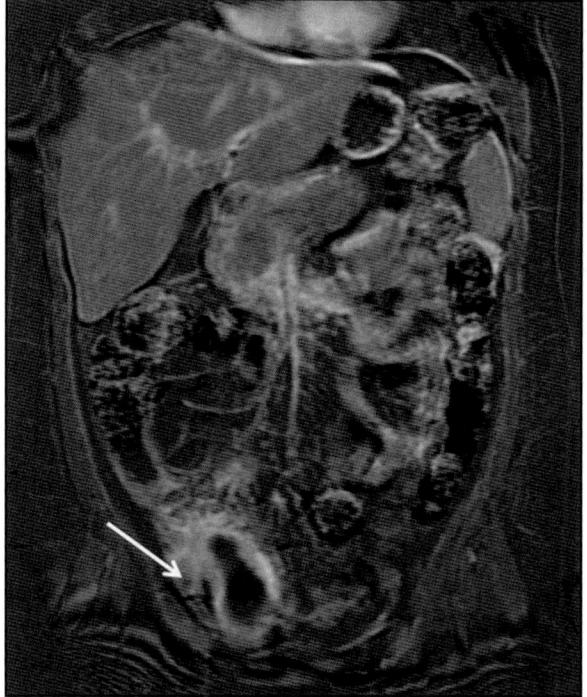

Figure A-2. Crohn's disease with thickening of the terminal ileum.

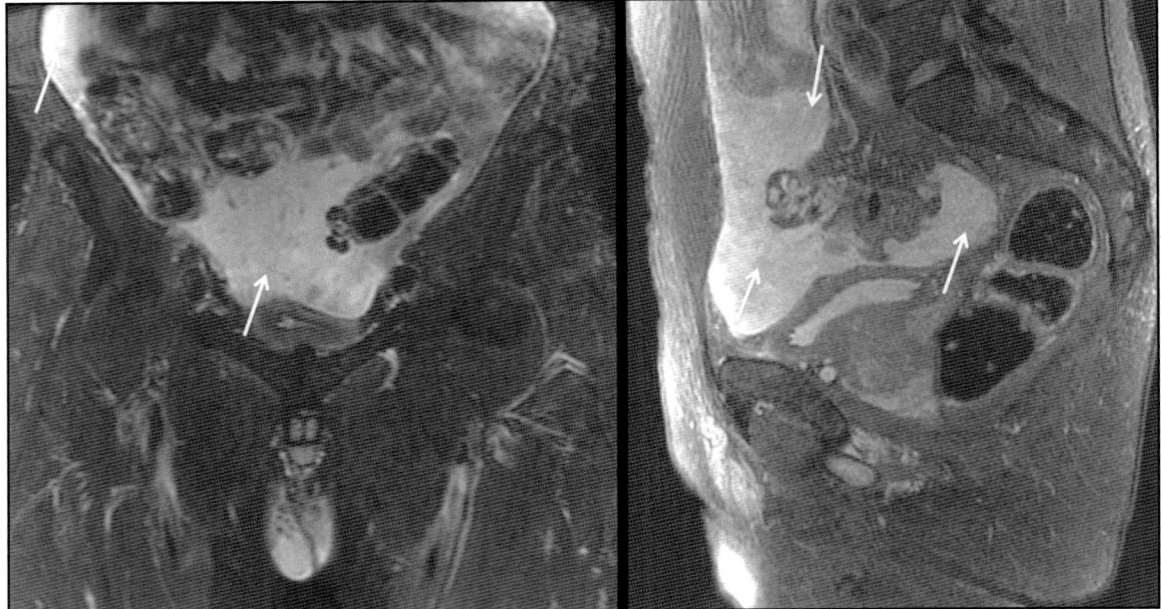

Figure A-3. Ascites.

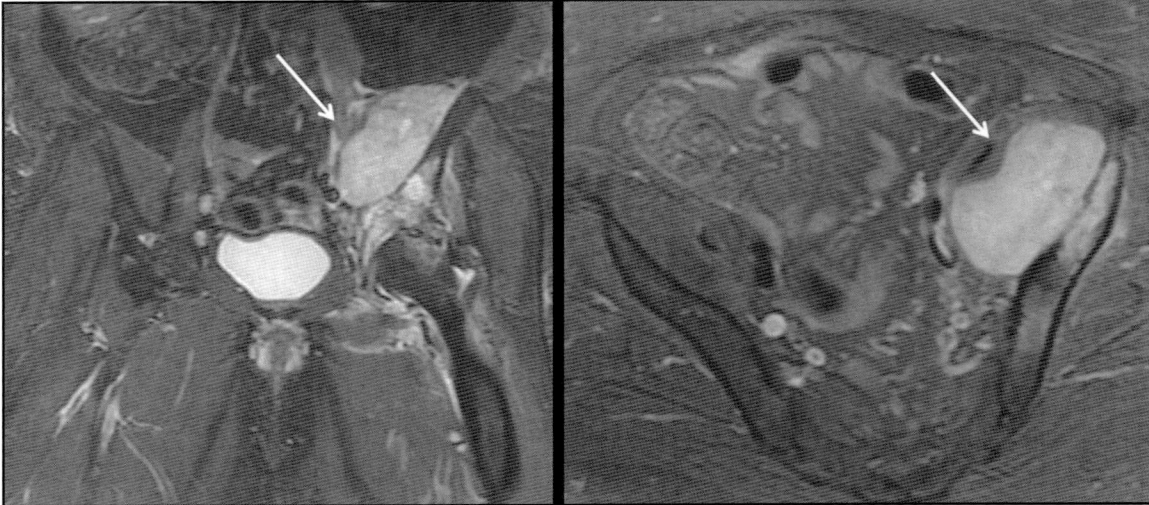

Figure A-4. Sarcoma of the iliopsoas mimicking a cyst.

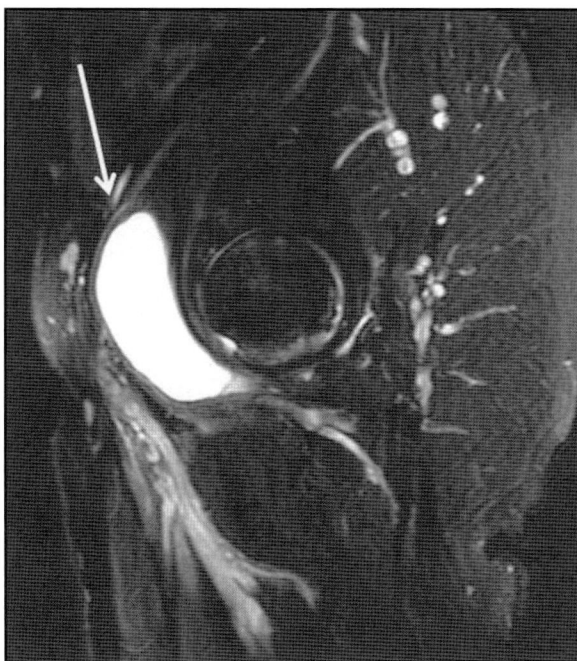

Figure A-5. Iliopsoas bursitis.

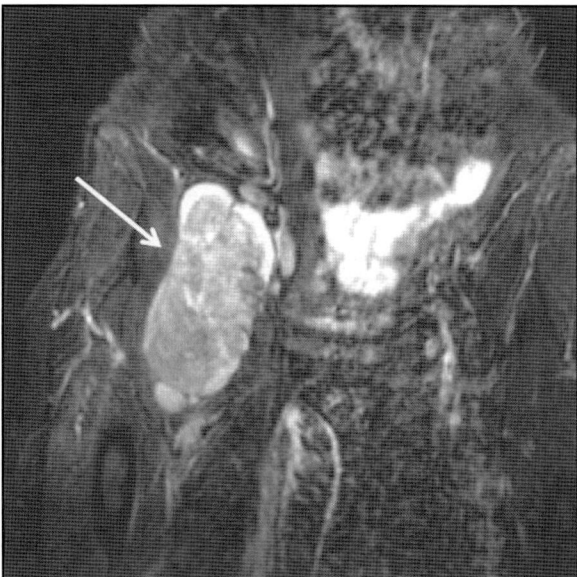

Figure A-6. Complex iliopsoas bursitis mimicking a tumor. (The term *tumor* refers to both true neoplasms and other mass lesions.)

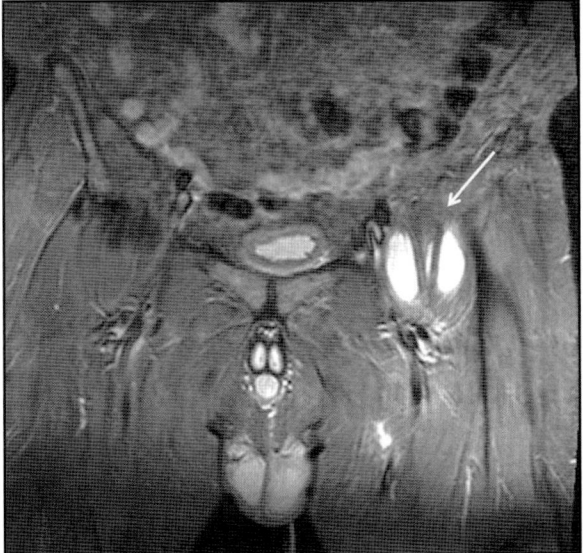

Figure A-7. Iliopsoas bursitis mimicking a tumor.

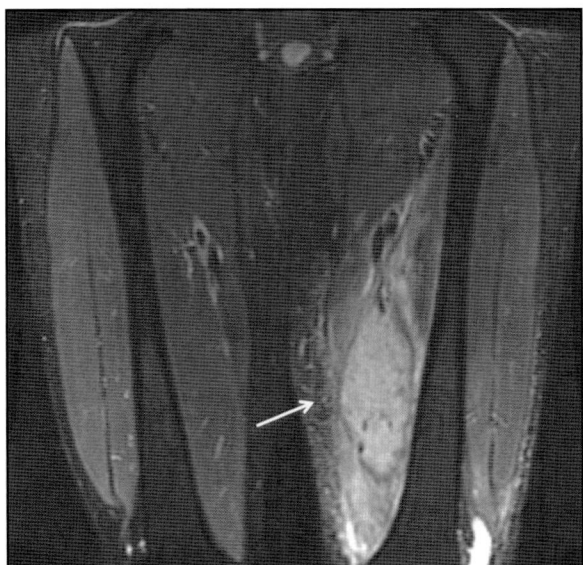

Figure A-8. Adductor/quadriceps tumor.

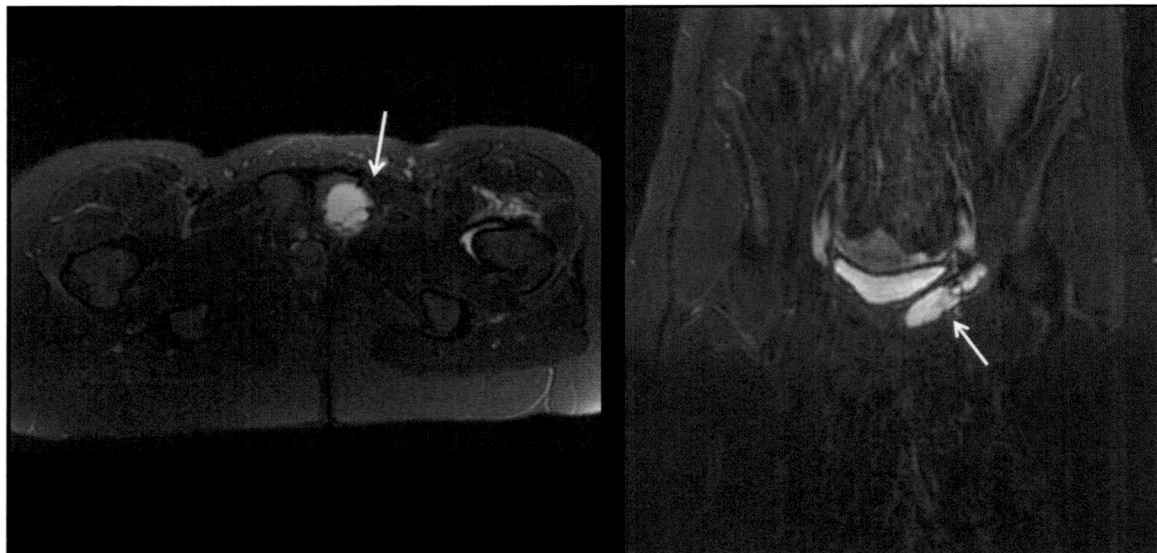

Figure A-9. Fibrous dysplasia (benign bone tumor) in the left pubic bone.

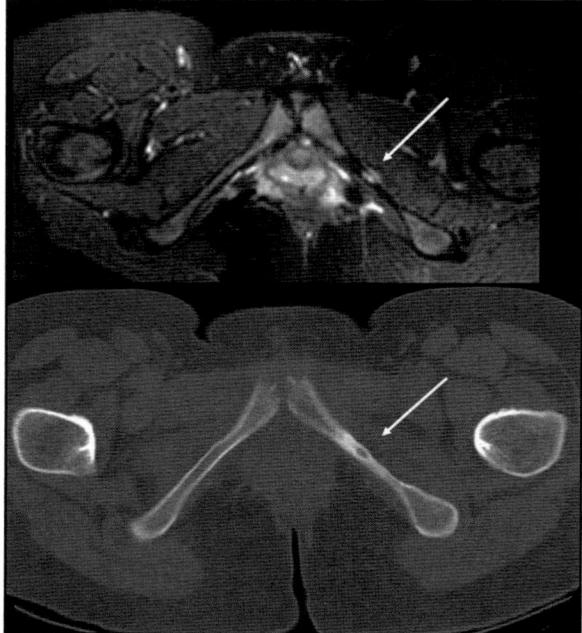

Figure A-10. Osteoid osteoma of the inferior pubic ramus.

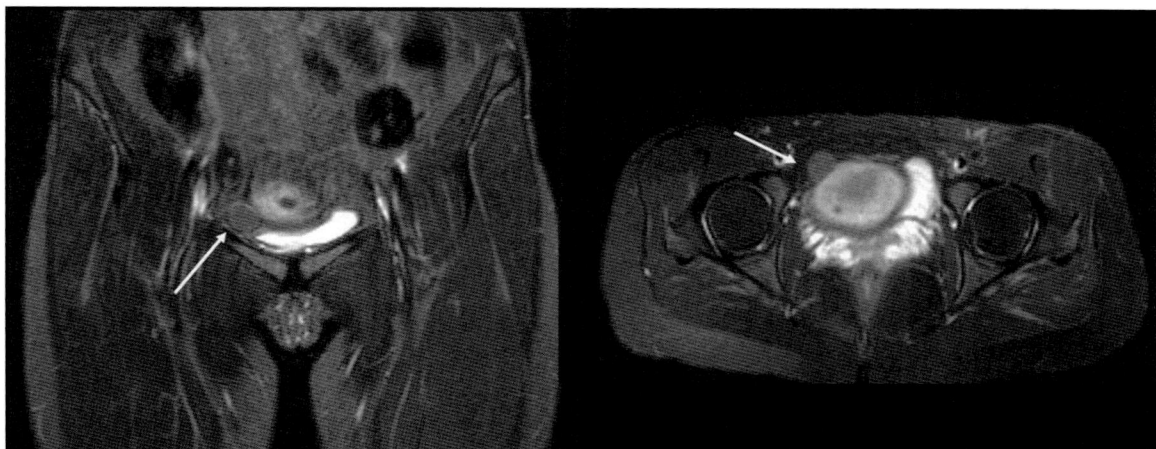
Figure A-11. Uterine fibroid.

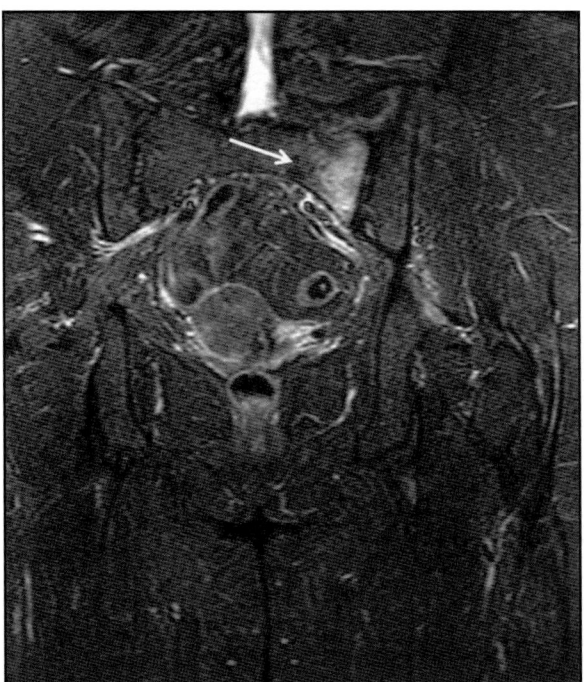
Figure A-12. Sacral stress fracture with inflammatory changes.

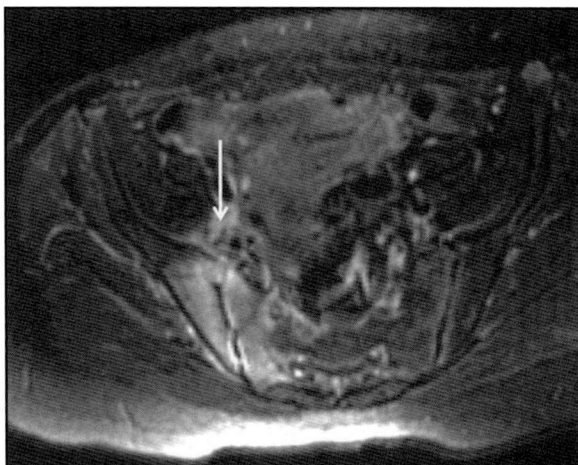
Figure A-13. Septic arthritis of the sacroiliac joint.

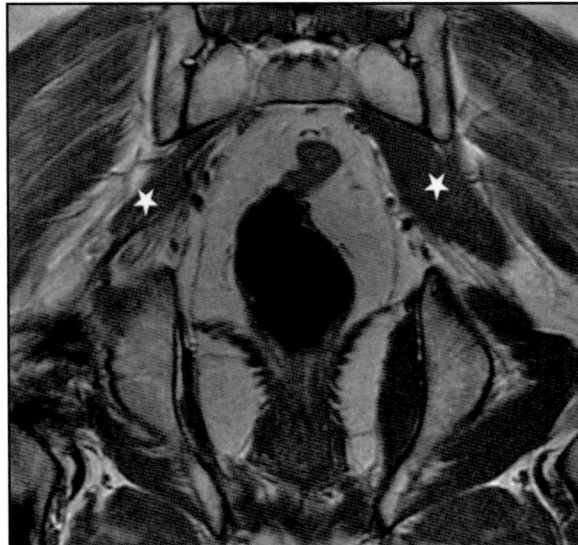
Figure A-14. Piriformis syndrome.

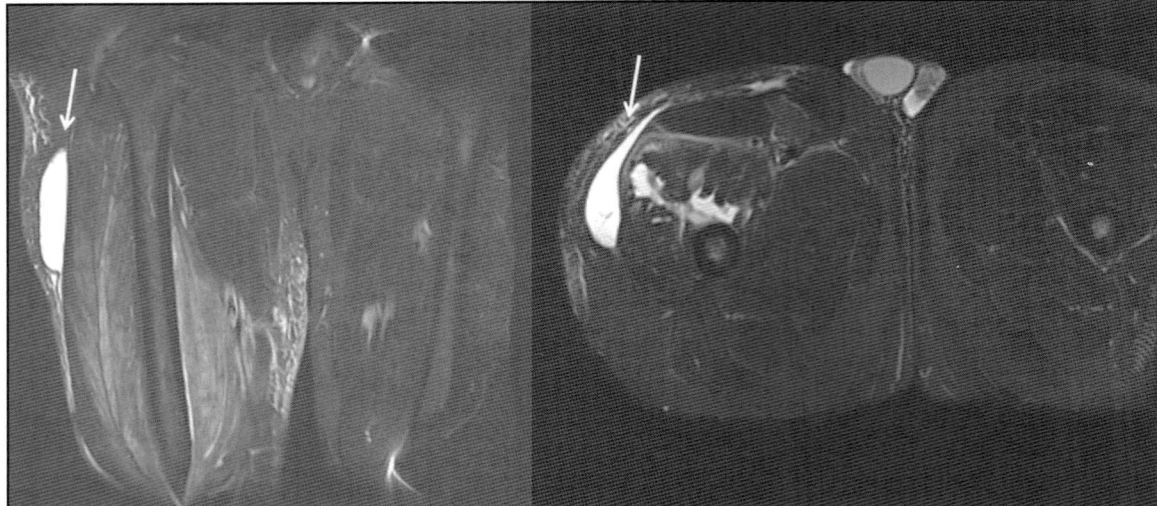

Figure A-15. Degloving quadratus femoris fascial injury.

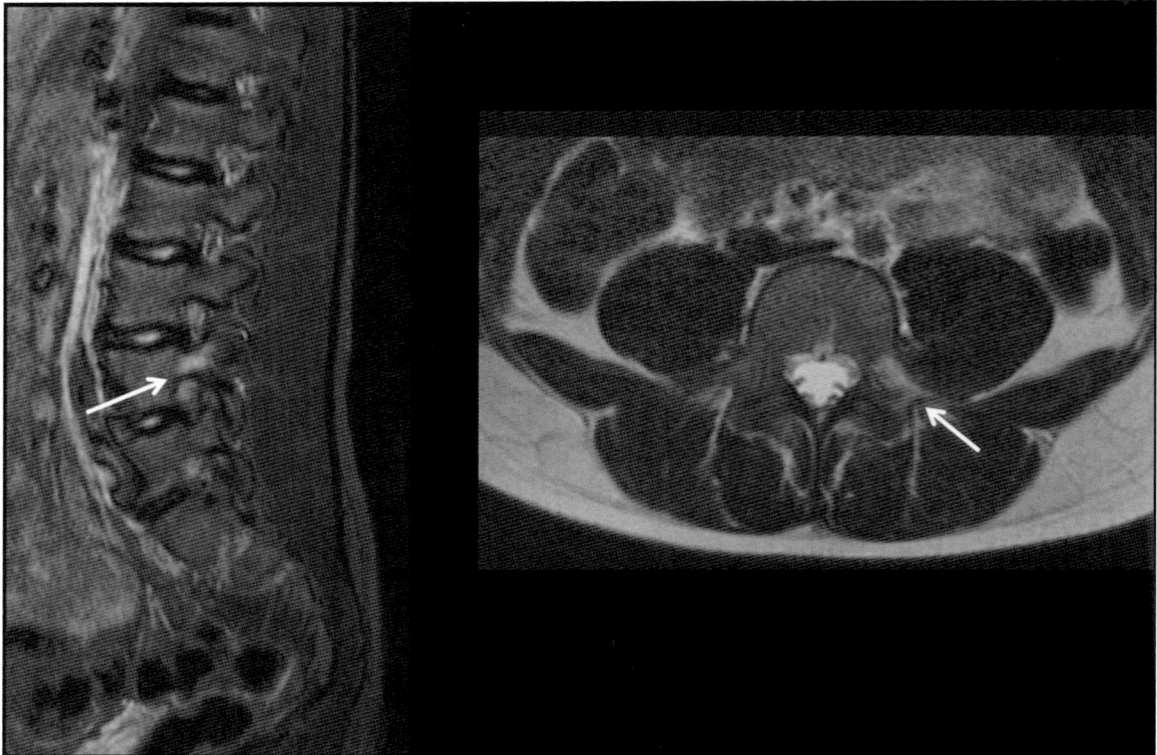

Figure A-16. L4 vertebral body stress reaction (pitcher's vertebral stress reaction).

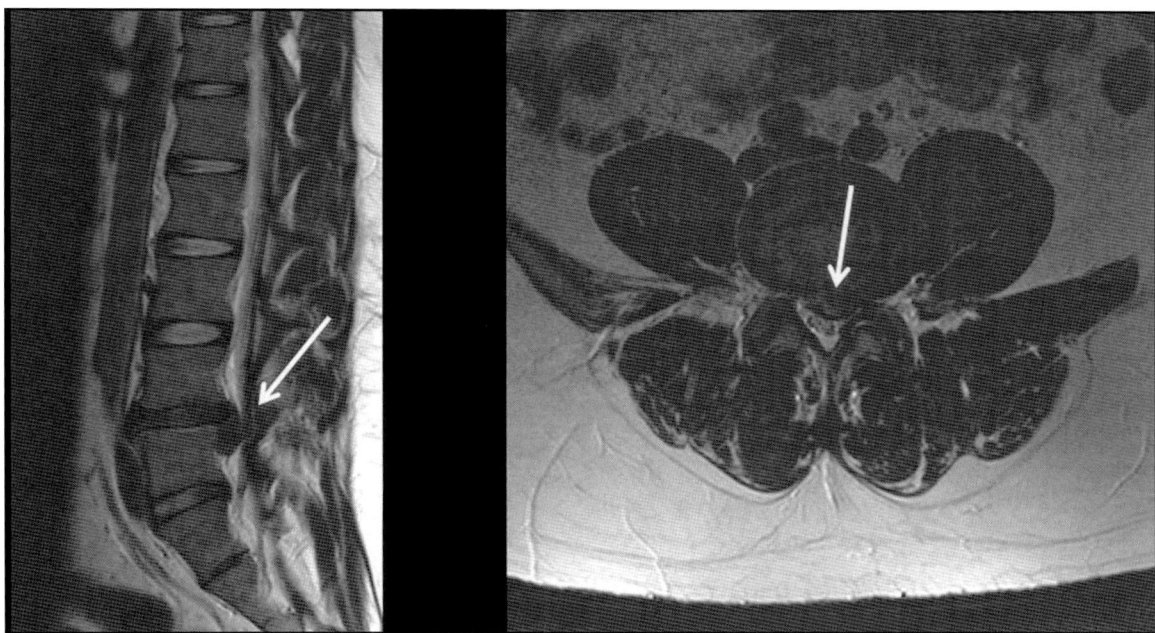

Figure A-17. L4-5 disc extrusion.

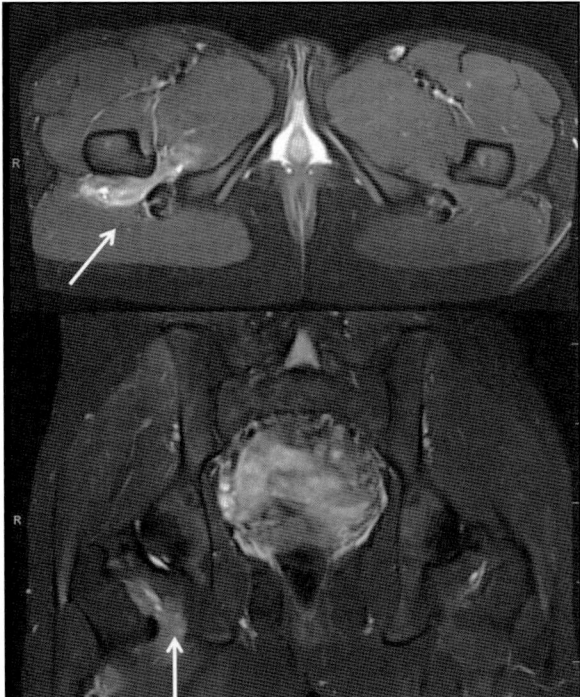

Figure A-18. Ischiofemoral impingement.

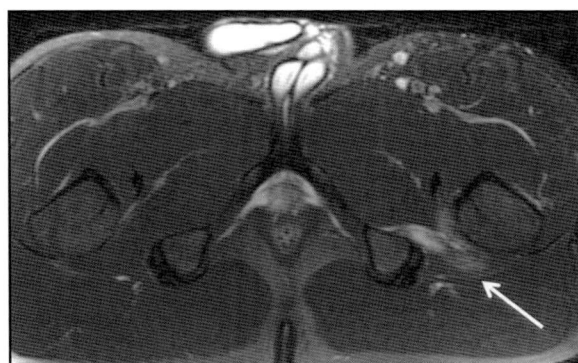

Figure A-19. Quadratus femoris strain.

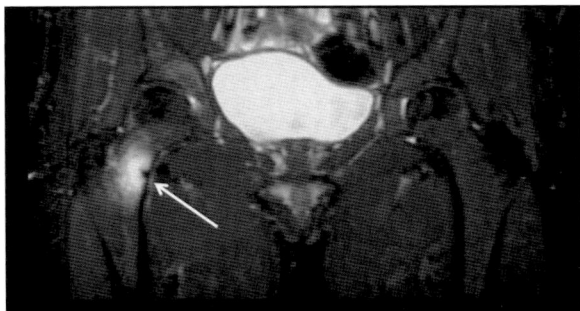

Figure A-20. Femoral neck stress fracture.

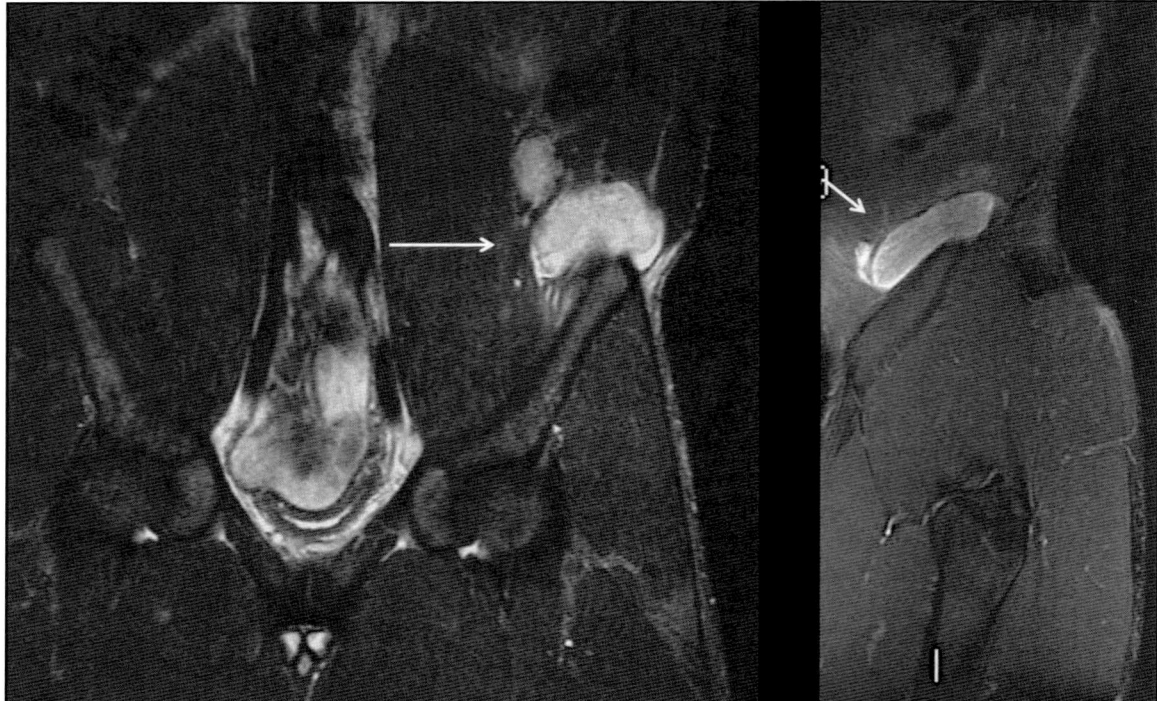

Figure A-21. Full-thickness avulsion of the abdominal obliques from the iliac crest.

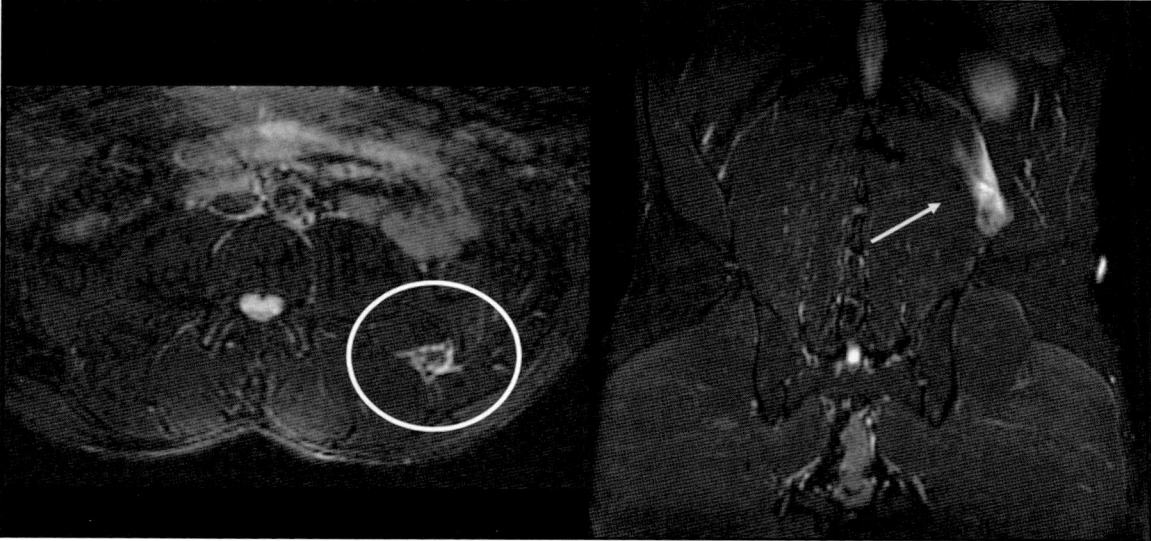

Figure A-22. Quadratus lumborum strain.

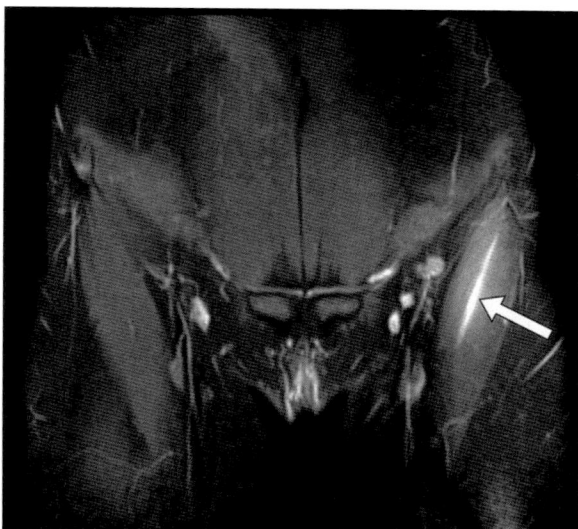

Figure A-23. Sartorius strain.

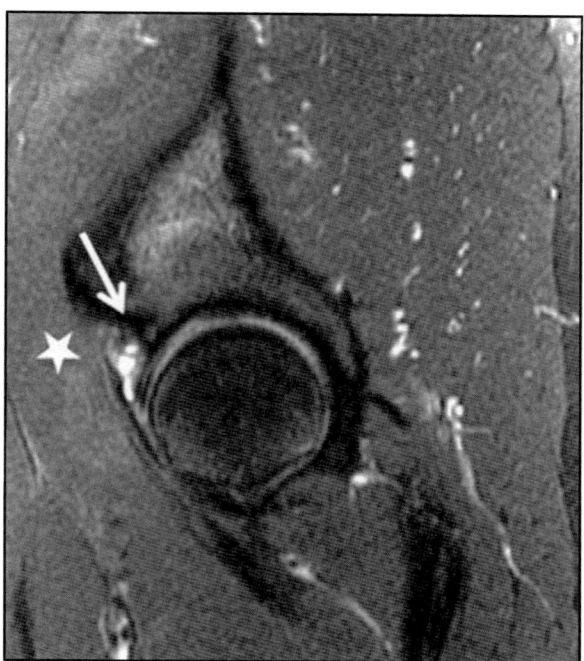

Figure A-24. Paralabral cyst with psoas irritation.

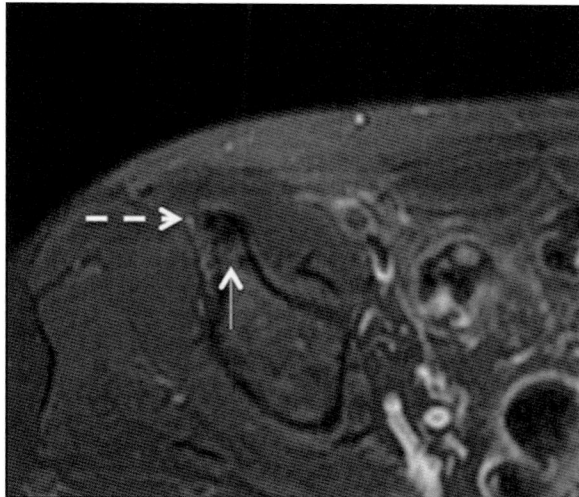

Figure A-25. Rectus femoris indirect head tear.

166　Atlas

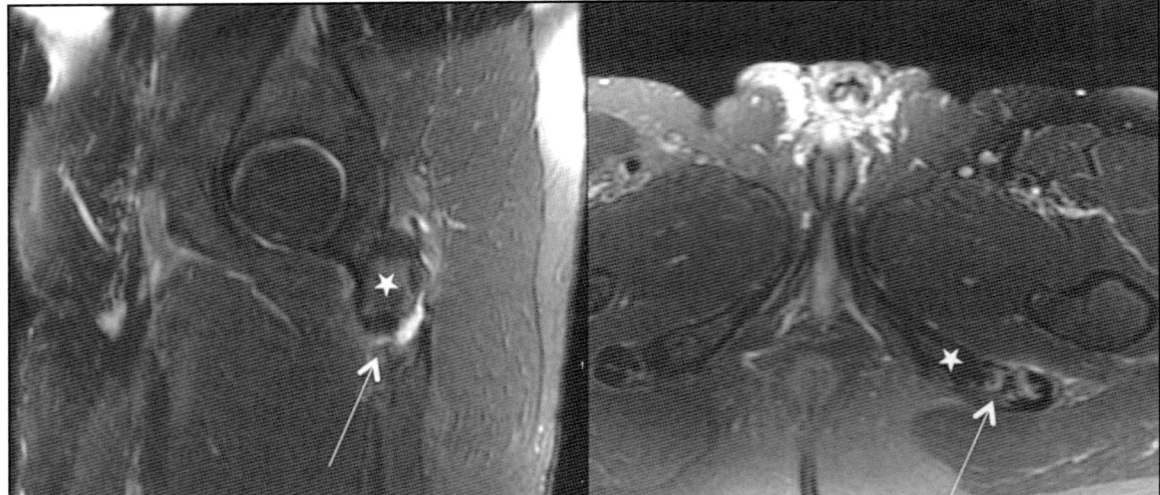
Figure A-26. Partial hamstring avulsion.

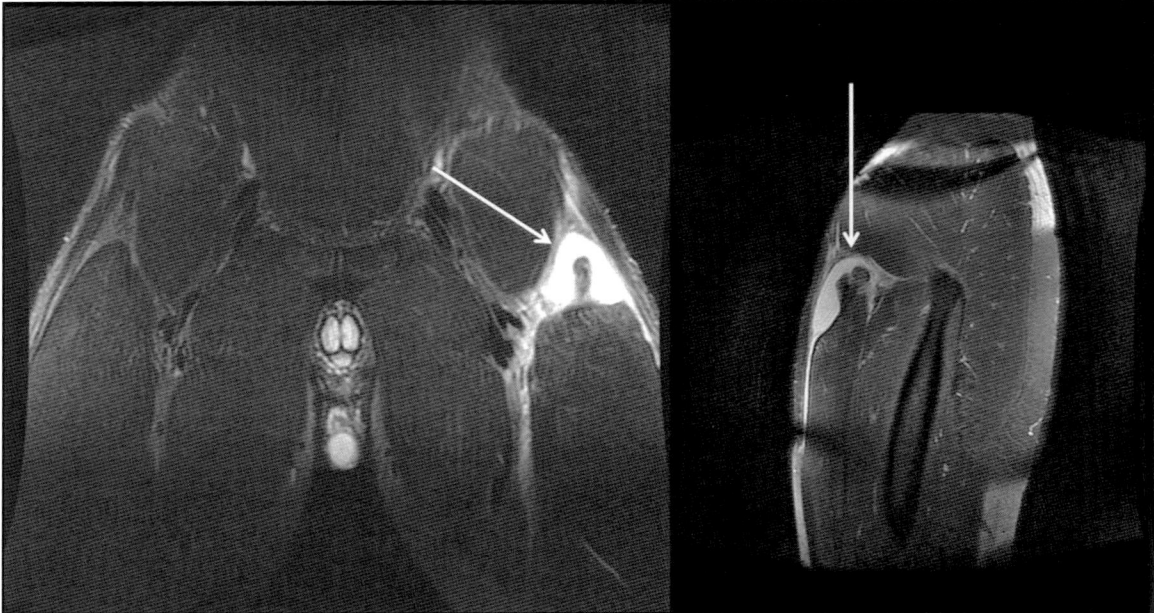
Figure A-27. Rectus femoris avulsion.

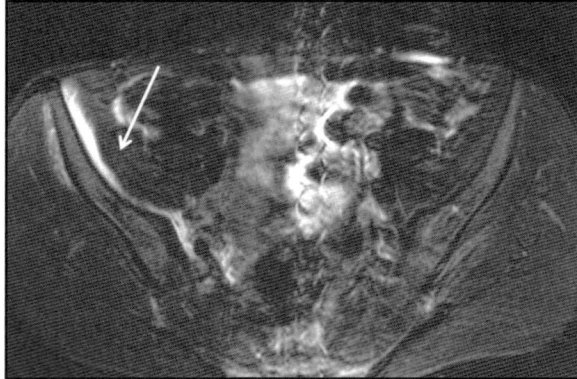
Figure A-28. Iliacus muscle strain.

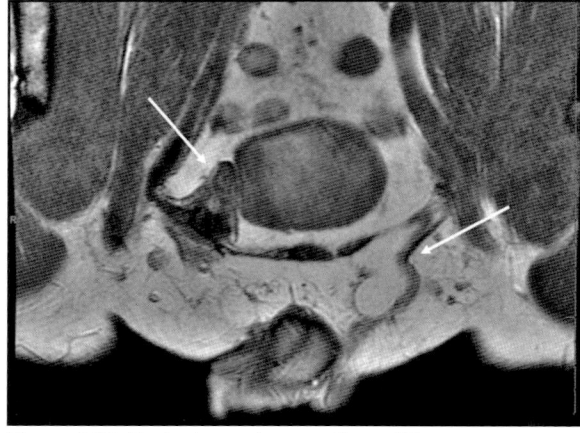
Figure A-29. Mesh plug and spermatic cord lipoma.

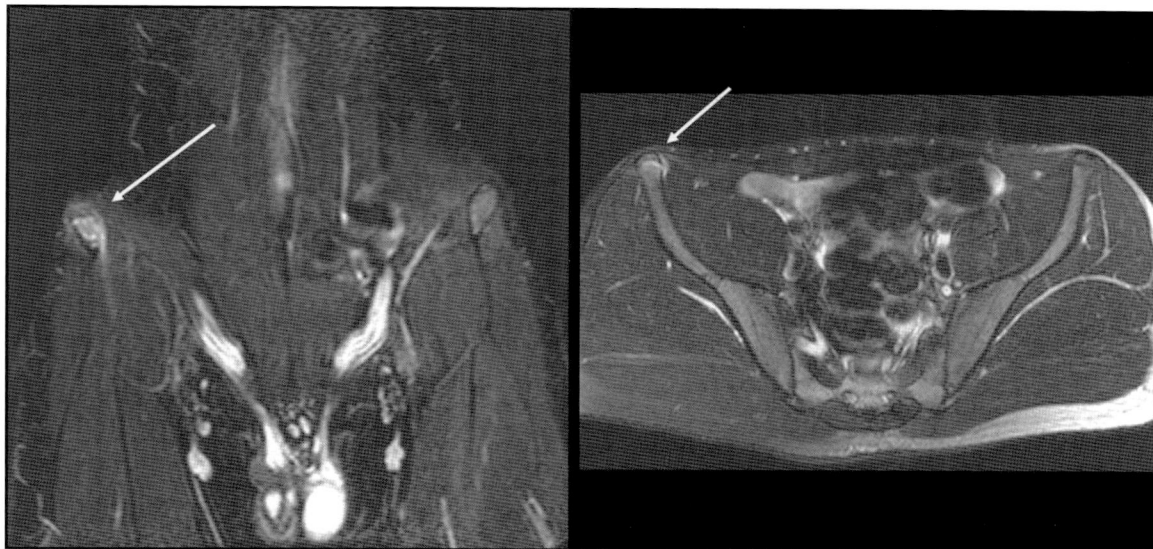

Figure A-30. ASIS apophysitis.

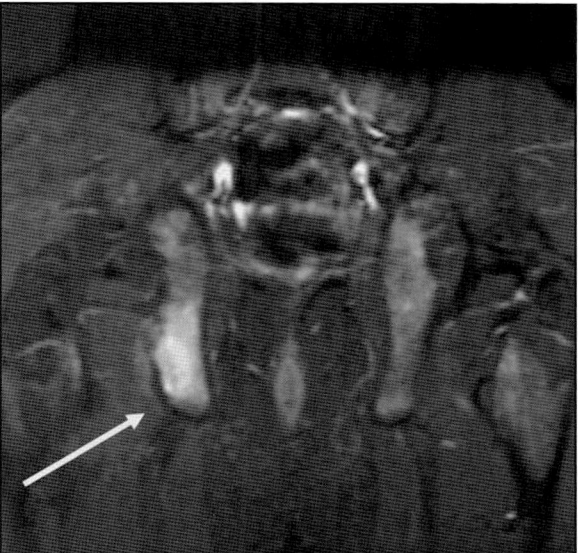

Figure A-31. Ischial tuberosity apophysitis.

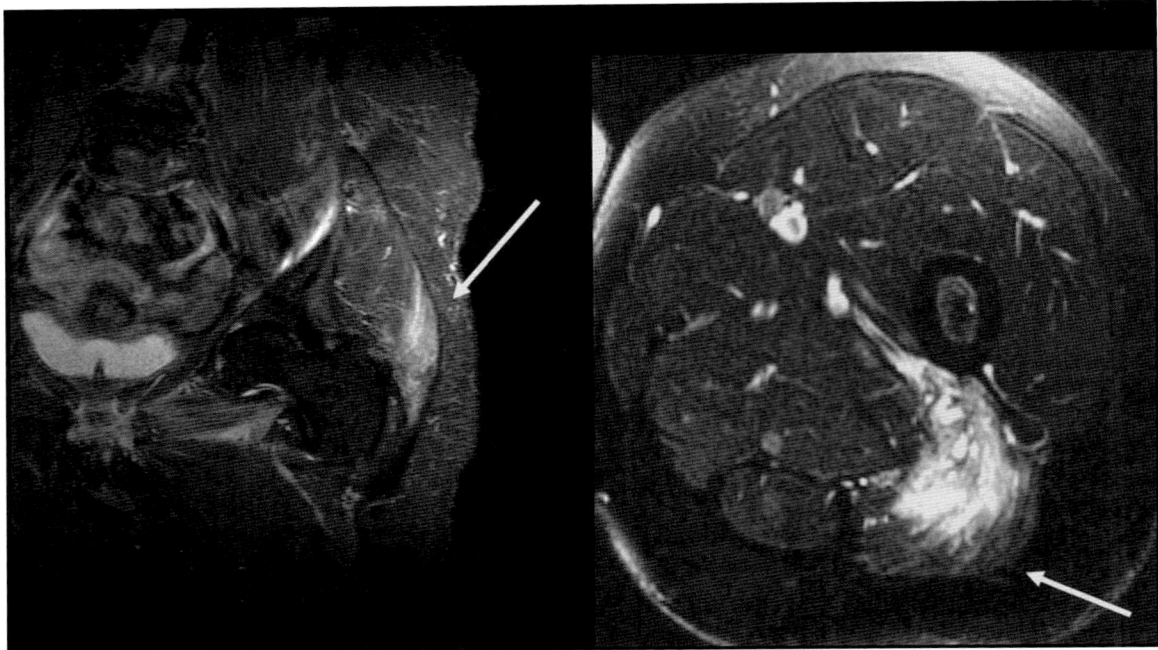

Figure A-32. Gluteus maximus tear.

Re-Entry

It is time to return to Earth. Hopefully, you had a pleasant journey. Two kinds of gravity await us. The next chapter addresses the ambushes that await us docs and athletic trainers within the core universe.

15

so, you want to become a **doctor**?
part **one**
diagnostic **ambushes**

Avoiding ambush begins with understanding what's out there [Figure 15-1].
—Current advice provided to Baltimore, Maryland, law enforcement officers.

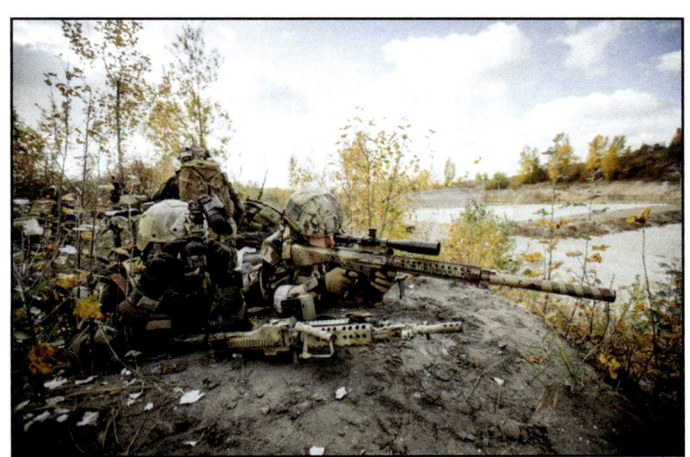

Figure 15-1.

So, you want to be a surgeon, do you? Well, it's not all red carpets, private planes, and yachts. Although most of it is! (Sarcasm.)

Consider the downside, like the orthopedic surgeon in Vermont who was conducting pelvic exams on women who were complaining about pain in the area. It made sense—except for the fact that he wasn't an OB/GYN doctor, and that several women complained that he had violated them.

We're talking about a very tenuous area here, especially for women. But while diagnosing the problem with some of the soft tissue around the hip isn't easy, the pain is very real. And a lot of it is found in people who aren't trying to stop a hockey puck from going into the net, drive a golf ball 300 yards, or dunk a basketball. People who sit often can have significant issues around their hips. Women can experience tremendous pain during sex.

A lot of this is quite new. We're just learning about some of the relationships between certain behaviors and the problems they can cause in this area. It's complicated and produces some odd complaints that lead to nontraditional diagnoses and outcomes. Of course, the more we investigate, the more we learn.

And the more Oscar parties we get invited to. (Sarcasm.)

Ideas that require people to reorganize their picture of the world provoke hostility.
—American journalist/author James Gleick, *Chaos: The Making of a New Science.*

THE WAY IT WAS

We already talked about the way things used to be (and to some degree still are) when it comes to these core injuries. The player/patient goes from specialist to specialist. Still no clear diagnosis emerges. The player quits or does not make the squad. The health administrator says: "We tried our darnedest to help you." The fact is, or was, that no one was smart enough to figure out the diagnosis.

That type of ambush was almost acceptable back then. Life was short. The player might even have been a malingerer. We knew no better.

THE WAY IT IS NOW

Look at things today, from the standpoint of the athletic trainer. The pressure mounts. The same athletic trainers and docs as yesteryear need a cure, for sure, for their star players. The athletic trainers are smart, they recognize a problem exists, yet they don't know exactly what the injury is, nor how much intervention may be necessary. They send the player to a hip surgeon or general surgeon.

At this point, various things happen. The quality of these consultations varies. It is easy for athletic trainers to be left "holding the bag." For the most part, coaches and general managers won't understand. They expect the athletic trainer and team doctor to come up with a definitive treatment or, in the least, a good plan. If the player doesn't do well, no matter the medical advice, the blame gets dumped on the athletic trainer. The coach thinks that, somehow, the athletic trainer either didn't get the player into good enough shape to begin with, or didn't inform the coach soon enough, or perhaps didn't pursue the right medical opinions. Somehow, the athletic trainer did something wrong.

So then, what keeps us from making the correct diagnosis? Why do so many patients continue to do badly with these types of injuries? Where are the ambushes?

No doubt, the biggest culprit remains in thinking these pelvic pains are "occult hernias." We've discussed this subject already. These traps come mostly from human glitches.

New ideas about pelvic pain in athletes (ie, the statement: "There is no such thing as a 'sports hernia'") force most people to reorganize their picture of the world. Just like Gleick said in the above quotation, paradigm-shift ideas provoke hostility.

Many types of ambushes loom with respect to this region of the body. Most traps relate to the narrowness in the way health care workers think (ie, the way we have been trained). Training of physicians dictates that we follow the empirical management rules handed down by our specialty predecessors—*Primum non nocere*. Doing things "that same way it always has been done" minimizes the chance of harm. Empiricism still dominates the way physicians are taught—"It works, so accept it."

THE WAYS WE GET AMBUSHED (TABLE 15-1)

We get ambushed in 2 ways:
1. By missing an important diagnostic possibility
2. By considering the right possibilities yet evaluating the patient badly

None of us are perfect, and this developing field is tricky. Thus, we are all ripe for ambushes.

As we get more experience, the ambushes shall decrease in number. We are amidst a learning curve. Hopefully, the curve shall soon be steep (steep curves are good; we may initially pay the price, but learn things quickly). Unfortunately, so far, the core learning curve has been gradual (which is bad). Misdiagnoses remain common. In fact, misdiagnoses still sometimes seem acceptable. Silly rationalizations abound. "After all, *I told you* there is no such thing as a sports hernia."

Let's not accept misdiagnoses or poor outcomes anymore. It is past time to bear responsibility for making every possible attempt to understand the anatomy and the potential anatomic problems in this region of the body.

TABLE 15-1
TYPES OF CORE AMBUSHES
1. Diagnostic
2. Evaluation

Type 1 Ambushes: Missing the Diagnosis (Table 15-2)

The most common ambushes come from:
1. **Not knowing the anatomy:** The number one ambush comes from not knowing the anatomy of the core muscles and hip. Even obvious clinical and MRI findings of muscular avulsion, pubic plate separation, and hip impingement problems still surprise people. The team doc recognizes some sort of adductor avulsion and presumes it will heal on its own. "Adductor releases are the way to treat these things anyway." Hopefully, this book will shrink the prevalence of this ambush type.
2. **Lack of experience:** Nothing substitutes for long-standing clinical expertise. No matter the type of training (eg, gastrointestinal surgery, physical therapy, athletic training, orthopedic sports medicine), nothing substitutes for just "having been around a lot" and observing the nuances of clinical situations. For example, recognizing that Crohn's disease and a huge paralabral hip cyst may cause similar pelvic signs and symptoms does not come from a book. It comes from experience. The overall problem here is that the core has not been recognized as deserving of a distinct specialty. Specialists are way too much in their silos and ordinarily don't immediately recognize the correct differential diagnosis may involve a totally different specialty. In the absence of a distinct specialty right now, experience is the only way to come up with the right diagnosis for many cases.
3. **The back:** This is a fun one. We've got to keep the hair up on our own backs to recognize some of these tricky diagnoses. Of course, back pain is extremely common in athletes—actually everyone. Over the years, all of us compress the cartilaginous padding between lumbar vertebrae, and no doubt repetitive pounding exacerbates the microtraumatic injuries and speeds up slipped discs and arthritis that inevitably ensue.

    Diagnosing such problems is okay when the pain lies in the back or follows certain radicular patterns down into the toes. The diagnosis is trickier when the only manifestation of a problem in the back is pain in the abdomen, pelvis, or thigh.

    Think about it. The nerves are all over the place and originate back at the spine. This is the anatomy... To quote Coach Belichick again, "It is what it is." The nerves make things confusing. Here are some pertinent details. Memorize them...just kidding.

    The seventh intercostal nerve arises from the T7 (T = thoracic spine) nerve root, runs below the seventh rib, and sends branches anteriorly below the rib cage. The anterior cutaneous branch of the 10th intercostal nerve ends at the umbilicus. The anterior cutaneous branch of the iliohypogastric nerve, from T12 and L1 (L = lumbar spine) spinal nerves, innervates the suprapubic region. L1 and L2 supply sensation to the groin, and the adjacent roots L3 and L4 may serve as additional possible groin pain culprits. Essentially, the same nerve roots innervate the internal organs. Branches shoot out from nerve tangles called *plexuses*. For example, the iliohypogastric nerve, the same one that signals pain in the suprapubic region, enters the spinal cord alongside the nerves that monitor the ovaries and fallopian tubes.

Table 15-2
Type 1—Diagnostic Ambushes

1. Not knowing the anatomy
2. Lack of experience
3. The back
4. Peripheral nerves
5. Complex regional pain syndrome and other neurological syndromes
6. Tumors
7. Benign gastrointestinal processes
8. Benign and malignant genitourinary puzzlers
9. Obstetric and gynecologic conundrums
10. Vascular challenges
11. Lymphatic enigmas
12. Pelvic floor disorders

Think about it some more. This same spinal nerve roots (from T7 to L4) keep watch over the internal organs, the skin, plus all the superficial and deep muscles and bones of the core. By their nature, nerves cross their signals routinely. What the heck? Talk about ambushes. How are we ever going to come up with an accurate diagnosis?

Again, the problem here comes from our specialty silos. Have orthopedic general or urologic surgeons ever been taught these neurological pathways? Again, we are talking about the experience and the learning curve thing.

The above discussion brings up one practical, and really important, pearl to avoid neurologic traps: The neurological anatomy has multiple ways it can fool us. Even when we think we know the nerve root involved, do not congratulate ourselves too early.

The following real example illustrates this warning. After an exhaustive search for a regional cause of a patient's groin pain, we decided to inject the spine. We injected a particular spinal nerve root with local anesthesia and the pain immediately and totally went away. We congratulated ourselves. The pain had to be coming from the back! We thought we had found the cause (ie, the spine). Did it turn out to be the spine? Not!

Remember, anesthetizing the spine does not mean the problem is in the spine. As we have mentioned, spinal roots innervate everything from the spine to the skin. Thus, the positive response showed that spinal injection would provide only a route for palliating the chronic pain and definitely did not solve the mystery. That ambush happened recently to the wife of one of our colleagues. A hip surgeon ordered a spinal injection. The pain went away totally, and he concluded, incorrectly, that her disc disease was the culprit. For 7 months, interventional treatment of the spine failed miserably. Don't worry, the ending turned out happily. Her pain totally and permanently went away after total hip replacement.

4. **Peripheral nerves:** This type ambush flows from the previous discussion of the back. Think about the many peripheral nerves that we run across in the pelvis: the "3" anterior inguinal nerves (iliohypogastric, ilioinguinal, and genitofemoral); the obturator, femoral, lateral and anterior femoral cutaneous, pudendal, and sciatic nerves. Let's make 3 ambush-prevention points.

   First, rarely are any of these a primary culprit. It is true that any can be pinched by adjacent anatomic structures, but then we have to figure out why (ie, what is the primary pathophysiologic culprit). Complete correction of a problem treatment rarely just involves just the freeing up or ablation of the nerves. Clues to a more central nerve impingement problem include profound weakness and/or atrophy. Surgeons frequently fall into traps like these. In just 1 month's time frame, we saw 4 patients with "obturator hernias" wrongly diagnosed by the same surgeon. Even to the general surgeon, diagnosis of an obturator hernia is a rare event. Indeed, all 4 patients had signs and symptoms that involved muscles innervated by the obturator nerves. The CT, MRI, and ultrasounds that supposedly showed the diagnoses all turned out to be baloney. All 4 patients had distinct core injuries that had nothing to do with hernias at all.

   Second, all of these nerves have considerable anatomical variability. For example, in the first paragraph of this section on peripheral nerves, we said there were "3" anterior inguinal nerves. We intentionally put the number 3 in quotation marks relating to the anterior inguinal nerves. While most anatomic textbooks say there are 3, just about any general surgeon will tell you that at inguinal exploration, there are often 4, 5, or more main identifiable nerve trunks.

   And third, remember that the pudendal and sciatic nerves lie posteriorly in the pelvis. Sometimes, people speculate that these nerves are injured during inguinal surgery. The only way that might occur anatomically is if somehow the pelvic bones dramatically shift. That's difficult to do in the absence of concomitant hip or other bony pelvic surgery. Watch out, on the other hand, when one works on the bones or dissects in the posterior pelvis. These nerves then do come into play. We should learn the gross anatomy of the latter-mentioned 2 nerves.

5. **Complex regional pain syndrome and other neurological syndromes:** Neurologists attribute many seemingly primary nerve problems to an entity called *complex regional pain syndrome* (CRPS). The problem supposedly has a real biochemical basis. Its pathogenesis relates to damage or malfunction initially of the peripheral nerves and then of the entire nervous system. The best prognostic scenario comes when there is a clearly delineated mechanical injury triggering the whole syndrome. If this mechanical injury can be corrected, the whole syndrome may go away. The first line of treatment for CRPS, therefore, may be to correct all structural damage that can be identified in regions where the pain seems maximal or to have begun. Dr. Robert Schwartzman, the guru of CRPS,[1] routinely states: "Without repairing the mechanical factors that trigger the pain, one has no chance to control the nervous system that has gone haywire."

    While most people consider CRPS a diagnosis of exclusion, it does not have to be. Even the most experienced of us diagnosticians see a lot of tricky patients. Never forget the possibility of CRPS.

    But also, do not dwell too much on the possibility of this diagnosis. Just entertaining the diagnosis sometimes sentences a patient to a lifetime of experimental therapy and pain clinics. Read more about CRPS and other neurological considerations in Chapter 18.

6. **Tumors:** Professional sports come full of stories about cancers and other tumors discovered in the unusual setting called sports medicine: Lance Armstrong,[2] Mario Lemieux,[3] Saku Koivu,[4] Eric Davis,[5] Jon Lester,[6] Billy Mayfair,[7] Darryl Strawberry,[8] and John Kruk[9]—to name a few. Remember that cancers do occur in the younger age groups and they occur more often in the core than other areas of the body. My first encounter with cancer and groin pain came in the late 1980s: a pro hockey goalie with a real muscle injury, but also with some extremely large superficial inguinal lymph nodes that turned out benign. Those lymph nodes, fortunately (so it turned out), were early harbingers of a rectal cancer that had metastasized to the liver. I remember this patient well because he was alive and well 28 years later, when he texted me to give me a hard time about the Philadelphia Flyers. I remember him also because, against medical advice, he played goalie in a pro playoff hockey game on the fifth postoperative day after a big (segment IV) central liver resection.[10] Here are a couple of MRIs of other tumors that we have picked up in our practice. The message here is to stay alert for this potentially devastating ambush, tumors tend to mimic core muscle injuries or hip problems (Figures 15-2 and 15-3).

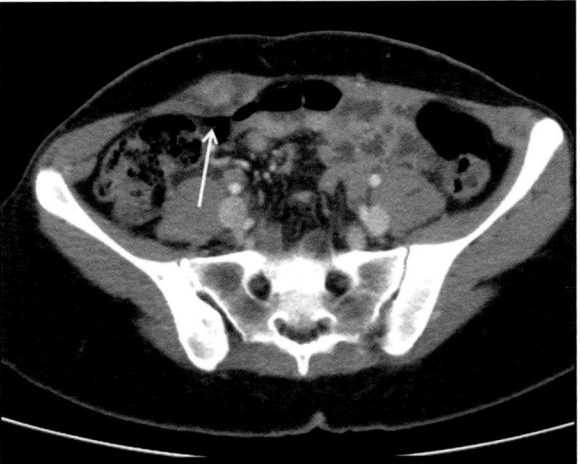

Figure 15-2. CT of an endometrioma of the right rectus abdominis muscle, a benign lesion mimicking a tumor in a female soccer player. The painful lesion was removed surgically.

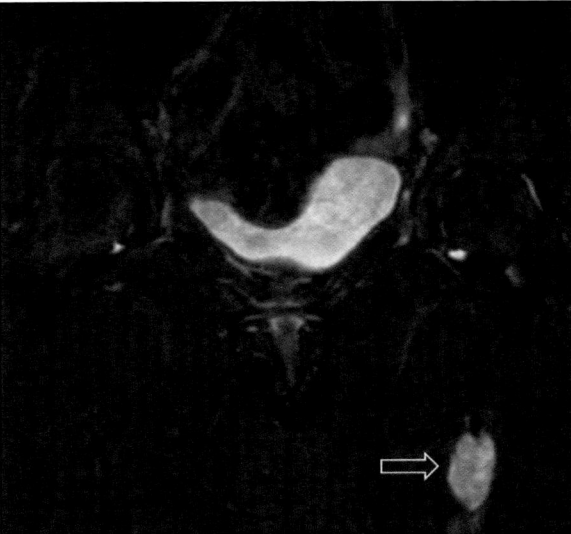

Figure 15-3. This vicious synovial sarcoma of the femoral sheath attacked a female volleyball player. We radically resected it, the patient received adjuvant radiation, and, fortunately, she remains alive and well, and now a journalist 10 years after all this. The tumor was pressing on the femoral nerve causing adductor pain and was initially thought to be an injury.

7. **Benign gastrointestinal processes:** There are a number of conditions to mention here including appendicitis. Of course, appendicitis comes into differential play almost exclusively with suspected acute injury. To complicate that statement, we did see one patient with long-standing pelvic pain due to an 18-inch-long appendix that encircled a floppy transverse colon. The most common gastrointestinal confusor in our experience is Crohn's disease (Figure 15-4).

8. **Benign and malignant genitourinary puzzlers:** Lots of things can happen here. First of all, testicular pain occurs frequently with core injuries. In our experience, the 4 most common causes of testicular pain have been (in order of decreasing frequency): hip, core muscle, mesh, and undetermined. Certainly, we have diagnosed a number of testicular cancers and benign cysts, and also true hernias and other problems. But these diagnoses were not in the top 4 of patients with testicular pain.

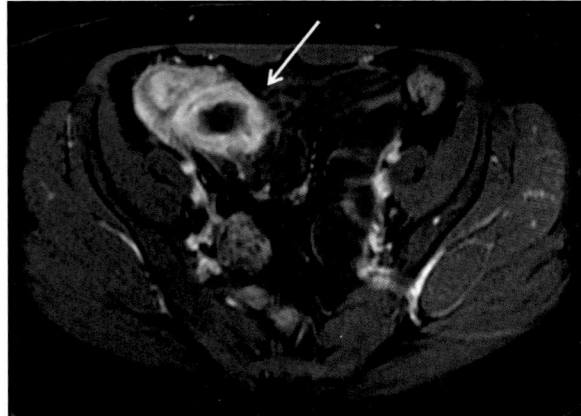

Figure 15-4. Crohn's disease with thickening of the terminal ileum in an athlete with groin pain.

The latter entities were not diagnostic puzzlers and required only a comprehensive physical examination and keeping one's eyes open and fingers equipped. Actual epididymitis, prostatitis, orchitis, and other infections have also been rare in our experience, although we have seen many patients who did not get better after having been treated by urologists for those conditions. Tenderness, certainly, is an important differentiator between local vs referred pain problems of the testicles.

9. **Obstetric and gynecologic conundrums:** Fortunately, obstetrics rarely enters into the overall diagnostic conundrum, although we often get asked about the ability to have children after core muscle surgery. The answer is "no problem." We have seen one case of ectopic pregnancy in an athlete with a suspected muscle injury. Plus, it always makes sense to think about pregnancy as one evaluates these patients owing to the possible needs for X-ray, surgery, and various medications. We have found cases of confusing groin muscular pain caused by ovarian cysts, infarcted uterine fibroids, and pelvic inflammatory disease.

The most common gynecologic mimicker of musculoskeletal pelvic pain is endometriosis. Endometriosis is the "tuberculosis" of the core. Just like tuberculosis, for years, has mimicked so many other conditions in the body, endometriosis ambushes us in the core in multiple ways. The implants can involve virtually any structure in the pelvis. A relatively easily diagnosable scenario is when one finds a tender round ligament in association with cyclically aggravated groin pain. Painful intercourse and other manifestations of pelvic floor syndromes are addressed in Chapter 23. Interestingly, Dr. Coleman and his colleagues have solved some long-time devastating pelvic floor chronic pain problems by hip arthroscopy.

Pelvic varicosities have received a fair amount of medical literature attention, but we have seen only one such case that might qualify for this distinction as a cause of pelvic pain. Perhaps our eyes are not open enough to recognize this problem, but we certainly have seen congested pelvic veins due to tumors, pelvic thrombophlebitis, and even endometriosis. It seems plausible that, just like varicose veins of the lower extremity, a similar process may occur in the pelvis and cause pain. We just haven't been able to diagnose this supposed entity with much certainty.[11]

10. **Vascular challenges:** One might think that arteriosclerotic vascular disease would mimic some of these athletic groin problems in older people. In fact, they can. Fortunately, when we have seen it, it has been easy to diagnose. We have not yet gotten ambushed thus far by this, as far as we can tell. On the other hand, we have seen a bunch of weird things, which have taught us to keep our eyes open for the unusual vascular problems. One such odd problem was epigastric artery pseudoaneurysm. Interestingly, we have seen 2 cases, not just 1. Both caused groin pain. We recognized both only at surgery, and did not see either on preoperative imaging. One was related to a laparoscopic tack used for mesh, and the other came after an open hernia surgery. In each case, we simply excised the aneurysm.

An important trap that may be extremely important to recognize is avascular necrosis (AVN) of the femoral head. This enters into the differential diagnosis mostly for patients with nagging and nonfocal pain in the acetabular, pubic, and adductor area and who often have uncertain findings on physical examination. Several times, we have also seen AVN appear several months postoperatively after femoroacetabular impingement surgery or even core muscle repair. The literature documents the problem to be associated with anabolic steroids as well as long-standing oral prednisone. We have not seen documentation that it comes from regionally injected catabolic steroids.[12-15]

11. **Lymphatic enigmas:** Fortunately, we have not seen too much of this. We had one patient with definite primary lymphatic ascites as part of the presenting groin pain. We have previously described the work-up and treatment of this.[16] Numerous lymphatic vessels exist in the pelvis and thighs. Most of these can't be seen with the naked eye. We have seen several lymphoceles complicate core muscle surgery. All resolved after drainage and patience. Two NFL football players played at full performance for over 1 month while still nursing external drains. The more visible lymph structures (eg, the thoracic duct and cisterna chyli) appear higher in the core and therefore are unlikely directly involved in these problems (Figure 15-5).

12. **Pelvic floor disorders:** While these disorders are mentioned earlier under OB/GYN ambushes, they are also listed here to highlight that they occur in men as well as women. Another syndrome often linked to this general category of disorders is interstitial cystitis. One theme that links the pelvic floor disorders is characterization by muscular weakness, spasm, and ligamentous instability, but the bottom line remains that they are not well-understood. Autoimmune and infectious causes have been implicated. Right now, we think of this category as containing mostly diagnoses of exclusion. Alternative modes of therapy follow the placement into this category.

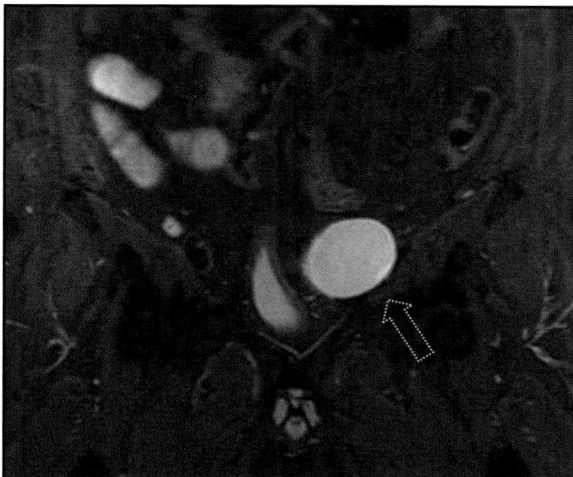

Figure 15-5. MRI of a postoperative retroperitoneal lymphocele (arrow) compressing the bladder. This appeared mysteriously after a straightforward rectus abdominis reattachment. It grew and caused pain, and eventually required surgical excision and external drainage for resolution.

Type 2 Ambushes: Evaluation Practices (Table 15-3)

Traps of this type come in various sizes, shapes, and locations.

For example, the core contains some private parts. We discussed this before and in Chapter 1 said simply: "Get over it." Well, that may be good advice for us, but it may not be so easy for the public to "get over it" as so poignantly illustrated by the aforementioned arthroscopic hip surgeon from Vermont accused of rape. His acquittal does not prevent everybody's nightmares.

Because this new field bridges so many specialties, soon we must draw new boundaries of patient care responsibility and establish fresh standards for proper behavior. Before long, we will also have to launch new operating room credentialing criteria. After all, either the orthopedist will routinely be operating on blood vessels, or heaven forbid, the general surgeon will be back fixing bone.

The credentialing scenario also brings to light the present-day health care reality of specialty boundaries creating vicious rivalries like no time before. Development of this new field crystallizes some challenges. That way it seems right to put some of these modern-day potential conflicts on the table, in another "ambush list" of why it has become so difficult to evaluate many of these patients properly.

Keep in mind that this just a list. And do not kill the messenger.

1. **Pelvic examinations:** The pelvis, of course, is one of the private areas. Even within an established doctor-patient relationship, examinations of this region may convey delicate stigmata. So, the question becomes who should do it? A gynecologist doesn't fit because he/she usually does not focus on the implications of musculoskeletal tenderness elicited via the vagina. The public would probably better accept a general surgeon doing the exam rather than an orthopedist. No matter who does it, it must be done in the right setting and with the highest ethical standards, in order to avoid any problems and to protect the patient.

   The fact of the matter is that, even in the specialized Vincera clinic, which focuses on problems of these types, we infrequently do pelvic exams in our female patients or rectal exams in our male patients. But we do do them, and almost certainly, we should be doing them more routinely. Logic shouts out that these tests should bring considerably more diagnostic information, and that more experience with these examinations shall contribute important knowledge. The fact is, however, that we cannot do these exams routinely right now. The fear of social stigmata prevents us. People will question us. That's the way it is.

2. **Locker room examinations:** For women and men, even less comprehensive core examinations can be embarrassing, owing to lack of control over who might be observing as well as other inherent limitations of the locker room environment. The set-up prevents completeness of the exam. It is even difficult to ask all the right questions. A limited exam is usually appropriate, but we must not accept this limited locker room examination as comprehensive. Relying on locker room examinations alone will produce errors of both diagnosis and management. Simply said, both the examiner and examinee need more privacy. Thereby, the locker room can easily be the site of an ambush (Figure 15-6).

3. **Suboptimal consultations:** GIGO: Garbage In, Garbage Out. An original computer science principle. This is also one of those "can't unsee" hurdles described in Chapter 4. The right core specialist needs to get involved. No longer should we be consulting a string of specialists focused only on what they have been trained to understand. Too often, the athletic trainer engages a general surgeon trained in hernias or a total hip replacement surgeon. The quality of the consultation depends on the experience and skill of the consultant.

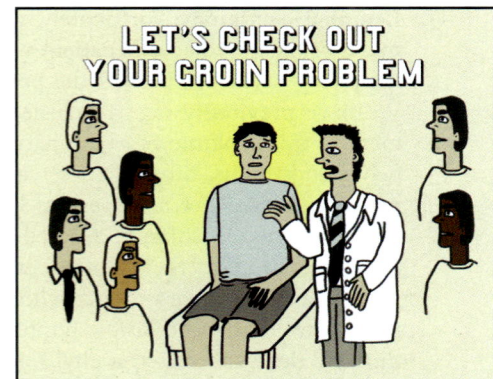

Figure 15-6. For obvious reasons, training and locker rooms are not ideal for comprehensive groin histories or physical examinations.

4. **Overconfident conclusions:** We all must guard against this. For example, as we have established, there is tremendous overlap between the various causes of pain in the core. We must remain open to the possibility of missing a simultaneously occurring important process. To the untrained core specialist, the last statement may seem non-Oslerian, but it is not. The core specialist will tell you that all parts of the core are involved in an important balance. Compensation happens all the time. I remember refereeing a fight between a general surgeon being "sure" the sports star's problem was hip impingement and the hip surgeon arguing fiercely that he had a "sports hernia." Both surgeons were blinded to the fact that the patient, in fact, had 2 related problems. Of course, both were wrong to be using that abysmal term. We must remain vigilant to the possibility of being wrong. We must quit staring each other down. We still have a lot to learn (Figures 15-7 and 15-8).

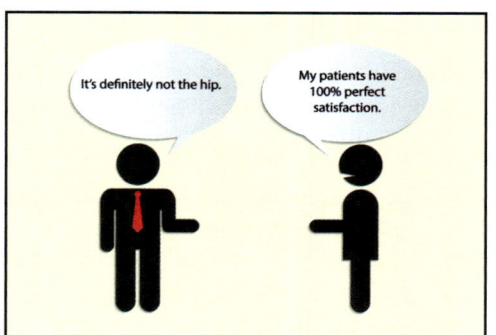

Figure 15-7. Overconfidence distracts from our understanding and treatment of this wide variety of injuries. We must stop saying (seeing) things so clearly.

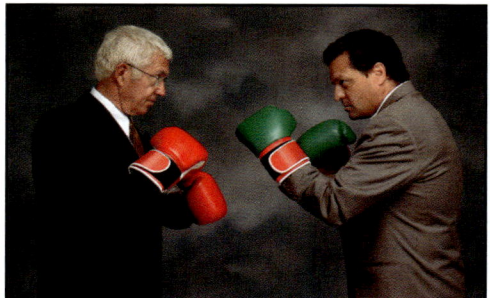

Figure 15-8. We also need to quit staring each other down. We still have a lot to learn.

Believe those who are seeking the truth. Doubt those who find it.
—André Gide, French author and winner of the Nobel Prize in Literature in 1947.

5. **Black-and-white interpretations:** As will be discussed in more detail in Chapter 21, a number of factors beyond the type and degree of injury enter into the decision-making processes. The desires to finish or not a season, contract or scholarship issues, and coaching or management decisions all influence best management of these injuries. Clinicians run into trouble by being too obstinate. The may come up with the right diagnosis pathologically but fail in diagnosing what others want or may be thinking.

6. **Insurance headaches:** We all recognize that insurance company decisions are based on a combination of maximizing quality, efficiency, and profit, not necessarily in that order. Those parameters may be interpreted in a variety of ways. Insurance guidelines and decisions for payment rely on panels of physicians and others hired by the company. That said, most leaders and innovators in medicine do not work for the insurance companies. New ideas and new procedures, therefore, do not readily get the endorsements of these panels. Patients, teams, and others get influenced by what the insurance companies do and do not endorse. Insurance companies ambush us in a variety of ways in this new and developing field of medicine.

TABLE 15-3
TYPE 2—EVALUATION AMBUSHES
1. Pelvic examinations
2. Locker room examinations
3. Suboptimal consultations
4. Overconfident conclusions
5. Black-and-white interpretations
6. Insurance headaches
7. Referral bias
8. Jealousy

For example, several insurance companies regularly label core repair surgery as experimental because of the absence of a randomized prospective controlled trial showing efficacy over nonoperative treatment.

Let's face it. The data are in: Surgery helps. Therefore, a star athlete will never accept a 50/50 chance of being in a nonsurgical control group when he/she hurts and can't play, and surgery is the only way to assuredly correct the problem. A proper randomized prospective controlled trial shall likely never take place.

7. **Referral bias:** One thing that everyone in health care develops is referral bias. Referral bias can play a huge role in the quality of care for core injuries. For a new field (ie, not standardly taught in medical school or residency), there is a high risk for referral bias to transform into an impending ambush. Referral bias by its definition means that the referral does not meet entry criteria. Entry criteria in the case of core injuries mean a sufficient knowledge base about these injuries.

As patients, we get forced by insurance companies, the institution for which we work, or even our doctors to see certain specialists, no matter what the medical problem may be. Often, we see the wrong type of specialist. Navigating the referral process is, by nature, difficult, and patients are often forced to take matters into their own hands. This developing field of core medicine only magnifies the number of ambushes that may take place within the existing systems.

8. **Jealousy:** Physicians are humans and personal disagreements also get in the way of good patient care. With this thought, it seems appropriate to restate the quotation from the beginning of this chapter: *Ideas that require people to reorganize their picture of the world provoke hostility.*

In life, some ambushes are easier to avoid than others. Some are nearly impossible to avoid. In this chapter, we have listed 2 sets of ambushes that presently plague this flourishing field. The core is complex and new, and the process of seeking and providing medical care today not simple. The best way to combat the ambushes lurking around us is to remain compulsive in our evaluations and transparent in our communications. We should recognize and treat the pathologies as we see them and to the best of our abilities, and in each case we must stay open to the possibility of being incorrect. As the field of core medicine grows, the ambushes will diminish. We must go through these growing pains because we are right. Many people suffer from these problems. As we hold to our principles, we shall set new standards.

Selected Readings

Sokol DK. "First do no harm" revisited. *BMJ.* 2013;347:f6426.
   An insightful commentary on how difficult it is to avoid doing harm in medicine. The perspective of a senior lecturer in medical ethics and law at King's College London.

Meyer AN, Payne VL, Meeks DW, et al. Physicians' diagnostic accuracy, confidence, and resource requests: a vignette study. *JAMA Intern Med.* 2013;173(21):1952-1958.
   An interesting study that demonstrates that physicians' confidence does not predict the likelihood of being correct.

References

1. Schwartzman RJ, Alexander GM, Grothusen J. Pathophysiology of complex regional pain syndrome. *Expert Rev Neurother.* 2006;6(5):669-681.
2. Armstrong L. Fighting cancer is everyone's obligation. *J Clin Oncol.* 2008;26(21):3473-3474. doi:10.1200/JCO.2008.18.6064.
3. Masisak C. Part 1: Lemieux's cancer comeback great sports story. NHL.com. https://www.nhl.com/news/part-1-lemieuxs-cancer-comeback-great-sports-story/c-658116. Published March 2, 2013. Accessed November 29, 2016.
4. Picard A. Koivu begins cancer treatment. The Globe and Mail Inc. https://www.theglobeandmail.com/life/health-and-fitness/koivu-begins-cancer-treatment/article763191/. Published September 13, 2001. Accessed November 29, 2016.
5. Montville L. Unbroken spirit. *Sports Illustrated.* 1998;March:46-48.
6. Petraglia M. Lester diagnosed with lymphoma. www.MLB.com. Published September 2, 2006. Accessed November 29, 2016.
7. Young B. PGA Tour's Billy Mayfair has more at stake than most. *USA Today.* https://www.usatoday.com/story/sports/golf/2013/08/15/billy-mayfair-pga-tour-wyndham-championship/2659143/. Published August 15, 2013. Accessed November 29, 2016.
8. Schmuck P. Yankee has colon cancer: Strawberry diagnosis stuns team. *The Baltimore Sun.* http://articles.baltimoresun.com/1998-10-02/sports/1998275015_1_colon-cancer-strawberry-eric-davis. Published October 2, 1998. Accessed December 2, 2016.
9. Smith C. When living for baseball is second; cancer gives Phillies first baseman a new perspective on the game. *The New York Times.* https://www.nytimes.com/1994/04/10/sports/when-living-for-baseball-second-cancer-gives-phillies-first-baseman-new.html. Published April 10, 1994. Accessed December 2, 2016.
10. Personal memories of William C. Meyers, MD, MBA about John Voss, a great friend and one of the great goaltenders in North American minor league professional ice hockey.
11. Borghi C, Dell'Atti L. Pelvic congestion syndrome: the current state of the literature. *Arch Gynecol Obstet.* 2016;293(2):291-301.
12. Weinstein RS. Glucocorticoid-induced osteonecrosis. *Endocrine.* 2012;41(2):183-190.
13. Yamamoto T, Schneider R, Iwamoto Y, Bullough PG. Rapid destruction of the femoral head after a single injection of corticosteroid into the hip joint. *J Rheumatol.* 2006;33:1701-1704.
14. Laroche M, Arlet J, Mazieres B. Osteonecrosis of the femoral and humeral heads after intraarticular corticosteroid injections. *J Rheumatol.* 1990;17:549-551.
15. McCarty DJ, McCarthy G, Carrera G. Intraarticular corticosteroids possibly leading to local osteonecrosis and marrow fat induced synovitis. *J Rheumatol.* 1991;18:1091-1094.
16. Rustgi AK, Rotolo FS, Peete WP, Vollmer RT, Meyers WC. Successful management of late-onset primary lymphatic hypoplasia. *Surgery.* 1985;97(6):714-720.

16
fifteen core principles

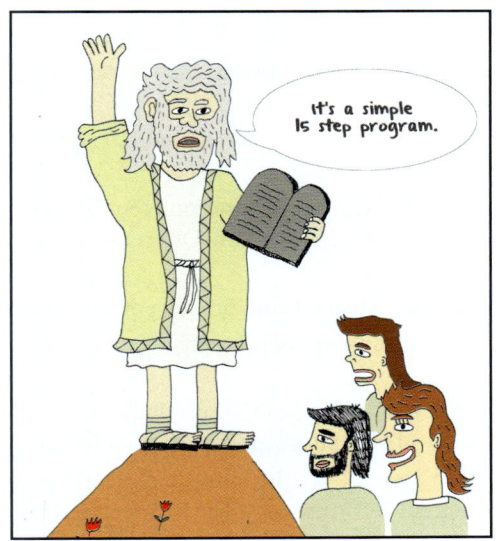

Figure 16-1. The 15 core commandments.

Okay, we diverted into clinical aspects and practicalities of the core for a while. Let's not get too far off track. Let's turn back, for a moment, to the anatomy and physiology of the core, the bottom-line subject of this book.

The 15 principles resonate (Figure 16-1).

THE WAY IT WAS

Remember that old Chuck Berry song, It Wasn't Me? There's a line in it that goes like this: "I met a German girl in England who was going to school in France."[VID 1]

Well, did you hear the one about the Russian hockey player who was playing for an NHL team in the United States and underwent 4 surgeries in different parts of the world and then suffered a fractured pubic bone and significant scarring that ended his career? Okay, it's not quite the same, but you get the picture.

Unfortunately, there are a lot of stories like that: people with core injuries treated by surgeons "fixing" the area with mesh or cutting sensory nerves,

179

then more serious problems. As hip and core specialists, we see new patients every day who just can't understand why their hernia repairs aren't working.

It's because they didn't have hernias.

People eventually will have to listen to the physicians and others studying this anatomy, physiology, and pathophysiology, so that they won't end up in the same situation as the Russian hockey star. Core injuries don't require mesh. They require precise expertise and know-how.

Right now, that may not be the most popular stance in the surgical world, but how badly should we feel about pointing out something that happens to be right? To a great degree, it is like lecturing at the barbershop convention that people don't need haircuts. Imagine declaring to the American Hernia Society that these injuries have nothing to do with hernias. It doesn't work. That happened. That pronouncement did not make this speaker the most popular guy in the room.

But Copernicus didn't have too many fans either when he said the Earth orbited the Sun. He just had to settle for being correct.

Okay, it's not quite the same, but you get the picture.

Near the sun is the center of the universe.

—Copernicus.

THE WAY IT IS—FIFTEEN CORE PRINCIPLES

By now, you should already appreciate the below-listed principles. Let this list serve as an interval summary. As you read on, implant these principles deep into your psyches. Here are the 15 core principles:

1. Think anatomy. Think in terms of the 4 parts of the core, and know that all 4 parts work together.
2. Think about the core's harness and the harness's communication with the brain and the bones and muscles.
3. Think of the central portion of the core as the axis for stability and athleticism. The pubic bone or an area just above the pubic bone is ordinarily the center of the core. That central focal point may change with injury and make things go off kilter. The hips and pelvis are a huge part of this central anatomy.
4. Think of the core as providing power and sense of balance for the upper and lower extremities.
5. Think of central core injuries as likely bad, and the more peripheral ones more likely to correct without surgical intervention.
6. Think with regard to protecting of the central core structures and building the power muscles and the rest of the peripheral core as protection for the central core.
7. Think of the kinetic chain as well as optimal order of sequential movements for developing strategies for improvement and maintenance of core integrity.
8. Think about the possibility of multiple sites of injury that might exist at the same time when serious central problems occur. This is a balance thing. To physicians, this concept may, on first glance, seem "non-Oslerian." In fact, when one considers the entire core as one body part, this concept is very Oslerian.
9. Think in terms of correction of central instability as all-important for optimal athletic function and performance.
10. Therefore, it follows that correction of central instability often requires a combination of primary repair and correction of compensatory defects.
11. Recognize that the systemic organs, blood vessels, nerves, and "everything else" (part 4 of the core) link anatomically to the bones and muscles of the core (eg, femoral vessels may actually affect the range of motion of the hip).
12. Think "out of the box" with respect to the possibility that visceral dysfunction affects the musculoskeletal function (eg, bladder irritation, Crohn's disease, sexual pain, or gastrointestinal dysfunction all may affect athletic performance).
13. Keep the bias that fitness, quality of life, and longevity all go together, but also remember that there remains controversy about this connection.
14. Don't think purely of bones and muscles when movement causes pain. In other words, do not miss the "more serious" stuff.
15. From our viewpoint, balance, fitness, strength, beauty, and stamina emanate from the core. Those are 5 good reasons to make core health a distinct medical specialty.

Memorize these 15 core principles. They will come in handy as we get back to more clinical stuff.

Okay, okay. You do not have to memorize them. Then, instead, read why we selected the 4 following readings for you.

SELECTED READINGS

Copernicus N. *De revolutionibus orbium coelestium* (*On the Revolutions of the Celestial Spheres*). 1543. Dictionary.com. Unabridged. Random House.
> *Of course, Copernicus's world-changing book has to be a selected reading. He laid the foundation for modern science when he propounded that his sun-centered model of the universe explained physical reality. Remember, at that time, this was truly heresy. He chose not to publish his book until he was near death.*

Kuhn T. *The Structure of Scientific Revolutions.* 2nd ed. Chicago, IL: University of Chicago Press; 1970.
> *In this landmark book, Thomas Kuhn destroys the concept that scientists search for truth. He substituted the goal of efficient puzzle-solving for a search for "scientific realism." "Normal scientific" research occurs within a paradigm. Puzzle-solving merely adds to the scope and precision with which the paradigm can be applied. The scientist, guided by the paradigm, asks questions that can be answered and that have an easily recognizable solution. Thus, the paradigm shapes both the questions and the answers. Normal science, as defined by Kuhn, is cumulative. New knowledge fills a gap of ignorance. But normal science does not permit for advancement by means of revolutionary theories. Inconsistent details threaten a paradigm. When enough inconsistent details concern a topic of central importance, science comes to a halt. Such a crisis requires scientists to reexamine the foundations of their science that they had been taking for granted. Copernicus's revolutionary new paradigm did just that. Therefore, Copernicus angered most everyone around him.*

Cohen IB. *Revolution in Science.* Cambridge, MA: Harvard University Press; 1985.
> *In his brilliance, my former professor Bernard Cohen, founder of the Department of History of Science at Harvard University, puts all this revolutionary stuff in perspective. He describes the stages that determine revolutions in science and how Copernicus, Galileo, Newton, and others fit into the overall picture. Alternate paradigms get proposed, usually by scientists who are young or new to the field and thus open-minded. Because different paradigms justify themselves with their own terminology and principles, one must actually jump into the paradigm in order to understand and accept it. Kuhn and Cohen use the word* faith *to describe the conversion.*

Voelker DJ. Thomas Kuhn: revolution against scientific realism. http://history.hanover.edu/hhr/94/hhr94_4.html. Accessed December 17, 2016.
> *In this editorial, David Voelker puts it all together. With a Bernie-Cohenian dialect, Voelker explains what Proust observed about real discovery requiring new eyes and not just seeing new landscapes ("The real magic of discovery lies not in seeking new landscapes, but in having new eyes"). A new paradigm requires jumping in and accepting, on faith, some new principles. One must jump in and accept these 15 new principles listed in this chapter, in order to understand the new paradigm for the core.*

VIDEO

1. https://www.youtube.com/watch?v=s_S3K0VzxN8

17

so, you want to become a **doctor**?
part **two**
history, physical examination, imaging, **and** other tests

You can't fit a square peg into a round hole.
—Idiomatic expression probably originating with Sydney Smith in a lecture entitled *On the Conduct of the Understanding*, on moral philosophy delivered at the Royal Institution in 1804: "If you choose to represent the various parts in life by holes upon a table, of different shapes—some circular, some triangular, some square, some oblong—and the person acting these parts by bits of wood of similar shapes, we shall generally find that the triangular person has got into the square hole, the oblong into the triangular, and a square person has squeezed himself into the round hole. The officer and the office, the doer and the thing done, seldom fit so exactly, that we can say they were almost made for each other."

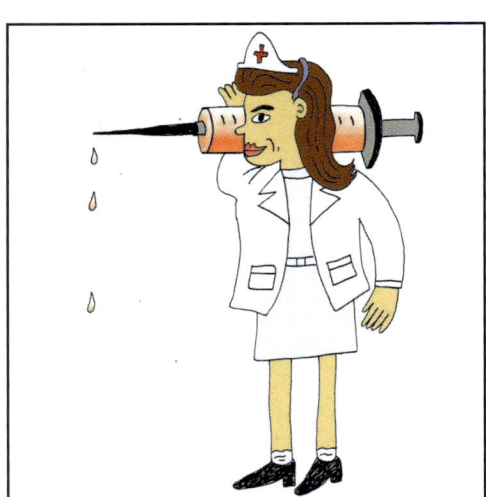

Figure 17-1.

THE WAY WE WERE
(AND WON'T BE IN THE FUTURE; FIGURE 17-1)

Let's take the perspective of the physician evaluating someone with groin pain. Depending on one's specialty training, a doctor is ordinarily going to try to wedge the constellation of symptoms and findings into a familiar diagnosis and something that has pertinence to his/her specialty, regardless of how well, or poorly, the history and findings fit that diagnosis.

The General Surgeon's Approach

When presented with a patient complaining of groin pain, a general surgeon immediately thinks of an inguinal, or other, hernia causing pain by stretching nerves in the inguinal canal. The general surgeon then sets out on a quest to prove the hernia's presence. He/She deftly maneuvers the tip of his/her finger into the external ring of the patient's inguinal canal, and perhaps other places, and asks the patient to strain and cough. If no familiar bulge reaches out to meet his/her fingertip, the good general surgeon undauntedly replaces his/her finger with an ultrasound probe on the belly. Thereafter, he/she relies on advanced technology to detect what his/her finger could not. If still no hernia is detected, he/she performs exploratory surgery, using a laparoscope or a direct incision to examine the natural weak points of the abdominal wall in case the hernia was so small that it could not be otherwise detected. Almost always, there is enough circumstantial evidence to justify placing a piece of mesh to reinforce the area of potential weakness. Usually very early after the doctor meets the patient, the focus of care has shifts from identifying the cause of the patient's pain purely to finding an elusive hernia.

The Orthopedic Surgeon

The orthopedic surgeon might already have been consulted on the same patient, but whether or not that has happened, usually little communication occurs between the orthopod and the general surgeon. The orthopedic surgeon, recognizing that occult groin pain can be due to a fracture, orders a series of X-rays and palpates over the pelvis. Any tenderness or inflammatory changes seen by the imaging are interpreted as consistent with a stress fracture and treated accordingly—with rest, sometimes physical therapy, and anti-inflammatories. Too often, the patients themselves are the only ones keeping track of the lessons learned from one specialist to the next, and they try to figure things out on their own.

Other Specialists (eg, Urologists, Gynecologists, Colorectal Surgeons, Physiatrists)

Other specialists get consulted, and just like the movie *Groundhog Day*, occurs over and over again. All specialists do what they do and send the patient home with certain instructions. The instructions often conflict. One of our patients saw 7 different specialists and amassed prescriptions for 7 different anti-inflammatories. The explanations become more and more inconsistent. Frustration intensifies.

THE WAY WE ARE (OR SHOULD BE)

Nomenclature

We have already established that we need to throw out all the terminology related to hernias and talk about the core. We shall apply the language introduced in the previous chapters to clinical practice.

History

We start this conversation by listening and then asking questions that pertain to the 4 parts of the core. As is hopefully obvious by now, suspected core injuries are best diagnosed by someone who is capable and comfortable addressing the entire core. Remember the boundaries of the core and everything within them: the muscles and pelvis bones, the ball-and-socket hip joint, the entire back with the thorax, hollow and solid organs, nerves, blood vessels, and other innards.

If this sounds complicated that is because it can be. The primary focus of evaluating someone with groin pain is to pinpoint the anatomy involved. If it is a core muscle injury, it is not enough to simply say that, we must hold ourselves to the standard of identifying, as exactly as we can, which of the 29 core muscles are involved if we are to have any hope treating folks. Table 17-1 lists the various clinical entities included under the umbrella term *core muscle injuries*. Pain that

Table 17-1
Some Diagnoses to Consider in the Evaluation of Core Pain(s)

The Core Muscles

- Harness muscle injury
- Individual vs multiple harness muscles
- Unilateral vs bilateral
- Pubic plate disruption
- Severe osteitis variant
- Power muscle injury
- Pelvic bone or apophysis injury
- Pure adductor syndromes
- Rectus femoris injury
- Primary vs secondary psoas injury or bursitis
- Baseball pitcher hockey goalie syndrome
- Pure rectus abdominis syndromes
- Spigelian or high rectus abdominis variants
- Female variant (medial disruption/lateral compensation)
- Round ligament syndrome
- Rower's rib syndrome
- Midline rectus abdominis variant
- Ischial tuberosity variants
- Adductor brevi/hamstring variants
- Pubic symphyseal disruption
- Gracilis injury
- Sartorius injury
- Dancer's variants (obturator externus/externus involvement)
- Tensor fasciae latae injury
- Iliotibial band issues
- Quadratus femoris syndrome
- Quadratus lumborum syndrome
- Gluteus syndromes
- Vastus syndromes
- Ischiofemoral impingement
- Other "deep derrière" impingements
- Calcification syndromes (eg, adductor, rectus abdominis, rectus femoris)
- Contracture syndromes (eg, adductor, iliopsoas, rectus abdominis)

The Hip

- Femoroacetabular impingement—unilateral vs bilateral, cam or pincer or both
- Pure labral tear
- Impingement syndromes without labral tear
- Ligamentum teres injury
- Arthritis
- Dysplasia
- Femoral neck fracture
- Avascular necrosis of the femoral head

Back Culprits

- Slipped disc
- Other nerve root compressions
- Pure peripheral nerve entrapments
- Sacroiliitis
- Sacroiliac "dysfunction"
- Vertebral facet joint problems
- Vertebral fracture
- Spondylolisthesis

Other Culprits

- Crohn's disease
- Other gastrointestinal disease
- Endometriosis
- Other identifiable gynecologic issues
- "Pelvic floor disorders"
- Bladder issues
- Vascular issues
- Lymphatic leakage
- Neoplasms

Combination Issues

- Hip causing core muscle involvement
- Core muscle causing hip involvement
- Can't distinguish between the above
- Core muscle or hip with back issues
- Combination of identifiable musculoskeletal defects with "other culprits"
- Complex regional pain syndrome

occurs only with exertion is likely to represent some degree of muscular injury, while relatively passive or postural pain is more likely from the hip.

A detailed history often rules out most of the "other" diagnoses. An in-depth discussion of the location and quality of the pain will get you started on the right path. Failing to identify correlations with gastrointestinal, genitourinary, or gynecologic issues is perilous. And this is easier than one might think. Understanding the movements and positions that produce pain provides important clues and opens up avenues to pursue during the rest of the work-up. This is not to say that we are Oliver Sacks, the famous neurologist and naturalist, making too-numerous-to-count detailed observations about our patients and how they compensate for their pain. Perhaps we should be Dr. Sacks, at least for some of our patients.

Physical Examination—An Open-Book Exam

While a comprehensive physical examination remains imperative, the most important tool in identifying the exact location of an injury or disease process is a focused physical exam. This involves a physical one-on-one interaction that leaves little room for modesty. It starts with inspection, when the bashful among us may become red in the face. Shyness cannot get in the way. All too often, people get treated for groin pain without anyone actually looking directly at the site of pain. We look for bruising, swelling, irregularities in the contours of muscles, and postural imbalances.

Physical Contact

After visual inspection, physical interaction involves pinpointing the exact locations of pain. The origins and insertions of different muscles often lie within millimeters of each other, as well as many other adjacent structures. Like anything else worth doing in life, a good exam requires good communication and physical contact. One may learn a lot by applying pressure to various sites. If one can reproduce the pain by pressing a specific spot, this may identify the whereabouts of an injury, but then we must separate out the many cases when tenderness reflects simply a byproduct of the inflammation associated with an adjacent injury. For example, severe inflammation of the periosteum of the pubic bone can yield false-positive hip signs. We feel or percuss for organomegaly, abdominal masses, boggy inflammation within soft tissues, dense scars along injured muscles, heat from a raging inflammatory process, popping when a tendon or cartilage is pinging over a bone, and subtle gaps where muscles once were and should be returned.

Active and Passive Testing (Figures 17-2 and 17-3)

Next we test the strength and function of various muscles in isolation, pausing to understand the exact location, triggering factors and clinical significance of any pain that is elicited. A complete hip exam is mandatory. One must have a detailed understanding of the anatomy of the hip and know the various normals of range of motion. Common pitfalls lie in wait for the naïve observer.

Inflammation of the pubis is common and can be one of the great mimickers of intrinsic hip pathology, as can be the psoas muscles or occasionally the rectus femoris. For example, long-distance runners, ultra-marathoners in particular, often continue extensive running despite severe core muscle injuries, and consequently develop tremendous inflammation between the pubic bone and its fibrocartilage plate. When pain finally sets off intolerable alarms, they have as much pain rolling their femoral balls around in their sockets as with resistance testing of the actual injured muscles, despite a relative absence of hip pathology. The Eminem muscle, love it or hate it, can mimic all of its anatomic neighbors, including the hip and adductors, which makes the differential diagnosis list of a psoas problem rather long. As mentioned in the Eminem chapter, psoas inflammation can simply represent a primary problem, or secondary psoas compensation for a hip or muscle issue. Often it is hard to tell. One thing for sure, the iliopsoas keeps things interesting.

The physical exam concludes after the muscle and hip examinations with a sweep of the entire body looking for signs of back issues, systemic disease, neurological signs, cardiovascular compromise, and everything else. While our focus of evaluation of these patients remains on the muscles and bones, our data show that one-third of the patients have "other" (ie, in the fourth part of the core) problems at the heart ("core") of their issues.[1]

At this point, we should have a pretty good idea of what's going on. Imaging confirms the suspected pathology and picks up clues to the primary pathology and related or coincidental pathologies.

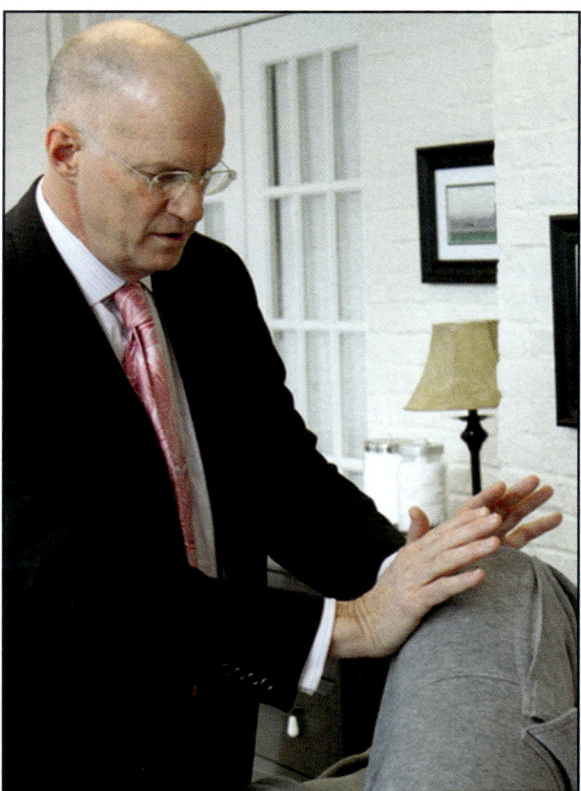

Figure 17-2. An active test on physical examination. This one is the pectineus resistance test.

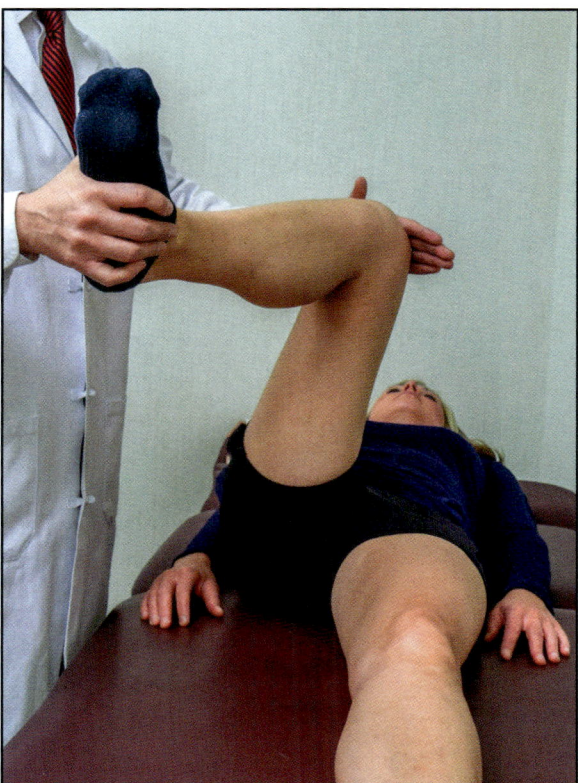

Figure 17-3. A passive test. Flexion, adduction, and internal rotation (FADIR test) is one hip circumduction test.

Imaging

In order of frequency of use, plain radiography, MRI, ultrasound, CT, and occasionally bone scans and other modalities complement the histories and physical examinations. With X-rays, we can see the gross bony structure of the pelvis and also calculate various measures of hip development and impingement, plus rule out obvious stress and other fractures and dislocations. Usually, the most important imaging remains a focused pelvic MRI using specific protocols correlating to suspected pathologies. One such MRI uses calculations to follow the slope of the pubic bone for precise identification of the muscular attachments to the pubic fibrocartilage ("baseball") cover. Often, patients have so much pain in one location they are unaware of the injury's extension. We use CT whenever we suspect one of the "other" diagnoses and can't see it on MRI. Three-dimensional CT is helpful for defining hip dysplasia.

Ultrasound has all kinds of uses including guiding injections. We get nauseated when someone says ultrasound is useful for the diagnosis "hernias." As we have said before, that notion has long been discounted. Worry about the knowledge base or motivation of the person who says that.

MRIs with the right techniques can show striking injuries that sometimes make it hard to believe that the outside MRIs missed the entire injury. We change the techniques for various suspected pathologies and in various postoperative settings. It is all a matter of where and how to look and the radiologist developing "new eyes." Figure 17-4 demonstrates what we are talking about.

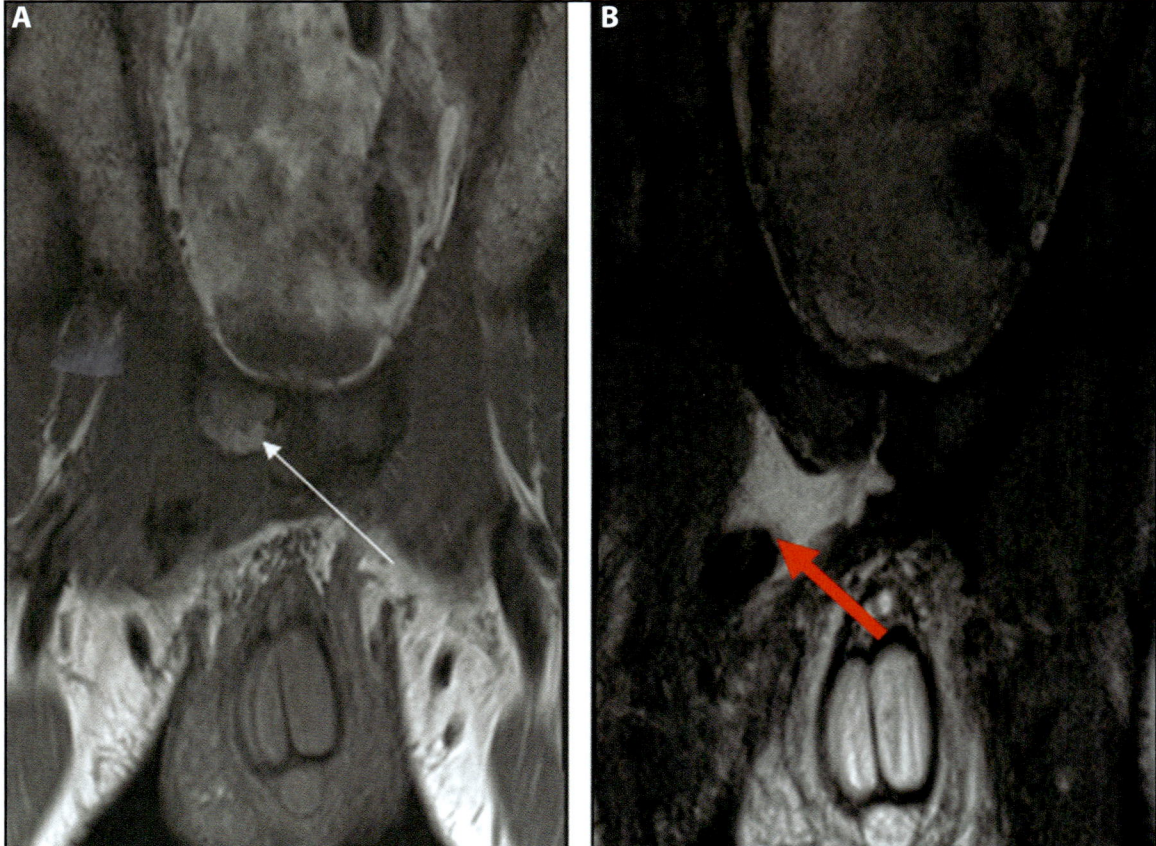

Figure 17-4. Technique matters. Both MRI images demonstrate a complete right-sided adductor avulsion. (A) One can barely see it on the first image using a traditional technique. (B) The second image, with a correct technique, shows the severe injury quite strikingly.

Take a look at Figure 17-4A, a coronal slice through the front of an athlete's body facing you. His head is above the image and feet below it. You may see subtle differences between the 2 sides of the body, with more white in the right pubic bone compared to the other side. The white arrow points to this. Now, look at Figure 17-4B. A red arrow points to the stump of the adductor muscles that have pulled completely off the bone. The white represents blood pooled within a now-empty space previously containing intact adductors. Now look at Figure 17-4A again. Now you can probably make out the stump and most of what looks like muscle is actually blood. Based on these fuzzy images, well-trained and well-intentioned professionals, who missed these injuries and diagnosed them as stress fractures and other things, have placed people on crutches for months. When you are looking for a fracture and all you see is some pubic inflammation, this becomes a logical conclusion.

Putting together images from the traditional and newer techniques, one can see how this case illustrates represents a "can't unsee" phenomenon. If you indeed see what we are pointing out, you now officially have new radiological eyes. Congratulations!

With these new radiologic eyes, let's revisit the concept of "osteitis pubis" (Figure 17-5). Note that we now use the terms *pubic plate separation* and *pubic bone marrow edema* preferentially since they are more descriptive. As discussed in Chapter 8, *osteitis pubis* refers to any kind of inflammation in or around the pubic bone. Plate separation refers to the beginning of the overall process of pubic inflammation (ie, when muscular or other injury causes the fibrocartilage cover to separate). Pubic bone marrow edema represents what happens with time. With continued pounding or other pressure, the fluid crosses the pubic bony cortex into the marrow, just as has been described in arthritis of other joints.[2]

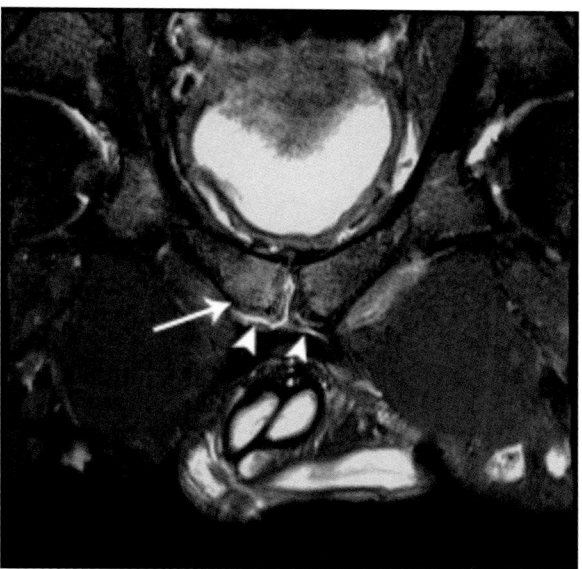

Figure 17-5. We call this MRI sequence "T2 axial obliques." Here, it demonstrates both the pubic plate separation (arrowheads) and pubic bone marrow edema (long arrow) that we just talked about. The patient's right side of the body is to your left and his left side is to your right. One does not see the main muscular injury. The continuous thin white line above the arrowheads extends into a cleft between the 2 sides of the pubic bone, forming an upside down "T." This white line is (inflammatory) fluid that fills the space between the fibrocartilaginous "baseball" cover (black tissue below the white line) and rest of the bony baseball (the white tissue above it). This fluid-filled space represents the "pubic plate" separation. The long arrow points to a mild amount of bone marrow edema within the right pubic bone. Whitish fluid in the darker tissue below the left pubic bone denotes a portion of an adductor injury.

"Clincher" Tests: "Little Pinches"

Often, a comprehensive history and physical examination augmented by excellent and appropriate imaging still does not yield the definitive cause(s) for the pain. When that happens, you can do what we call "clincher tests." This means to anesthetize the anatomic locations suspected to be culprits, with or without steroid, and find out, by pain relief or not, how much each area seems to contribute to the symptoms. If you do these clincher tests, then it may also be worth having the patient try to aggravate the pain first (eg, by doing specific exercises). For example, if one is trying to distinguish between muscle pain and hip impingement or a "combined" muscle/hip problem, then one might send the patient up to physical therapy and have the therapists try to aggravate the pain by simulating what has caused it before.

Following the attempt to make the pain more pronounced, one then injects local anesthetic and contrast first into the hip, examines the patient again, and then gets an MR-arthrogram. Following that, one may inject various muscles, the pubic plate, or other areas in the core, and reexamine the patient additional times. Accurate interpretation of pain relief takes into account potential roles of inflammation and the various neural pathways. One should also recognize that aggravation, rather than relief, of pain might also represent a positive test. These clincher tests may provide the practitioner and patient a better understanding about both the origin of the various pains, as well as the relative contributions of identified sites.

We call this whole process *differential injections*.[3] It is important to recognize that even though we may call these *clincher tests*, differential injections are rarely, in fact, clinching. In other words, rarely do they reveal truly definitive diagnoses. One must take into account all the variables for any patient. Tremendous subjectivity enters into virtually all conclusions. The precise injection techniques matter, as do the roles of eagerness to come up with a definitive diagnosis, on the part of both the patient and practitioner.

IT'S ALL ABOUT HIGH-FIVING

Many of the patients we see come with months or years of puzzlement, fear, and frustration about their pain. We regard the whole investigatory process as tremendous fun—from reading what patients wrote on their forms to performing the history and physical examinations, then interpreting the imaging, and, lastly, doing the clincher tests. We love to high-five when we solve a patient's problem.

One of the most gratifying things in medicine is solving a mystery, then making the pain get temporarily better, and, finally, definitively fixing the underlying problem. This developing field of core medicine has all that, in spades. All one has to do is learn the anatomy and apply that knowledge cleverly. We venture to say that most patients in this world with severe, undiagnosed chronic pelvic pain have definitive answers just waiting there for us to find. We believe that with more study, we will find distinct and definitive pathophysiological answers to the disorders still out there in mystery land (eg, pelvic floor disorders).

Let's stop here and allow you to congratulate yourselves on your new eyes. Hopefully, the new eyes and new expertise will enrich your journey in health care and/or fitness worlds and bring more satisfaction.

Selected Readings

Zoga AC, Kavanagh EC, Omar IM, et al. Athletic pubalgia and the "sports hernia": MR imaging findings. *Radiology.* 2008;247(3):797-807.
We were convinced that MRI would show most of these injuries, so created the techniques to do so. The specificity turned out to be over 90%. The techniques described in this paper came by doing MRI on fresh cadavers.

Meyers WC, McKechnie A, Philippon MJ, Horner MA, Zoga AC, Devon ON. Experience with "sports hernia" spanning two decades. *Ann Surg.* 2008;248(4):656-665.
This article describes many diagnostic and therapeutic advances that occurred over 2 decades. Now, over a decade later, a lot more has changed.

McCarthy E, Hegazy TM, Zoga AC, et al. Ultrasound-guided interventions for core and hip in athletes. *Radiol Clin North Am.* 2016;54(5):875-892.
An introduction to the concept of differential injections with ultrasound guidance.

Sacks O. *The Man Who Mistook His Wife for a Hat and Other Clinical Tales.* New York, NY: Summit Books; 1985.
Even if we never acquire Dr. Sacks's superhuman powers, his stories inspire us to observe more closely.

References

1. Meyers WC, Kahan DM, Joseph T, et al. Current analysis of women athletes with pelvic pain. *Med Sci Sports Exerc.* 2011;43(8):1387-1393.
2. Simkin PA. Bone pain and pressure in osteoarthritic joints. *Novartis Found Symp.* 2004;260:179-186; discussion 186-190, 277-279.
3. McCarthy E, Hegazy TM, Zoga AC, et al. Ultrasound-guided interventions for core and hip in athletes. *Radiol Clin North Am.* 2016;54(5):875-892.

18

nerves in the **core**
a "**fifth dimension**"

Enrique Aradillas, MD

Editor's Note: *Once the understudy of Dr. Robert Schwartzman, the undisputed guru of complex regional pain syndrome, Dr. Enrique Aradillas has taken over top billing. When he retired, Dr. S. had a patient waiting line of over 6 years long. Patients actually waited that long to see him. With his youth and vigor, Enrique has shortened that line considerably. Graciously, Dr. Aradillas volunteered to write this chapter.*

By now, this book has drilled into you the importance of a healthy core for both simple and complex movements, from vacuuming the carpet to specialized athletic performance. A healthy core requires normal execution of all the core's parts. The neurological system monitors and, in a sense, governs that execution. Pain affects the core's normal execution in so many ways. We need to know more about the mechanisms involved, as well as the various interpretations of the various sensations that occur there.

No one has yet addressed, in any kind of comprehensive way, the nervous system of the core. This newly identified, important section of the body has an intricate and pretty well-identified forest of nerves. This chapter addresses the subject. The aim is to help everybody understand 3 simple things as they pertain to the core: (1) what pain really is, (2) how pain gets "perceived," and (3) how pain gets misperceived. The brain's interpretation of pain often leads to alterations of normal movement and cognition. We need to know more about those mechanisms and malfunctions.

Don't worry. Read on. We will make it simple.

First, we shall go through simple concepts about anatomy and physiology of the "pain system." Then we shall finish with several neat examples. The patients described are real, and all have had successful therapy, at least up to now.

I write this chapter so as to make things understandable for non-neurologists. I hope I have not made it too simple. In some sections, I poke fun at us neurologists who, I know, come across at times as arrogant because we tend to speak a different language of our own. I do so in good humor, and hope that I do not offend. I have tremendous respect for my colleagues and the science of neurology.

Reality is neurology, and is not absolute.

—David Cronenberg, talking about his book *Consumed.*

THE ANATOMY OF PAIN (FIGURE 18-1)

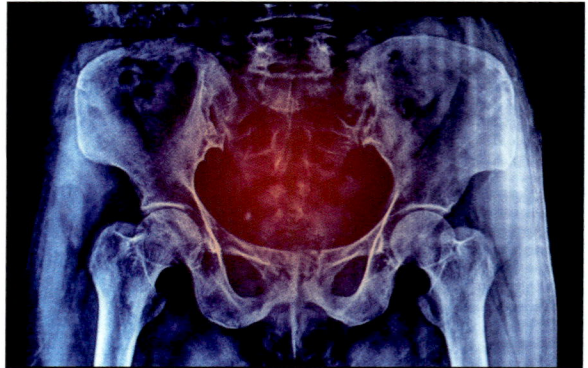

Figure 18-1. A painful pelvis.

It's time to talk reality and neurology. People who know us neurologists might think the latter statement an oxymoron; many other specialists in medicine joke about reality and neurologists not necessarily being compatible. They also consider all of us neurologists eccentric.

So, in the spirit of eccentricity, let's talk about trees. Bear with me for a few moments while I articulate this. At first, this will get weird, but then it will get less weird. Think about a tree. A tree has roots, then the roots come together and form a trunk, then the trunk divides into branches and the branches keep dividing over and over again. The more the branches divide, the smaller the branches get, right?

Well, our nerves are exactly like that. We have nerve roots, these roots come from the spine (not the ground), and they come together and form a trunk. Since we neurologists are also a little arrogant, we give these trunks fancy names. We call each trunk a *nerve plexus*. Then the plexus divides into branches (peripheral nerves) as each enters the face, arm, or leg. The nerve branches keep dividing over and over again; the more they divide, the smaller they get. Here we go, the forest and the trees thing again. LOL.

Now think of the nerves as wires, and the whole tree as an electrical circuit. If you don't know what an electrical circuit looks like, again think of it like a tree. In fact, you don't have to think of the nervous system as like an electrical circuit. It is an electrical circuit. The nervous system circuit transmits continual electrical messages to and from the brain via the spinal cord. To make it simpler, think of the spinal cord as an extension of the brain. Think of the brain and the spinal cord as 2 parts of the same thing—the central nervous system. Think of the nerves as "wires." That is because they are wires. And these wires, in fact, do transmit electricity.

Our neurological or electrical tree has 3 major trunks, which we neurologists call *plexuses*. Of course, we neurologists are also not too bright. The plural of plexus should be, according to Latin derivation, *plexi*. So, you may conclude, correctly, from the above few paragraphs that we neurologists are a little weird, arrogant, and stupid. That's okay. We take these insults as compliments. Here are the 3 plexuses:

1. The cervical plexus: The face and head trunk, from cervical nerve roots 2 through 4 (C2-C4)
2. The brachial plexus: The arm trunk, from cervical nerve roots 5 through 8 (C5-C8) and the upper thoracic roots (T1-T2)
3. The lumbosacral plexus: The leg and pelvic tree, from all the low back nerve roots

MORE ANATOMY AND THE FOUR CRUCIAL NEUROPHYSIOLOGICAL CONCEPTS (TABLE 18-1)

As the nerve branches advance through the arm, leg, or face, they divide more and more and become smaller and smaller, and ultimately the sizes of nerves reach the limits of microscopes. We call the tiny-sized wires *nerve fibers*.

Table 18-1
Four Crucial Concepts
1. Nerve fibers cover every part of our body.
2. Only branches, and not fibers, transmit electrical messages.
3. Small branches may travel back to widely different areas of the body.
4. The neural system commonly recognizes more than one injury at a time.

Here comes our first crucial concept. The nerve fibers literally cover every little part of our body. In general, most electrical messages originate from these fibers. This is where messaging transmission to and from the brain both begins and ends. Two types of little branches exist: ones that go from the body to the brain and ones that go from the brain into the body. The brain analyzes the messages that come to it, and then translates the messages into "feelings" or "sensations" with such names as "soft touch," "cold," "hot," "shakiness," and—drumroll—a sensation called "pain."

Okay, got it? Let's see what happens when we hit our thumb with a hammer (Figure 18-2).

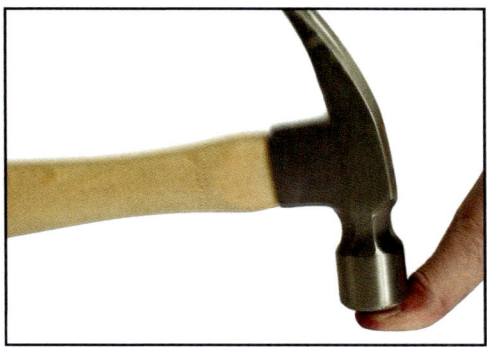

Figure 18-2. Ouch!

Pretend you are the message. The injury propels you, the message, to move within your nerve fiber and quickly travel through it and away from the thumb. You then journey toward the wrist in a tiny vehicle, a nerve wire, and there bundle up with other little wires. These fibers join and become a peripheral nerve. You continue your journey through the forearm and then the arm. The peripheral nerve continues to bundle with other bigger wires until it forms the "trunk" or the nerve plexus. Right before the trunk enters the spine, something happens. The vehicle splits back into new models of message vehicles. The messages may actually get mixed up or even travel in new vehicles as they become roots.

Here comes the second crucial concept. You must remember that the branches are larger than the fibers and branches are the ones that deliver the message to the brain. Only the branches, and not the fibers, transmit electrical messages that the brain can interpret and translate into sensations, pain included. Such electrical messages can come from any sized branches or trunks or roots. Let's explain the issue with an anatomic example.

You damage the ball-and-socket hip joint, and you send a message via fibers to a branch that travels the above route to the brain. Many other potential messages from the ligaments, muscles, and other nearby soft tissues may utilize the same branch pathway. Your brain translates the message to pain, but your brain cannot tell for sure where the pain originated.

Okay, you got the first 2 crucial concepts? The first is the concept of nerve fibers and how they initiate messages. The second is that only the branches, and not the fibers, are capable of delivering the messages.

Here's the third crucial concept. Small nerve branches may travel back to widely different areas of the body. For example, a message that the brain sees may travel back to the hip, muscle, or testicle, you name it! Consequently, because of this sharing, similar messages from those different areas may travel in either direction, to the brain or back from it. For example, pain in the right groin may represent pathology in the right sacroiliac joint or the right hip joint (or even the first sacral nerve root itself). Why should that be? The simple answer: Both joints have many branches from the same first sacral nerve root. The skin overlying the inguinal region may also connect. So, an injury in any of those 3 places (the 2 aforementioned joints or the first sacral nerve root) may easily send similar pain messages and the brain may easily translate it as groin pain remote to any of 3 real areas of injury. And to make clinical diagnosis even more difficult, the remote injury may even produce pain to direct palpation (ie, inguinal tenderness). These are real exceptions to the rule that direct tenderness reflects a local cause for the pain.

Okay, how much pain do you have now? Just thinking about all this electricity? Are you ready for the fourth crucial concept? Too bad if you are not…here it is: Keep in mind that the patient may have more than one injury at the same time. As we have said before, simultaneous injuries happen frequently in the core. There are real mechanical reasons for this (eg, the simultaneous occurrence of hip and sacroiliac joint problems, hip and core muscle injuries). Remember the 2 injuries, separately or together, may send the exact same ultimate pain message to the exact same location. In other words, one distinct type of pain in one precise spot may be coming from 2 different injuries at the same time. In these cases, you can't cure the pain by fixing just one of the injuries. You have to fix them both. An important clinical correlate is that you may fix one obvious mechanical injury successfully, and still not cure the pain. Think of yourself as a surgeon. If you understand this fourth crucial concept, then you will not kick yourself hard if the patient does not get better if you know there is another injury anatomically right next door. Instead, you may go ahead and fix the second injury, or even a third, if absolutely necessary.

STEREO PAIN

Sometimes, the pain gets "out of control." This is a real pathophysiological condition. Don't let people say, "The patient is a crock." The precise mechanism remains unknown. Several events appear to be necessary. Researchers (us included)[1-3] have shown that pain messages can trigger a vicious cycle when it reaches the brain/spine, such that the initial pain message triggers spontaneous and unstoppable pain messages. While good evidence suggests correcting the initial biomechanical generator for the pain, the pain messages may remain even if no lesion is identifiable after repair.

Think of this pain as a pain stereo system. The stereo only plays pain tracks. You hit your thumb with the hammer over and over again. Plus, you can't turn the throbbing song off. Instead of the stereo turning off when you press the on/off button, you keep hammering your thumb. The initial pain from the hammer was physiological, but at some point it should have turned off. Eventually, the pain stereo becomes so loud that the patient loses other cognitive senses. We call this process *central sensitization*.[4,5] Keep this process in mind as a possibility when you see a patient whose pain seems too much or out of control. This syndrome is complex regional pain syndrome (CRPS); many still call it by its old name, reflex sympathetic dystrophy (RSD).[6,7]

Don't dwell on this syndrome too much when you evaluate patients with unrelenting pain. Most patients have diagnosable lesions. CRPS fits only a minority of patients. And it is not like there is an easy solution to CRPS; a misdiagnosis of CRPS may sentence the patient to needless years of experimental therapy.

Anytime somebody is absolutely certain about something, he/she is almost always absolutely wrong.

SO, WHERE IS THE PAIN REALLY COMING FROM?

The previous section describes the complexity of using pain as the only guide for making a precise diagnosis. That said, the symptom pain remains immensely helpful. To do this, you have to ask 3 main questions:
1. What spots in the core commonly cause pain?
2. What are the common and uncommon pain characteristics for each spot?
3. How does one prove or disprove a spot from where the pain is suspected to originate?

Once you know the first 2 questions and go on to the third, remember the words of Sherlock Holmes: "Never guess. It is a capital mistake to theorize before one has data. Insensibly one begins to twist facts to suit theories, instead of theories to suit facts." In other words, when you suspect a spot, go after it and prove it if you can.

Suppose a patient complains of right groin pain. Once you think it comes from either the hip, the sacroiliac joint, or the first sacral nerve root, direct the rest of your history toward differentiating between the 3 possibilities. Don't get sidetracked. Target your physical examination the same way. And if your hypothesis still holds up, be thinking about injecting each spot with local anesthesia in a way that would prove or disprove things.

What Spots in the Core Commonly Cause Pain?

As you read this section, remember this is a neurologist talking, not someone who fixes the muscles or bones. I think in terms of 5 regions. My thinking corresponds pretty well with Dr. Meyers's "4 parts" of the core described in Chapter 5. On the other hand, we are talking the neural tree as a new dimension. So, you may think of it this way. The core has 4 dimensions already. Length, width, and depth are the first 3. Time, which really means movement, is the fourth dimension. The nervous system then becomes the fifth. Here are the 5 parts or dimensions:

1. **The ball-and-socket hip joint.** This joint allows us to move the leg in ALMOST any direction! The muscles that move this joint are better understood if we talk about how they help to do the "Hokey-Pokey": internal rotation (you put your right foot in), external rotation (you put your right foot out), flexion-extension (you put your bottom in, you put your bottom out), abduction-adduction (then you turn yourself around), and all movements together (then you shake it all about, you do the "Hokey-Pokey," and that's what it's all about!)
2. **The core skeletal muscles.** Think of these in a room with a floor and front, back, and side walls. These include both the large skeletal muscles and the muscles of what gynecologists call the *pelvic floor*. This room is "built" on top of a foundation called the *bony pelvis*.
3. **The "back."** This includes much more than just the spine. It contains the sacroiliac joints, the lumbar and thoracic facet joints (between the spine bones), the discs (the jelly-like stuff in between the vertebrae), and finally the joints between the thoracic spine bones and the ribs (the ones that allows us to breath).
4. **The pelvic and abdominal organs systems.** The gut, kidneys, bladder, connecting tubes, and both male and female reproductive systems.
5. **And—oh yes—the nerves.** Think about the whole tree. Small branches, bigger branches, trunks, and roots go to each of the above structures. Roots come from the thoracic, lumbar, and sacral regions. Let's just talk about the lumbosacral region. Think of the 5 lumbar vertebrae as having 6 roots on each side, and the sacrum having just 5 on each side. The lumbar region includes the last thoracic (usually T12) vertebra. Each root corresponds in number to the vertebra above it. The lumbar roots send out usually 6 identifiable branches: iliohypogastric, ilioinguinal, genitofemoral branch, lateral femorocutaneous, obturator branch, and femoral. The 6 sacral branches are the sciatic branch, pudendal, coccygeal, inferior gluteal, superior gluteal, and posterior femoral cutaneous.

What About the Pain Characteristics?

Here are the questions you should ask during both the history and physical examinations. Go over them time and again, make them second nature.
1. Where does it hurt? This important question may lead you to a precise diagnosis, but it may also not. Remember what we talked about previously.
2. How does it hurt? The quality of the pain helps distinguish between muscle injury and joint injury and the other bafflers. But remember that one injury does not exclude another simultaneous nearby injury, or occasionally even something remote.
3. Where does the pain go? If present, pain radiation really helps localize the nerve that is involved.
4. How and when did it start? Know the specifics. They often help.
5. How bad is the pain? Most clinicians use the visual analogue scale, the 1 to 10 system with 1 representing no pain and 10 the worst pain ever. The answer must come from the patient, not the clinician, and the question must be asked in 3 different ways: while at rest, while exercising, and while performing the movement or activity that specifically aggravates the pain. We usually categorize the answers as "best pain level," "average pain level," and "worst pain level."
6. What makes it better? The question is especially useful if position or movement improves the pain.
7. What makes it worse? The same thing goes as for the previous question.
8. Are there any other symptoms other than pain? Specifically, weakness in any part of the body, tingling, numbness, pins and needles, difficulty urinating, difficulty evacuating, difficulty with sex.

So, How Do We Neurologists Come Up With the Right Diagnoses? How Do We Generally Think?

We guess, of course.
We use our knowledge of neural anatomy to come up with likely diagnoses based on 3 things:
1. The location of pain or other neurological issue
2. The likely nerve tissue involved
3. The most likely diagnostic culprits

Table 18-2 provides a cheat sheet for mysterious pains within the anatomic region we call "the core."

Table 18-2
Neurological Cheat Sheet

Core Site	Nerve Tissue	Keep in Mind
Low back	Lumbar facet, sacroiliac joint, torn disc	Muscle tear, referred pain from kidney
Low abdomen	Muscle, pelvic organ (bladder, ovaries, gut, etc)	Referred pain from a "pinched" nerve, most often the fifth lumbar root or the first sacral segment
Perineum (woman)	S1 nerve root, pudendal nerve	Pelvic floor muscle tear, hip, core muscle injury
Perineum and testicles (men)	L5 nerve root, pudendal nerve or S1 nerve root	Testicular problems, hip, core muscle or pelvic floor muscle injury
Clitoris	Genitofemoral nerve/pudendal nerve	Local injury, hip or deep derrière problem
Penis	S1 nerve root/pudendal nerve	Local injury, hip or deep derrière problem
Groin	Hip joint, sacroiliac joint, S1 nerve root	Core muscle injury, first lumbar nerve root
Top of the thigh	L4 nerve root	Muscle injury
Side of the thigh	L5 nerve root, if it continues beyond the knee; greater trochanter, if it stops at the knee	Lateral femorocutaneous nerve
Back of the thigh	S1 nerve root, if it continues beyond the knee; sacroiliac joint, if it stops above the knee	Muscle injury
"Private area" pelvic pain	For men: pudendal nerve, obturator nerve, prostate, rectum; for women: uterus, pudendal nerve, obturator nerve	Bony pelvis for both, osteitis pubic, muscle injuries
Lower chest (under the breast)	Brachial plexus injury, the intercostobrachial nerve	Right side: gall bladder; left side: heart
Upper abdomen	Muscle injury, pinched thoracic nerve root	Abdominal cavity organs, stomach, pancreas, liver, etc

And How Do We Neurologists Generally Classify Characteristics of the Pain With Neural Anatomy?

Again, we have cheat sheets in our head. Table 18-3 is an example of what we think when we hear certain characteristics of the core pain.

Table 18-3
Pain Characteristics Cheat Sheet

Type of Pain	Think
Burning, electrical, pins and needles	Nerve issue
Ache, sharp, bruising, well-localized	Not primary nerve issue (eg, muscle, joint, tendon, bones)
Improves with movement	Joints
Worsens with touch	Nerve issue
Pain beyond the knee	Nerve root
Worsens with inactivity	Joints
Worse at night (eg, burning, cramps, spasms)	Nerve issue

Using Your Savvy

Here are 3 real case examples of how we super-smart neurologists use our savvy and provide incredible diagnoses. (I still don't understand why people call us arrogant!)

Case 1. Back Pain in a World Champion Barrel Racer

A 19-year-old woman, a world champion horseback barrel racer, comes with "pain in my lower back." She points to her lumbar region.

Remember that this region includes consideration of the sacroiliac joints, lumbar and thoracic facet joints, and the discs between the bones in the spine.

Next question: How and when did it start?

The pain began immediately after falling off her horse and landing directly on her rear end. She actually already had some pain there, but this had been mild. The pain worsened with the fall.

Okay, so horseback barrel racing is a very demanding and energetic occupation. The most common cause of pain in any joint is wear and tear. For the joints in the low back, this is also true. Lumbar facet joints are also easily affected by bending over, picking up something heavy with the arms, and twisting. It is virtually guaranteed that she already has some sort of a lumbar facet joint injury.

Next question: How does it hurt?

The pain is deep and aching, almost like if she was "punched" and had a bruise all over her low back.

This is really good! Any joint-related pain from any reason will be deep and aching and feel as though the joint was bruised. Other questions you may ask that might bring out a facet joint problem: Is the pain worse after not moving it for a while? Does it get better when the joint is gently manipulated or worsen if the joint moves too much? Positive answers usually go along with a joint problem—facet, hip, or sacroiliac.

Next question: Any other symptoms with the pain?

She has "numbness" in the same region of the back, but no weakness anywhere nor "pins and needles" or anything else.

Next questions: What makes it better? What makes it worse?

The worst time is when she initially wakes up in the morning. This goes along with a prolonged duration of not moving. Her pain gets better after she gets out of bed and starts to move. This goes along with mild joint pain relief with minimal movement. But when she sits or stands for a while it hurts again. Obviously, positions alter things…again you are thinking joint. She feels good when she begins to ride, but after about 10 minutes, the pain gets much worse. She is using her joint too much.

Perfect. This looks more and more like a joint problem in her lower back.

Next question: Where does the pain go?

One side is no worse than the other. Her pain does not go beyond her buttocks, and on the right side the pain does not reach the buttocks.

This also is very helpful. Usually, pain from either the facet or sacroiliac joints does not go into the legs. It never goes distal to the knee. If it does, you think of other things. In this case, it does not, so your working hypotheses are still operative. Remember also that the disc must be torn to cause localized back pain. If the disc is not torn and instead just bulging or herniated, then the disc-associated symptoms should radiate down the legs.

Next question: How bad is the pain?

Her pain averaged a 5; at best a 2, and at worst a 9.

This is a straightforward documentation of her pretreatment baseline. This will help in assessing the efficacy of diagnostic tests and treatment.

Final question: What has been done so far, and did those things makes things better or worse?

Many other doctors have evaluated her and tried medications that did not work. Anti-inflammatories had equivocal relief, low-dose Elavil (amitriptyline) as an anti-pain medication helped a little bit. An intra-articular hip injection did not help at all. Sacroiliac joint injections also did not help. Actually, she may have had very mild, temporary relief from the latter, but they were not worthwhile even in the short term.

So, we have found there obviously might be an inflammatory component to her pain. The hip injection was done after she provoked her pain by exercise. So, the test was a good one; the pain is unlikely to be coming from her hip. Her partial, but basically insignificant relief from sacroiliac injections probably goes along with chronic wear and tear, and does not mean too much. You are thinking facet joints.

What next? The physical examination, of course.

Physical exam: We did a compulsive bony, muscular, and neurological back examination (of course), in addition to a comprehensive physical examination. She had a normal recent pelvic examination by a gynecologist, and her gynecological history had revealed no suspicious elements. The core muscle and hip specialists in our clinic had already seen her and had been treating her. Our going diagnosis, as we mentioned, was a facet joint problem.

There was only one simple thing left to do to distinguish a lumbar facet joint problem from many other things: a lumbar facet weightbearing test. This test is not foolproof, but in experienced hands, it can lead to the correct diagnosis.

The patient stood up and placed her feet comfortably apart, and then simply twisted her shoulders first to the right and then to the left. We asked the patient to hold her position for 5 seconds, in the end stage of twisting to each side. BOOM!! It was the facet joints! On each side, she could not help but to cry out in pain. None of the other tests reproduced her pain. I was convinced. A recent MRI had showed pronounced thickening of tissue near her facet joints. A new MRI of the lumbar spine revealed unequivocal wear and tear at the last lumbar facet joint on each side.

She then underwent a surgical procedure and is back doing her barrel racing at her previously high level.

Case 2. Groin Pain in an Avid Cyclist

A 56-year-old, well-preserved man comes with: "The darndest pain in my left groin."

Localization: He pointed to a precise area in his mid-superior thigh, probably deep to his adductors.

The patient used exact anatomical terms, and was just a little bit off in his anatomy. He was close, but not quite accurate. Many patients do that. He was right about the term *groin*, but wrong about *adductors*, *hip flexors*, and *sartorius*. Watch out. This is a trap. Patients come to you for your answers, not the other way around. Take their anatomical terms with a grain of salt. In his case, he pointed anatomically to a location that easily could have represented 4 structures: the hip, the sacroiliac joint again, the first lumbar nerve root, or the first sacral nerve root. The latter diagnosis is a real diagnosis and new to this differential diagnosis.

Pain characterization: The pain began about 4 to 5 months ago, a day or two after finishing a 40-mile, cross country bicycle race. Initially, the pain was mild; over-the-counter anti-inflammatories made it tolerable. The pain worsened. He had stopped racing because the pain became unbearable after the bicycle competitions.

So, exercise worsens the pain. Exercise has variable effects on nerve root compression pain. The pain is usually maximal at its onset, and in this man's case, the history does not quite fit. Plus, usually with nerve "pinching," one gets other symptoms such as pins and needles, weakness, and radiation down a specific route (called a *dermatome*) according to the nerve root affected. For this to be nerve root compression, he should have something else.

Other symptoms: He had nothing…nada.

Okay, it has to be the joint. We seem to have a solid case for that. The question now, which joint?

A few more questions: He described the pain as constant, deep, and achy, "as if I had a broken bone." His pain improves minimally while working out or at the beginning of a race, but then grew gradually worse again. He was stiff initially in the morning, then it got "looser." Sitting was worse than standing.

In general, nerve root problems get worse with position, especially when the leg is straight. The pain also usually improves with bending of the knee. The increased pain with more activity and also with certain positions like sitting goes much more along with joint problems. The sitting pain almost clinches hip vs sacroiliac pain.

It seems obvious now that the pain is coming from a joint. The question is to be as sure as we can as to which joint, always keeping in mind that he could still have a nerve root problem. Nothing in medicine is 100%.

Physical exam: Time for the "Hokey-Pokey" again.

We think in terms of 3 main hip tests. Of course, none of these tests are specific to the hip. Plus, there are many other tests including gait analysis. But I leave those more sophisticated tests to the hip arthroscopy pros.
1. The FABER test: flexion, abduction, and external rotation
2. The FADIR test: flexion, adduction, and internal rotation
3. The rest of the range of motion

All these tests were abnormal in this man. We confirmed the diagnosis by hip injection (complete relief after it) and MR-arthrography (a big floppy labral tear, severe cam impingement and a loose body, and little arthritis). Hip arthroscopy cured his pain. He is back cycling and winning senior races.

Case 3. Lower Abdominal Pain After Vomiting at a Wedding

A 33-year-old man, a recreational ice hockey player, comes in saying: "My lower abdomen hurts all the time."

When prompted to localize his pain he points to the entire right lower quadrant of his abdomen.

It began when he started vomiting severely the morning after a wedding. "Food poisoning," he called it. This was about 6 months ago; since that time, it got much worse.

Okay, think about the mechanism of "injury." Vomiting increases intra-abdominal pressure and flexion and extension of the chest, abdomen, and pelvic muscles. We begin asking, Is this really a muscle injury or is there something else the Valsava maneuvers could be affecting? Or, are we missing something inside—the gastrointestinal system or something?

The answers to other questions reveal no continued gastrointestinal symptoms. He does describe a vague sense of "numbness" or "tingling" in the skin of that area. He also mentions that his left leg seems a little "weak." He adds, "And... er...my testicle sometimes burns."

Yes...we got it, nerves must be involved! That gets us into the electrical tree stuff. Remember, nerve problems happen anywhere within the tree: roots, trunks, branches, or twigs. Our anatomical headlight starts to shine. Like all good neurological athletes, we remember that pinching the fifth lumbar root shoots pain into the lower abdomen and below. The same fifth lumbar root also has branches to the testicles. A portion of the L5 dermatome goes to those areas as well as to the lower leg and foot.

Eureka! We have found it. Or have we? We remember that L1 does some of the same things. Branches of that root contribute to the ilioinguinal, genitofemoral, and lateral femorocutaneous nerve branches. Knowing all you ask more questions.

You ask if the pain travels anywhere else. It turns out the patient has foot pain as well.

Now we are really onto something. Pain that goes beyond the knee is most likely from neurologic compression. Think about the specific pain "map" of the fifth lumbar nerve root: It starts at the belt line, travels to the lateral buttock, then the top side of the thigh, then the knee, then the top of the shin, and finally the top of the foot and big toe. You ask about other symptoms in the map and bet he has them. The patient also noticed that lying down with his legs straight worsened the symptoms, while bending the knee improved it.

The additional questions clinch the diagnosis. Remember, though, that other people do not have all the symptoms on the map. Some may have only groin pain, yet nerve root compression may still be the cause. Yes, it's tricky. But it is not so tricky if you keep your eyes open and your antennae up.

Interestingly, this patient had an inguinal hernia repair 2 months previously. A surgeon diagnosed this purely on the basis of inguinal pain and that coughing, sneezing, or straining aggravated the pain. Of course, that surgery did not work.

You think you have the diagnosis already and go on to the physical exam.

Physical exam: We examine the sensory maps (dermatomes) for specific nerve roots as well as the motor maps (myotomes). We tease out pain from a possible pinched nerve root (eg, the straight leg raising test) vs maneuvers to test for other causes.

The physical exam sensory map of the fifth lumbar nerve root follows the symptoms map. We usually test pain and light touch. The fifth lumbar root "motor map" gets more precise as it gets into the leg, foot, and big toe. We test for weakness and the inability to do things. For example, we ask the patient to bring his toes to his nose (dorsiflex) while we push down on the foot trying to break the movement. Also, we might passively flex the big toe and ask the patient to extend it. Remember, the patient may be "locked" and can't move the toe in certain ways and lead you to think there is not weakness. In other words, you can be fooled by these tests if you don't do them right.

The straight leg raising test is exactly the way it sounds. One simply raises a straight leg (ie, locked in extension at the knee). A positive test occurs only if you evoke pain, numbness, or another neurological deficit and are convinced the deficit travels through the entire sensory map of a particular nerve root.

This patient had a positive straight leg raising test. An MRI of the lumbar spine showed a "pinched" L5 nerve root. Well-directed cortisone injections and physical therapy cured the pain, which has not come back yet. It has been over a year.

THE ELECTRICAL TREE (FIGURE 18-3)

In conclusion, think of the pain system as a holiday tree with lights. The core is the tree itself and is covered throughout with an intricate and organized lighting system. Pain is an electrical message. Think of the circuitry within which the message originates, travels, and gets interpreted, as a big electrical tree—with roots, trunk, and branches called "nerves," and then the tiny, barely discernible twigs called "fibers." Pain messages initiate, often in fibers, anywhere within or near the tree, including muscles, joints, bones, organs, etc. The fibers are everywhere. Only nerves, and not fibers, transmit the pain messages to the spinal cord and brain, regardless of where they started. In thinking about the core's 4 components, add to it a fifth one—this electrical tree. The electrical magic happens whenever injuries occur within any of the core's first 4 components—the ball-and-socket hip joint, back, core muscles, and organs. The site of injury sends signals to our newly adopted fifth part. The tree starts to glow.

Watch out when the tree glows too much. Pain occasionally magnifies way beyond what's normal. We're using, of course, our mixed metaphor—"stereo" pain (ie, CRPS) and its loud, burning glow.

Let's go back to the pure tree analogy. We ought to be able to diagnose most of the glows within the tree, where the pain resides and its possible causes. Usually, we can figure out ways to stop or minimize the various types of glows. All it takes is a good knowledge base. Of course, we arrogant neurologists prefer to call it our amazing clinical savvy.

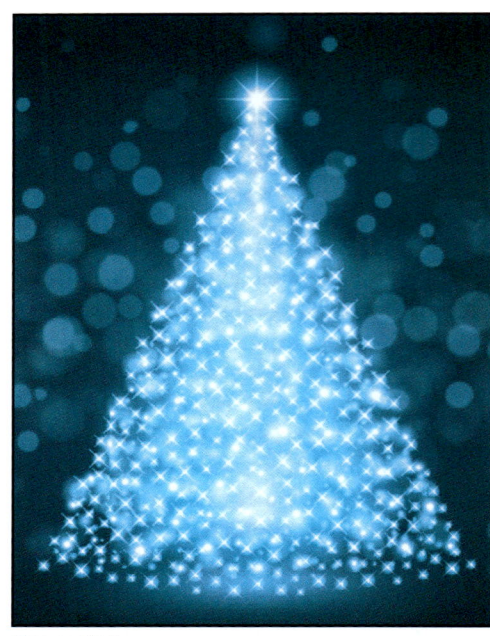

Figure 18-3.

Nothing beats a good history, you only need the patient's age and chief complaint to make the correct diagnosis...there is no need for any extra tests (MRIs, CT scans, nerve studies, etc) because they will only prove that you were right to begin with, the only electricity you need to diagnose anyone is the electricity in your brain.

—Robert J. Schwartzman, widely considered the guru of complex regional pain syndrome and Founding Chairman of the Drexel University College of Medicine Department of Neurology.

SELECTED READINGS

Koes BW, van Tulder MW, Ostelo R, Kim Burton A, Waddell G. Clinical guidelines for the management of low back pain in primary care: an international comparison. *Spine (Phila Pa 1976)*. 2001;26:2504-2513; discussion 13-14.
   This is the most comprehensive set of guidelines that exists for low back pain. It is written for primary care doctors and is easy to read for any clinician.

Freynhagen R, Baron R. The evaluation of neuropathic components in low back pain. *Curr Pain Headache Rep*. 2009;13:185-190.
   This review represents a great evaluation tool for suspected "nerve tree" injury in conjunction with low back pain.

Verwoerd AJ, Peul WC, Willemsen SP, et al. Diagnostic accuracy of history-taking to assess lumbosacral nerve root compression. *Spine J*. 2014;14(9):2028-2037. doi:10.1016/j.spinee.2013.11.049.
   An excellent review of neural anatomy and how this anatomy translates into "pinched nerve" clinical scenarios.

REFERENCES

1. Schwartzman RJ, Erwin KL, Alexander GM. The natural history of complex regional pain syndrome. *Clin J Pain*. 2009;25:273-280.
2. Schwartzman RJ, Alexander GM, Grothusen J. Pathophysiology of complex regional pain syndrome. *Expert Rev Neurother*. 2006;6:669-681.
3. Harden RN, Bruehl S, Perez RS, et al. Validation of proposed diagnostic criteria (the "Budapest Criteria") for complex regional pain syndrome. *Pain*. 2010;150(2):268-274.
4. Costigan M, Scholz J, Woolf CJ. Neuropathic pain: a maladaptive response of the nervous system to damage. *Annu Rev Neurosci*. 2009;32:1-32.
5. Schwartzman RJ. Systemic complications of complex regional pain syndrome. *Neuroscience & Medicine*. 2012;3(3):225-242. doi:10.4236/nm.2012.33027.
6. Edinger L, Schwartzman RJ, Ahmad A, et al. Objective sensory evaluation of the spread of complex regional pain syndrome. *Pain Physician*. 2013;16:581-591.
7. Wolanin MW, Schwartzman RJ, Alexander G, et al. Loss of surround inhibition and after sensation as diagnostic parameters of complex regional pain syndrome. *Neuroscience & Medicine*. 2012;3(4):344-353.

19

the universe of diagnoses

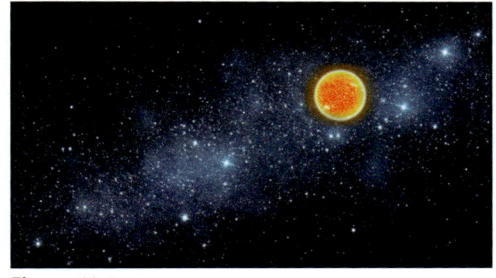

Figure 19-1.

Okay, let's get literal for a moment. Solar system, galaxy, universe… What's the difference (Figure 19-1)? The standard answer is that the solar system consists of the sun and its orbiting planets, along with moons, asteroids, comets, rocks, and dust. Our sun is just one star among the hundreds of billions of stars in our Milky Way galaxy. The universe consists of billions of galaxies.

Then astronomers talk about the most distant reaches of "the observable universe."[1] Are there, indeed, other universes? Copernicus had it simple. He dealt only with the Earth and Sun and a few other planets. His was a pretty simple conceptual universe.

You got it?

Man is not born to solve the problem of the universe, but to find out what he has to do; and to restrain himself within the limits of his comprehension.
  Johann Wolfgang von Goethe, 18th-19th century German writer and statesman.

The attitude reflected in Goethe's quote might also partially explain physicians' hesitancies to explore the core and find out what's there and how the different parts of the core interrelate. Just thinking about seemingly endless possibilities can be exhausting. The medical literature reflects these physician hesitancies. You can see this attitude with your own eyes, if you Google key words such as *chronic pelvic pain* and *gynecology*.

THE CORE UNIVERSE

Copernicus's comparatively simple "universe" is the one we shall go with for this book (Figure 19-2). The point here is that the pubic bone sits in the center and its harness or bridle communicates with the brain and other core muscles (see Chapters 6, 7, 8, and 16). The core is vital for optimal musculoskeletal function of the head, neck, and upper and lower extremities.

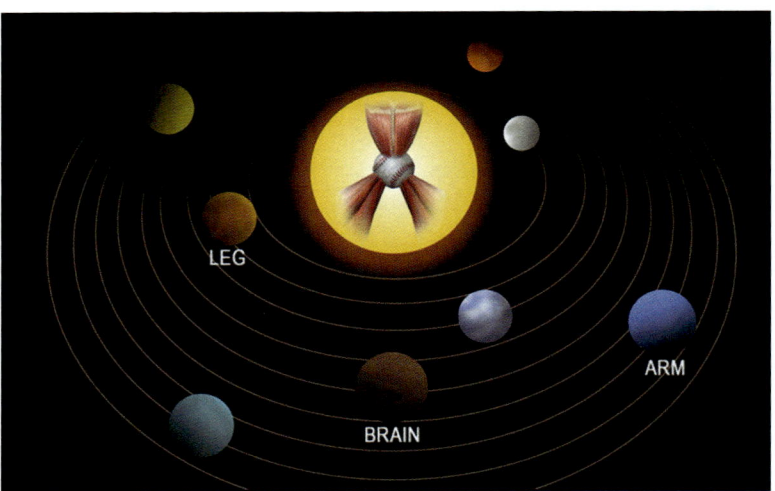

Figure 19-2. The pubic bone, with its "harness" or "bridle" muscles, at the center of the body's universe.

THE DIAGNOSIS UNIVERSE

The anatomic region we call the core—nipples to knees—contains a huge number of anatomic and physiological systems known to physicians for centuries. The item left out of physicians' understanding is the musculoskeletal system. That absence, therefore, calls for a whole new understanding, particularly when one considers how many people in this world have undiagnosed pelvic pain of one sort or the other. Now that we have some handle on some of the causes of these pains, it is time to look at this region as a whole new universe. In the past, physicians and other physical specialists have siloed their knowledge. No specialty has taken on responsibility for all the possible causes and answers. This chapter is a call for appreciating the magnificent number of diagnostic considerations that reside here. Appreciate the beauty of this all. Be aware of all the system's planets as well as the many comets, meteorites, and rocks that can both help and harm us.

Get on your space suit, wander outside your ship, and take in all the heavenly bodies afloat in varying orbits around the pubic bone and everything else. Be ready to hurl yourself backward to avoid getting hit—by planets, comets, and other asteroids that dart into view. Diagnoses with common themes inhabit each object. See the gastrointestinal planet and the neurologic dust. Occasional wandering comets streak onto the scene. Nomads harboring rare diagnoses may wreak havoc unless we prepare for their possible arrival. Farther out, nebulae appear. Wonder if these clouds of apparent dust are developing concepts or practical knowledge just beginning to coalesce into forms.

Try to name the planets directly in front of us. Let's find the right appellation for a planet populated by muscular problems and another crawling with disorders of the skeleton. Not surprisingly, those 2 planets rotate closely around each other as they follow what seems to be the same orbit. A planet hovers nearby, full of gastrointestinal issues, and 4 others for genitourinary, neurological, lymphatic, and vascular disorders. Comets flash across the view bearing malignancies, autoimmune processes, and toxins. Distant clouds of stardust contain rapidly developing understandings of how physical training influences the shapes of hips and why brains stop functioning normally when the core muscles are damaged (Figure 19-3).

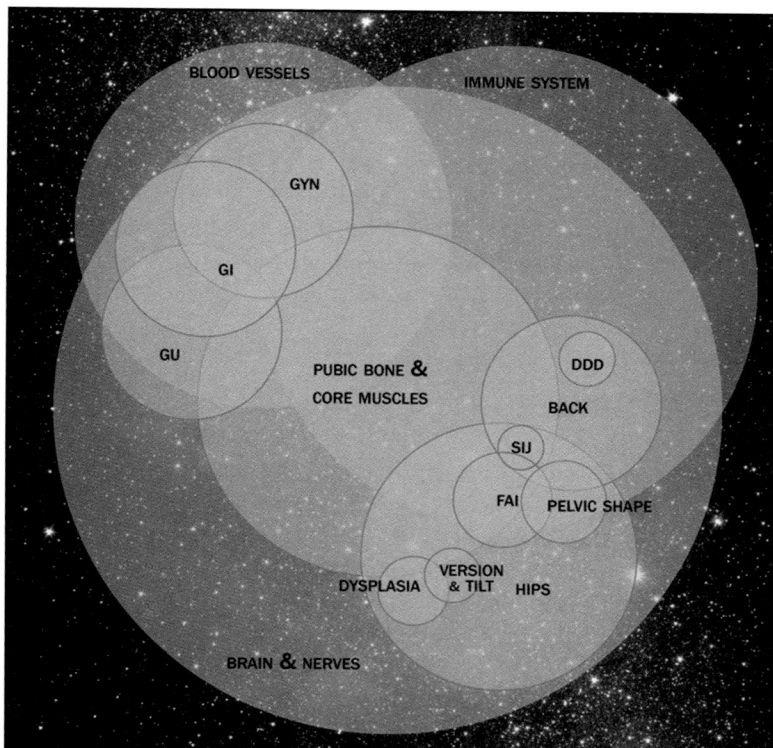

Figure 19-3. The universe of core diagnoses. Venn planets represent the diagnoses within each system as well as the overlap in diagnoses. DDD=degenerative disc disease, FAI=femoroacetabular impingement, GI=gastrointestinal, GU=genitourinary, GYN=gynecologic, SIJ=sacroiliac joint.

Take closer looks at each planet as we fly by, briefly skimming each planet's atmosphere. Catch a view of the center of the universe (ie, the pubic bone), tightly bound by Saturn-like rings that resemble core musculature.

Inhabitants of this bright, hot pubic planet include 4 muscles that attach directly to the pubic bone and many others from mid-chest to mid-thigh. They form symmetrical rings around what looks like a baseball cover of the bone. Planets that look like the hip and back join the core muscles in an inner ring with their own orbital paths. Femoroacetabular impingement dominates the terrain of the hip planet. Nearby independent states resemble hip dysplasia, abnormal rotations, version, and tilt. We see fractures, all shapes of cartilage loss, and then a lot of arthritis. The back planet contains degenerative discs, fractures, nerve root compression, and scoliosis. Some planets seem to have more force than others and affect the orbits of other planets in this region.

As we speed farther away from the pubic bone, we encounter the planets of the outer orbits, and a sign that says, "Entering 'Everything Else' Space." A GI planet exhibits constipation, Crohn's disease, other inflammatory bowel diseases, incarcerated and strangulated intestine, and appendicitis. The GU planet seems infested with urinary tract infections, prostate problems, testicular torsion, and epididymitis. The GYN planet exposes fields of endometriosis, disorders of the round ligament, ovarian cysts, uterine fibroids, and pelvic varices.

Even farther out are seemingly huge pockets of dust, like clouds on the horizon. In some cases, the dust seemingly diffuses throughout the solar system. Their gravitational pulls overlap. Some of the pockets resemble planets. One really looks like a planet and comprises brain and all shapes of nerve bundles. We see CRPS and other chronic pain syndromes, tangles of nerve entrapments. The nerve planet overlaps gravitationally with the back.

Another giant dust-pocket planet carrying immune system particles travels by. This immune planet exerts extremes of gravitational pull on everything, the entire universe. Complex processes abound on the immune planet. These include autoimmune disorders, lupus, and uncontrolled inflammation. Blood vessels predominate within another planet. The blood vessel planet also influences all the other planets via thrombosis, embolus, aneurysm, or pseudoaneurysm. We see a potentially sinister partnership between blood vessels and the hips: a combination of injury and toxins blocking blood flow supplying the head of the femur. Avascular necrosis can look similar to the signs and symptoms of femoroacetabular impingement and arthritis. Something labelled "PRP" is conniving with the immune system to create heterotopic bone.

Still traveling outward, we leave the realm of planets and enter an even newer dominion with extreme outliers and still-forming figures. Unlike the regular appearances of the comet predicted by Edmond Halley,[2] malignancies turn up without predictable pattern and lurk in the shadows of other nearby planets.

The Most Outward Dominion

Not everything in the way-outer layers is sinister. In this periphery lie substances destined to become planets in the future. Some are practicing new sequences of body movement that will prevent musculoskeletal core injuries in the future. We see some seemingly well-formed large land masses with mixtures of bladder and bone, the femoral triad and hip, and nerve forms, brain, and bone. We see yoga postures containing viscera and muscle, and we see one large planet in formation with all kinds of new magnetic imaging, ultrasound, and other imaging techniques that we have never seen before.

These undiscovered or new coalesced planets are exciting. We gain confidence that our curiosity shall be rewarded as our vision gets better and better.

Looking Forward

Okay, you found us out. We are imagining (some of) these travels. The point is that the core represents a whole new world of discovery. New planets are forming. Philosophies of osteopathy, ancient yoga,[3] and other alternative treatments—despite the distrust of us docs—are coming to scientific realization. Discoveries abound. Our heightening awareness of the new entities arise from a tacit understanding that the thigh is not separate from the abdomen, back, and innards and that our harness muscles, basically, speak to our brain, bones, and other muscles.

This new world emerges from what we are learning about femoroacetabular impingement, core muscle function, and other incipient knowledge—planets actively coalescing data that look like stardust.

Selected Readings

Klasko SK, Shea GP. *The Phantom Stethoscope: A Field Manual for Finding an Optimistic Future in Medicine.* Franklin, TN: Hillsboro Press; 1999.
   Klasko, an MD/Wharton MBA, and Shea, a PhD health care consultant, cleverly use a combination of science fiction and industry expertise for people to see the light in health care. Their principles apply as well to discovery of new fields in medicine. Permit our imaginations to wander when we don new eyes and see the incredible alignment of anatomical structures within the core.

Klasko SK, Shea GP, Hoad MA. *We CAN Fix Healthcare: The Future Is NOW.* New Rochelle, NY: Mary Ann Liebert; 2016.
   Again, science fiction provides the methodology to lead our health care system into an optimistic future. Employing a no-blaming conversation, Democrats and Republicans collaborate successfully on 12 disruptive transformations. Klasko, now head of the transformative Thomas Jefferson University/Jefferson Health System, beats on the theme of discarding old dogmas. Likewise, stubborn medical and physical practitioners need no-blame discussions about anatomy and function of the core. Discovery awaits this collaboration.

References

1. Luciani TB, Cherinka B, Oliphant D, et al. Large-scale overlays and trends: visually mining, panning and zooming the observable universe. *IEEE Trans Vis Comput Graph.* 2014;20(7):1048-1061.
2. Rivas-Ruiz R, Pérez-Rodríguez M, Palacios L, et al. Clinical research XXI. From the clinical judgment to survival analysis. *Rev Med Inst Mex Seguro Soc.* 2014;52(3):308-315.
3. Mustian KM, Sprod L, Peppone LJ, et al. Effect of YOCAS yoga on circadian rhythm, anxiety, and mood: a URCC CCOP randomized, controlled clinical trial among 410 cancer survivors. *J Clin Oncol.* 2011;29(15 suppl):9034.

20

how the core universe forms

All growth is a leap in the dark, a spontaneous unpremeditated act without the benefit of experience.
— Henry Miller,[1] famous American author known for breaking with existing literary formulae. For example, his book *Tropic of Cancer* led to a series of obscenity trials that tested laws on pornography in front of the Supreme Court.

WHEN DOES THE CORE DEVELOP?

Fifteen-year old lacrosse players aren't supposed to worry about their cores. They have more important things on their minds, like whether their hair is long enough to produce a suitably cool "bro flow" out the back of their helmets. But when one visited Dr. Meyers with some hip issues that he couldn't explain, the focus went from style to substance.

It seems the young laxman had torn some muscles in his core a couple years earlier. Everything seemed all right in that area, but there was that hip problem. Could the 2 issues be related? Hmmm.

The answer, of course, is that nobody knows.

What we do know, however, is that adolescence is a time when core muscles and the hips are still developing, and that it's important to teach young people the right way to optimize their strength, balance, and function from an early age. Granted, nothing makes a 10-year-old's eyes glaze over more than a curt, "Stand up straight" from his/her mother. But it's damn good advice. Proper posture is vital for children to develop healthy cores.

The things we do during our childhood and adolescent years can determine how the hip socket and core are shaped. The trick is figuring out exactly what to do. Too much emphasis on flexibility can compromise strength. Devote extra attention to power, and elasticity might suffer. It's hard to know what the keys are, especially since everybody's frame is different, but we do know that any compromise early will lead usually to some consequences later on.

Take the 17-year-old athlete with the big labral tear from impingement. He had complaints as well in the adductor region, and his hip had to be repaired, along with the adductor.

The moral? It is important for young people to minimize their exposure to future trouble by finding a balance between flexibility and power. A contortionist may be able to bend in every direction, but how much strength does he/she have? And while a person with tremendous musculature might be able to hoist a car over his/her head, stiff hips may not allow him/her to load up and move explosively.

It's not always easy to prepare a young person for a life of good core health, because he/she isn't sure what his/her goals are going to be. The optimal balance is elusive, because different pursuits require varied amounts of strength and power.

It turns out that Henry Miller, in the opening quote, is wrong. Growth is not all "un-premeditated," at least not for the core. We can influence it. With proper training, we can likely affect how our bony and muscular structure forms. Development does not solely happen in utero. Yes, a lot happens there. But a great deal also transpires during childhood, early adolescence, and adulthood. The latter development, in fact, may have the most impact later on. As you read, think of the terms *growth* and *development* as slightly different. Growth, by definition, involves enlargement. Development involves growth to some extent, but does not require it. The latter term refers to improving (or worsening) the structure we already have. Like poker, your hand enlarges as the dealer deals more cards. You then rearrange your cards and make them, hopefully, better.

The Beginning (Figure 20-1)

No matter the part of the body, human growth and development involves a lot of moving parts. "Moving" in 2 senses: (1) actual bodily movement, transferring from one position to another (ie, the meaning that this book mostly tackles) and (2) in the sense of growing or developing. Both meanings incorporate a timeline as an important element. For the former, time involves very short durations; for the latter, time periods can last way longer. In this chapter, we shall talk more about the latter meaning, rather than the former. Pay particular attention to the fact that, as we grow, our head gets smaller relative to the rest of our body. We go from a head-prevailing physical state of being to a core-dominant existence.

In this chapter, we shall sprinkle out a few facts that have long, seemingly, held true. Most of these facts relate to hip development. We shall proclaim a few "facts" that have probably not been decreed facts before. Notice that we shall not address the all-important elephant-in-the-room question: why. That question is way, way too deep for us country doctors to comprehend.

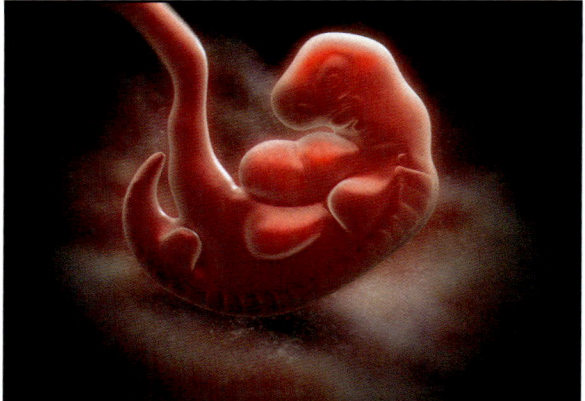

Figure 20-1. Early embryo.

Here are the nuts and bolts of why that deeper question is way too profound for us. Consider that many regions of our body far away from each other (eg, the feet and hands) grow at the similar rates, while other regions very close to each other (eg, the hip and rest of the bony pelvis) grow at different times and at different rates. The cascades of growth and development occur essentially everywhere with independent clocks. Plus, every individual seems to have a different biologic growth clock and different set of modulators. And also consider the question, once growth or development turns on, what stops it? It's all way too deep for us to understand.

As we said, for the purpose of this book, we shall totally give up trying to answer why these things happen. We shall not try to make sense of the different sequences of growth and development. A higher power probably understands that and has a perfectly explainable rationale. Maybe that rationale shall be revealed in the after-life. It won't be right here. Instead, we shall leave this paragraph with the following ecumenical statement: The processes of growth and development begin in utero and continue well into our 20s, 30s, and maybe beyond.

THE FEMUR AND OTHER PELVIC BONES

Let's start out with bits and pieces of what we do know. Time to yawn a little bit. Yes, we are talking about embryology, and many of us found that subject, at least in medical school, unbearably boring. The subject *was* the answer for lack of sleep. Here goes. Bear the pain. As my pediatrician used to say, "This will be just a pin-prick."

Think of the bones as the core's growth lattice. Once bone formation (ossification) occurs, softer structures "fall" into place. Here are some isolated facts. The femur, along with the clavicle, is our first bone to ossify. The femoral head and greater trochanter form separate ossification centers with something called the *femoral neck isthmus growth plate* that lies between them. The whole complex develops so that the femoral head is offset from the femoral shaft. A somewhat cartilaginous environment allows flexibility at the hip joint. The shape of the femoral neck depends on coordinated growth. It angles 35 degrees forward at birth; this angle reduces to 15 degrees as we become adults. (See Figures 20-2 and 20-3.)

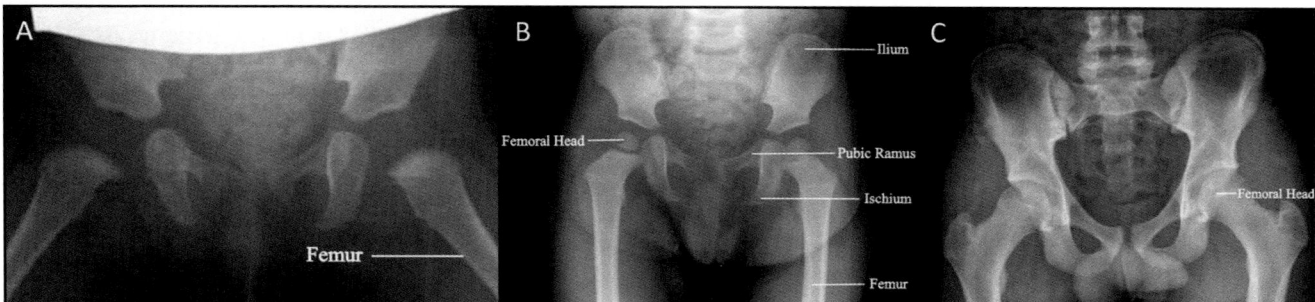

Figure 20-2. Three stages of femoral head ossification: (A) before calcification of the femoral head, (B) after femoral head calcification, (C) after femoral head and acetabular fusions.

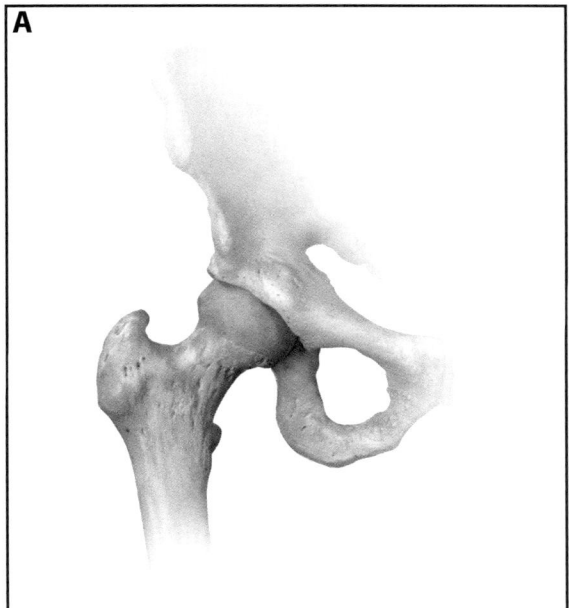

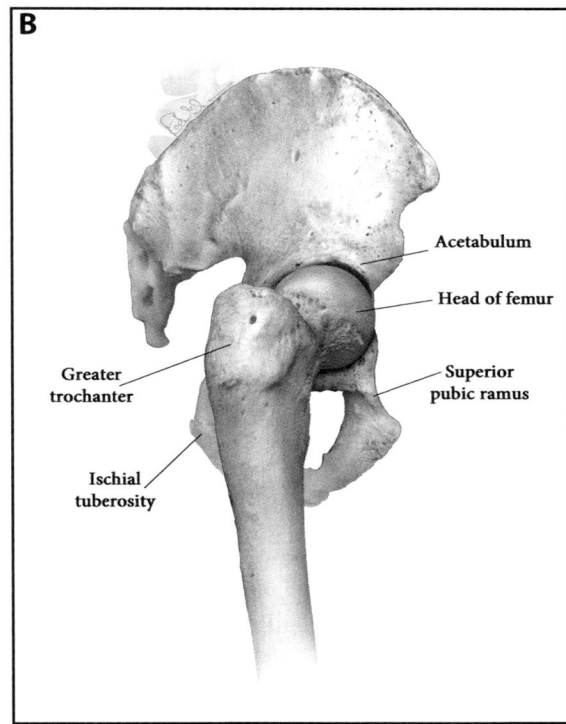

Figure 20-3. Compare Figure 20-2 with Rob's (A) frontal and (B) sagittal views of a normal adult human hip.

The proximal end of the femur articulates with the os coxa of the acetabulum. As Fares Haddad notes in his brilliant description of hip embryology, the development of a normal hip joint requires well-balanced growth of the multifaceted acetabulum and a centered, spherical femoral head.[2] Without the presence of the femoral head, the acetabulum fails to deepen and the cartilage atrophies. Without appropriate acetabular coverage, the femoral head fails to develop spherically. We know that anatomic variations of the hip, regardless of other influences, place individuals at increased risk for hip problems.

The proximal femur develops in concert with the acetabulum, a complex structure that represents the extensions of 3 bones of the pelvis: ilium, ischium, and pubis. The 3 extensions fuse before adulthood. The ilium, an ancient name for Troy, is said to be "war-like"—superior and broad—and extends upward from the acetabulum. The ischium, not so war-like, yet is the lowest and strongest portion of the bone, proceeds downward from the acetabulum, expands into a large tuberosity, and then curves forward and forms, in conjunction with the pubis, a large aperture called the *obturator foramen*. Our friend the pubis extends medially and downward from the acetabulum and articulates in the middle line with the bone of the opposite side. The articular surface of the acetabulum ends up being made of hyaline cartilage. The fibrocartilaginous "labrum" extends from the margins of the bony acetabulum. In its development, the labrum appears to increase the depth of the acetabulum and perhaps contribute to vacuum-type suction as it becomes continuous with the joint capsule, periosteum, and femoral ligaments.

Ossification of the ball and socket utilizes input from 8 ossification centers and takes 20 years to complete. Just in case you want to know more about these ossification centers, here's some more information. They are 3 "primaries" (the inferior ileum, ischium, and pubis) and 5 "secondaries" (the iliac crest, anterior inferior spine, ischial tuberosity, pubic symphysis, and the acetabular bottom). And here is the way they form: At birth, the 3 primary centers are quite separate. The crest, bottom of the acetabulum, ischial tuberosity, and inferior rami of the ischium and pubis remain cartilaginous. By the seventh or eighth year, the inferior rami of the pubis and ischium unite with bone. By year 13 or 14, the 3 primary centers have extended their growth into the bottom of the acetabulum. They remain separate but connect via a Y-shaped "tri-radiate" cartilage plate. The os acetabulum, the small piece of bone at the anterior acetabular edge, appears between the ilium and pubis at about 12 years of age and fuses around 18 years; that os forms the "pubic" part of the acetabulum. Then the ilium and ischium join, and lastly the pubis and ischium. Slowly, the tri-radiate "cartilage" is no more. At puberty, ossification begins to replace remaining portions of cartilage, and the whole process does not finish until 20 or 25 years of age.[3]

The whole process, though, really extends into our 70s and 80s. Think about our ultimate loss of hip articular cartilage, arthritis, etc. Isn't this just part of a normal development process? Can we affect the progression of arthritis as we get older? You bet we can. Staying in good shape fends off arthritis and its ravages, not only in the hip, but also in the knee and other joints.

If we can prevent the progression, why not begin this progression during adolescence or earlier? That's one of our main points!

Bad or Beneficial?

Whether or not you have read each detail of the previous paragraphs, it is now obvious that the complexity of femur and adjacent bone development explains the many variations of hip anatomy. In this book, we talk a lot about femoroacetabular impingement. These particular abnormal hip morphologies develop throughout those years. Commonly, femoroacetabular impingement categorizes into 2 broad groups: femoral head/neck protrusions (cam impingement) and acetabular overcoverage (pincer impingement). Both cause abnormal contact between the femur and the acetabulum. A cam lesion refers to a prominence of the anterosuperior aspect of the junction of the femoral head and neck that can pinch off the labrum and rip underlying articular cartilage. The end product is severe arthritis. The term *acetabular undercoverage* does not specifically refer to femoroacetabular impingement, but rather a form of dysplasia or lack of development of the hip socket.

But also think about the possible advantages of impingement or dysplasia. With some padding, bone rubbing against bone is not necessarily bad; it gives you more leverage. Think about the tightness of the hips of a power hitter in baseball or a running back in football. Have you ever wondered about those butterfly ice hockey goalies out there? How amazingly deft they appear when they swing around their pads over their heads? How do they do that? Under-coverage of the hips, of course! In fact, that does explain it. Some of these goalies have real hip dysplasia. Others have broken through their nuisance acetabular ossification by years of training. Yes, both sets of goalies are more likely to get hip replacements in the future.

There is also scientific evidence that survival advantages of certain hip morphologies also predispose to injury. Hogervorst et al described 2 stereotypical mammalian hips (ie, coxa recta and coxa rotunda) as likely adaptations in response to the running (coxa recta) and climbing and swimming (coxa rotunda). The manuscript goes on to explain that coxa rotunda represents an evolutionary conflict between upright gait and the birth of a large-brained fetus within the female pelvis; somehow that explains pincer-type impingement.[4]

Pathologic aspects of these variations have been appreciated since the 1970s. Only recently have we understood that subtle morphologic aberrations and variations in the way we train, and at the ages when we train, likely influence the development of hip problems. For example, intense training in a high-impact sport (such as soccer, ice hockey, and basketball) at the physeal closure development phase likely promotes the cam bump on the femur. The cam enhancement possibly comes from high shear stress applied to the femoral head.[5,6]

But not all athletes with cam lesions develop hip problems. In a study of asymptomatic non-athletes undergoing hip imaging for medical conditions unrelated to the hip, 53% of the population had femoroacetabular impingement.[7] The correlation between the bump on an athlete's femoral head and intense high-impact training leads to a variety of interesting questions. Are cam lesions already more common among those participating in intensive training? Is that what makes them participate in athletics and play at a higher level in the first place? Are there other variations that predispose the athletes to cam development around puberty? Could cam or associated inflammatory changes in that anatomic region be a marker for overtraining? Some athletes, including some great shot-putters, for example, with cam lesions have dramatically decreased hip range of motion (eg, decreased decline of the pelvis during a squat).[8] Let's leave this paragraph with one more question: Might cam development or symptomatic cam also result from variations in flexibility of surrounding core muscles and soft tissue?

WHAT ABOUT THE CORE MUSCLES?

Okay, that's it for the bones. No one knows much about growth and development of the core musculature, as we have defined this second of the 4 parts of our core. We have some information about certain isolated muscles, but know next to nothing about differences in core muscular function from the embryo to adult. We shall not discuss, in any sort of depth, the growth and development of the other 2 parts of the core—the back and the "other" systems (eg, gastrointestinal, genitourinary, gynecologic). We already know a whole heap about the latter subjects. Let's walk—pun intended—through what we know about the core muscles, and what likely transpires.

Stability of the active hip joint comes mostly from tension provided by the muscles and the other soft tissues surrounding the joint. That stability works additively to the intrinsic stability within the hip's immediate environment with its bony and cartilaginous structures. Of course, nobody has studied hip stability within the early developmental stages of life. We don't know which muscles are initially involved. Hip instability (see Chapter 14) and other hip problems result from, among other things, bad hip morphology, a variability of static hip load types, and the mechanics of the surrounding musculature.[9] Sporting activities involving repeated axial loading and rotation, such as gymnastics, football, tennis, ballet, martial arts, and golf, influence the development of focal laxity and increase risks. Muscles in the same vertical plane as the hip (eg, gluteus minimus, quadratus femoris, gemelli, obturator internus and externus, iliocapsularis, and iliopsoas[10]), as well as other core muscles (rectus abdominis, adductor magnus[11]), grow at similar rates as the hip, so likely provide an increasingly dynamic stabilization of the femoral head with the acetabulum.

Embryologically, the rectus abdominis muscle forms from the ventral longitudinal column of the ventral hypomere, which, in turn, develops from the lateral plate of the paraxial mesoderm. The ventral longitudinal column divides into the 2 heads of origin for each hemi-abdominal rectus abdominis muscle, attaching at the pubic symphysis and tubercles medially and the upper border of the pubic crest laterally.[12] They run side by side caudo-cranially to broaden out as they reach their superior insertions at the fifth to seventh costal cartilages.

A few additional, perhaps less boring, anatomical tidbits: The attachments of the rectus abdominis onto the fibrocartilaginous plate of the pubis must form after fusion of the pubic symphysis. The pubic rami muscular attachments to the pubic rami likely develop after the central attachments and origins of the thigh adductor muscles.[13] The adductor longus and rectus abdominis tendons coalesce to form the symphyseal capsule of the pubic symphysis as a non-synovial diarthrodial joint between the pubic bodies.

Each articular surface somehow gets covered by hyaline cartilage, and, presumptively, at about the same time, the symphysis separates from the fibrocartilaginous plate. Probably in early adolescence, the plate joins more tightly to the underlying pubic periosteum via fibrocartilage/bony spicules. Generous potential spaces remain, so that injuries, produced by opposing forces, detach the plate and fluid accumulates within those spaces. Nobody yet knows from where the fluid comes; it makes sense that some of it comes from a disrupted symphyseal joint. That's what it looks like radiologically.

For a moment, let's go up to 30,000 feet. And put on some new eyes and see what happens evolutionally (monkey to human) as well as embryologically (fetus to 2-year-old). Let's compare the 2 processes. The processes have some striking similarities.

One extraordinary similarity "stands" out, doesn't it? Before we say it, see if you can guess that process that we are talking about. It is obvious. This same progression goes on in both growth and evolution.

In both the evolutionary and embryological processes, we progress from 4-legged or crawling creatures and end up as upright adult human beings. The progression process turns out to be similar in the 2 dramatically different scientific worlds. That said, what happens in this process? How does the anatomy change? There must be something to learn here. This process must involve both hips and the muscles. A few paragraphs ago, we speculated about the hips. What about the muscles? (See Figure 20-4.)

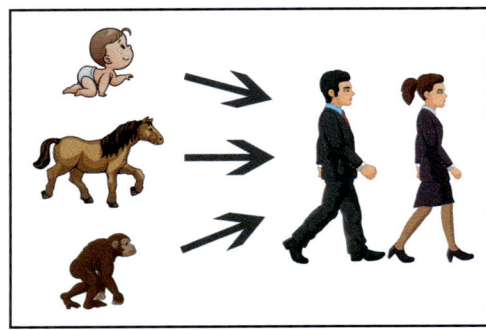

Figure 20-4. The core links 3 subjects: human growth and development (represented by the crawling baby), comparative anatomy (the horse), and evolution (the monkey). The anatomical similarities are striking. The rectus abdominis, adductors, and psoas muscles take center stage in the transformation from the quadrupedal to the bipedal pose.

Think about the anatomy we have learned so far in this book. Now think about how, in God's name, this change—going from 4 to 2 legs—might come about...and so smoothly? Assuming few changes in the actual muscles and bones, what muscle or muscles would have to undergo the biggest anatomic alterations, and the largest shifts in forces to go from 4-legged to upright? Assume, up here at 30,000 feet, that this process within the 2 worlds—evolution and embryology—is one and the same. The 2 life marvels have such extraordinary similarity. There must be something profound in this question.

The answer turns out to be high definitionally obvious. Two sets of muscles are crying out they are the ones, the ones who undergo the most change going to upright postures. These "victims," of course, are the iliopsoas and the rectus abdominis/adductor muscles. Think about it. These flexor/adductor/rotational muscles have to adapt the most. Those movements of the core improve and must have survival advantages. With so much added extension, abduction, and rotation that the upright posture demands, certain muscles have to change the most. Those 2 sets of muscles have to change the most as the hip changes their orientations. They are positioned right in front of the hip and the pubic bone. No wonder they are shouting out. Think about how comfortable and relaxed those muscles must once have been, relatively relaxed underneath the flexed hips of a dog, horse, or baby. They were so comfortable, just lying around all day unstressed, enjoying, every now and then, a few stretches. That utopia is no more. Think about how those muscles felt within an early, 4-legged caveperson or 6-month-old baby. They greatly enjoyed their relative anatomic safety. (See Figure 20-5.)

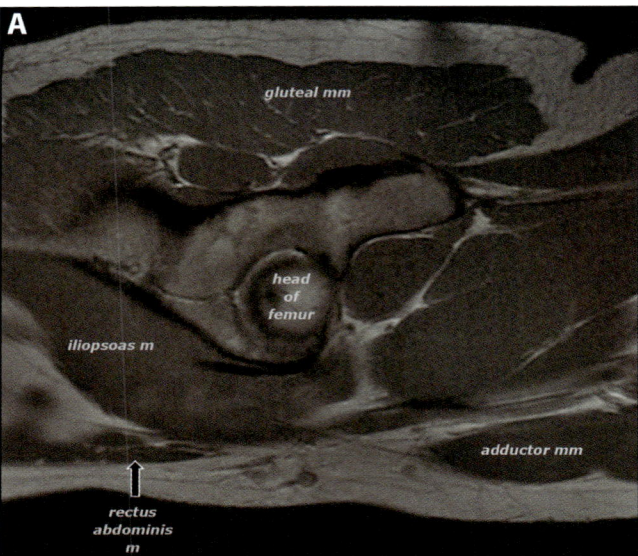
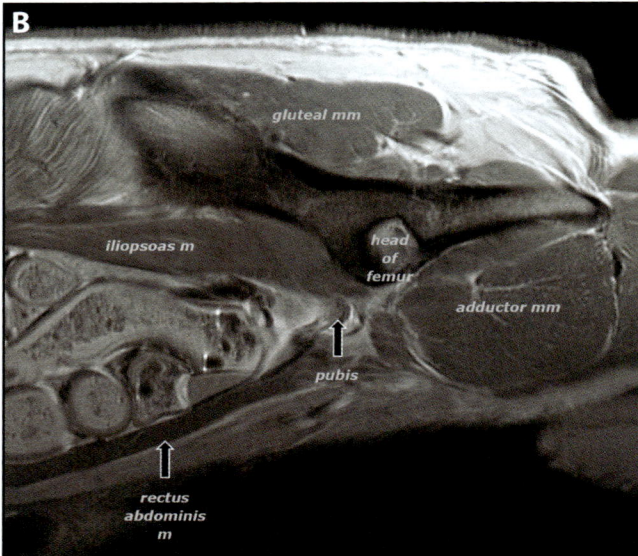

Figure 20-5. Sagittal MRIs of the (A) human and (B) dog. ([B] Reprinted with permission from Dr. Thomas F. Fletcher, University of Minnesota.) Stare and compare.

Then, reality hits.

Let's explore the possible consequences when these 2 muscle complexes each assume the progressive process (ie, crawling to walking, 4-legged to 2-legged). Consider the psoas first. No doubt, the relative hyperextension might account for its role as a generator of "hip" pain and its association with pathological labral abnormalities. Internal snapping hip syndrome describes the snapping of the iliopsoas tendon over deeper structures within the pelvis.[14] Under the increased extensory stretch, the tendon seems more likely to snap and to pull the anterior labrum right off, particularly in the company of impingement anatomy. Remember the psoas's nickname—Eminem (see Chapter 12). You either love him or hate him. Either way, you know the psoas is important.

Now think again about the rectus abdominis/adductor. What happens there? Remember the pubic bone and its baseball cover and how those muscles connect (ie, the harness concept)? Think about the new stress forces there that have to emerge with the new uprightness posture. This area has to become much more susceptible. Increased length and tension must create more susceptibility to imbalance and the wrath of opposing forces. The pubic plate must become more likely to pull away. Think about it. How many horses or dogs suffer from groin pain?

How many groin injuries have you ever seen on the weekly Greyhound Races Injury List?

None. How much more proof do you need?

THE INJURY PREVENTION THEME

No matter what muscles or joints we are talking about, repetitive stressful action creates accrual of microtraumatic injury. Consider also that the world of athletics has changed dramatically over the past 2 generations.

Dr. Edward Wojtys describes his perspective as an athlete and orthopedic surgeon in the changing landscape of adolescent sports in a recent commentary published in *Sports Health*. "Over the past 40 years or so, there has been a significant change in the direction of amateur sports in the United States. Way back when, participating in several sports (baseball, basketball, football, or track) was the goal of many high school athletes. If you could letter in three, especially before your senior year in high school, that was quite impressive. Those who achieved this goal in their sophomore or yet freshman years were the top of the class. High school sports were the pinnacle for most, with a few going on to college careers. There were no travel teams, and there were limited opportunities outside of high school sports except for summer leagues."[15]

Today, earlier sport specialization and increasingly rigorous training predispose athletes to different types of injuries. There has been a migration from acute injuries to overuse injuries.[16] In 2005, more than 3.5 million children aged 14 years and younger were treated for sports injuries. Nearly half of all injuries sustained by middle school and high school students during sports were overuse injuries.[17] Musculoskeletal overuse injuries can result in a significant loss of time from sport and/or threaten future sport participation. These include certain stress fractures, physeal stress injuries, osteochondritis dissecans, and apophyseal injuries.[18] While specialized training allows young athletes to achieve expertise at an earlier age, this practice predisposes to injury and contributes to imbalances between hypertrophic muscle groups and immature tendons and epiphyses.[19]

Understanding that developing athletes are at an increased risk for overuse injuries, as specialized training becomes the norm, there is a great deal of research addressing how child athletes train with an eye toward injury prevention. There is evidence that, for example, providing feedback on certain elements of movement can improve core stability and body mechanics.[20-22] Physical therapists have developed screening tools such as the Functional Movement Screen, which aims to identify poor movement patterns (that develop as compensatory mechanisms for lack of strength or flexibility in a joint or muscle) and to differentiate athletes who are at increased risk for injury.[23,24]

QUESTIONS

We have so many questions left to answer with respect to growth and development of the core. Let's end this chapter by framing one overall cardinal (now ornithology?) question. Let this one question be the stimulus to a decade of research. Here it is:

If a large of part of the core's development occurs after birth, then what and how should we train in order to both: (1) perform maximally at sports or other endeavors, and (2) at the same time, preserve our joints and bodies for the short and long terms?

To answer this question satisfactorily, we have to recognize that we have, as President Trump says, "yuge" basic science knowledge gaps.

Let's leave the chapter with 6 necessary questions:
1. How can we influence hip development within the embryo or after birth?
2. How do we know when the hip really stops developing?
3. How do muscles influence development of the hip?
4. What really are the best exercises? Do "best" exercises change as we grow?
5. Are there ways to keep the hip "fit" besides focusing on muscles?
6. What can we do to prevent problems in the core or core development?

Growth and development are continuous processes that begin in the fetus, reach additional levels of dynamism in childhood and adolescence, and then alter their forms dramatically as we mature and age. It makes sense, therefore, that the methods involved in staying in good physical shape might influence these processes anywhere along the way. The next chapter brings up those methodologies, how we should be thinking about them, and when to intervene.

SELECTED READINGS

Haddad FS, ed. *The Young Adult Hip in Sport*. London, United Kingdom: Springer-Verlag; 2014.
   Perhaps a definitive text on the subject of hip development and adolescent hip joint pathology.

Hogervorst T, Bouma H, de Boer SF, de Vos J. Human hip impingement morphology: an evolutionary explanation. *J Bone Joint Surg Br*. 2011;93(6):769-776.
   An evolutionary perspective on the observed patterns of femoroacetabular impingement and their prevalences in our species.

REFERENCES

1. Miller H. *The Wisdom of the Heart*. New York, NY: New Directions Publishing; 1941.
2. Haddad FS, ed. *The Young Adult Hip in Sport*. London, United Kingdom: Springer-Verlag; 2014.
3. Gray H. *Anatomy of the Human Body*. Philadelphia, PA: Lea & Febiger; 1918.
4. Hogervorst T, Bouma H, de Boer SF, de Vos J. Human hip impingement morphology: an evolutionary explanation. *J Bone Joint Surg Br*. 2011;93(6):769-776.
5. Leunig M, Beaule PE, Ganz R. The concept of femoroacetabular impingement: current status and future perspectives. *Clin Orthop Relat Res*. 2009;467(3):616-622.
6. Lindberg H, Roos H, Gardsell P. Prevalence of coxarthrosis in former soccer players: 286 players compared with matched controls. *Acta Orthop Scand*. 1993;64(2):165-167.
7. Jung KA, Restrepo C, Hellman M, et al. The prevalence of cam-type femoroacetabular deformity in asymptomatic adults. *J Bone Joint Surg Br*. 2011;93B:1303-1307.
8. Lamontagne M, Kennedy MJ, Beaulé PE. The effect of cam FAI on hip and pelvic motion during maximum squat. *Clin Orthop Relat Res*. 2009;467(3):645-650.
9. Bedi A, Kelly BT. Femoroacetabular impingement. *J Bone Joint Surg Am*. 2013;95(1):82-92.
10. Retchford TH, Crossley KM, Grimaldi A, Kemp JL, Cowan SM. Can local muscles augment stability in the hip? A narrative literature review. *Musculoskelet Neuronal Interact*. 2013;13(1):1-12.
11. Montgomery WH 3rd, Pink M, Perry J. Electromyographic analysis of hip and knee musculature during running. *Am J Sports Med*. 1994;22(2):272-278.
12. Milloy FJ, Anson BJ, McAfee DK. The rectus abdominis muscle and the epigastric arteries. *Surg Gynecol Obstet*. 1960;110:293-302.
13. Palisch A, Zoga AC, Meyers WC. Imaging of athletic pubalgia and core muscle injuries: clinical and therapeutic correlations. *Clin Sports Med*. 2013;32(3):427-447.
14. Nunziata A, Blumenfeld I. Snapping hip: note on a variety. *Prensa Med Argent*. 1951;38(32):1997-2001.
15. Wojtys EM. Sports specialization vs diversification. *Sports Health*. 2013;5(3):212-213.
16. Jones SJ, Lyons RA, Sibert J, Evans R, Palmer SR. Changes in sports injuries to children between 1983 and 1998: comparison of case series. *J Public Health Med*. 2001;23(4):268-271.
17. Jayanthi N, Pinkham C, Dugas L, Patrick B, Labella C. Sports specialization in young athletes: evidence-based recommendations. *Sports Health*. 2013;5(3):251-257.
18. DiFiori JP, Benjamin HJ, Brenner JS, et al. Overuse injuries and burnout in youth sports: a position statement from the American Medical Society for Sports Medicine. *Br J Sports Med*. 2014;48:287-288.
19. Mersmann F, Bohm S, Schroll A, Boeth H, Duda G, Arampatzis A. Evidence of imbalanced adaptation between muscle and tendon in adolescent athletes. *Scand J Med Sci Sports*. 2014;24(4):e283-e289.
20. Parsons JL, Alexander MJ. Modifying spike jump landing biomechanics in female adolescent volleyball athletes using video and verbal feedback. *Strength Cond Res*. 2012;26(4):1076-1084.

21. Herman DC, Oñate JA, Weinhold PS, et al. The effects of feedback with and without strength training on lower extremity biomechanics. *Am J Sports Med*. 2009;37(7):1301-1308.
22. Wouters I, Almonroeder T, Dejarlais B, Laack A, Willson JD, Kernozek TW. Effects of a movement training program on hip and knee joint frontal plane running mechanics. *Int J Sports Phys Ther*. 2012;7(6):637-646.
23. Cook G, Burton L, Hoogenboom B. Pre-participation screening: the use of fundamental movements as an assessment of function: part 1. *N Am J Sports Phys Ther*. 2006;1(2):62-72.
24. Garrison M, Westrick R, Johnson MR, et al. Association between the functional movement screen and injury development in college athletes. *Int J Sports Phys Ther*. 2015;10(1):21-28.

21
optimizing and fixing the core muscles

I was a great athlete until I was 7. Then I took time off. Now I can beat most of my friends in tennis because they have artificial hips and knees.
—David Rubenstein, Co-Founder and CEO of The Carlyle Group.

LIFE IS A CONTINUOUS PROCESS

David Rubenstein's quote says it all. Life subjects the body to all kinds of stresses that may not be good for us. Sports or other strenuous activity exposes muscles and joints to continuous microtrauma. Unequivocally, wear and tear eventually gets us. We call low-grade deterioration *degeneration* or, more euphemistically, *interstitial tearing*, and the more serious harm *injury*. Injury is inevitable when we perform the same activity repeatedly or hard enough. Athletes routinely experience the paradox of preparing themselves for short-term gain vs sacrificing their bodies in the long term. Simply said, fitness ultimately leads to injury.

Not only does staying in great shape stress our bones and soft tissues, it challenges our heart, brain, and longevity.[1-3] Is exercise good or bad for us? Believe it or not, the subject is controversial. Cardiologists and fitness specialists have argued about this for years,[4-7] the risk of sudden death, etc. The recent pandemonium about concussions represents the controversy's latest chapter.

As you read on, keep in mind that the editors of this book are biased. We subscribe to the point of view that staying in shape is good, that life creates a wear and tear called the *aging process*. We, as therapists, truly believe we can affect this aging process. No matter how good we may be at minimizing age effects on muscles, bones, and joints, we must recognize that our opinions represent a bias. We could be wrong—staying in shape may really be bad for us. Some really smart people believe that staying in great shape is not a good thing.[8]

TWO IMPORTANT QUESTIONS

This chapter addresses how to answer 2 questions (Table 21-1):
1. How good a shape do we need or want to be in?
2. When we truly do injure something…when, why, and how should we fix it?

With regard to Question 1, you should know by now that the core is the "engine room" for getting into shape. Most of this chapter focuses on answers to Question 1.

Before getting too far into the first question, let's concentrate for a moment on Question 2. One must consider certain practicalities with regard to Question 2. Consider the practicality that if you ask almost any physical trainer if he/she knows much about the core, virtually all of them will tell you yes. They will go on and tell you they are experts. Realize that, in fact, only a few of them really are. The same thing is true in spades about surgical treatment of the core. For example, more and more hip arthroscopists are being trained. Yet, almost everyone in the field will say that the more experienced you are, the better are your results. Plus, only a few surgeons yet understand the principles of core muscle surgery, and truly know how to fix those injuries.

TABLE 21-1
THE TWO BASIC QUESTIONS—REPHRASED
1. What do we mean by "good shape"?
2. When, why, and how should we fix an injury?

That is because there is no formal recognition of this new field, which we call the core, in medicine. Most physicians don't understand it. The functional anatomy is not taught in medical schools. None of the core muscle anatomy, pathophysiology, or procedures has been incorporated into medical schools or residency training programs. And many insurance companies refuse to pay for the surgery. Instead, the executives label any such surgery as "experimental."[9] Therefore, surgeons who dabble in this region of the body list the procedures under existing codes (eg, hernia repair, tendon division). The code "hernia repair," in fact, oftentimes represents the procedure that the surgeon is doing. The problem is that the diagnosis and treatment is wrong. But with that false mindset, the surgeon will say, "Why not code the procedure this way?"

In turn, the billing/insurance problem perpetuates that old mindset and ancient eyes. Because many of the procedures are unsuccessful, those results add fuel to the insurance companies calling the procedures experimental. Consequently, the inaccurate coding and terminology perpetuate the term "sports hernia." All this cultivates the insurance companies' argument against new procedures. Because they see many of the failures, their arguments become stronger and have more ammunition for a demand for a randomized prospective study, which they know will never be accomplished. How do you ask a star athlete with a muscular avulsion to subject him-/herself to a 50/50 chance of not getting the surgery?

The result is a vicious cycle, a Catch-22 so to speak. If you call a new procedure by an appropriate name, you just don't get reimbursement. The consequence of all the above factors is that surgeons, for the most part, become more likely not to do the right procedures. Much of the surgery presently going on is predictably unsuccessful. The answers to Question 2—when, why, and how to fix the injuries—presently depend on how aggressive or knowledgeable the patients or caretakers are with respect to seeking out optimal treatment. (See Figure 21-1).

This chapter brings together the principal factors that should enter decision processes for the above 2 questions. It provides guidelines for how to answer the questions. It does not provide the actual answers. Chapter 30 gets into more specifics about how to fix things, but still offers only guidelines. The present chapter is short and sweet. Therefore, please allow the main themes to marinate in our brains, so that they infuse smoothly into our psyches. Like other walks of life, the questions "when" and "why" eclipse the queries "how" and "what." The rest of this chapter focuses on the answer to Question 1.

Optimizing and Fixing the Core Muscles 219

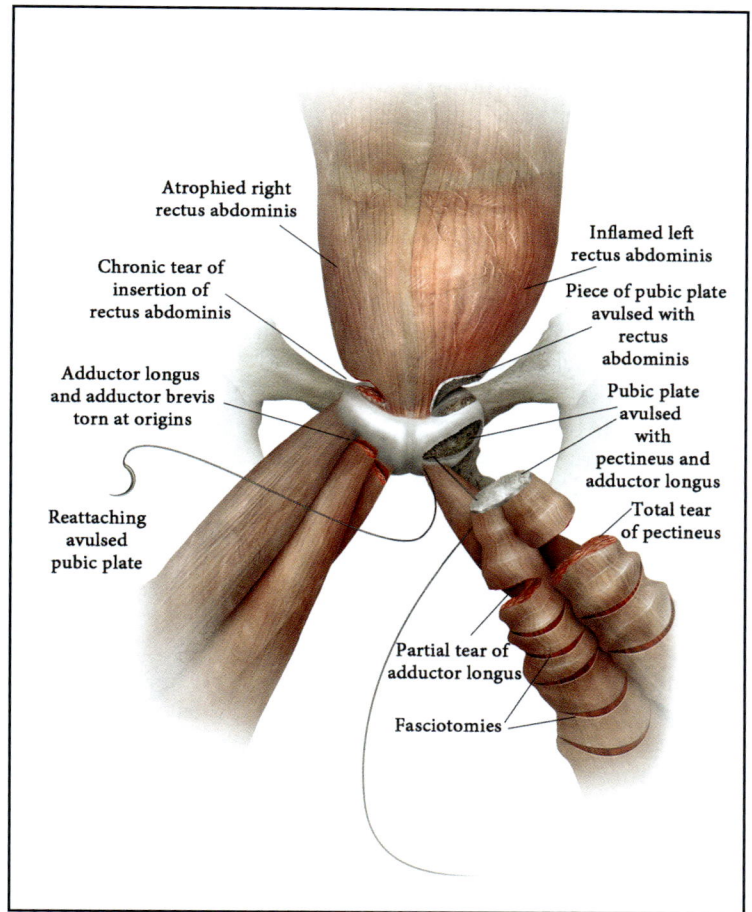

Figure 21-1. Surgical repair of a severe core muscular injury.

If it ain't broke, don't fix it.
—This expression is commonly attributed to T. Bert Lance, Office of the Management of the Budget Director in the 1977 Jimmy Carter administration. In fact, this is an old Southern proverb. My grandfather, a carpenter from South Carolina, delivered this exact same advice to me way back in the 1950s.

WHAT DO WE MEAN BY "GOOD SHAPE"?

The above proverb sounds like medical school's cardinal principle: Primum non nocere—first, do no harm. This principle brings up another apparent paradox. If getting someone into the best shape means having to cause deterioration in his/her joints and muscles, doesn't that go against medicine's cardinal principle?

Well, get over it. We must get over that paradox. We have already admitted bias. We believe staying in shape is good for us. Let's modify our goals and ask: How good a shape should we get people into? Plus, let's ask a corollary to that question: How do we best prevent injury or disability in the short or the long run?

Getting into shape is sort of like drinking wine. They say drinking a glass of wine a day is good for you and some studies say drinking 2 glasses a day is even better. When does that stop? How many glasses does it take to cause harm? What's the right number of glasses?
—Paul Tiffany, Berkeley and Wharton business strategy professor, made similar declarations about loans, credit ratings, and how much money a business should optimally borrow.

Therefore, we shall define the term *fixing* in this chapter to mean "optimizing the body for desired performance." This definition may apply to *either* the short term or the long term, or *both* short and long terms.

Think in terms of 3 categories of clients/patients/athletes (Table 21-2):
1. Those seeking to be in the best shape for short-term performance almost no matter what (eg, preparing for the NFL Combine or the upcoming season, making a team) to "feeling good" or to "look more attractive"
2. Those genuinely looking to get into or "back into" shape for far-reaching health purposes
3. Those with mixed motivations (eg, some veteran athletes, patients with lawsuits, and, in some cases, worker's compensation claims)

Of course, we all run across various blends of the above categories. Basically, we treat the 3 categories differently. For the first, it is all about various professional, personal, or social contracts. Short-term performance goals dwarf long-term injury concerns.

One needs to keep in mind, nonetheless, that the patient/client in this first category has only chosen the moment and, for the most part, ignores the long-term consequences. Hence, in this first category, it is imperative that the therapist achieve complete trust. The trust comes from an unwritten conspiratorial pact that the therapist will bring the athlete right to the edge of the cliff but won't let him/her go over it. The other 2 categories do not mandate the same degree of collusion.

Table 21-2
Three Categories of Clients
1. Short-term purpose
2. Health purpose
3. Mixed purpose

The second category characterizes for most of us what should be the right balance of short-term success and body preservation. The creepy third category heralds all sorts of murky interactions that shall most likely lead to many frustrations related to conflicting agendas.

Provided the therapist has the right skill sets, it should be relatively easy for therapists to deal with people in any of the 3 above relatively uninjured categories. They all just want to get into optimal physical shape. As mentioned, optimal shape means different things depending on the motives. For the most part, the transactions involve just 2 parties, the patient/client and the therapist. Of course, one may argue the latter point with respect to the creepy third category. Nevertheless, therapy programs all come down to identifying and uniting goals.

Whatever the case, in all 3 categories, therapists must be extremely careful. We see many core muscle injuries that result from therapists being too aggressive with both the ultimately in-shape bodies as well as the ridiculously out-of-shape bodies. We also see frustrations and dissatisfaction related to therapists not being nearly aggressive enough.

The "perfect-storm for core injury" comes when a previously in-shape athlete gets out of shape over several years while beginning a family or working hard at his/her regular job, and then becomes determined to pursue, purely on his/her own, an aggressive P90X-type workout program. Talk to the receptionists at the Vincera Institute. They will tell you how common this perfect storm scenario is. Based on their initial phone conversations with new patients, they will tell you that this perfect-storm scenario is really common. Likewise, it is so easy for us as therapists to get caught in the same "enthusiasm trap" and work out these individuals way too aggressively. It is so tempting to do so. They are so highly motivated and enthusiastic. We therapists just have to be careful.

Let's now go to the more complicated Question 2.

Fixing Actual Injuries

If it is broke, fix it. When, why, how?

Let's get into how to go about answering the 3 parts to the question, assuming an unambiguous diagnosis of a specific core muscle injury has already been made. First, let's itemize possible variables that might be important for the decision-making, then list general guidelines, and, finally, provide a few real case examples. Understand that we are talking about either athletes or everyday people like us.

Decision-Making Factors

Begin by thinking comprehensively about all possible variables that might be important for management decisions. Think about 5 categories of variables:
1. The injury itself
2. The patient
3. Other people involved
4. The goals
5. The environment

Don't worry, you will soon understand what we are talking about.

The **injury** must have many characteristics. Here are some of the questions that have to be asked. What specific muscle or muscles are involved? Is there a primary injury and one or more compensatory injuries? What part(s) of the muscle is (are) injured and how severe is the injury? Is it a central or a more peripheral injury? Does it involve harness or power muscles? What about the hip, is it involved? What about other new or pre-existent injuries? Is this an acute or chronic injury or a combination of the two?

The **patient** never quite fits into a precise, preordained category. The variables are numerous. There are the standard patient demographics, such as age, gender/sex, location, insurance status, etc. What is the general physical condition? Is this an athlete? How good an athlete? Is the injury important in terms of functioning in one's job or everyday life? What sport or sports does he/she play or participate in? Are we talking about a professional or top amateur? Is this a recreational athlete? How important is that sport or are sports in general to the person? How important is staying in shape in general to that person? I bet you can think of many other questions that could be asked.

Others involved can mean many people (eg, for professional or top amateur athletes) or no other people (eg, for the pure recreational athlete). In the latter case, management decisions become more purely a matter of what the patient wants. Think about the number of folks who might be involved with a top athlete: the team's management—general manager, head coach, other coaches, athletic trainers and physical therapists, the athlete's personal therapists, the agent, family, entourage, and even sometimes the public, the list goes on… All might become part of the decision-making tangle.

The **goals** of each of the various parties may be drastically different from the others. The team may be in a playoff race and management wants the player back at all costs, the agent may not want the player to return because it is near the end of the season and the agent sees the downsides of not playing well and no upsides of playing well. It may be the contract year, in which case the motivations of the various parties usually differ drastically. A spouse may want the veteran athlete to quit. The player may already be thinking retirement. Numerous scenarios arise.

Finally, let's discuss the **environment**. This is a miscellaneous category that captures all the other factors that may contribute, such as when did the injury occur (eg, during or after the season)? Did the athlete play with injury all year? Does he/she want it fixed so that it doesn't bother him/her during the next season? Or, consider the scenario: there is one remaining NFL playoff-determining game, it is the player's contract year, and the player knows he won't play well in below-zero weather.

Or consider the "university" situation. What do the financial decision-makers at a given university understand about the nature of these injuries? Will the university require the player to have a "hernia repair" at its own local hospital where they have a good financial deal? Many kinds of scenarios come into play; thus, we have this miscellaneous category of decision-making variables.

Fifteen Guidelines

These 15 are listed purely as general principles to shape thinking with respect to decision-making and not as absolutes. This is a selected list (Figure 21-2). Numerous exceptions exist for each of the "guidelines."

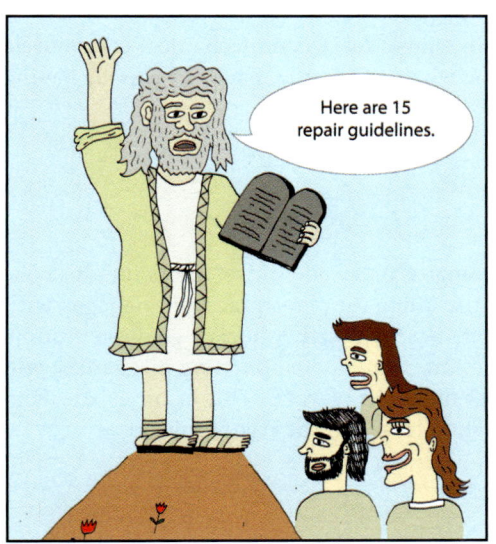

1. Every muscle of the core is subject to injury, so therapeutic decision-making depends on a precise diagnosis as well as the severity of the possible disability. Core pain can be caused by many muscles, the hip, and other entities. Many of these causes do not need surgery.

2. The more central the core muscle injury, the more likely it is to need surgical correction. Think sort of like for the anterior cruciate ligament of the knee. This is a very central ligament and if torn it is unlikely to mend on its own. The rest of the knee just can't stay still enough for the floppy ends to find their way to get together and heal without surgery. The same is true here; once the pubic fibro-cartilage starts to slip severely, it is difficult to stay still enough for these central muscles to heal without surgical help.

3. Injury to the harness usually needs surgical correction. This is a corollary to Guideline 2. Of course, the need for surgery depends on the severity and degree of disability, but these injuries almost always progress with time.

Figure 21-2.

4. Likewise, the more peripheral the muscular injury, the more likely it will heal on its own. As you probably have guessed, the more central stability is preserved, the more peripheral the muscular injury. The parallel again is the knee and the collateral ligaments. There are exceptions, of course. Huge tears, for example, of the adductor longus muscle belly may not heal without surgery. Size of the tear does matter here. The same is true of huge tears of the collateral ligaments of the knee.
5. Injury to the power muscles usually do heal on their own. Again, this is a corollary principle to Guideline 4.
6. The more central the injury, the more likely there will be compensatory injuries. In other words, for large muscle tears of the rectus abdominis or pectineus at the pubic plate, it is extremely likely that the other rectus abdominis and adductors will get involved. The involvement may be a simple compartment type syndrome or the muscle itself may pull off.
7. Central avulsions should be repaired acutely if possible. Most of these involve the plate and other muscles and create pubic or core instability over the long run. One can also compare the return times of athletes with these type injuries. It is usually a 6- to 8-week process without surgery and the performance success after return remains marginal. Surgery continues as the likely necessary option. Plus, when the player does return, he/she is subject to injury (eg, concussions) due to pain or tentative type straight-line running and loss of cognitive awareness or even anterior cruciate injuries due to general loss of core stability. Return to play after surgery is usually 6 weeks (ie, shorter than for the non-operative attempt).
8. Complete rectus femoris avulsions usually should be repaired. In contrast, injuries to the indirect head usually do not have to be repaired.
9. Steroid injections into core muscles and the region of separation of the pubic plate and bone have about an 80% chance of temporary return to play and adequate performance. The injections work by decreasing inflammation and they do not heal the injury, which will almost certainly progress. In these cases, the success rate for surgery after the season remains statistically the same as being done sooner.
10. Platelet-rich plasma injections, on the other hand, do not seem to be effective as a temporary or permanent solution and carry with it the risk of heterotopic ossification.
11. Most core muscle injuries in athletes co-exist with hip pathology and vice versa (ie, core muscle injuries accompany most hip impingement problems in athletes).
12. In the above cases (Guideline 11), the decision whether surgery is required for the hip should usually be made independently of the decision for core muscle surgery. That is not to say that the 2 pathologic processes are independent. And sometimes, neither of the sets of signs and symptoms will correct unless both pathologies are corrected.
13. Also, sometimes the hip signs and symptoms will correct after performance of just the core muscle surgery alone. Conversely, peripheral core muscle problems will usually correct after hip surgery, but central core muscle injuries usually do not.
14. Osteitis pubis is a reactive process to core muscle injury and sometimes hip impingement alone and only rarely an independent pathologic process. Those rare cases of primary osteitis usually occur in nonathletes and are probably associated with yet-unidentified systemic diseases.
15. Complex regional pain syndrome (CRPS) is a great mimicker of core injury. Yet, when mechanical core muscle and/or hip injury is identified, it often should be repaired because the whole syndrome may get better by having corrected the mechanical "trigger" for the pain.

Actual Case Examples

- The star pitcher for the Houston Astros develops an acute adductor longus injury about two-thirds into his contract year while pitching a no-hitter in Yankee Stadium. With the Astros still in the playoff race, his manager, with whom he is close, wants him to finish out the year. The injury, a severe baseball pitcher hockey goalie syndrome type, will eventually need surgery. The pitcher heroically risks arm injury from altered pitching mechanics, and pitches fairly well the rest of the year. Unfortunately, the Astros don't make the playoffs. This example attests to the great character of a star athlete who goes against financial logic and plays with the risk of injury.

- A 61-year-old dean/provost of a medical school decides to get "back" into better physical shape after years of little activity. He hires a personal trainer. While doing a vigorous isolated adductor "leg press," he feels a "pop" and severe pain and develops an immediate large hematoma. MRI shows an acute avulsion of the entire left pectineus, adductor longus, and rectus abdominis with the fibrocartilage plate. He chooses to undergo immediate reconstruction on a day that he had already decided to take off for research and does not miss a single administrative meeting. He began physical therapy on day 1 postoperatively, the drains were removed on postoperative day 7, and he returned to full physical training but with a different trainer after 6 weeks. This relatively speaking non-athlete makes the personal decision, against some advice from friends, to go ahead and have his core muscles reattached repaired despite his age, etc. These decisions are often highly personal. (See Figure 21-3.)

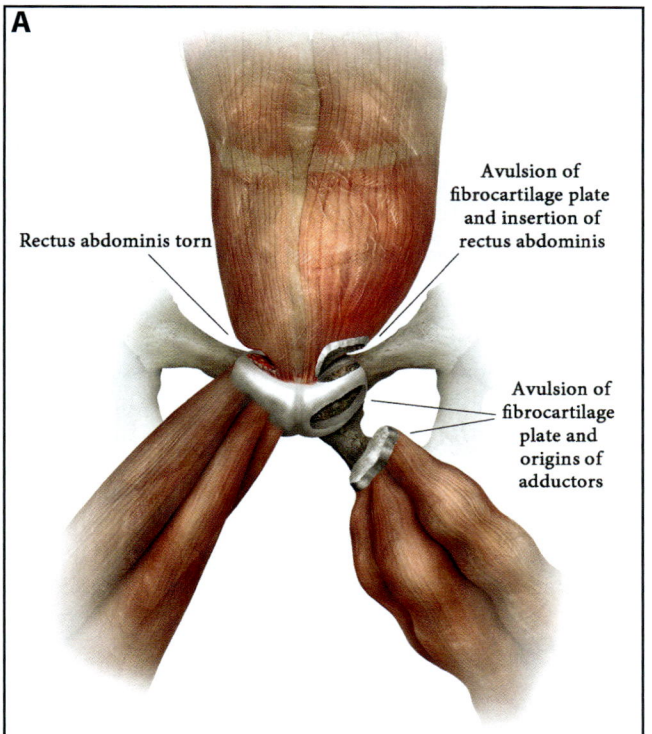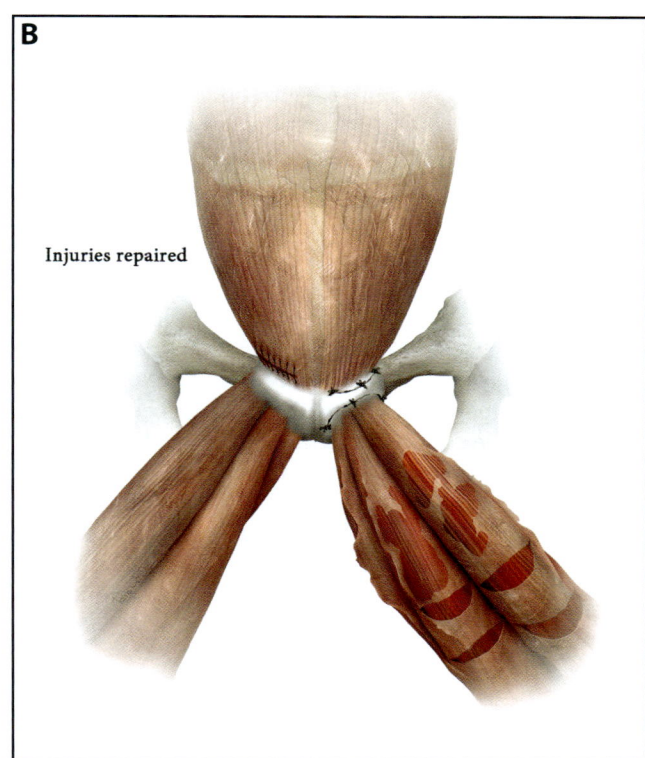

Figure 21-3. Complete adductor harness (A) avulsion and (B) repair. Note the "de-accordianization" and creation of muscle length.

- A star linebacker for an NFL team develops more severe core muscle pain halfway through the season and plays after a steroid injection despite the severe limitation. He had been playing through pain for the past 2 years and a laparoscopic mesh hernia repair had not helped and gave him an additional new pain related to intense fibrosis around the mesh. His team did well that year and made it to the Super Bowl. The linebacker came to the clinic a month after the end of the season and had 3 different areas of severe pain: the original core muscle injury, mesh pain, and severe hip impingement problem on the same side. The hip pain was the most severe, yet he chose to have only the first 2 problems corrected so that he could make it to the next season's training camp. He played well that next year with only the hip pain improved by injections. The linebacker elected for hip surgery right at the end of that following season, and he has played well again for 2 more years. This NFL star took matters into his own hands, worked through complicated variables, and made successful decisions that preserved his career.

- An NHL player develops severe deep groin pain just before the playoffs and is told he has a "sports hernia" and because of so much pain is advised to miss the playoffs and have it fixed. He seeks out another opinion and turns out to have partially torn a deep pelvic internal rotator with severe associated inflammation. He undergoes an ultrasound-guided injection and returns and plays well in the first playoff game, 3 days after the injection, and remains without problems for the past 3 years. This player aggressively sought out another opinion, which preserved his season and helped the team as well as his career. (See Figure 21-4.)

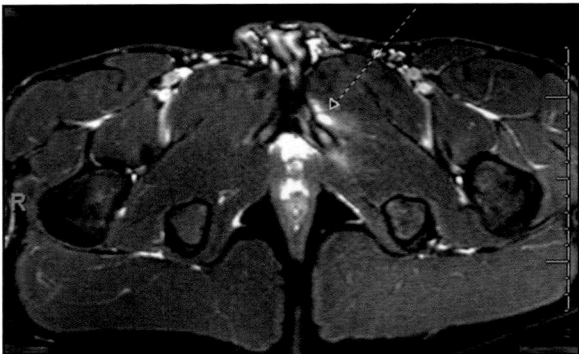

Figure 21-4. Deep strain and associated inflammation of the obturator externus muscle (thin arrow/arrowhead). The NHL player underwent a steroid injection and returned to the playoffs 3 days later.

- A college basketball star has severe deep abdominal and groin pain at the beginning of the season and cannot play. He has a small pubic plate injury on MRI. On exam, he has mild right lower quadrant tenderness and objective guarding. The tenderness had been going on for a month. He turns out to also have chronic intermittent diarrhea and then definite Crohn's disease after an accelerated gastrointestinal work-up. He gets treated with medications as well as undergoes laparoscopic interposition of omentum underneath a thickened, exudative loop of small intestine where it had been attached to the pelvis and undoubtedly the source of pain. The treatment returned him to full play 3 weeks later, and his team went far in the NCAA tournament. This case shows the complexity of the diagnoses and how clinical savvy enters into decision-making. In this case, the head athletic trainer at the school and his athletic administration facilitated the efficient work-up, successful return to play, and multiple levels of satisfaction.

It's paradoxical that the idea of living a long life appeals to everyone, but the idea of getting old doesn't appeal to anyone.

—Andy Rooney.

ATHLETIC WISDOM

Athletic wisdom refers to the quality of having experience, knowledge, and good judgment in sports. It applies to both the athlete and the therapist. Age and wisdom are sometimes dependent and sometimes independent processes, for both the athlete and therapist. Athletic wisdom is a necessary part of athleticism, which refers to abilities of a great athlete that include balance, strength, and power.

In practicality, 3 "organs" get involved in both athleticism and athletic wisdom: the brain, the heart, and the core. The most important of the 3 is the brain. The brain can see, hopefully, the limitations of the core, plus overcome, whenever necessary, the far-reaching desires of the heart to surmount those limitations. The brain's job is to help accomplish what's best for the whole person. The therapist's wisdom generates knowledge from the same 3 organs, plus the experience of having seen what usually works and what customarily does not.

In this chapter, we inspected numerous factors that play into optimal formulae for core muscle injury prevention as well as therapeutic decision-making. Age, wisdom, and heart emerge as the top 3 variables that enter into a wide range of formulae. All 3 link closely to the patient, the therapist, and the exact circumstances.

The number of anatomic variables are about to grow exponentially. In Section Three, we jump to the hip joint. The hip joint adds a whole other layer of anatomic complexity. Do not fear. We shall continue to keep it simple.

SELECTED READINGS

Paffenbarger RS, Blair SN, Leeb I. A history of physical activity, cardiovascular health and longevity: the scientific contributions of Jeremy N. Morris, DSc, DPH, FRCP. *Int J Epidemiol.* 2001;30(5):1184-1192.
   These authors report on the fascinating logic involved in Dr. Morris's adaptation of classical infectious disease epidemiology to "non-communicable diseases," and conclude that exercise is good for longevity.

Morris JN, Heady JA, Raffle PA, Roberts CG, Parks JW. Coronary heart-disease and physical activity of work. *Lancet.* 1953;265:1111-1120.
   Dr. Morris' sentinel paper on improved health metrics among active bus drivers compared to sedentary compatriots.

Dijkstra HP, Pollock N, Chakraverty R, Ardern CL. Return to play in elite sport: a shared decision-making process. *Br J Sports Med.* 2017;51(5):419-420. doi:10.1136/bjsports-2016-096209.
   The authors report on the complexity of return-to-play decision-making. The numbers of variables increase exponentially with decisions such as surgery.

REFERENCES

1. Middleton N, Shave R, George K, et al. Left ventricular function immediately following prolonged exercise: a meta-analysis. *Med Sci Sports Exerc.* 2006;38:681-687.
2. Thompson PD, Funk EJ, Carleton RA, Sturner WQ. Incidence of death during jogging in Rhode Island from 1975 through 1980. *JAMA.* 1982;247:2535-2538.
3. Lane NE. Exercise: a cause of osteoarthritis. *J Rheumatol Suppl.* 1995;43:3-6.
4. Thompson PD, Franklin BA, Balady GJ, et al. Exercise and acute cardiovascular events placing the risks into perspective: a scientific statement from the American Heart Association Council on Nutrition, Physical Activity, and Metabolism and the Council on Clinical Cardiology. *Circulation.* 2007;115:2358-2368.
5. Eijsvogels TM, Fernandez AB, Thompson PD. Are there deleterious cardiac effects of acute and chronic endurance exercise? *Physiol Rev.* 2016;96(1):99-125.
6. Morris JN, Heady JA, Raffle PA, Roberts CG, Parks JW. Coronary heart-disease and physical activity of work. *Lancet.* 1953;265:1111-1120.
7. Rauramaa R, Halonen P, Vaisanen SB, et al. Effects of aerobic physical exercise on inflammation and atherosclerosis in men: the DNASCO Study: a six-year randomized, controlled trial. *Ann Internal Med.* 2004;140:1007-1014.
8. Paffenbarger RS, Blair SN, Leeb I. A history of physical activity, cardiovascular health and longevity: the scientific contributions of Jeremy N. Morris, DSc, DPH, FRCP. *Int J Epidemiol.* 2001;30(5):1184-1192.
9. Athletic pubalgia surgery. Aetna. http://www.aetna.com/cpb/medical/data/700_799/0750.html. Accessed December 29, 2016.

section three
hip hop movement*

*from the subculture that formed in the early 1970s in the South Bronx

22

the **hip**
how **far** we have come!

J. W. THOMAS BYRD, MD

Editor's Note: *In the first chapter of this section, Thomas Byrd reflects on the state of the field of hip arthroscopy. Tom seems the best person to do this. Soon after Jim Glick performed the first therapeutic arthroscopy in the early 1990s, Thomas followed with a series of patients and stands as the first true popularizer of this field. For many years, Thomas's panache, fresh perspective, and generous supply of technical pearls has facilitated the launch and acceptance of hip arthroscopy. No doubt, Thomas would win, or be in the top 2 or 3 of, a vote for "Most Respected" among the hip surgeons in the world today.*

Tom was also one of the first to recognize that hip and core muscles injuries occur together. I remember a phone call from him in the early 1990s. He was excited. "I have a player with both sets of injuries, Bill. There's got to be a connection. I am convinced of it!" Tom described a star freshman ACC football player destined to go to the NFL. "Why don't you do your surgery first? Then, we get him through the season. I will do mine [hip arthroscopy] at the end of the season." We did that. The player exceeded expectations, and went in the top 5 of the draft 2 years later.

Tom and I began seeing a number of high-level athletes together in a cross-country way. Initially, ice hockey exceeded all other sports in terms of numbers of patients with the combined injuries. We speculated a "skate blade" theory. The hockey players repeatedly jump and land on thin blades. We speculated that somehow the thin blades transmitted powerful forces along narrow, vertical vectors directly into the balls and sockets; the muscle injuries came as a consequence to that. Then we saw at least one player in whom, seemingly, the complement sequence occurred. The latter star NHL defenseman initially ripped off all the adductor muscles plus his rectus abdominis muscle on one side off the pubic plate. Two years later, hip symptoms and new hip MRI pathology ensued on that same side. Possible reasons for the co-existence of the 2 sets of injuries are discussed more in other chapters.

Okay, enough chat. Let's hear Thomas's thoughts and reflections. As you read Thomas's words, keep in mind that his spoken words flow effortlessly in a Southern accent. Don't be afraid to smile. Read and listen closely. You will hear his happy Tennessean drawl resonating within carefully written words.

Overview

Three factors led to the current exponential recognition of sports-related hip disorders. Arthroscopists began looking in the hip, identifying and addressing joint damage that previously went unrecognized and untreated. Meyers published his work on athletic pubalgia as a prelude to current understanding of core muscle injuries. Then, Ganz described femoroacetabular impingement (FAI) as the etiology of many joint problems.

FAI with accompanying joint damage and core muscle injuries often co-exist. This necessitates skillful clinical diagnostic acumen to differentiate the various components and a multidisciplinary approach in the treatment that includes both surgical and non-surgical strategies.

Knowing the history of the evolution of our understanding of sports hip disorders gives an appreciation for how far we still have to go. This understanding is incomplete and our treatment strategies imperfect.

Exponential Recognition of Sports Hip Disorders: Influence of Three Independent Forces

There has been an explosion of interest and attention to sports-related hip disorders in both the lay press and scientific publications. It raises the question of whether this is hype, are we overdiagnosing these problems, or is it a real entity? If it is real, why has there been such exponential awareness?

From this author's perspective, it is real and can be explained by 3 independent forces that were at work in the world. First, in the 1990s, a few enthusiasts began looking more into the hip joint with the arthroscope, recognizing the existence of numerous disorders that historically had gone unrecognized and untreated.[1-3] Previously, athletes were simply resigned to living within the constraints of their affliction, often with no explanation as to the source. Frankly, with the poor understanding of these hip disorders, frequently the athlete's motivation and character would be called into question when he/she could no longer excel for unexplained reasons.

Second, in the first month of this millennium, Bill Meyers et al published their landmark article on athletic pubalgia.[4] Groin disorders and their treatments in athletes have been recognized for decades on other continents where football meant soccer. It was a common affliction, but it was Meyers who put all of this together, especially in North America.

Third, in 2003, Professor Reinhold Ganz and his colleagues, the Bern Group, published the landmark article on FAI as a cause of joint damage in the native hip.[5] Previously, it had been described only as an iatrogenic phenomenon with overcorrection of acetabular dysplasia.[6] Impingement was not a new concept.

Cheilectomy for removing the bump associated with sequelae of childhood slipped capital femoral epiphysis was described in the German literature 100 years ago (Figure 22-1).[7] Smith-Petersen, in his 1936 article, illustrated reshaping the acetabulum and the proximal femur in a pattern that, although primitive, is strikingly similar to what is described with today's open techniques (Figure 22-2).[8] Bill Harris et al, in the 1970s, advocated that there was no such thing as primary osteoarthritis of the hip; all osteoarthritis occurred secondary to something, and they wrote back then about the pistol grip deformity of the proximal femur (Figure 22-3).[9] However, it was Ganz and his colleagues who tied all of this together with our current understanding of FAI with pincer, cam, and combined patterns.

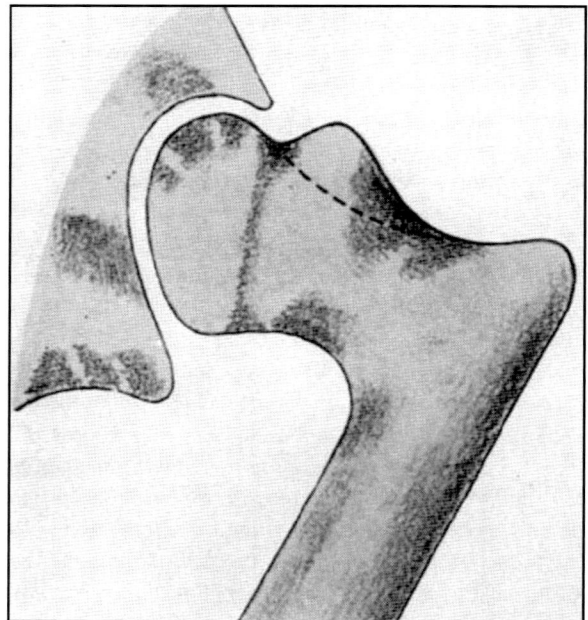

Figure 22-1. This illustration by Vulpius and Stöffel, published in 1913, illustrates cheilectomy for slipped capital femoral epiphysis. The bone above the curved dotted line is removed to relieve the obstruction to motion at the rim of the acetabulum. (Reprinted from Vulpius O, Stöffel A. *Orthopäadische Operationslehre*. Stuttgart, Germany: F. Enke; 1913.)

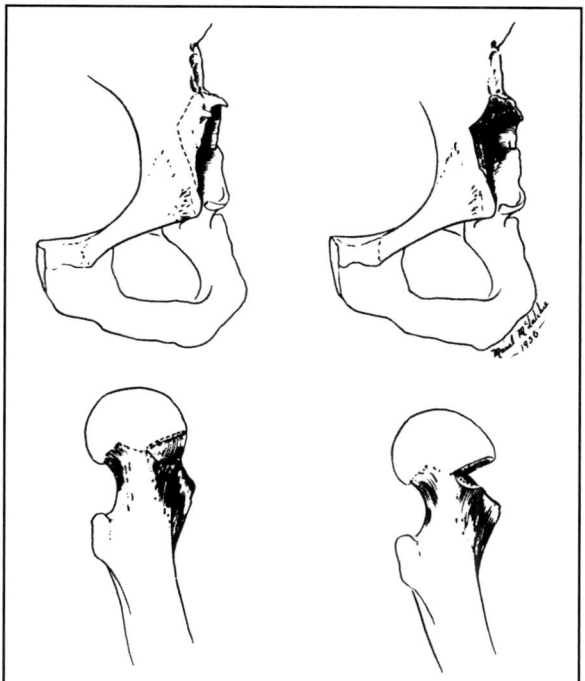

Figure 22-2. Diagrams illustrating early efforts at reshaping the acetabulum and femoral head for improved range of motion. (Reprinted with permission from Smith-Petersen MN. Treatment of malum coxae senilis, old slipped upper femoral epiphysis, intrapelvic protrusion of the acetabulum, and coxa plana by means of acetabuloplasty. *J Bone Joint Surg Am.* 1936;18:869-880.)

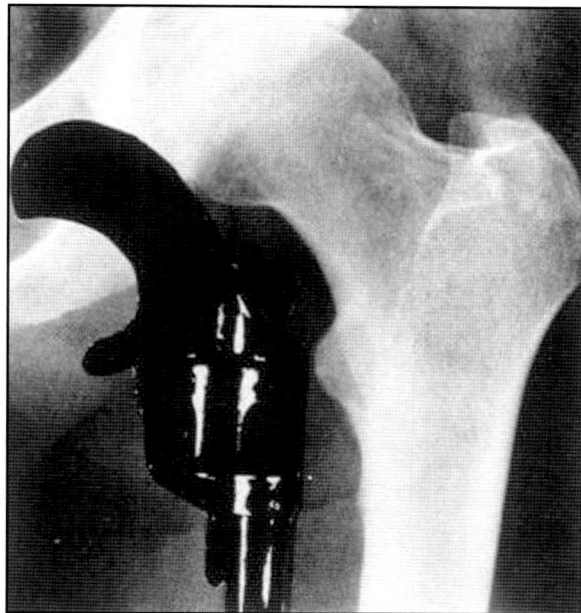

Figure 22-3. This image illustrates pistol grip deformity of the proximal femur associated with secondary osteoarthritis. (Reprinted with permission from Stulberg SD, Cordell LD, Harris WH, Ramsey PL, MacEwen GD. Unrecognized childhood hip disease: a major cause of idiopathic osteoarthritis of the hip. *Otto E. Aufranc Award Paper in the Hip, Proceedings of the Third Open Scientific Meeting of the Hip Society.* St. Louis, MO: CV Mosby; 1975:212-228.)

EVOLVING UNDERSTANDING OF FEMOROACETABULAR IMPINGEMENT

Keep in mind that the understanding of FAI is still too simplistic. We are just starting to scratch the surface to understand all of the contributing factors, including femoral version, pelvic orientation, and lumbar lordosis/kyphosis, just to mention a few. It is likely that many individuals with radiographic features of FAI have long active lifestyles, never developing pathological sequelae. How are some people lifelong compensators? These are the questions for which we need better answers. Pathological FAI is like a perfect storm where there are numerous factors that come together just wrong, leading to joint breakdown, pain, and dysfunction. We may never identify all of the factors, but if we can identify enough to reach critical mass in effective treatment including surgical and non-surgical strategies, that may be the best for which we can hope.

It is unusual to observe symptomatic FAI in adolescents and young adults unless they are involved in athletic activities.[10-12] These are individuals pushing their bodies beyond the reduced physiologic limits imposed by the altered morphology of FAI. Thus, the joint starts to break down with activities better tolerated by teammates and competitors with more normal joint morphology. This is a big problem in our athletes today, and stating that it is of potential epidemic proportion is not a severe overstatement. John Bergfeld, a legendary NFL team physician who evaluates many retired NFL players, commented that osteoarthritis of the hip is the most common disorder with which these retired players are plagued. Less active individuals just present in middle age with what used to be described simply as early age onset osteoarthritis.[10]

Evolution of Hip Arthroscopy

This author performed his first hip arthroscopy in 1990 armed only with a single article by Jim Glick from the 1988 Instructional Course Lectures publication.[13] Jim described the lateral position, but we opted for supine just for simplicity, trying to mirror how we would manage a hip fracture. The case was a teenager with loose bodies for whom we chose to try arthroscopic removal as a less invasive alternative to a conventional arthrotomy (Figure 22-4). It worked, and over the ensuing 2 years, we did 2 more cases of loose body removal.

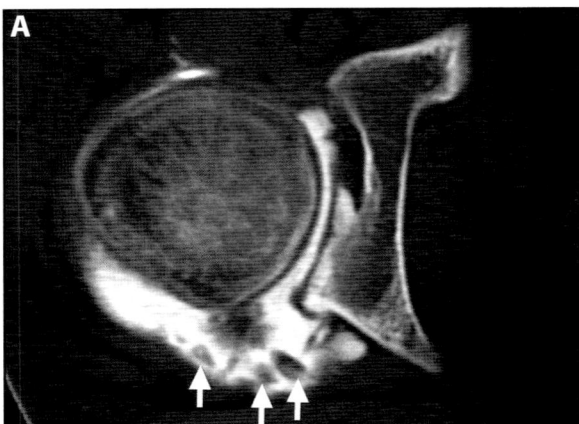
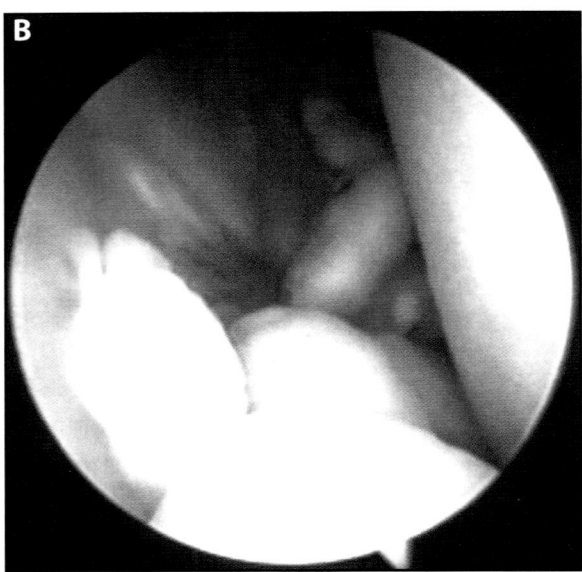

Figure 22-4. A 17-year-old boy with mechanical right hip pain, 2 years following closed treatment of a posterior column fracture of the acetabulum. (A) A double contrast arthro-CT scan confirms the presence of multiple loose bodies (arrows) represented by the filling defects posteriorly. (B) Arthroscopic view reveals several of the representative loose bodies between the femoral head and acetabulum. (© J. W. Thomas Byrd, MD.)

Then the physical therapist who oversaw the rehabilitation in these cases presented his brother with a 14-year history of locking, catching, and giving way of his hip following a motorcycle accident. All studies were unremarkable, but we suspected he might have some type of elusive radiolucent loose body. With protracted symptoms, the idea of considering at least a diagnostic arthroscopy seemed logical. At arthroscopy, he had a bucket-handle tear of his labrum, which was excised with prompt resolution of his symptoms after 14 years of difficulties (Figure 22-5). We will complete this story later in the chapter, but this sparked awareness that there were joint problems poorly detected by conventional imaging that could be a significant source of disability and might potentially benefit from arthroscopic intervention.

In 1994, the supine position technique was published, and it has become a mainstay in the field of hip arthroscopy (Figure 22-6).[1] In 1997, this author and Howard Sweeney composed the first Arthroscopy Association of North America hip arthroscopy course at the Orthopaedic Learning Center in Chicago, Illinois. It was well-received, and a second course was planned for the following year but had to be cancelled because no one registered. It was felt that perhaps everyone interested in hip arthroscopy had been taught. But, undeterred, another course was planned for 1999. That course filled, and the number grew from 2 to 3 courses annually, with each one being oversubscribed.

In 2001, the first scientific article on hip arthroscopy in athletes was published.[3] An important piece of data was that 60% of this group was treated for an average of 7 months before it was recognized that the joint might be the source of symptoms. Hip problems were poorly recognized. At this stage, the evolution of hip arthroscopy was strikingly different than other joints like the knee or shoulder. In those joints, conventional open procedures for recognized forms of pathology evolved to less invasive arthroscopic methods. Most hip problems benefiting from arthroscopy evolved from no treatment at all. As noted, most of the problems that could potentially benefit from arthroscopy were going unrecognized and untreated. Rarely was arthrotomy a consideration for these elusive disorders. Thus, a particular challenge of hip arthroscopy was trying to identify and treat the pathology at the same time that we were still trying to distinguish normal anatomy and its variations, while also having little understanding of the underlying etiology of the disorders we were treating.

The Hip—How Far We Have Come! 233

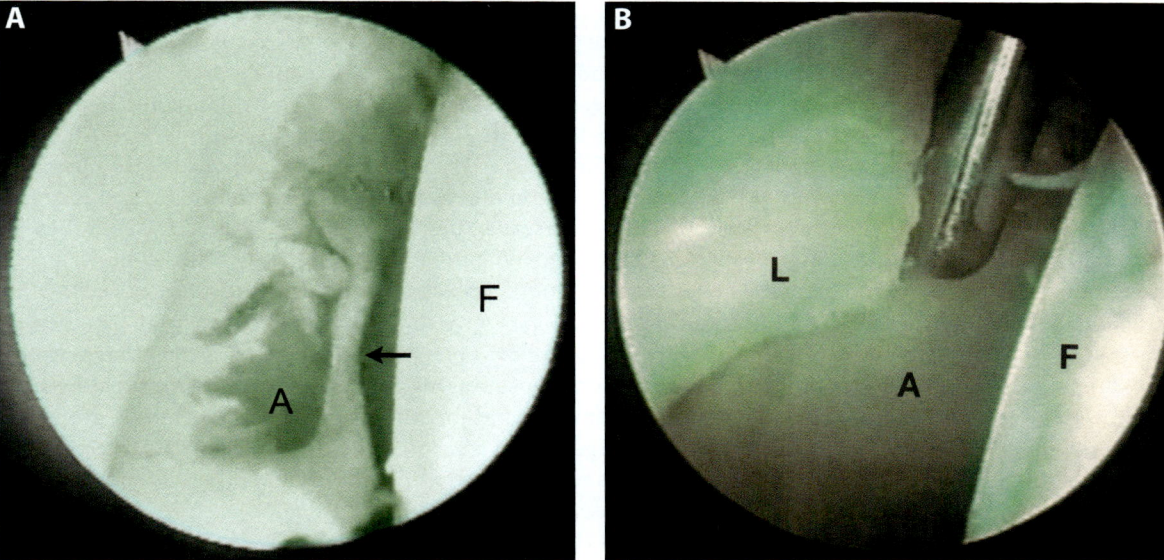

Figure 22-5. A 32-year-old man with a 14-year history of intermittent pain, catching, and giving way of his right hip. (A) Arthroscopic view of the right hip from the anterolateral portal demonstrates extensive tearing of the acetabular labrum (arrow) displaced into the joint obscuring view of the acetabulum (A). The femoral head is on the right (F). (B) View from the posterolateral portal as the tear is debrided back to the normal labrum (L) better exposing the acetabulum (A). (© J. W. Thomas Byrd, MD.)

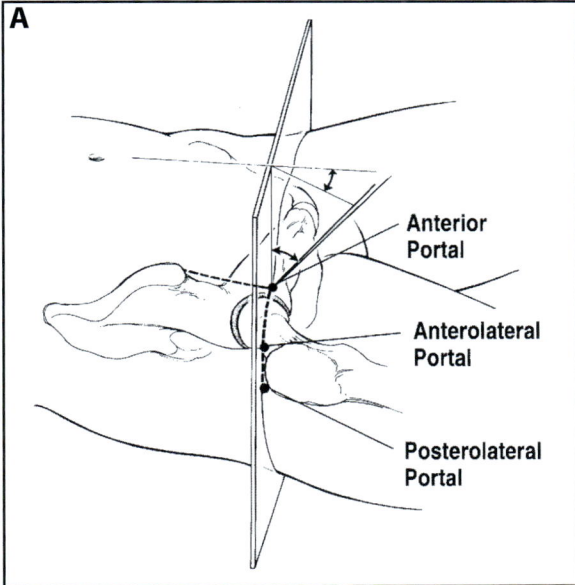

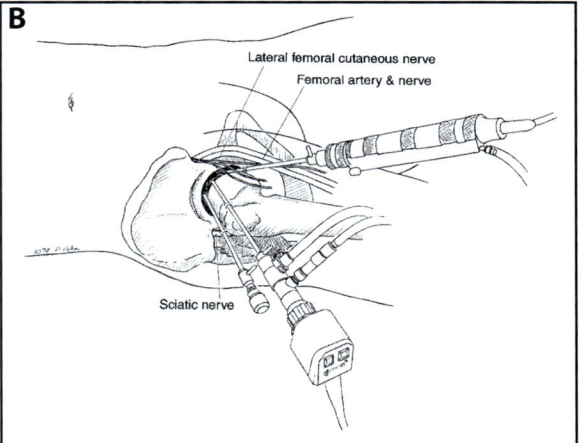

Figure 22-6. Illustrations from a 1994 publication on supine technique illustrate (A) topographical landmarks and (B) relationship of the major neurovascular structures. (© J. W. Thomas Byrd, MD.)

The evolution of hip arthroscopy changed with Professor Ganz's landmark 2003 article on FAI.[5] Although, perhaps, the understanding of the etiology of FAI was incomplete, it was well mapped out with reliable methods of correction with open surgical dislocation. Quickly, arthroscopy began to find its role as a less invasive alternative. For a while, there tended to be a clash of arthroscopic vs open management of FAI and other similar disorders. Over time, this has equilibrated, understanding that it is not either/or, but simply a matter of where each method exists on a spectrum of options available in the comprehensive management of hip disorders. Many are amenable to arthroscopic intervention, but there are numerous problems that can only be completely addressed with open methods.

Hip arthroscopy is different than other joints such as the knee or shoulder or even the elbow. For these joints, portal placement is a given, and it is the finer points of the operative procedures that are emphasized. Portal placement in the hip is both more challenging and more critical for the safety and the efficacy of the procedure. Atraumatic access is a challenge because of the constrained ball-and-socket architecture, limited distractibility due to the non-compliant capsule, and dense surrounding soft tissue envelope. These same features lead to limited maneuverability within the portals, and thus precision in placement is equally important to be able to effectively carry out operative procedures. Despite these challenges, operative hip arthroscopy has evolved from simple resection procedures to repair, restoration, and reconstructive techniques. The hope is, and the evidence suggests, that these can lead to more durable results.[14,15] However, these innovations have not come without some cost to the patients entrusted to our care. With more sophisticated complex procedures, we encounter new complications and obligate these patients to more sophisticated rehabilitation strategies.[16,17]

As we look at these innovations, it is important to keep in perspective that not everything we've done in the past has been done poorly. Looking at labral debridements with 10-year follow-up, 83% did well if they did not have clinical findings of arthritis at the time of the index procedure.[18] That sounds encouraging, but younger and younger patients are being encountered who already have significant secondary joint damage and for whom simple debridement is unlikely to be a viable long-term answer. Also, the patient population undergoing hip arthroscopy 2 decades ago was different. Typically, arthroscopy was only considered as a last resort for patients with protracted symptoms and otherwise healthy-appearing joints. If early radiographic features of degenerative disease were present, they were usually told to simply hold on until they needed an arthroplasty. Thus, the hips selected for arthroscopy had already proven to be quite durable. Now, we are recognizing many young adults and even adolescents whose joints are less durable and may not withstand years of benign neglect before considering corrective intervention.

Some things we've done in the past have worked pretty well. Our hope is that with more sophisticated procedures, they can do better. Along with this evolution, we must still be thoughtful to weigh the consequences of these more advanced procedures, and hopefully avoid some of the pitfalls that have been encountered in other joints.[19] Keep in mind that that first bucket-handle tear excised in 1992 is still doing well more than 20 years later. He remains asymptomatic with normal radiographs (Figure 22-7).

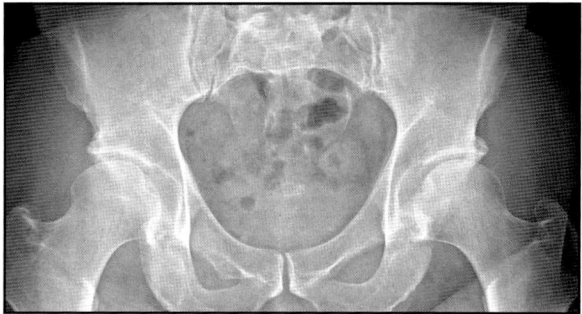

Figure 22-7. AP radiograph of a man, now 53 years old, and 21 years following arthroscopic labral debridement of the right hip reveals good joint space preservation and no significant secondary osteoarthritic changes. He remains asymptomatic and unrestricted in his activities. (© J. W. Thomas Byrd, MD.)

FEMOROACETABULAR IMPINGEMENT AND CORE MUSCLE INJURIES: HOW THEY COME TOGETHER

There is a growing body of evidence to support the association between FAI and what was previously described as athletic pubalgia, but now better understood as a component of core muscle injuries.[20,21] The association is not hard to understand, especially in athletic populations. Diminished hip motion associated with FAI is compensated by increased pelvic motion, putting more stress on the pelvic stabilizers, eventually leading to breakdown of these structures. Like other forms of overuse tendinosis, the damage and the treatment exist on a spectrum ranging from simple activity modification to strengthening, to judicious use of various injectables, to surgical repair. There is pretty compelling evidence that the core dysfunction occurs secondary to FAI, and sometimes correcting the FAI may result in spontaneous resolution of core dysfunction. Obviously, core surgery will not solve the underlying FAI. However, there are circumstances where breakdown due to core dysfunction exposes the hip, making the underlying FAI more symptomatic. Thus, correcting the core dysfunction, whether through conservative or surgical methods, may restore an individual's ability to compensate and improve the hip, although still not solving the FAI.

Meyers et al also noted that the results of treatment of core muscle injuries are superior in athletes compared to nonathletes.[4] This makes sense. Among athletes, these injuries are the result of excessive force on normal muscle structures that possess good healing capacity, especially if the underlying FAI is corrected. Among less active individuals, these types of muscle injuries imply an element of intrinsic muscle disease and likely less effective healing capacity.

A growing understanding is being gained regarding the negative role that hip disease can play in the complex kinematic linkage, extending far beyond just the pelvis. Interplay of hip and lumbar spine disease has been well recognized in sports where rotational velocity is a premium, such as golf and baseball. As one area breaks down, the athlete may lose his/her ability to compensate for the other. Recognizing this is important when outlining a comprehensive treatment strategy. However, this negative interplay can be even further up the kinetic chain. In one study of high-level baseball players, 75% of major league pitchers having undergone hip arthroscopy also had concomitant ulnar collateral ligament surgery in their throwing elbow.[22]

SUMMARY

Presently, we have come just far enough to appreciate how far we have to go. Much remains to be learned on how to best restore a damaged joint. We are just scratching the surface on understanding the complex interactive nature of the etiology of these disorders and how to address these with a multidisciplinary approach. Lastly, we are expanding our awareness of how hip dysfunction plays into the kinetic chain of the human body and how it can both negatively influence and be negatively influenced by other compensatory disorders.

REFERENCES

1. Byrd JWT. Hip arthroscopy utilizing the supine position. *Arthroscopy*. 1994;10(3):275-280.
2. Byrd JWT. Labral lesions, an elusive source of hip pain: case reports and review of the literature. *Arthroscopy*. 1996;12(5):603-612.
3. Byrd JWT, Jones KS. Hip arthroscopy in athletes. *Clin Sports Med*. 2001;20(4):749-762.
4. Meyers WC, Foley DP, Garrett WE, Lohnes JH, Mandelbaum BR. Management of severe lower abdominal or inguinal pain in high-performance athletes. PAIN (Performing Athletes with Abdominal or Inguinal Neuromuscular Pain Study Group). *Am J Sports Med*. 2000;28(1):2-8.
5. Ganz R, Parvizi J, Beck M, Leunig M, Notzli H, Siebenrock KA. Femoroacetabular impingement—a cause for osteoarthritis of the hip. *Clin Orthop Rel Res*. 2003;417:112-120.
6. Myers SR, Eijer H, Ganz R. Anterior femoroacetabular impingement after periacetabular osteotomy. *Clin Orthop Rel Res*. 1999;363:93-99.
7. Vulpius O, Stöffel A. *Orthopäadische Operationslehre*. Stuttgart, Germany: F. Enke; 1913.
8. Smith-Petersen MN. Treatment of malum coxae senilis, old slipped upper femoral epiphysis, intrapelvic protrusion of the acetabulum, and coxa plana by means of acetabuloplasty. *J Bone Joint Surg*. 1936;18:869-880.
9. Stulberg SD, Cordell LD, Harris WH, Ramsey PL, MacEwen GD. Unrecognized childhood hip disease: a major cause of idiopathic osteoarthritis of the hip. *Otto E. Aufranc Award Paper in the Hip, Proceedings of the Third Open Scientific Meeting of the Hip Society*. St. Louis, MO: CV Mosby; 1975:212-228.
10. Byrd JWT, Jones KS. Arthroscopic "femoroplasty" in the management of cam-type femoroacetabular impingement. *Clin Orthop Rel Res*. 2009;467(3):739-746.
11. Byrd JWT, Jones KS, Gwathmey FW. Arthroscopic management of femoroacetabular impingement in adolescents. Proceedings of AAOS 2014 Annual Meeting, New Orleans, Louisiana.
12. Byrd JWT, Jones KS, Gwathmey FW. FAI in adolescent athletes. Proceedings of the American Academy of Orthopaedic Surgeons 2015 Annual Meeting, Las Vegas, Nevada.
13. Glick JM. Hip arthroscopy using the lateral approach. *Instr Course Lect*. 1988;37:223-231.
14. Larson CM, Giveans MR, Stone RM. Arthroscopic debridement versus refixation of the acetabular labrum associated with femoroacetabular impingement: mean 3.5-year follow-up. *Am J Sports Med*. 2012;40(5):1015-1021.
15. Krych AJ, Thompson M, Knutson Z, Scoon J, Coleman SH. Arthroscopic labral repair versus selective labral debridement in female patients with femoroacetabular impingement: a prospective randomized study. *Arthroscopy*. 2013;29(1):46-53.
16. Souza BGS, Dani WAS, Honda EK, et al. Do complications in hip arthroscopy change with experience? *Arthroscopy*. 2010;26(8):1053-1057.
17. Coplen EM, Voight ML. Rehabilitation of the hip. In: Byrd JWT, ed: *Operative Hip Arthroscopy*. 3rd ed. New York, NY: Springer; 2012:411-439.
18. Byrd JWT, Jones KS. Hip arthroscopy for labral pathology: prospective analysis with 10-year follow-up. *Arthroscopy*. 2009;25(4):365-368.
19. Collins HR, Hughston JC, Dehaven KE, et al. The meniscus as a cruciate ligament substitute. *J Sports Med*. 1974;2:11-21.
20. Larson CM, Pierce BR, Giveans MR. Treatment of athletes with symptomatic intra-articular hip pathology and athletic pubalgia/sports hernia: a case series. *Arthroscopy*. 2011;27(6):768-775.
21. Hammoud S, Bedi A, Magennis E, Meyers WC, Kelly BT. High incidence of athletic pubalgia symptoms in professional athletes with symptomatic femoroacetabular impingement. *Arthroscopy*. 2012;28(10):1388-1395.
22. Byrd JWT, Jones KS. Hip arthroscopy in high level baseball players. *Arthroscopy*. 2015;31(8):1507-1510.

23

private eyes on the hip
sometimes a culprit in pelvic pain and pelvic floor disorders

STRUAN H. COLEMAN, MD, PHD

Editor's Note: Dr. Byrd's wonderful historical perspective in the previous chapter pointed out clearly at least 5 things:
1. The field of hip arthroscopy is still in its infancy. Therefore, the thinking within the field remains pretty basic. Current practice focuses on intrinsic activities within the ball and socket, and not on extra-articular contributing factors, such as femoral version, pelvic tilt, or lumbar curvature.
2. Right now, hip arthroscopists see different groups of people. At one extreme, people have lots of radiological impingement but no symptoms. At the other extreme, people exhibit severe signs, symptoms, and progressive disease. What defines these differences? It is doubtful that the answer is solely athletics. It may be like a perfect storm, with multiple factors at play, such as pelvic orientation, muscle anatomy, the person's specific movements. The best ultimate answers may come from the question: How do some people compensate so well life-long with such severe apparent misalignments?
3. It is unusual to observe symptomatic femoroacetabular impingement (FAI) in adolescents and young adults unless they are involved in athletic activities.
4. We are getting better at hip arthroscopy, but the answers are not all in. Hip arthroscopists are onto something good.
5. But our knowledge base is nowhere close to perfect. The correlation of the hip with core muscular anatomy is a prelude to future understanding.

The ensuing chapters go into various aspects of new clinical and anatomic understandings of the hip. In this chapter, Struan Coleman, head of hip arthroscopy at the Hospital for Special Surgery in New York City, describes the development of his special expertise in hip arthroscopy for women or men with pelvic floor pain. He has become the best-known surgeon in this expanding clientele of patients. Also a gifted sports orthopedic surgeon and team physician for the New York Mets, Struan has dramatically good results with this complicated group of patients. In the chapter, Struan becomes Sherlock Holmes. He regards the patients with severe, chronic pelvic pain sitting (or, more accurately, standing because it is too painful to sit!) in uro-gynecologic offices as great mysteries. He writes the chapter like Sir Arthur Conan Doyle. His gynecology colleagues play the role of Watson.

Not Just Another Day at the Beach (Figure 23-1)

By way of introduction, I am a sports medicine orthopedic surgeon working in New York City. I have a particular interest in disorders of the hip in young people. In 2008, Sarah, a 26-year-old athletic woman, came into my office complaining of groin pain for more than 2 years. Sarah described a dull ache in the groin with occasional "catching, locking, and popping." Sarah experienced this groin pain with sitting, getting in and out of a car, and with all activities involving rotation of the hip joint. Sarah had completed multiple rounds of physical therapy and activity modifications without relief. Sarah's pain was getting worse and was now interfering with most of her daily activities. I asked Sarah about some of those activities. I was to learn that I did not ask about the important ones.

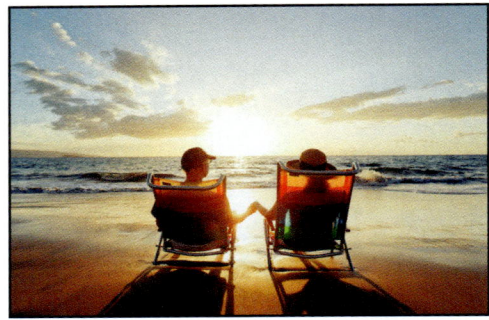

Figure 23-1.

After examining Sarah, I concluded that Sarah was suffering from a hip disorder. I sent Sarah for a number of imaging studies: X-rays of her hip and pelvis, an MRI, and a 3-dimensional CAT scan of the hip. At her second visit, I explained to Sarah that she had a condition called *femoroacetabular impingement*, or FAI, in which excessive bone next to the ball of the hip joint was rubbing on the rim of the socket. Moreover, the impingement had torn her labrum, an "O-ring" that runs around the rim of the bony socket and creates a seal with the ball. I recommended a surgical procedure using an arthroscope (a tiny camera introduced into the joint) to repair the torn labrum and remove the excess bone at the top of the femur. After discussing potential risks and benefits of the procedure, Sarah set a date for the surgery and left my office. Two months later, Sarah underwent the surgical procedure. At the time of the surgery, it was noted that her psoas tendon was red and excessively tight and so we performed a psoas lengthening in addition to the other procedures.

Three months after the surgery, during her second postoperative office visit, Sarah reported that her hip symptoms had completely resolved and that she had returned to her daily activities without pain. Later that day, I received a call from Sarah's gynecologist, Dr. Deborah Coady, who had surprising news. In addition to her hip pain, Sarah had been suffering for more than 4 years with another type of pelvic pain, a condition called *vulvodynia*. Vulvodynia is characterized by continuous burning pain of the external genitalia, and often associated with spasms of the pelvic floor muscle, painful intercourse, and bowel and bladder dysfunction. Dr. Coady was amazed. All of those symptoms had resolved as well following her hip arthroscopy. What had I done during the hip procedure that could possibly have affected Sarah's vulvodynia? The truth was: I had no idea.

The Quest

This phone call with Dr. Coady sparked the start of a fascinating journey, namely, a quest to understand the association between impingement of the hip and pelvic pain.

I spent the next few months reading about pelvic floor pain and discussing these issues with Dr. Coady; her partner, Dr. Deena Harris; and Stacy Futterman, an extraordinary "internal" physical therapist, who had been treating patients with pelvic pain for many years. Over those few weeks, I learned about the extraordinary prevalence of vulvodynia in the United States; it affects 8% to 16% of women within their lifetimes. The problem leads to diminished physical, sexual, and emotional function in millions of women.[1-4] Vulvodynia is difficult to cure due to both insufficient understanding of the causes of pelvic floor dysfunction and the presence of co-morbidities.[5] Treatment options for vulvodynia include specialized internal massage, intravaginal injections, topical medications, and, as a last resort, surgical procedures such as vestibulectomy (ie, removing parts of the external genitalia).

My treatment of Sarah swiftly generated optimism for Dr. Coady and her colleagues. For some of their patients with vulvodynia, there was hope. A relationship between the hip and "their" pelvic floor dysfunction would mean that treating the hip problem might resolve the pelvic pain. At the time, this seemed like a Eureka moment. But…there was more work to be done. The key was to understand the association between the hip and the pelvic floor.

We know that there is a close anatomical relationship among the hip joint, the pelvic floor, and the pelvic girdle. So, it was not too surprising that chronic inflammation inside the hip joint and surrounding structures might produce a variety of signs and symptoms within other areas of the pelvis.[6,7] We surmised that branches of the pudendal nerve may become irritated by an inflamed hip and/or iliopsoas tendon. Of course, we did not have all the answers, but advances in imaging, particularly MRI, together with the newer arthroscopic techniques, seemed likely to reveal some answers. Since 22% to

55% of all women have some sort of unexplained, chronic pelvic pain,[8] certainly the hip might have something to do with the pain of at least some of these people.

Read just about any chapter of this book, and you know that hip impingement can refer pain into the groin as well as a variety of other regions around the hip. "Shared" muscles, such as the iliopsoas, obturator internus, and other pelvic floor musculature, plus the interweaving, regional connective tissue, make it obvious that all these musculoskeletal structures are connected. If you remain unconvinced of the Machiavellian nature of this region, go back and reread Dr. Aradillas's chapter on the nerves of the pelvis. The bottom line: There are numerous anatomic pathways by which the hip can potentially interact with the pelvic floor.

Moreover, we knew that hip impingement leads to nonoptimal movement patterns or, more specifically, a change in the body's normal kinetic chain.[9] We considered this change in the movement of the pelvis in the setting of hip pathology. Certainly, it could result in spasm and dysfunction of pelvic floor musculature and eventually myofascial and/or neural (pudendal) vulvodynia. Read about the "generalized vulvodynia subtype."[10] This form of vulvodynia fit directly into our hypothesis.

Initial successes with Sarah, plus a second very similar patient a few months later, led us to construct an algorithm for the diagnosis and management of the "combined problem"—vulvodynia and hip impingement. We first identified suspected "combo patients" and screened them for hip pain, vulvodynia, and pelvic floor dysfunction. We obtained both a detailed gynecological history and physical exam and then a detailed musculoskeletal core history and physical examination. Specifically, we asked about both pelvic or groin pains or other symptoms associated with hip impingement: locking, catching, sitting, and getting in and out of a car. The most impressively overlapping symptoms were painful sex (dyspareunia) and painful sitting. The ones designated as combo patients then went for X-rays and MRIs of the hip and pelvis. When the history, physical exam, and radiographic findings all intertwined and pointed to pelvic floor dysfunction and hip impingement, we got ready to do more tests or treat them.

Let's take a step back and go more clearly through our thinking. One of our hypotheses was that iliopsoas muscle irritation, secondary to the underlying hip impingement, caused the spasms and generalized pelvic floor dysfunction. Over time, irritation of the pudendal and other nerve branches then triggered the vulvodynia, bladder and rectal pain, and dysfunctions. We stopped at different points in the testing and performed selective injections.

Selective injections of local anesthetic and cortisone are used commonly in orthopedics and other medical specialties to determine which precise anatomical site(s), joints, or areas around joints might be causing pain. Sometimes we even use these sorts of techniques as definitive treatments for the pains. For these patients, we used the differential injections technique quite liberally. We felt this critical for the evaluation, plus to confirm (or not) involvement of the hip joint. After we injected the hip joints, we then waited designated time intervals in order to assess the results. (See Figure 23-2.)

Three main possibilities emerged in terms of results:
1. No apparent effect; therefore, it seemed the hip was not involved
2. Partial or complete resolution of most of the hip pain but no effect on the vulvodynia
3. Relief of both the presumptive "hip" pain and the vulvodynia

Result 3 was obviously the strongest indicator to proceed with hip arthroscopy. Result 2 usually generated another injection, this time in the region of the iliopsoas tendon. This additional injection might either diminish or flare up the pelvic pain. In either event, we would presume the iliopsoas to be involved, and this, too, would become an indication for hip arthroscopy, with the additional procedure during surgery of lengthening the iliopsoas tendon. If we could not demonstrate any sort of relief (or aggravation) of the pain by the injections, we would not operate, unless the patient had reasons other than vulvodynia to do so.

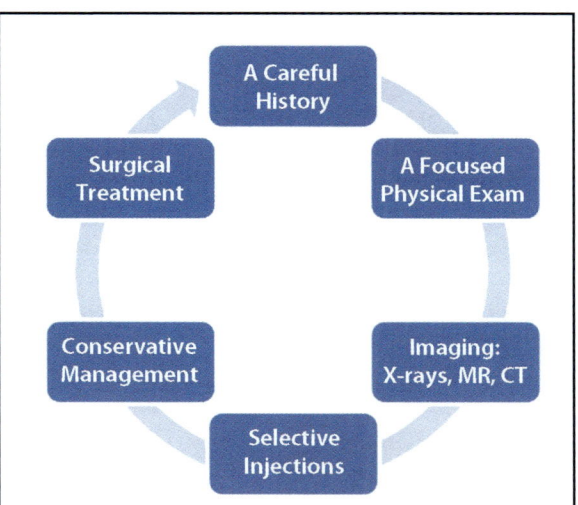

Figure 23-2. Diagnosis management flow chart for vulvodynia and hip impingement.

Even when patients were thought to have a combined problem, we put them through more "combined physical therapy" before surgery was performed. That meant both internal and core muscle work. Surgery was offered when everybody agreed that physical therapy failed to resolve the symptoms.

Of course, we would not guarantee that arthroscopy would bring success and rid the patients of any or all their pains. This is an important point as patients with severe vulvodynia are desperate to find a cure for their condition and will try everything. Therefore, it is critical the work-up is exhaustive and that, when surgery is indicated, we do our best to manage expectations.

The surgical procedure for hip impingement in patients with combined hip and pelvic pain involves traction to the hip joint by pulling the leg against a post positioned in the perineum. One of our early fears was that compression on this region of the pelvis, in close proximity to the pudendal nerve, would exacerbate the vulvodynia. Fortunately, we found that the traction was safe in these patients. We then introduce a camera into the hip and carefully inspect the distracted joint, and then address the pathology. We usually repair torn labra with "anchors" and shave away the "pinching" bone on the head and/or neck of the femur (hip "ball") and/or from the acetabular socket. In selected cases, we also lengthen slightly the psoas tendon. Following surgery, patients walk with crutches until their gait normalizes as they go through a strict postoperative physical therapy program. Pre- and postoperative gait and movement analyses sometimes help determine certain aspects of the postop rehabilitation program and may be useful for assessing progress.

So, we were almost set. The hip seemed a culprit. All we needed was proof.

THE SET-UP

So, this is what we did. A subgroup of patients with combined vulvodynia and hip impingement failed conservative treatment with physical therapy and underwent hip arthroscopy between November 2008 and August 2010. Surgery was followed by a 3- to 6-month course of hip and pelvic floor physical therapy following a standard postoperative protocol in which the focus is on strengthening the muscles of the core and the abductors (ie, gluteal muscles), in addition to the ongoing therapies for vulvodynia.

In September 2013, 36 to 58 months after surgery, we did a follow-up analysis of the outcome of arthroscopy for the treatment of combined hip impingement and vulvodynia. Patients were considered to have improved clinically if they no longer required ongoing evaluation or treatment for vulvodynia, and had developed no other ("co-morbid") type pelvic pain. The co-morbid conditions were carefully defined and labeled as painful bladder syndrome/interstitial cystitis, irritable bowel syndrome, or endometriosis. We also followed the patients' numerical rating score (NRS), an 11-point pain scale ranging from 0 (no vulvar pain) to 10 (worst vulvar pain imaginable), as a self-reported average compared to the preceding month. The scores were categorized for tabulation as mild (1 to 4), moderate (5 to 6), or severe (7 to 10). The grade of 11 was reserved for patients already self-assessed at 10 and who said the pain then became "worse." Most recent scores were compared to preoperative scores. We considered 2-point reductions in score to be clinically important.[11,12]

In addition, we asked 3 questions by phone or email:
1. On a scale of 0 (no pain) to 10 (worse pain imaginable), what has been your average vulvar pain level over the past month?
2. How satisfied are you with the results of your hip surgery on your vulvar pain, on a scale of greatly (3), moderately (2), mildly (1), or not satisfied (0)?
3. Would you recommend this surgery to another person in the same situation, who has both hip and vulvar pain? (Answer yes or no.)

Of course, we got institutional review board approval for all this.

THE EVIDENCE

It turns out we were good but not perfect. The hip was sometimes the culprit, and sometimes was not—or more accurately stated, "sometimes maybe was not." *Maybe* refers to the fact that most of the patients who didn't improve or improve much were older or had vulvodynia for a longer period of time. During that 26-month period, 72 patients fit into the vulvodynia-FAI hip group. They were 21 to 63 years old (mean: 39.7), and the duration of their vulvodynia ranged 1 to 21 years (mean: 5.5). Nine patients, all over 35 years, were "fully disabled" by their vulvar pain and, as a consequence, received Social Security disability benefits. Twenty-nine had had specific hip injuries in the past, all reported to disability agencies. One of the injuries, interestingly, occurred at the time of labor and delivery, and another occurred in the early postpartum period, while lifting twin newborns. All injuries preceded onset of vulvodynia.

All 72 patients had had 3 to 6 months of pelvic floor and hip physical therapy. Many also had had other nonsurgical vulvodynia therapies such as oral and topical medications. The majority of patients experienced satisfactory improvement or stabilization in hip pain preoperatively, and so did not undergo hip arthroscopy.

Twenty-six patients underwent arthroscopy for symptomatic FAI after failed conservative management during the 22 months from November 2008 through August 2010. The procedures consisted of pincer or cam bone resections or a combination of the two, labral repair with or without iliopsoas release. This surgeon made those technical decisions. Interestingly, most of the disabled patients underwent arthroscopy, and those patients had vulvodynia on an average of over 6 years. The arthroscopy group was also older than the non-operative group. Hip pain and pelvic floor dysfunction improved in all but one patient after arthroscopy. (See Table 23-1.)

Also note that this turned out to be an exceedingly complex group of patients. The table displays their characteristics and compares 2 subgroups: those with sustained improvement vs those without that. The patients suffered from 3 specific types of vulvodynia: diffuse (generalized) vulvodynia alone (16 patients), clitorodynia or localized vulvodynia (8), or diffuse vulvodynia with groin pain (2). It turns out—and this is something I certainly didn't know before visiting this Soho clinic—that the most common type of vulvodynia is localized vestibulodynia. Ten patients had co-morbidities, most commonly the painful bladder syndrome kind.

Only 6 patients had dramatic and sustained improvement in their vulvodynia and no longer required surveillance or treatment. The patient with the localized vestibulodynia was in this group. Her diffuse pain went completely away, and she later underwent excision of her vestibule. Intercourse has been totally normal for several years. The mean age of these 6 patients was 25 years, with a range of 22 to 29 years. They had all been suffering for 4 years or less. In fact, only 1 patient younger than 30 years did not improve.

A bunch of other interesting things happened. Fourteen patients had striking initial improvement, but this was not sustained. No patient over 33 years old had anything that we could interpret as dramatic and sustained improvement. One of the 2 patients with diffuse vulvodynia plus groin pain later underwent surgical removal of ilio-inguinal neuromas on both sides of the vulva, which completely eliminated her pain for the past 3 years. None of the disabled patients reported sustained improvement in their vulvodynia. This was also true of the non-operative group of patients on disability. They all reported no improvement.

Fascinatingly, over half of the arthroscopic patients said they would recommend hip arthroscopy to friends with similar clinical symptoms. Those recommenders included patients who reported no improvement and ones in the disability categories.

YAY OR NAY

Our conclusion was that some of the patients with a clear combined hip impingement/vulvodynia problem got better on both fronts with surgery. A small number had no improvement. The largest group of hips remains suspect. The best patients were those who were young women with less than 5 years of generalized vulvodynia or clitorodynia and who did not improve with physical therapy. Most of the other hips remain at large and under investigation. One thing is for sure: The hip plays a role in the pelvic pain for most of those patients.

MORE WORK NEEDED

Our work adds to a growing knowledge base connecting pelvic floor dysfunction and pain sensations in the vulva, with the musculoskeletal structures in the core region.

As discussed earlier, the biomechanical consequences of hip impingement may lead to vulvar pain by several mechanisms.[6] Therefore, we can speculate that the gluteus (abductor) muscles, often weakened by hip impingement, trigger overcompensation, shortening, and sustained contraction within the pelvic floor muscles. Resultant dystrophy, spasm, and other dysfunction stimulate pain receptors (nociceptors), and irritate or compress branches of the pudendal nerve. It should not be surprising, therefore, that most patients with generalized vulvodynia and/or clitorodynia describe their pain as "burning" (ie, just like most other peripheral neuropathies).[13,14] (See Chapter 18.)

Table 23-1
Vulvodynia Outcomes After Hip Arthroscopy (N = 26)

	Improvement (n = 6)	No Improvement (n = 20)	P[a]
Mean age at arthroscopy (years)	25.2	47.1	< .001
20 to 29, no. (%)	6 (100)	1 (5)	
30 to 39, no. (%)	0	5 (25)	
40 to 49, no. (%)	0	5 (25)	
≥ 50, no. (%)	0	9 (45)	
History of hip injury, no. (%)	0	8 (40)	.13
Disabled,[b] no. (%)	0	7 (35)	.15
Mean duration of vulvodynia (years)	2.5	5.7	.015
1 to 2, no. (%)	2 (33)	2 (10)	
3 to 4, no. (%)	4 (67)	7 (35)	
5 to 10, no. (%)	0	11 (55)	
Type of vulvodynia			
Generalized vulvodynia, no. (%)	3 (50)	13 (65)	.64
Clitorodynia, no. (%)	3 (50)	5 (25)	.33
Generalized vulvodynia with groin pain, no. (%)	0	2 (10)	1.00
Comorbidities,[c] no. (%)	2 (33)	8 (40)	1.00
Preoperative mean NRS[d]	6.7	6.7	.99
Mild (1 to 4), no. (%)	1 (17)	3 (15)	
Moderate (5 to 6), no. (%)	3 (50)	7 (35)	
Severe (7 to 10), no. (%)	2 (33)	10 (50)	
Postoperative mean NRS[d]	3.4	4.8	.026
None (0), no. (%)	0	1 (5)	
Mild (1 to 4), no. (%)	6 (100)	5 (25)	
Moderate (5 to 6), no. (%)	0	6 (30)	
Severe (7 to 10), no. (%)	0	8 (40)	

[a] P values comparing patients with improvement vs without improvement in vulvodynia.
[b] Disabled from paid employment due to vulvodynia.
[c] Comorbidities = Painful bladder syndrome/interstitial cystitis, irritable bowel syndrome, or endometriosis.
[d] Numerical rating score "average vulvar pain level in past month," values from 0 to 10.
Adapted from Coady D, Futterman S, Harris D, Coleman SH. Vulvodynia and concomitant femoro-acetabular impingement: long-term follow-up after hip arthroscopy. *J Low Genit Tract Dis*. 2015;19(3):253-256.

We should be assessing more comprehensively patients with vulvodynia for hip pathology and vice versa. Again, this poses a potential dilemma for the orthopedic surgeon as most patients don't expect to be asked about pelvic pain when seeing a hip specialist. However, we believe that it is an important part of the history. The physical exam of the hip, utilizing maneuvers such as the FABER test, have been well studied and reported.[6-9] If pelvic floor dysfunction is suspected, the patient should be referred to an appropriate specialist for further work-up. A digital vaginal exam may reveal pain at specific anatomic hip landmarks, tender myofascial restrictions, hypertonicity, shortening, and asymmetries in the superficial and/or deep pelvic floor muscles. The vaginal exam may also provoke burning along the distribution of branches of the pudendal nerve.[13,15]

Therapies directed at both the vulvar/pelvic floor to treat vulvodynia and the core muscles surrounding the hip joint to treat FAI may "normalize" muscular, fascial, or other soft tissue abnormalities[13,16] and may, in some cases, help to avoid surgical intervention for one or both of these conditions.[17]

To our knowledge, there have been no previous studies correlating hip arthroscopy for the treatment of FAI with resolution of vulvodynia. Based on our evidence to date we can say that some patients with both FAI and vulvodynia respond to both non-operative and surgical modalities. It also seems likely that, for some patients, vulvar pain originates from or is exacerbated by hip impingement.[7-9,17-19]

Since the subgroup of patients suffering with vulvodynia for a mean of 6 years did not do as well as the group who suffered for less than 3 years, it seems likely that long-term myofascial and neural injury contributes to establishment of a more central pain component that can be challenging to treat.[20] This should put pressure on us as health professionals to recognize vulvodynia early and to identify those patients in whom there may be any underlying musculoskeletal cause. Early identification would likely improve outcomes. We therefore encourage hip specialists, and orthopedists in general, to familiarize themselves with the various review articles on this subject.[6,13,14,21,22]

Despite some success among our patients with combined vulvodynia and hip impingement, more studies are needed to develop interventions that will prevent the chronic refractory vulvar pain that many of our patients continue to experience. Some alternative therapies provided inconsistent relief for these patients; these included neuropathic pain medications, opioid pain relievers, behavioral therapies, and interventional procedures such as injections, regional analgesia, spinal cord stimulation, and pudendal nerve surgery. Recent studies are suggesting that centralized pain may be helped by mind-body therapies such as yoga and meditation, which have benefited some of our patients.[23] Plus, we may ponder the benefits of therapy such as ketamine infusions, as performed for complex regional pain syndrome.

Despite the shortcomings of our current understanding and treatment, individualized, patient-centered, integrative approaches, with a focus on discovering potential underlying causes, and early referral to professionals with specific expertise in vulvar pain will improve outcomes and decrease the burden of suffering for women with vulvodynia.[24,25]

SUMMARY

There is no question that the hip plays an important role in some of these complicated patients with pelvic floor dysfunction and vulvar pain. By nature, these problems and patients are complex. We have to consider all the various patterns of pain and possible musculoskeletal abnormalities involved. Our studies highlight the importance for health professionals to know more about all aspects of the core.

Think of all the parts of the core that we know are involved in this particular issue of the hip and vulvodynia: the pelvic girdle, the core muscles, the nerves, as well as the genitourinary, gynecologic, and gastrointestinal systems. We have not even discussed the smaller contingent of male patients with hip pathology and pelvic floor dysfunction, including pudendal nerve pain patterns. How about the blood and lymphatic systems? Are they involved? What other physiological systems are we missing?

Perhaps then, the most important send-home message from this chapter comes in 2 parts:
1. We must think more "outside of the box."
2. The core deserves to be a distinct medical field, with its own distinct considerations and specialists.

SELECTED READINGS

The following 4 articles should be read in order for a more in-depth understanding of the anatomy, pathophysiology, and current terminology of pelvic floor dysfunction. Together, they provide a distinct perspective on possible pathophysiological associations among vulvodynia, pelvic floor anatomy, and the hip joint.

Prather H, Dugan S, Fitzgerald C, Hunt D. Review of anatomy, evaluation, and treatment of musculoskeletal pelvic floor pain in women. *PM&R*. 2009;1:346-358.
   This article represents one of the standard reads on this subject.

Coady D, Futterman S, Harris D, Shah M, Coleman S. The relationship between labrum tears of the hip and generalized unprovoked vulvodynia. *J Low Genit Tract Dis*. 2009;13:S7-S8.
   This was our first publication on the association between hip pathology and vulvodynia.

Coleman S, Donegan S, Futterman S, Shah M, Coady D. The relationship between femoroacetabular impingement and chronic pelvic pain. Presented at the International Society of Hip Arthroscopy meeting; 2014; Rio De Janeiro, Brazil. ***This abstract from a presentation contains data on both the operative and nonoperative groups of patients with vulvodynia.***

Dellon AL, Coady D. Vulvar and pelvic pain terminology review: implications for microsurgeons. *Microsurgery.* 2015;35:85-90. doi:10.1002/micr.22298.
This is an excellent review of current terminology.

REFERENCES

1. Harlow BL, Kunitz CG, Nguyen RHN, et al. Prevalence of symptoms consistent with a diagnosis of vulvodynia: population-based estimates from 2 geographic regions. *Am J Obstet Gynecol.* 2014;210:40.e1-e8.
2. Reed BD, Harlow SD, Sen A, et al. Prevalence and demographic characteristics of vulvodynia in a population-based sample. *Am J Obstet Gynecol.* 2012;206:170.1-170.9.
3. Harlow BL, Stewart EG. A population-based assessment of chronic unexplained vulvar pain: have we underestimated the prevalence of vulvodynia? *J Am Med Womens Assoc.* 2003;58(2):82.
4. Arnold LD, Bachmann GA, Rosen R, Kelly S, Rhoads GG. Vulvodynia: characteristics and associations with comorbidities and quality of life. *Obstet Gynecol.* 2006;107:617-624.
5. Reed BD, Harlow SD, Sen A, Edwards RM, Chen D, Haefner H. Relationship between vulvodynia and chronic comorbid pain conditions. *Obstet Gynecol.* 2012;120:145-151.
6. Prather H, Dugan S, Fitzgerald C, Hunt D. Review of anatomy, evaluation, and treatment of musculoskeletal pelvic floor pain in women. *PM&R.* 2009;1:346-358.
7. Hunt D, Clohisy J, Prather H. Acetabular labral tears of the hip in women. *Phys Med Rehabil Clin N Am.* 2007;3:497-520.
8. Groh M, Herrera J. A comprehensive review of hip labral tears. *Curr Rev Musculoskelet Med.* 2009;2:105-117.
9. Burnett S, Della Rocca G, Prather H, et al. Clinical presentation of patients with tears of the acetabular labrum. *J Bone Joint Surg Am.* 2006;88(7):1448-1457.
10. Moyal-Barracco M, Lynch PJ. 2003 ISSVD terminology and classification of vulvodynia: a historical perspective. *J Reprod Med.* 2004;49:772-777.
11. Dworkin RH, Turk DC, Wyrwich KW, et al. Interpreting the clinical importance of treatment outcomes in chronic pain clinical trials: IMMPACT recommendations. *J Pain.* 2008;9:105-121.
12. Li KK, Harris K, Hadi S, Chow E. What should be the optimal cut points for mild, moderate, and severe pain? *J Palliat Med.* 2007;10:1338-1346.
13. Hartmann D, Sarton J. Chronic pelvic floor dysfunction. *Best Pract Res Clin Obstet Gynaecol.* 2014;28(7):977-990. doi:10.1016/j.bpobgyn.2014.07.008.
14. Tu FF, Hellman K, Backonja M. Gynecological management of neuropathic pain. *Am J Obstet Gynecol.* 2011;205:435-443.
15. Neville CE, Fitzgerald CM, Mallinson T, Badillo S, Hynes C, Tu F. A preliminary report of musculoskeletal dysfunction in female chronic pelvic pain: a blinded study of examination findings. *J Bodyw Mov Ther.* 2012;16:50-56.
16. Fitzgerald MP, Payne CK, Lukacz ES, et al, for the Interstitial Cystitis Collaborative Research Network. Randomized multicenter clinical trial of myofascial physical therapy in women with interstitial cystitis/painful bladder syndrome and pelvic floor tenderness. *J Urol.* 2012;187(6):2113e8.
17. Hunt D, Prather H, Hayes MH, Clohisy JC. Clinical outcomes analysis of conservative and surgical treatment of patients with clinical indications of prearthritic, intra-articular hip disorders. *PM R.* 2012;4:479-487.
18. Krych AJ, Thompson M, Knutson Z, Scoon J, Coleman SH. Arthroscopic labral repair versus selective labral debridement in female patients with femoroacetabular impingement: a prospective randomized study. *Arthroscopy.* 2013;29:46-53.
19. Prather H, Hunt D, Fournie A, Clohisy JC. Early intra-articular hip disease presenting with posterior pelvic and groin pain. *PM R.* 2009;1:809-815.
20. Hampson JP, Reed BD, Clauw DJ, et al. Augmented central pain processing in vulvodynia. *J Pain.* 2013;14:579-589.
21. Brooks AG, Domb BG. Acetabular labral tear and postpartum hip pain. *Obstet Gynecol.* 2012;120:1093-1098.
22. Gyang A, Hartman M, Lamvu G. Musculoskeletal causes of chronic pelvic pain: what a gynecologist should know. *Obstet Gynecol.* 2013;121:645-650.
23. Villemure C, Ceko M, Cotton VA, Bushnell MC. Insular cortex mediates increased pain tolerance in yoga practitioners. *Cereb Cortex.* 2014;24(10):2732-2740. doi:10.1093/cercor/bht124.
24. Nguyen RH, Turner RM, Rydell SA, Maclehose RF, Harlow BL. Perceived stereotyping and seeking care for chronic vulvar pain. *Pain Med.* 2013;10:1461-1467.
25. Stockdale CK, Lawson HW. 2013 Vulvodynia guideline update. *J Low Genit Tract Dis.* 2013;18:93-100.

24

traps in hip arthroscopy

JOHN P. SALVO JR, MD
KEVIN O'DONNELL, MD

Editor's Note: *John Salvo, a trusted colleague and Rothman Institute partner, has one of the busiest sports orthopedic practices in the Philadelphia area. He does many hip arthroscopies and keeps a keen eye out for medical and surgical traps. It seemed appropriate for John and his fellow Kevin to write this chapter.*

Here's the rest of the story.

—Paul Harvey, the famous conservative American ABC radio broadcaster.

AN ARCHETYPAL TRAP—HIP DYSPLASIA

Everyone looked up to Becky, a model student and captain of the cheerleading team in her senior year in high school. No one knew she was suffering, and now taking an occasional narcotic to fight off the growing pain in her right groin. Simple walking was becoming difficult, let alone jumping from a pyramid.

The pain started her junior year, a barely uncomfortable "popping" deep in her groin. She had joked with her cheerleading mates about the loudness of it since ninth grade. She thought little of the popping then. It was definitely not painful. So, this school year, she initially discounted the new slight ache. Then the ache began to travel deeper and into her buttock, and then got so bad, she stopped competing. The cause of the popping, she was told, was a simple tear in her labrum, some loose cartilage in her hip, and something called *femoroacetabular impingement* (FAI). It would all be addressed via a hip scope, by shaving off a bump of bone, "debriding" cartilage, and "releasing" her psoas muscle. She understood that the psoas muscle traveled intimately close to and in front of her hip, rubbing against it and causing the popping.

Becky did not do well, to say the least, after the arthroscopic surgery. At 4 months, she could no longer take even a few steps without severe pain. "My hip is coming out of joint," she conveyed to everyone. Becky could not do simple tasks, let alone return to cheerleading. Frustrated, she and her family sought another opinion.

From plain X-rays done in the clinic, Becky's problem became clear. She had, what the new hip surgeon announced, hip dysplasia, a more serious problem than simple impingement. A portion of her hip socket had never developed so she was prone to hip instability. The growth development problem was only "moderate," but the combination of the reduction in bone, the loss of more of her labrum, and the surgical psoas detachment had created a new problem, called *hip instability*. That was why she walked with so severe a compensatory tilt. Her pelvis was shifting and altering the direction of forces in order to minimize the pain. She was told by the second hip surgeon that treatment might, fortunately, be relatively straightforward. At this point, she knew there was no guarantee. Becky underwent the second hip arthroscopy, at which time tissue was taken from her leg and a new labrum created. At the time, she also underwent "repair" of her hip capsule. Nothing could be done, she was told, about the psoas release.

Two days after surgery, Becky felt she had been "cured." Her preoperative pain was no longer present. She stopped all her pain meds and felt normal. At 14 days, she discarded her crutches and walked without a limp. Becky did well for the next 4 years. As Paul Harvey used to say, here is the rest of the story.

She never did return to cheerleading or other vigorous activities. She graduated from nursing school and then became a certified nurse practitioner. Five years out from surgery, she developed similar pains and eventually underwent a periacetabular osteotomy operation. This procedure involved intentional fracture and reorientation of her hip socket. At the present time, 2 years after the third surgery, she has no pain whatsoever again. She is aware, though, that she may require total hip replacement in the not-too-distant future.

Hip Arthroscopy Remains New

Unfortunately, Becky's story is not unique. Whether or not her end result was inevitable is debatable. But, in a nutshell, she represents the sorts of potential ambushes that hip arthroscopists face every day. We must continually remind ourselves that we live still in the formative years of a new field.

The whole field developed in the late 1990s and early 2000s. Techniques have sprouted from simple removal of loose bodies, to labral debridement, and then to applying the discoveries of Ganz. No matter how experienced any of us are, we all remain on a learning curve. The curve is extremely steep initially and, at different points for each of us, becomes more gradual. There are numerous ledges on that curve where we may fall. The trick is to avoid as many of those ledges as possible. All within this field continue to experience traps prowling out there. (See Figure 24-1.)

Becky's initial surgical team encountered at least 2 ambushes: Certainly, they missed the hip dysplasia, and the psoas release likely contributed to her hip instability. But who really knows if the latter is true? Perhaps, they shaved away too much bone or reduced a critical amount of intrinsic vacuum with the labral debridement. We shall never know

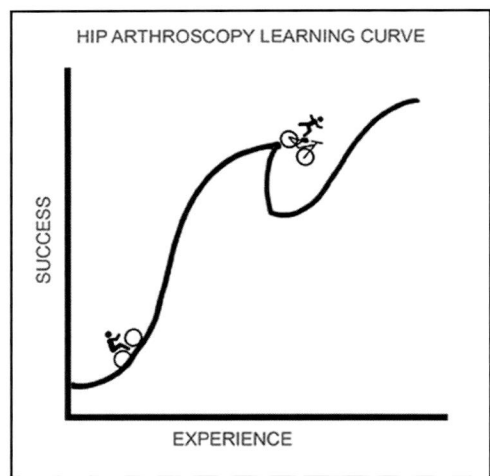

Figure 24-1.

exactly. Surely, 1, 2, or all of those 3 factors contributed to the arrival of hip stability in this preoperatively stable, yet already dysplastic, hip. By definition, a dysplastic hip teeters on instability. It does not take much to tip this type of hip into instability. Chapter 25 discusses developmental hip problems in much more depth.

What we shall go through here is a top 15 list of the traps in hip arthroscopy. More traps loom out there, ready to pounce on us "innocent" hip arthroscopists, athletic trainers, and other fitness experts. We can't play innocent sheep much longer.

A little dreaming is dangerous, the cure is not to dream less but to dream more, to dream all the time.

—Marcel Proust.

THE MINEFIELD

The Usual Femoroacetabular Impingement Work-Up

Okay, so we have made a lot of progress in hip arthroscopy. And we await more progress. As mentioned previously (see Chapters 1 and 2), one of the great things about medicine is empiricism. And, as stated before, one of the really bad things about medicine is empiricism. Empiricism brings a certain safety to physicians' decision-making. But it also blinds us. By doing only what we have been taught, we can only extend the horizons of our eyes rather than put on new eyes. Remember our lead quote from Marcel Proust in Chapter 2.

Think about the new Marcel Proust quote listed above. The dreams and imaginations of Ganz, Byrd, Villar, and others are what put hip arthroscopy on the sports medicine map. Hip arthroscopy seems now well incorporated into training programs. But we have to ask ourselves, isn't this too soon for hip arthroscopy to be thus so much incorporated? Many of us in the field have barely moved off the steep part of the learning curve. Isn't it too soon for the work-up and treatment of FAI to become written into stone?

We physicians have a lot of pressure on us to provide cookbook medicine, black-and-white stuff that residents-in-training can follow and pass their boards and get credentialed. From a patient safety standpoint, routine may seem good. But is it good during the development of a new field? Routine may benefit some patients, but how many? Is it possible that routine stifles our imaginations, shuts down our dreams? Routine is certainly not good for all patients. It protects us in some ways, but does it also somehow close our eyes? Remember hip arthroscopy remains relatively new. How can we mandate things when we don't yet know what to mandate? We must not close our eyes already. Keeping our eyes wide open will help us avoid the many traps out there.

The work-up and treatment of FAI may have already become too demarcated at this point. Let's go through what has become routine. The usual initial work-up for FAI includes a series of plain radiographs, usually an "AP pelvis," "AP and cross table lateral of the hip," a "modified Dunn view,"[1] and a "false profile view of the affected hip."

Several radiographic measurements detect the presence of FAI and further classify the type of FAI (eg, cam, pincer, or a mixed lesion). Knowing the type of FAI helps us formulate the plan of surgical attack and to "stay out of trouble." Typically, the measurements include the alpha-angle, lateral center edge angle, anterior center edge angle, and the sourcil angle. We should also look for coxa breva, coxa magna, coxa profunda, or protrusio acetabuli. Plus, we should also look for hip dysplasia or acetabular undercoverage. And, oh yes, we should look for arthritis. If the patient has "too much" arthritis, sometimes we should "stop right there." Phew, that's a lot to look for. We are only human. Ask yourself if it is possible for the hip arthroscopist to miss something?

Add to this insurance companies entering into the clinical arena and requiring certain hip angles for them to pay for surgery.

Here's the rest of the story. Following the plain radiographs, we order MRIs and MR-arthrograms. We argue about using 3 vs 1.5 Tesla MRIs. We look for such things as chondral damage, stress fractures, or associated psoas and abductor muscle problems. We may get 3-dimensional CT scan reconstructions.[2] We also may inject a local anesthetic or corticosteroid for diagnostic or therapeutic purposes. Algorithmic decisions often depend on response to injections, physical therapy, and even alternative therapies. Again, insurance companies now play big roles in our decision-making processes.

Let's go on. Hip arthroscopists then focus on the type of FAI, precise location of the impingement, and degree of pathology. We decide what to do among the various available procedures and choose among ones we have been trained to do (eg, labral repairs, grafting, acetabuloplasty, femoroplasty, microfracture, psoas lengthening, abductor repair). Granted, the algorithm has been vetted with consistent good-to-excellent short- and mid-term outcomes, but sometimes we still need to think outside the box to allow our success to expand.

Keeping the Dream

Before careers of young hip arthroscopists even start, so much unproved, mandated information packs their brains. What about a good history and physical examination? Add perhaps some plain X-rays and maybe an MRI, and some savvy clinical judgment? How about talking to colleagues and find out if a specific clinical situation has ever been faced before and how it was handled? How does one value savvy and clinical experience? With today's clinical care yielding so much to regulatory pressures, we are forced to follow algorithms and care maps. Fear replaces the desire to accumulate experience. Many patients, miserable with hip pain, remain out there, outside the guidelines and who can be corrected.

New hip arthroscopy fellowship–trained surgeons can't help but follow suit, stick to their training, and make decisions based on what seems best, what has been done before, and whatever it takes to follow the mandated "guidelines." With so much (yet so little) in our heads, of course, young hip arthroscopists shall follow guidelines to the hilt. The confidence of experience never arrives, at least in the right way. Success with several straightforward cases may generate cockiness, but that's not the right confidence. They shall miss opportunities to cure patients because of growing fears of going outside of the guidelines. They shall miss subtleties in many individual patients. They won't take a chance and cure the patient who does not fit the mandated guidelines. That said, it remains remarkable that we do as well as we do.

The traps come in many categories, not just patient selection, under- or overtreatment, or misdiagnosis and operative mishaps. Here are a few questions that provide the camouflage for ambush: What guidelines should be followed in deciding how much bone to remove? How should we treat articular cartilage damage? When should we employ microfracture or the use of intrinsic or extrinsic substances to help hip arthritis? Let's face it, thus far, hip arthroscopy remains as much an art as a science.

"Thirty" has been suggested as the number of cases that a hip arthroscopist must do to become "proficient."[3] What about the patients who are those 30 cases? What about after that? The truth is that the whole world of hip arthroscopy is evolving. This world is fast-paced and a process of learning and improving. The exact number of cases is immaterial. Right now, we've got to keep our senses keen and deflect the noise of regulatory mandates. Right now, we learn from every case we do. Experience has no competitor.

A dream doesn't become reality through magic; it takes sweat, determination, hard work, and experience.

—Colin Powell, American statesman and retired 4-star US Army general.

FIFTEEN TRAPS (TABLE 24-1)

1. **Denying the learning curve.** The learning curve is not the trap. Learning curves accompany everything we do in medicine. The trap is the denial of the existence of a learning curve or the mistaken belief that you are beyond it. That denial creates the setting for error. The setting causes the lumping of multiple patients into a same category and treating them exactly the same, when they are, in fact, subtly, meaningfully different. In this hazardous setting, subtle distinctions in pathology may elude detection. The fact is the learning curve never ends.

2. **Denying the eligible patient.** Clinical guidelines from any source (eg, training, teaching courses, mentorship, or insurance companies) often sway decisions in terms of selecting patients for surgery. The net effect ends up on the side of not operating on patients with real, life quality–diminishing symptoms and curable hip pathology. Most guidelines are set purposefully conservatively (ie, to prevent unnecessary surgery or surgery to be done by inexperienced surgeons). That reasoning is solid. But the fact is that patients don't come with labels on them saying their symptoms come from hip impingement, and many patients remain miserable on account of those guidelines. We should consider this trap inherent to any type of surgical intervention.

3. **Shaving too little or, more unfortunately, too much.** Speak to any busy hip surgeon. More "redo" hip arthroscopy is occurring than ever before, usually the result of inexperience and missed areas of bony impingement. Experienced surgeons can tell you the most common regions of the femur or acetabulum (or both) that are missed. Fortunately, they do report remarkably good results after the subsequent corrections.

Certainly, immediately preoperative X-rays and intraoperative fluoroscopy help plan the angles, boundaries, and depths of bony resections and direct endoscopic observation of the impingement while varying flexion, abduction, and rotation help steer the surgeon. But that does not tell the whole story. Inadequate bony resection commands the top spot for revision arthroscopic hip surgery, accounting for 79% to 97% of cases.[4,5]

Less common, but often oh-so-much-more devastating, is removing too much bone. "Chomp trap" appears in 2 different forms: femoral neck fracture or hip instability. No doubt falls and too-early weightbearing contribute to postoperatively appearing femoral neck fractures. Certain anatomic arrangements (eg, acetabular undercoverage < 25 degrees) factor into the risk for hip instability.

4. **Missing what to do with the labrum.** Correct selection among a spectrum of techniques for the labrum requires experience, of course. The spectrum ranges from minimal debridement, repair and total resection, and complete grafting. There are a few common denominators with respect to traps in this category. The most prominent relates to the early days of arthroscopy, when simple debridement was often all that was done. Of course, our new knowledge holds true; many of these patients have subsequently needed bony resections. The most experienced hip arthroscopists have identified fairly firm visual criteria for when the labrum needs to be reconstructed with a graft.

5. **Under- or overestimating arthritis.** Don't say, if you can help it, "arthritis" to a hip arthroscopist. The word incites pallor and fear. The fear arises from possibly accelerating arthritis. No doubt that occurs. But certainly things need to be kept in perspective.

   Chondral damage is incredibly common in the setting of labral tears. Up to 73% of patients with labral tears have some element of associated chondral damage.[6] Degenerative tears are, by nature, ubiquitous and part of the normal aging process. They represent 90% of specimens in cadaveric studies.[7]

   The fear that evoked from the mention of "arthritis" comes from a small number of cases. And the most cited paper in the literature just notes 8 patients.[8] Plus, most hip arthroscopies in the presence of arthritis are being performed as "salvage" procedures in the first place (ie, last attempts to "save" the hip from replacement). Add to that the longer experience with knee arthroscopy and poor outcomes in the face of severe arthritis, and the reasoning for caution with hip arthroscopy for the comparable problem becomes clearer.

   We may never be able to eliminate the pallor response. But we can administer sugar to lessen that vagal response.

6. **Discounting the core muscles.** This is a large part of what this whole book is about. About 15% of Dr. Meyers's cases are now done as combined (hip arthroscopy and muscle repair) procedures. That stat tells us to be aware of associated core muscle injury. Most such combined injuries involve the rectus abdominis, adductors, and/or rectus femoris.

   Another important factor to keep in mind for most hip patients is the important protective function of the harness adductors. This important set of muscles usually tightens as a consequence of long-time compensation for the hip. Therefore, when bone is shaved, range of motion consequently increases, and tight adductors become more subject to pain and more injury. If you want, reread the earlier chicken-and-egg discussion in the book (see Chapter 5) regarding bidirectional explanations for the simultaneous or sequential appearance of the 2 types of injury.

   You, the astute reader, may have picked up a seeming redundancy below. Two other sets of core muscles, the iliopsoas and glutes, create distinct other types of traps so have separate categories below.

7. **Hip dysplasia.** As mentioned in the sentinel case for this chapter, this condition represents an archetypal trap for hip arthroscopists. Sometimes a distinct advantage in sports (eg, the butterfly ice hockey goalie), acetabular undercoverage, by its nature, produces a limited contact area for the femoral ball and the rest of our body's weight. Therefore, large forces pound continuously the same specific acetabular locations. Not surprisingly, this congenital set-up predisposes to sharp impingement syndromes in specific locations and intra-articular cartilage damage. It does not take much injury to throw the whole joint off kilter. That is why so many of these people end with total hip replacements so early. It is also not clear whether or not the disruptive periacetabular osteotomy pelvic bone shift procedure alters the ultimate outcomes.

   Plus, one has to recognize the risk of creating hip instability with minimal femoroplasty or psoas release.

8. **Doing too much (or too little) to the psoas.** The mystery that shrouds the Eminem muscle brings shudders to experienced hip arthroscopists. Diagnosing a tight or painful psoas brings certain pride because one has to utilize a fair amount of clinical savvy. As discussed in the psoas chapter, a psoas strain or bursitis can occur by itself just related to particular activities. But often those entities accompany a real hip or core muscle problem. When it accompanies hip impingement, then one has to decide what to do with it. Will simple removal of a bump of bone—or, for that matter, a total hip replacement—make the psoas problem better or worse? Will the surgeon have to lengthen or partially release the psoas to make the patient better? What's the best way to do that technique without risking loss of psoas function or creating a new kind of pain related to proximal retraction of the psoas? Is there a particular anatomy that shouts out to stay away from doing a psoas release (eg, femoral anteversion)?[9] These are issues for which solutions remain mysterious. The Eminem muscle, again, lives up to its name.

9. **Underestimating balance issues.** To understand this trap, ask an experienced hip arthroscopist how many times has he/she "fixed" one hip and then the "good" side starts hurting.

TABLE 24-1
FIFTEEN TRAPS
1. Denying the learning curve
2. Denying the eligible patient
3. Shaving too little or, more unfortunately, too much
4. Missing what to do with the labrum
5. Under- or overestimating arthritis
6. Discounting the core muscles
7. Hip dysplasia
8. Doing too much (or too little) to the psoas
9. Underestimating balance issues
10. Underestimating the roles of tilt and version
11. Ischiofemoral impingement and other "tweeners"
12. Heterotopic ossification and other unanticipated complications
13. Missing the glute injury
14. Missing the ligamentum teres injury
15. Missing the stupid stuff

10. **Underestimating the roles of tilt and version.** This is easy to do because nobody really understands what the exact roles are with respect to performance and injury. Of course, there is consensus that these orientation dynamics are very important. This agreement seems based on a rationale of "These exist; they must be important," rather than distinct biomechanical data that demonstrate real pathophysiology. The Philippon and Kropf chapters go into this more. The bottom line here is that consensus shouts that these orientation factors represent traps for hip arthroscopists.

11. **Ischiofemoral impingement and other "tweeners."** Read through the literature of Hal Martin[10] and you shall appreciate the many "tweeners" that can cause traps. In other words, we usually think in terms of either the hip and/or the core muscles that have been mentioned as causing the patient's pain. What about when one has fixed perfectly both the hip core muscle injuries and the patient still has pain? Of course, there remains a whole world of other anatomy in the pelvis that has not been considered (eg, the deep posterior core muscles, the varying routes of the sciatic nerve, impingement caused by bone rubbing just adjacent to the ball-and-socket hip joint [ischiofemoral impingement]). And it turns out there may interventional fixes for some of these things, such as endoscopic resection of bone near the lesser trochanter for the latter problem(s).

12. **Heterotopic ossification and other unanticipated complications.** Virtually all experienced hip arthroscopists have (or should have) seen postoperative heterotopic ossification (HO). HO's postoperative appearance can be innocuous but usually creates frustration. The hip arthroscopist may kick him-/herself, wondering why and how it could have been prevented. It is usually recognized because of the pain it causes related to recreating impingement problems. One may remove the HO and often relieve the pain, but then the huge question arrives: How does one prevent it for the future? Indomethacin and other anti-inflammatories have been tried, and with some success. Keep in mind also that HO can cause the original hip impingement (eg, HO that complicates non-repair of a rectus femoris avulsion; see Chapter 11).

Other unanticipated, yet usually preventable, postoperative traps include traction injury, iatrogenic intra-articular injury, and portal injury. The most common traction injury is nerve damage (neuropraxia). The neuropraxias are of 2 types: compressive and distractive. The most common compressive injury is to the pudendal nerve, from the intraoperative post that provides stabilization of the pelvis as the leg is pulled away to open up the hip joint space for arthroscopic visualization. The patient feels numbness and erectile dysfunction in the private areas. The most common distractive neuropraxias are to the femoral, peroneal, and sciatic nerves. All these neuropraxias, fortunately, usually resolve spontaneously. The optimal strategy to prevent these is more padding and less traction time.[11]

The articular surface of the femoral head and the labrum are prone to injury simply by inaccurate placement of needles and other instruments. An air arthrogram using the initial spinal needle may provide some additional joint distraction and prevent inadvertent penetration of the labrum or scuffing of the articular surface of the femoral head.

Portal placement refers to the process of placing trocars into the hip joint, through which instruments for the surgery are introduced. The most common nerve injury with portal placement is to the lateral femoral cutaneous nerve. In second place, and much less common, is injury to the sciatic nerves. The lateral femoral cutaneous nerve lies in close proximity to the usual anterior portal site. One should place the trocar medial to the anterior iliac spine to minimize the chance of that injury. Posterior portals place the sciatic nerve at risk. Internal rotation of the hip during placement of these trocars helps prevent the latter.

13. **Missing the glute injury.** As we go back and review the preoperative MRIs, glute injury, usually the gluteus medius, often accompanies hip impingement. This may be an isolated or a compensatory issue. It could even be a causative factor in terms of why the impingement symptoms began in the first place. Whatever the case, this is another potential trap, for which we don't have definitive answers. If one repairs all these at the time of surgery, we certainly will be doing a lot of extra surgery, since they are so common.
14. **Missing the ligamentum teres injury.** Hip arthroscopists tend to minimize the importance of the ligamentum teres in hip stability. Ricky Villar, one of the great pioneer hip arthroscopists, has pointed out articulately how occasionally this ligament can "bite" us, either as a cause of pain or impingement or as a postoperative complication.[12]
15. **Missing the stupid stuff.** Okay, the stupid stuff. We define "stupid" as an event that causes us to call ourselves stupid. Here are a few: not realizing that the hip distraction table does not fit a 7-foot NBA basketball center, not releasing the hip distraction device when there is an obvious delay in surgery, not having the right assistant.

SELECTED READINGS

Gawande A. *Complications: A Surgeon's Notes on an Imperfect Science.* New York, NY: Metropolitan Books; 2002.
 An accomplished surgical oncologist and author, Dr. Gawande explores how and why good surgeons end up getting blindsided and causing mortal harm to their patients.
Kahneman D. *Thinking, Fast and Slow.* New York, NY: Farrar, Straus and Giroux; 2011.
 This best-seller delves into the mechanics of overconfidence and why our predictions are often so off base.

REFERENCES

1. Clohisy JC, Carlisle JC, Beaulé PE, et al. A systematic approach to the plain radiographic evaluation of the young adult hip. *J Bone Joint Surg Am.* 2008;90(suppl 4):47-66.
2. Beaulé PE, Zaragoza E, Motamedi K, Copelan N, Dorey FJ. Three-dimensional computed tomography of the hip in the assessment of femoroacetabular impingement. *J Orthop Res.* 2005;23:1286-1292.
3. Konan S, Rhee SJ, Haddad FS. Hip arthroscopy: analysis of a single surgeon's learning experience. *J Bone Joint Surg [Am].* 2011;93-A(suppl 2):52-56.
4. Heyworth BE, Shindle MK, Voos JE, Rudzki JR, Kelly BT. Radiologic and intraoperative findings in revision hip arthroscopy. *Arthroscopy.* 2007;23:1295-1302.
5. Philippon MJ, Schenker ML, Briggs KK, et al. Revision hip arthroscopy. *Am J Sports Med.* 2007;35:1918-1921.
6. McCarthy JC, Noble PC, Schuck MR, et al. The Otto E Aufranc Award: the role of labral lesions to development of early degenerative hip disease. *Clin Orthop.* 2001;393:25-37.
7. Seldes RM, Tan V, Hunt J, et al. Anatomy, histologic features, and vascularity of the adult acetabular labrum. *Clin Orthop Relat Res.* 2001;382:232-240.
8. Byrd JW, Jones KS. Hip arthroscopy for labral pathology: prospective analysis with a 10-year follow-up. *Arthroscopy.* 2009;25(4):365-368.
9. Ricciardi BF, Fields K, Kelly BT, Ranawat AS, Coleman SH, Sink EL. Causes and risk factors for revision hip preservation surgery. *Am J Sports Med.* 2014;42(11):2627-2633.
10. Hatem MA, Palmar IJ, Martin HD. Diagnosis and 2-year outcomes of endoscopic treatment for ischiofemoral impingement. *Arthroscopy.* 2015;31(2):239-246.
11. Papavasiliou AV, Bardakos NV. Complications of arthroscopic surgery of the hip. *Bone Joint Res.* 2012;1:131-144.
12. Bardakos NV, Villar RN. The ligamentum teres of the adult hip. The ligamentum teres of the adult hip. *J Bone Joint Surg Br.* 2009;91(1):8-15.

25

special considerations in **adolescents**

FARES S. HADDAD, MD (RES), FRCS (ORTH),
DIP SPORTS MED, FFSEM
FERAS YA'ISH, FRCS (ORTH), MBBS
KONSTANTINOS TSITSKARIS, MSc, MRCS, FRCS (TR & ORTH)

Editor's Note: *The fact of the matter is that there are special considerations for children and adolescents who have pain in the "hip" region. We all need to be aware of these conditions. I called on Fares Haddad and his colleagues in his world-leading adolescent hip orthopedic group to identify and simplify some of these conditions.*

You see what you look for and recognize what you know.
—From an article on diabetes (Harkless LB, Dennis KJ. You see what you look for and recognize what you know. *Clin Podiatr Med Surg.* 1987;4[2]:331-339.)

WHAT WE ARE TALKING ABOUT

A 15-year-old athletic, but slightly overweight, boy had pain in the right "hip area" for about 6 weeks. He saw his primary care physician, who got an X-ray that was interpreted as normal. Figure 25-1 shows the X-ray. The yellow lines are ours; they were not there during the initial radiologic evaluation.

To any practitioner aware of the diagnosis, this is no-brainer—slipped capital femoral epiphysis (SCFE).

The point is that parents should know to whom the patient is being referred. So many times, particularly with these core, or "black box" problems, the person is sent to a "specialist" in this area and the resultant diagnosis is absolutely useless. It is possible for the specialist to just happen to come up with the right diagnosis, but it is by chance. More likely, this turns out to be a fishing expedition without a fish finder. With hip area pain, the patient might see a general surgeon, urologist, gynecologist, colorectal surgeon, or general orthopedist. They will only rule in or out only the diagnoses with which they are familiar. (See Figure 25-2.)

From the symptoms, this young boy could have had a variety of things. The fact of the matter is that the diagnosis is obvious from the X-ray. Note the difference in lengths of the heads and necks of the 2 sides. The yellow lines are called Klein's lines. The right side is much shorter, and you can see the ball looks compressed.

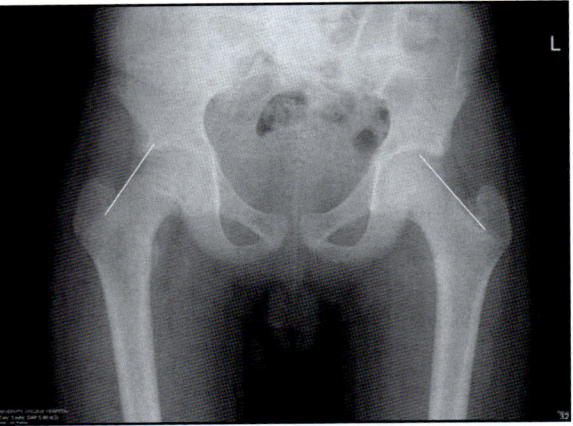

Figure 25-1. Foreshortened right hip. Note the shortened and deformed hip (yellow lines) on the right side on this AP X-ray of the pelvis, compared to the left side. This was the actual X-ray taken at the time.

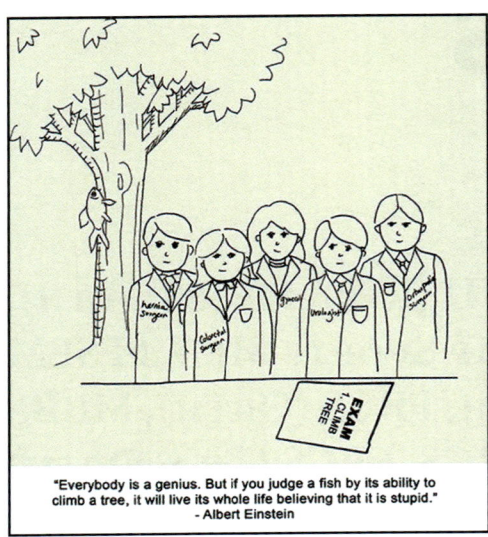

Figure 25-2.

Any good pediatric orthopedic surgeon will have tales to tell about misdiagnoses in this region of the body, and usually dramatically bad outcomes. In fairness to the physicians who missed this diagnosis, no one has the ability to diagnose a condition or spot a sign he/she is not aware of. Coxa saltans and hip impingement are 2 diagnoses that many pediatric orthopedic surgeons missed just a few years ago.

Awareness of the hip conditions that can affect the adolescent hip can prevent detrimental, lifelong complications. The primary care doc and radiologist who missed the above case did not need to know details of the staging or controversial management of SCFE. All that was needed was to be mindful of such a diagnosis, and then one is prepared to identify the pathology and initiate appropriate care.

The Way It Was

Until just the past decade, "active neglect" was the name of the game when it came to treating hip deformities in adolescents. We ignored the adolescent patient in the room with all the symptoms while the doctor-patient relationship flourished, and we chose to treat all deformities such as residual hip dysplasia or from Legg-Calvé-Perthes disease (LCPD) or SCFE, without surgery, until such degenerative changes occurred that we had no choice. Any kind of snapping or impingement was simply dismissed. We had no awareness of the pathology or potentially available treatments.

Evolving understanding of these disorders and the consequences in adult life of not doing anything during childhood, combined with revolutionary, new corrective techniques, have changed everything. Direct targeting of the underlying pathology has abolished the classical "active neglect" or what was euphemistically called the *conservative* approach in many cases. Identifying applicable abnormalities in a timely manner can have such a wonderfully positive effect on the adolescent's future.

The Way It Is

Pediatric surgeons are busy now operating on cases that, not too long ago, used to be treated non-operatively. The new orthopedic subspecialty of "young adult hip surgery" has become real and addresses many of the deformities. We correct residual acetabular dysplasia with periacetabular osteotomies. We sometimes correct SCFE directly intra-articularly, or just "pin" the problems in situ to prevent progression. We can correct residual deformities from either LCPD or SCFE with proximal femoral and/or acetabular osteotomies. And of course we can arthroscopically correct impingement and labral disorders. One problem deserves special mention—apophyseal avulsions. These injuries are increasingly recognized, and early aggressive treatment is sometimes warranted based on new understandings of the pathology and possible bad consequences if these are left untreated.

We need to make all relevant practitioners aware of all this new knowledge. The revolution in treatment is real, and we are developing a whole new field. The field of adolescent hip conditions is huge. Continuous education of all relevant parties involved in youth sports need to be aware of these newly recognized understandings about adolescent hip disorders.

Nomenclature

- *Slipped capital femoral epiphysis (SCFE):* Posterior and inferior slide of the proximal femoral physis over the femoral neck through the physeal interface. This can result in abnormality of the shape of the head, leading to future complications, such as impingement and arthrosis or, more dramatically, avascular necrosis of the head.
- *Legg-Calvé-Perthes disease (LCPD):* Avascular necrosis of the proximal femoral head epiphysis, resulting in deformity and loss of femoral head sphericity. This is a childhood condition resulting in disruption of the blood supply to the femoral epiphysis, followed by collapse, revascularization, and remodeling. The amount of restoration of normal femoral head shape determines the clinical outcome.
- *Developmental dysplasia of the hip (DDH):* Multifactorial, developmental disorder that results in abnormal shape of the head of femur and/or acetabulum. The term *congenital dysplasia* misrepresents the condition, since the condition may develop after delivery, as late as adolescence. The acetabulum is usually shallow with a steep (open) angle (inclination angle), seen on the anteroposterior radiograph. The condition commonly occurs with femoroacetabular retroversion and a thin anterior bony wall. The femoral head can sublux proximally or be uncovered laterally. The femoral neck can be in valgus and relatively anteverted.

Clinical Experience

We are diagnosing adolescent hip disorders more commonly. We know more about them, and more young individuals are competing at high levels earlier in life. With better diagnostic acumen,[1] hip problems now represent 10% to 24% of all athletic injuries in children. These are most common in ballet dancers, runners, martial artists, hockey, football, and rugby players.[2]

Certainly, the increase in hip diagnoses in this patient group could be due simply to increased awareness. One hypothesis for the large number of hip injuries is accelerated growth and a resultant mismatch between limb length and body mass that impairs coordination and muscular flexibility. The hamstrings and hip flexors are implicated in one study.[3] Open physes are at their highest risk for fractures and avulsions during the growth spurts and closures. Compared to adults, adolescents have stronger ligaments, which exert strong loads to the physeal region, likely rendering it more prone to injury.[4]

In addition, athletic activities may unmask neglected or missed childhood hip disorders (eg, DDH, SCFE), and these patients may develop their first symptoms during adolescence. Sometimes, diagnosis is essential before those patients should be allowed to return to their sports.

The Doctor-Parent-Child Triad

We feel compelled to harp on proper communication within this important medical triad. Communicating with adolescents may be a challenge in itself. In early childhood, the communication and ultimate decision-making usually lies primarily with the parents. With young adults, of course, the individual decides for oneself. The adolescent lies very much in the middle. He/She, obviously, is the focus, yet there may be heavy reliability on the immediate family to assist with the history and decision-making even despite being encouraged by everybody to participate actively in the process.[5] Managing the parents may be tricky as well. They are usually anxious and burdened by the decision-making responsibility. They may not say it, but they also may be worried about their own difficulties in life (eg, financial concerns, single parent issues, immigration status, language difficulties). The parents may also have high, even unrealistic expectations (eg, a professional athletic career). Sometimes grandparents get involved.[6]

One must also be careful whether the main complaint is truly just a parental concern rather than the patient's complaint. When that is recognized, the medical decision-making is easy compared to your interaction with the parent and child. The child may feel compelled to go along with the parent, so addressing both firmly and with conviction turns out to be key in these circumstances. Mercer Rang has written: "Paediatric visits are particularly challenging in requiring that the physician engage in a dance with not one but at least 2 partners—parent and child—and that the physician be able to lead at times and follow at others."[5]

The child's participation in the medical conversation is influenced by many factors, including the communicative behavior of the doctor and the parents. The child's engagement and perception of bodily function also varies with age, sex, family background, and cognitive development. Communication with the child is more complex than with the adult. The language may involve multiple modalities—verbal, electronic, and body, and even the surrounding environment. Innocent-appearing factors may influence the relationships, and sometimes shape the child's future attitude toward health providers.

The treating doctor needs to invite the child's input as well as maintain a balance between the child's and parents' rights and the doctor's view of the patient's best interests.

The History and Physical Examination

Owing to its communal anatomy with nearby structures, the hip shares symptoms with the lower spine, sacroiliac joint, muscles, and organ systems.[7] The initial symptoms may also seem far away from the hip, such as the low back or knee. The experienced diagnostician may quickly narrow the list of potential diagnoses.

The history should include presenting symptoms, precise location, duration, radiation, aggravating and relieving activities, related injuries, previous surgery/injuries, pain at rest vs exertion, and associated symptoms anywhere considering the body's various functions (eg, gastrointestinal, genitourinary, gynecologic, vascular, and neurologic). Probing carefully the past medical history or even perinatal history may provide clues to LCPD or DDH. The precise site of pain, if identifiable, may be immensely helpful. Table 25-1 describes what orthopedists have commonly thought about with respect to some pain patterns. These descriptors are inherently imprecise and sometimes deceiving.

Table 25-1
Common Hip-Related Symptoms and Their Common Etiology

Symptom	Common Etiology
Groin pain	Intra-articular etiology
Lateral pain	Extra-articular etiology
Isolated posterior hip pain	Lumbosacral spine, sacroiliac joint
Painful popping/clicking	Hip instability, coxa saltans (psoas or iliotibial band), chronic avulsion fractures
Increasing groin pain with increasing/repetitive activities (eg, running)	FAI

We conduct the hip examination similar to the way we do it in adults. Particular attention needs to be paid to the rotational profile, limb length, and alignment. Screening for knee and spine abnormalities as well as neurovascular compromise are inherently necessary, especially when concomitant spine or knee problems exist. Focused hip examination is performed in multiple positions: standing, walking, sitting, supine, lateral decubitus, and prone.

The standing position helps the assessment of posture (ie, hip and lower spine), alignment in the weightbearing status, limb positional attitude (ie, foot/patella rotation), muscular atrophy, scars, and obvious limb length discrepancy. The latter assessment demands attention to shoulders, anterior-superior-iliac-spines, knees, and heels. We do the Trendelenburg test before or after gait assessment. Resting unilateral or bilateral foot external rotation may indicate underlying SCFE, and internal rotation abnormal femoral anteversion. Limp shortening sometimes signposts severe or neglected SCFE. Excessive spinal lordosis, with or without fixed hip flexion (ie, tight hamstrings), may indicate spondylolisthesis or another spinal disorder.

The sitting position helps assess hip internal/external rotation in 90 degrees of flexion. Because much hip pathology exhibits signs in the sitting position, this portion of the exam, with the pelvis fixed by body weight,[8] may be particularly helpful.

Gait patterns are usually easily identifiable and further guide the diagnostic thinking. Table 25-2 lists common gait patterns and common underlying pathology. Infrequently, complex patterns require formal gait analysis.

Table 25-2
Common Gait Patterns and Their Common Underlying Hip Pathology

Gait	Common Hip Pathology
Trendelenburg	Weak abductors (neurological/mechanical), painful inhibition, abnormal hip biomechanics (DDH, LCPD)
Antalgic	Pain on weightbearing
Short limb dip	Apparent/true limb shortening, iliotibial band pathology
Excessive external rotation	Femoral retroversion, excessive acetabular anteversion, hip effusion, SCFE
Excessive internal rotation	Excessive femoral anteversion, acetabular retroversion
Pelvic rotational wink	Intra-articular pathology, flexion contracture

Most of our important information comes from the supine position. The examination is performed bilaterally and includes the Thomas test for fixed flexion, limb length assessment, rotational profile, and range of motion in both flexion and extension. Compromised or painful internal rotation often indicates articular hip pathology.[9] Obligatory external rotation in flexion often suggests SCFE. Localizing tenderness also may aid in the clinical diagnosis.

Special tests include McCarthy's[10] flexion-extension maneuvers for anterior impingement, FABER (flexion-abduction-external rotation), leg roll, and Ober's. These all help differentiate intra- vs extra-articular pathology. Remember that the FABER test (aka Patrick's test) can also localize sacroiliac joint pathology. The test classically includes pressing down on the knee in certain positions, which may result in either low back or groin pain. The former relates to the sacroiliac joint and the latter to intra-articular pathology.[11]

The lateral position allows easier palpation of lateral and posterior structures, as well as assessment of gluteal muscles and iliotibial band strength and tightness (Ober's test).[12]

The prone position permits easier palpation of posterior structures, such as the ischial tuberosity and sacroiliac joint. This position also allows the Duncan-Ely test[13] for a tight rectus femoris.

Radiologic Assessment

Standard for proper evaluation of the adolescent hip are plain anterior pelvic radiographs and lateral views of the hips. Frog lateral views are important for diagnosing SCFE. CT scan may identify occult fractures and unusual bony anatomy. MRI remains the investigation of choice for soft tissues, osteonecrosis, and labral and articular cartilage. Intra-articular and occasionally intravenous contrast may enhance its diagnostic accuracy.[14]

Slipped Capital Femoral Epiphysis

Defined by posterior and inferior slippage of the proximal femoral physis over the femoral neck through the physeal interface, SCFE occurs in 10.8 per 100,000 children and most commonly in boys 10 to 16 years of age.[15] The etiology is multifactorial and not completely understood, and probably associated with factors that increase stress on the physis or that render the physis vulnerable to stress, such as obesity, accelerated growth, or hormonal imbalance. Examples of accelerated growth are the adolescent growth spurt and growth hormone abnormalities. Hormonal imbalances include hypothyroidism, hypopituitarism, and hypogonadism. Endocrine disorders should be suspected in age groups outside the usual one mentioned previously and when there is bilateral disease. Mechanical factors such as proximal femoral retroversion and vertical physis are also risk factors.[16]

Loder classifies SCFE into "stable" or "unstable" slips.[17] The patient is able to ambulate in the former but not in the latter, even with crutches. The unstable slip is perilous and associated with a high risk of avascular necrosis. It needs urgent treatment.[18]

A high index of suspicion is the only way to make this diagnosis. Most commonly, the young person has a limp with pain vaguely localizing to the hip. Fifteen percent have knee pain.[19] Physical findings depend on classification, duration, and severity of the slip. It may be normal with an early slip. Classical findings include limited internal rotation, obligatory external rotation on flexion, and, in late cases, shortening. Comparing the normal side to the painful side is quite important both on physical and radiographic assessment. Contralateral hip SCFE may be observed in as many as 25% of the cases, and is seen most commonly, as suggested above, with underlying endocrine or growth disorders.

Radiographic assessment includes AP pelvis and bilateral frog lateral views. A line along the lateral neck cortex (Klein's line) normally overlaps a portion of the lateral physis, and does not in SCFE.[20] Other signs include widened and irregular physis in the early stage, reduced epiphyseal height, and the relative displacement of the epiphysis over the metaphysis (neck) on the frog lateral view. We use Wilson's classification[18] to grade the relative displacement: 1 = less than one-third, 2 = one-third to one-half, and 3 = more than one-half.

Patients with SCFE should be immediately referred to or discussed with an orthopedic surgeon with pediatric interest. Treatment principles include gentle closed **or** open reduction and internal fixation for unstable slips. Stable ones may undergo in situ pinning, open reduction, or periarticular osteotomies depending on the situation. In situ pinning has been heralded as standard treatment,[21] but this can lead to residual deformity and degeneration.[22] Open reduction greatly reduces the latter worry. Prophylactic pinning of the contralateral hip may be somewhat controversial, but we recommend this for patients with underlying endocrine or growth disorders.

Patients with neglected, missed, or residual treated SCFE deformities may develop anterior hip impingement, usually caused by anterolateral prominence at the head-neck junction. Functionally, this leads to cam impingement, a common consequence even in mild deformities. The severity of the slip/deformity correlates with degenerative changes.[22] The anterolateral, metaphyseal prominence leads to labral damage from impact at the acetabular rim. Forced flexion even in mild deformities allows the head to lever and allow the prominence to come into play, which can cause considerable acetabular chondral damage.[23]

Radiographic signs for residual SCFE deformity include the α-angle, femoral head ratio, and the anterior femoral head-neck offset ratio.[23] The former 2 are performed on both anteroposterior and lateral views, and the latter on the lateral. The α-angle seems to be the most predictive.[23] Chronic SCFE deformities resulting in impingement can be treated by restoring head morphology and congruent head-acetabulum coupling. This may be achieved via proximal femoral osteotomy. The osteotomy may be subcapital, basi-cervical, intertrochanteric, or subtrochanteric. The more proximal the osteotomy the greater the potential for correction, but a higher risk of osteonecrosis and chondrolysis.[24]

Legg-Calvé-Perthes Disease

This disorder results from avascular necrosis of the proximal femoral head and subsequent deformity and loss of head's sphericity. Again, the etiology is not fully understood and likely multifactorial and involving both genetic and environmental factors.[25] The prevalence is 1 in 10,000 children under the age of 15. The onset is usually between the ages of 2 and 14 years, most commonly between 4 to 8 years.[26] Classically, LCPD occurs in hyperactive boys with delayed skeletal maturity. Other risk factors include a positive family history and low birth weight. Pathologically, one sees osteonecrosis of the femoral head, revascularization and resorption. Pathologists call this *creeping substitution*.

Functional remodeling occurs more completely in individuals who develop the disorder under 6 years of age.[27] Treatment during the active disease process focuses on pain relief, maintenance of range of motion, and "head containment" (ie, prevention of lateral subluxation of the flattened femoral head out of the acetabulum). Those principles theoretically allow molding the head into a spherical shape by the growing acetabulum. Various different options have roles.

These include physiotherapy, orthosis, femoral osteotomy, and pelvic osteotomy. Severity and age at onset matter in the selection of modality of treatment.

Residual deformities can result in adolescent hip pain.[24] The resulting abnormal femoral head shape, disturbance of the physis, and acetabular dysplasia can result in femoroacetabular impingement (FAI), hip instability, or a combination.[28] The acetabular dysplasia in LCPD is due to retroversion, remodeling process, or following innominate pelvic osteotomy. Intra-articular impingement can result from abnormal head morphology, similar to SCFE, or by creating a lateral hinge between the head and the superior rim of the acetabulum. Extra-articular impingement results from the short neck, which leads to prominence of the greater, or less commonly lesser, trochanter and bony collision against the hemipelvis.

Surgical treatment of residual LCPD deformities aims to restore joint congruency, reduce impingement and instability, and increase range of motion. This can be achieved by proximal femoral osteotomy (intertrochanteric, subcapital, or trochanteric distal advancement). Periacetabular osteotomies may also be required for the accompanying acetabular dysplasia or retroversion. Sometimes a combined approach is necessary.

Adolescent Hip Dysplasia

This is DDH, developmental dysplasia of the hip. The primary abnormality here is a malformed acetabulum. This leads to unconventional weightbearing and instability of the femoral head. It may also be associated with other anatomic disorders, such as acetabular retroversion, femoral anteversion, coxa valga, and abnormal anterolateral head neck offset. The problem often ends up with FAI, instability, and joint degeneration.

Adolescent DDH comes from a completely missed DDH of infancy, a partially treated infancy DDH, or even a DDH that develops during adolescence.[29] As mysterious as it may be, the latter form has a higher rate of bilaterality and ultimate hip arthroplasty.[29] Severe untreated hip dysplasia routinely leads to severe osteoarthritis. The natural progression for mild dysplasia is certainly more variable.[30-32]

Many of those patients are initially asymptomatic. Classical symptoms are groin or anterolateral pain sometimes associated with coxa saltans. The patients may exhibit impingement signs or positive apprehension tests.

Imaging includes routine AP pelvic X-ray and lateral radiographs. A whole gamut of measurements can be done, including acetabular index, inclination, Tönnis angle, and anterior and lateral center-edge angles. A "cross-over sign" and/or a prominent ischial spine may indicate acetabular retroversion. CT helps with bony anatomy, direct contrast MRA with the identification and significance of intra-articular pathology.

The aim of surgical treatment is primarily to restore anatomy and presumptively minimize the progression to arthritis. Symptomatic patients with severe dysplasia and minimal degeneration seem the ideal candidates for surgery. It is not clear whether or not asymptomatic patients with mild dysplasia should undergo surgery, although there is a recent trend to do that.[32] Patients with severe degenerative changes probably should undergo arthroplasty when it seems inevitable.[33]

Surgical treatment usually means a focus on correcting the acetabulum, usually with what's called a *Ganz periacetabular osteotomy*.[34] Arthroscopy may be added for intra-articular pathology. Hip arthroscopy shouldn't be done when there is severe dysplasia without a corrective acetabuloplasty. Otherwise, it may create instability of the hip and acceleration of arthritis.[33] The proximal femur may have to be addressed if it is deformed or if a previous osteotomy has altered the anatomy enough to require it. Several more complicated osteotomies may also play roles in correction, such as a triple "steel," Chiari, or shelf osteotomy. These procedures involve such things as intentional leg shortening, bone augmentation, or enhancing the lateral hip with other tissue.[35]

Apophyseal Avulsions

The adolescent hip is particularly prone to growth plate fractures. The "open" growth plate—or physis—has an inherent weakness. With the normal process of growth, limb length may increase disproportionately compared to the whole mass of the limb. With this musculoskeletal imbalance, repetitive tensile stresses to the epiphyseal plate and open physis then account for the relatively common occurrence of apophyseal avulsion fractures.[3,4] These injuries can appear acutely as a traumatic avulsion or more indolently related to overuse, most commonly with athletes and sports that involve rapid acceleration and deceleration, such as skating or skiing. Table 25-3 lists the potential anatomical sites of the apophyseal avulsions around the hip and their reported prevalences.

Most commonly, the patient will provide a history of sudden onset of well-localized pain after a non-contact trauma. The patient may describe a "pop" and even have trouble walking. Patients often experience tenderness at the relevant part of the hip or hemipelvis, and symptoms or signs may be aggravated by passive stretching or resisted contraction of the muscle group involved in the avulsion fracture.

Table 25-3
Common Sites of Avulsion in the Hip and Pelvis

Apophysis	Muscle or Muscle Group	Relative Prevalence
Anterior inferior iliac spine	Rectus femoris muscle	22%
Anterior superior iliac spine	Sartorius and tensor fasciae latae muscles	19%
Iliac crest	Abdominal muscles	1%
Ischial tuberosity	Hamstring muscles	54%
Pubic tubercle	Hip adductor muscles	3%
Lesser trochanter	Iliopsoas muscle	Rare
Greater trochanter	Hip abductor muscles	Rare

Plain radiographs of the pelvis are important. They may confirm the diagnosis and magnitude of displacement or rule out SCFE or proximal femoral fractures. The diagnosis of apophyseal avulsions may require CT scan, which is in general excellent at detailing bony anatomy. MRI may differentiate a true apophyseal avulsion fracture from a nagging but less urgent apophysitis.

The initial management of apophyseal avulsion fractures is usually non-operative (ie, rest, cryotherapy, elevation, analgesia and protected weightbearing [eg, crutches]). Physiotherapy begins with gentle passive range of motion and stretching followed by progressive strengthening as the pain resolves.[36] Return to sport is usually not advocated until the patient is pain free and radiographs show excellent healing.

Surgery is generally reserved for displaced ischial tuberosity avulsions, symptomatic non-unions, unrelenting pain, or persistently impaired function.[37,38] Some people have used displacement greater than 15 mm as an indicator for surgery. That much displacement for an ischial tuberosity avulsion fracture is certainly an indication. It is risky to leave that much displacement alone. It is a set-up for fibrous non-union and an ischial prominence that causes chronic buttock pain and sciatic nerve impingement. Some young athletes with this may complain simply of indolent ache, decrease in hamstring strength and endurance, with suboptimal performance.[37] Even normal healing callus after a mildly displaced fracture sometimes leads to chronic pain, irritation on sitting position, and sciatic nerve symptoms. Perhaps we should be intervening more for less displaced fractures.

Table 25-4
Classification of Apophyseal Avulsion Fractures

Type I	Undisplaced fractures
Type II	Displacement up to 2 cm
Type III	Displacement > 2 cm
Type IV	Symptomatic non-unions or painful exostosis

McKinney et al[39] have recommended probably the best classification for these avulsion fractures (Table 25-4). This provides an imperfect guide for their treatment. According to them, operative intervention should be considered for all type III and type IV injuries, and more selectively for type II.

Labral Tears

Labral tears may occur after a single traumatic event or repetitive mechanical stresses. With respect to labral tears and the adolescent hip, you have really 3 things to think about.

1. Did the tear occur by itself, simply as a result of excessive flexion within an otherwise normal anatomic hip? This is more likely to occur in the adolescent compared to the adult hip.
2. In the vast majority of the cases though, one still sees an underlying bony FAI impingement deformity on the radiographs. The question here, of course, is: Does this impingement matter in these young hips?
3. Perhaps most importantly, what roles do the developmental abnormalities of the hip mentioned (SCFE, LCPD, and DDH) play in the individual's problem? Of course, FAI may either share the same pathophysiology just like an adult or be a consequence or anatomic accompaniment of a developmental disorder.[24]

The adolescent with a labral tear may have more anterior hip or groin pain or more "catching" or "locking." The symptomatology is more commonly than in the adult just related to activity and not present at rest. Clinical examination usually reveals findings such as a positive test with flexion, adduction, and internal rotation (the FADIR test). Other tests, of course, may also be positive, such as the FABER test. Like with adults, plain radiographs of the pelvis and the affected hip, MRI, and MRA are the best imaging tests. MRA has up to 87% sensitivity.[40] Three-dimensional CT may be important to understand whether or not to consider treatment for an underlying developmental abnormality.

The initial management of labral tears may be rest, cessation of sporting activities and analgesia. These initial measures may be followed by physiotherapy aimed at improving the strength and flexibility of the core muscles and the major muscle groups around the hip and pelvis. Modern surgical management of isolated labral tears involves arthroscopic repair or debridement.[41] Of course, the bony abnormalities of FAI and the developmental abnormalities may also have to be addressed.

Femoroacetabular Impingement

Just as for adults, FAI is also recognized as a cause of hip pain in adolescents.[24] The basic mechanisms by which impingement can occur is the same, namely cam type, pincer type, or mixed cam/pincer type. Underlying childhood hip disorders can also lead to FAI, as discussed previously. In addition to the anterior symptomatology, the patient may also have pain in the gluteal area, especially with pincer impingement and a postero-inferiorly directed force on the femoral head, leading to overload and damage of the postero-inferior acetabular cartilage (contrecoup injury). The patient may exhibit the classic "C sign." He/She may identify the pain by cupping the anterior and posterolateral aspects of the thigh between the thumb and the index finger (C sign).

Imaging should always begin with plain radiographs, both in order to facilitate the diagnosis of the type of impingement and also to exclude other, more urgent bony deformity, such as SCFE. Beyond the plain radiographic investigation, MRA and CT are commonly used in the diagnosis of FAI. MRA provides very high diagnostic sensitivity for labral pathology, but has variable sensitivity for articular cartilage pathology (generally 50% to 90%) and significant limitations in detecting acetabular cartilage delamination.[40,42] CT has the benefit of providing 3-dimensional surface renderings of the proximal femoral and acetabular bony anatomy, providing detailed information for surgical planning, especially useful in arthroscopic surgery.[43] The major drawback of using CT in adolescents is the substantial radiation exposure. Furthermore, there are limitations in terms of the provision of information on soft tissue pathology, which is typically inferior to MRA.

The main goal of treatment for FAI is to improve the clearance during hip movements, by eliminating the abutment of the femoral head-neck junction to the acetabular rim. This is aimed at primarily achieving relief of symptoms and return to activities in a group of patients who are typically very active. The secondary aim is to help prevent the potential progressive degeneration of the hip joint and early onset of osteoarthritis.[44] Both open and arthroscopic techniques have been proven to be safe and successful in adolescents.[45] Hip arthroscopy is currently the most commonly employed technique for FAI, with complication rates equivalent to those found in adults.[46]

Snapping Hip Syndrome (Coxa Saltans)

Snapping hip syndrome is defined purely by an audible snap or pop during range of motion of the hip. A lot of people have this, and it is not important if there are no symptoms or another associated more serious issue. When it is a problem, the phenomenon is usually exacerbated by sporting activities. Think simply here. Think in terms of 3 principal anatomic types that may produce noise (Table 25-5).

1. Coxa saltans externa (or iliotibial band syndrome): Snapping of the iliotibial band (or nearby structure) over the greater trochanter when the hip goes from flexed to extended (iliotibial band syndrome)
2. Psoas snap (or internal type): Snapping of the iliopsoas tendon over the iliopectineal eminence or actual femoral head
3. Intra-articular type: Clicking or clacking from any kind of intra-articular pathology

The location of the pain or sound and reproducibility of it on physical examination can help distinguish the different types of snapping hip. For coxa saltans externa, the snapping sensation and discomfort are over the greater trochanter during flexion and internal rotation. For both the internal snapping hip and the intra-articular type, the pain and sound are localized in the groin and anterior hip during flexion and a combination of adduction and abduction. The more distal the psoas sound, the closer it is to the lesser trochanter and the easier it is to diagnose.

TABLE 25-5
CLASSIFICATION OF COXA SALTANS

Types of Coxa Saltans	Etiology
Coxa saltans interna	Iliopsoas tendon
Coxa saltans externa	Iliotibial band, anterior border of gluteus maximus muscle
Intra-articular coxa saltans	Labral tears, loose bodies, cartilage flaps

Treatment depends on symptoms and whether the problem is occurring in isolation or associated with another underlying problem. One must also recognize that these sounds may be so common that they may be confused with a nearby real problem. So, one has to be careful not to jump to the conclusion that a loud snap signifies the cause of the patient's problem.

Initial treatment of the isolated, symptomatic coxa saltans usually is oral nonsteroidal anti-inflammatory drugs (NSAIDs) and/or corticosteroid injection with physical therapy. The focus of the physical therapy depends on the type of snapping hip. Surgical treatment may be considered when non-operative management does not relieve the symptoms. The surgical approach can be open or arthroscopic, and aimed at lengthening the offending structure (eg, iliotibial band or iliopsoas tendon) or repair of the underlying problem (eg, intra-articular pathology).[47-49]

Other Hip Area Considerations in Adolescents

Table 25-6 provides a brief overview of the other pathological processes near the hip. Some of these are discussed elsewhere in the book. One needs to consider all conditions that affect the bony skeleton or adjacent soft tissues, whether or not they are trauma related. Of course, they may be benign or malignant.[50] One also needs to consider all the conditions of the core that may mimic the musculoskeletal conditions.

TABLE 25-6
OTHER CONSIDERATIONS IN ADOLESCENTS

Traumatic	Nontraumatic
• Physeal hip fracture • Non-physeal hip fracture • Subtrochanteric femoral fracture • Pelvic fracture • Hip dislocation • Stress fracture of the femoral neck • Iliacus hematoma syndrome	• Meralgia paresthetica • Abdominal cutaneous nerve entrapment syndrome
Benign	Malignant
• Bone cysts • Osteoid osteoma • Eosinophilic granuloma • Fibrous dysplasia • Exostosis	• Ewing's sarcoma • Osteosarcoma

Special Considerations in Adolescents   263

ILLUSTRATIVE CASES/STUDIES

The following cases portray a spectrum of the problems:

Case 1 (Figures 25-1 and 25-3) is our sentinel case for the chapter. This is what happened subsequently. Four weeks after going to the general practitioner, the 15-year-old athlete desperately seeks help for his persistent pain at an emergency department. Similar X-rays are taken. The emergency staff consults pediatric orthopedic surgeons, who get more detailed X-ray views and note a widened and irregular growth plate (physis). The Klein's line on the right (one of the yellow lines on the X-ray) does not cross the epiphysis. The orthopedists describe "a physis overlap and postero-inferior displacement of the epiphysis over the metaphysis." The new radiographs demonstrate progression of the slip, and the patient undergoes in situ hip pinning the next day. Fortunately, he did well despite the initial delay in diagnosis.

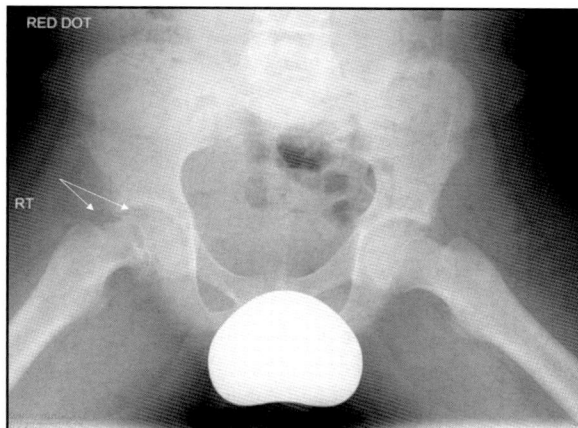

Figure 25-3. Foreshortened femoral neck and head of SCFE. Frog-leg lateral view of both hips, 10 weeks after onset of symptoms. You can see how closely the right femoral neck abuts the acetabulum (arrows).

Case 2 (Figures 25-4 and 25-5) is a 14-year-old athlete with essentially the same SFCE problem as Case 1, except involving an even later recognition and a worse outcome. We saw him 1 year after a soccer injury when he ended up with continuous pain, after an attempt at pinning. At that time, he had severe shortening of his left leg. We had to do a total hip replacement (see Figure 25-5). This unfortunate young man, together with Case 1, displays the value of recognizing these entities promptly, plus including the right expertise early.

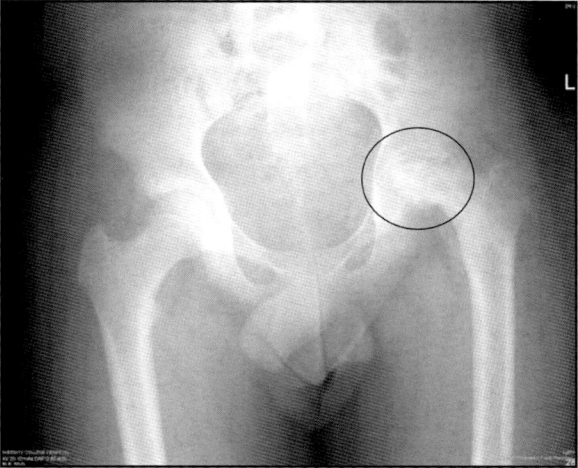

Figure 25-4. Fourteen-year-old athlete with left "hip" pain. Avascular necrosis (ie, destruction due to loss of blood supply) of the left femoral head after surgical attempt to save the hip from SCFE. Note high-riding left hip (circle).

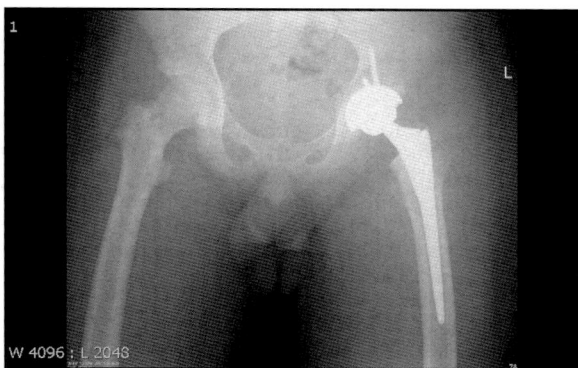

Figure 25-5. X-ray of the same 14-year-old athlete after total hip replacement.

Case 3 (Figure 25-6) is a 39-year-old man after bilateral childhood LCPD. The right hip had already been treated with total hip arthroplasty. X-rays show the severe loss of sphericity and "mushroom appearance" of the now symptomatic left femoral head. Subsequently, he underwent a similar procedure on the left.

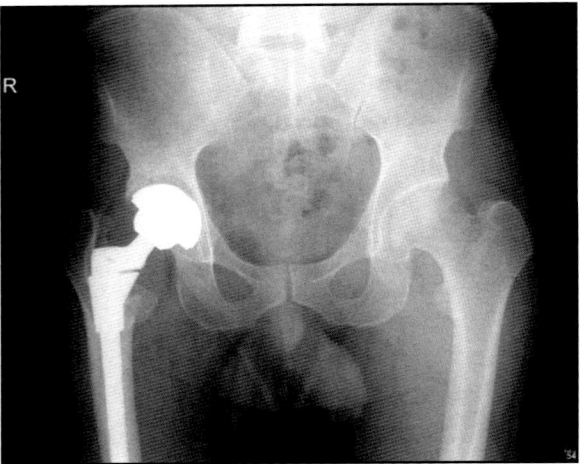

Figure 25-6. In this AP X-ray of the pelvis, focus on the left hip, the one without the hardware. Note the loss of sphericity and "mushroom" appearance. The same LCPD problem is now occurring on the other side.

Case 4 (Figure 25-7) is a 16-year-old female dancer with an avulsion fracture of the ischial tuberosity (ie, adjacent to and part of the acetabulum). Displaced inferiorly and posteriorly, the avulsed fragment was mobilized, reduced, and stabilized using 2 screws. Fortunately, she resumed full activity within 8 weeks. This problem can be devastating if not picked up and treated promptly.

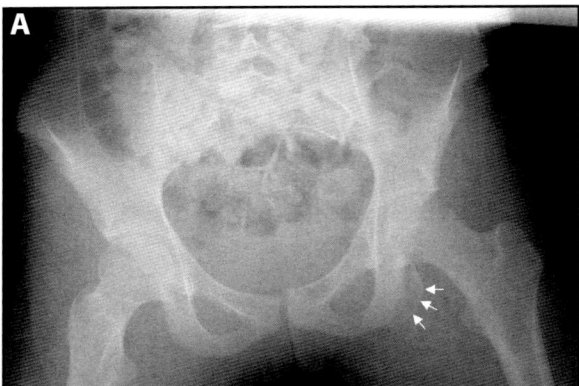
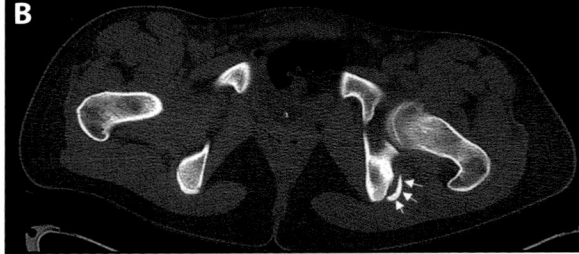
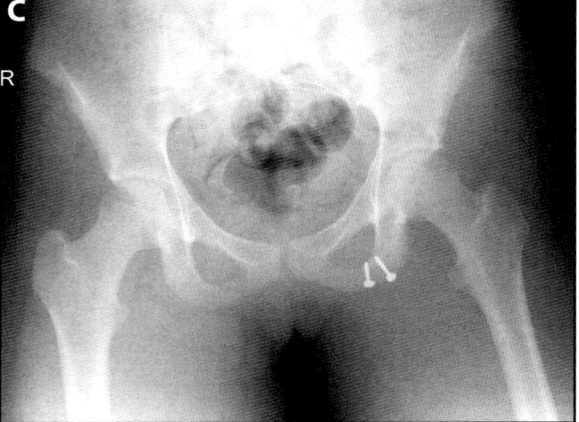

Figure 25-7. Pre- and postoperative imaging of a dangerous avulsion fracture. (A) Arrows designate the large bony avulsion fracture near the inferior aspect of the left acetabulum. (B) CT scan of the same (arrows). (C) Postoperative X-ray shows excellent reduction of the fragment with 2 fixation screws. Note no avulsed piece of bone (ie, no arrows).

Special Considerations in Adolescents 265

Case 5 (Figure 25-8) is a 15-year-old figure skater with deteriorating bilateral hip pain, worse on the right side, due to developmental dysplasia. The patient underwent a periacetabular osteotomy. This is a big surgical procedure that encompasses breaking pelvic bones and reorienting the acetabulum. Her symptoms improved substantially after the periacetabular osteotomy, and she is due to have a similar procedure on her left side.

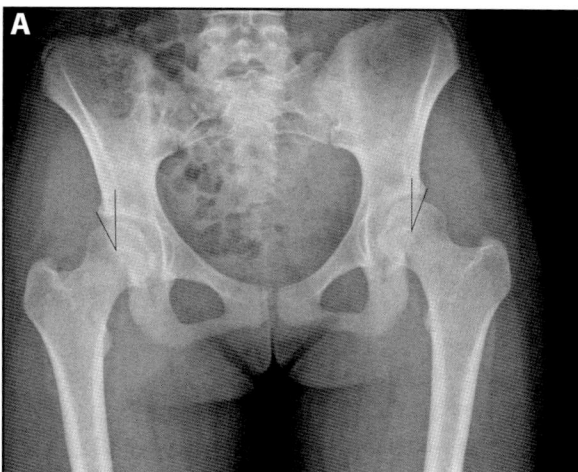 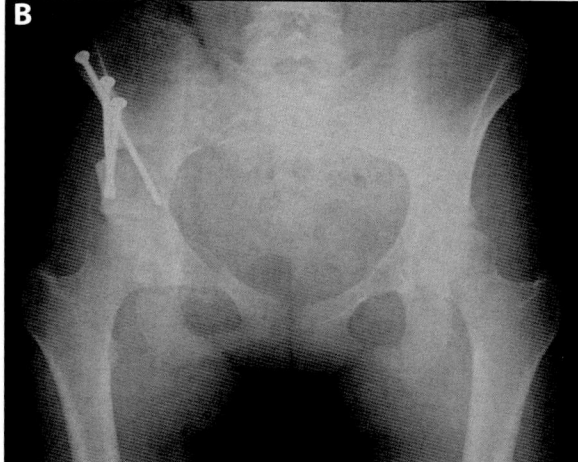

Figure 25-8. Pre- and postoperative pelvic X-rays of a figure skater showing (A) bilateral reduced lateral center edge angles. In her case, the angles were way less than 20 degrees and diagnostic of DDH. (B) Postoperative radiograph showing 3 large screws and acetabular reorientation of the right hip.

Case 6 (Figure 25-9) is an 18-year-old male, multisport athlete who experienced difficulty with right groin pain over 2 years, to the point that he could no longer play. He turned out to have a mixed cam/pincer type FAI. After diagnosis, he underwent (1) arthroscopic resection of the os acetabuli and a portion of the acetabular rim, (2) repair of the labrum, and (3) femoral reshaping. He returned fully at 6 months.

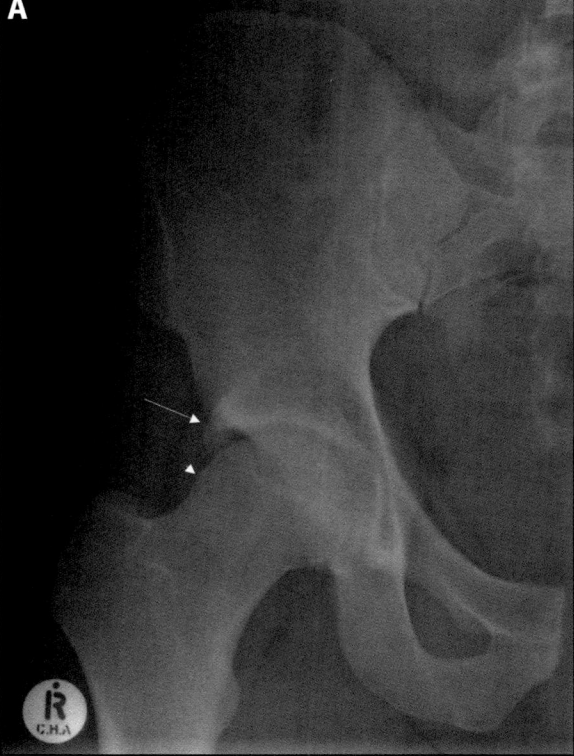 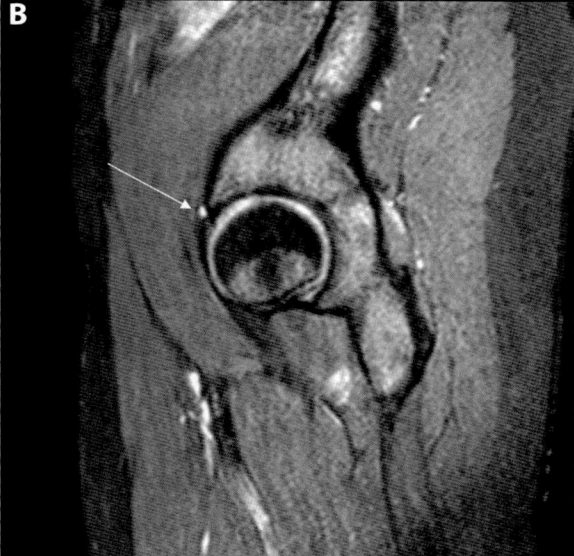

Figure 25-9. Pre- and postoperative images of a young, multisport athlete with mixed-type FAI. (A) Preoperative plain radiograph showing the os acetabuli of pincer (arrow) and the pistol grip deformity of cam (arrowhead). (B) Preoperative MRI with arrow pointing to joint fluid outside the hip, indicating a labral tear. *continued*

Figure 25-9 (continued). Pre- and postoperative images of a young, multi-sport athlete with mixed-type FAI. (C) Postoperative radiograph of the same patient showing the os acetabuli and cam to have vanished.

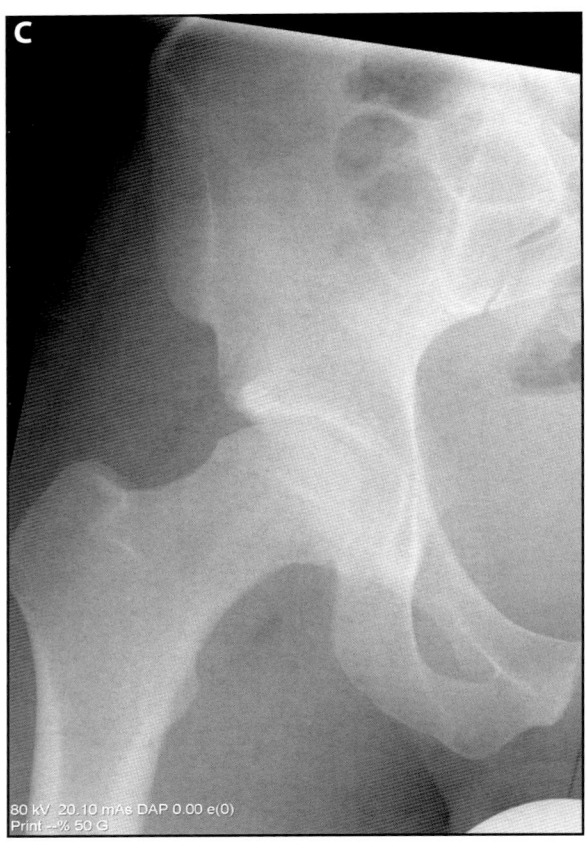

SUMMARY

Adolescents can have age-specific disorders, such as SCFE, that need urgent pediatric orthopedic attention, as well as disorders similar to adults. Missed or residual deformities sometimes turn up in adolescence or adulthood, and factor into FAI or hip instability. Adolescents also seem more prone to certain conditions, such as apophyseal injury and benign or malignant skeletal tumors. Successful diagnosis and management require awareness of the various disorders and thorough clinical assessments by appropriate health care teams.

SELECTED READINGS

Purvis JM. The challenge of communicating with pediatric patients. AAOS Now. http://www.aaos.org/news/aaosnow/feb09/clinical5.asp.
   An excellent and brief guide to the challenges in communicating with children as patients.
Braly BA, Beall DP, Martin HD. Clinical examination of the athletic hip. *Clin Sports Med.* 2006;25:199-210.
   A detailed reference for athletic hip examination.
Loder RT, Dietz FR. What is the best evidence for the treatment of slipped capital femoral epiphysis? *J Pediatr Orthop.* 2012;32:S158-S165.
   An update on the most recent evidence for management of such condition.
Ramachandran M, Azegami S, Hosalkar HS. Current concepts in the treatment of adolescent femoroacetabular impingement. *J Child Orthop.* 2013;7:79-90.
   Excellent review of adolescent FAI with overview on underlying childhood causes.
Kim HK. Pathophysiology and new strategies for the treatment of Legg-Calvé-Perthes disease. *J Bone Joint Surg Am.* 2012;94(7):659-669.
   Excellent update in management of a poorly understood disease.

REFERENCES

1. Coaching our kids to fewer injuries: a report on youth sports safety (April 2012). Safe Kids Worldwide. https://www.safekids.org/sportsresearch. Accessed May 9, 2018.
2. Boyd KT, Peirce NS, Batt ME. Common hip injuries in sports. *Sports Med.* 1997;24:273-288.
3. Hawkins D, Metheny J. Overuse injuries in youth sports: biomechanical considerations. *Med Sci Sports Exerc.* 2001;33(10):1701-1707.
4. Perron AD, Miller MD, Brady WJ. Orthopedic pitfalls in the ED: pediatric growth plate injuries. *Am J Emerg Med.* 2002;20:50-54.
5. The Easter Seal Society. *The Easter Seal Guide to Children's Orthopaedics: Prevention, Screening and Problem Solving.* Toronto, Ontario, Canada: Mercer Rang; 1982.
6. Purvis JM. The challenge of communicating with pediatric patients. AAOS Now. http://www.aaos.org/news/aaosnow/feb09/clinical5.asp. Accessed January 16, 2019.
7. Brown MD, Gomez-Martin O, Brookfield KF, et al. Differential diagnosis of hip disease versus spine disease. *Clin Orthop.* 2004;419:280-284.
8. Margo K, Drezner J, Motzkin D. Evaluation and management of hip pain: an algorithmic approach. *J Fam Pract.* 2003;52:607-617.
9. Ilizaliturri VM Jr, Martinez-Escalante FA, Chaidez PA, Camacho-Galindo J. Endoscopic iliotibial band release for external snapping hip syndrome. *Arthroscopy.* 2006;22(5):505-510.
10. McCarthy JC, Busconi B. The role of hip arthroscopy in the diagnosis and treatment of hip disease. *Orthopedics.* 1995;18:753-756.
11. Reider B, Martel JM. Pelvis, hip and thigh. In: Reider B, Martel JM, eds. *The Orthopaedic Physical Examination.* Philadelphia, PA: WB Saunders; 1999:159-199.
12. Braly BA, Beall DP, Martin HD. Clinical examination of the athletic hip. *Clin Sports Med.* 2006;25:199-210.
13. Marks MC, Alexander J, Sutherland DH, Chambers HG. Clinical utility of the Duncan-Ely test for rectus femoris dysfunction during the swing phase of gait. *Dev Med Child Neurol.* 2003;45:763-768.
14. Schoenecker PL, Clohisy JC, Millis MB, Wenger DR. Surgical management of the problematic hip in adolescent and young adult patients. *J Am Acad Orthop Surg.* 2011;19(5):275-286.
15. Lehmann CL, Arons RR, Loder RT, Vitale MG. The epidemiology of slipped capital femoral epiphysis: an update. *J Pediatr Orthop.* 2006;26(3):286-290.
16. Munchow R. Slipped capital femoral epiphysis: an update on the current management and outcomes. *Curr Orthop Prac.* 2013;24:612-616.
17. Loder RT, Richards BS, Shapiro PS, Reznick LR, Aronson DD. Acute slipped capital femoral epiphysis: the importance of physeal stability. *J Bone Joint Surg Am.* 1993;75(8):1134-1140.
18. Dunn DM, Angel JC. Replacement of the femoral head by open operation in severe adolescent slipping of the upper femoral epiphysis. *J Bone Joint Surg Br.* 1978;60:394-403.
19. Matava MJ, Patton CM, Luhmann S, Gordon JE, Schoenecker PL. Knee pain as the initial symptom of slipped capital femoral epiphysis: an analysis of initial presentation and treatment. *J Pediatr Orthop.* 1999;19(4):455-460.
20. Mitchell SR, Tennent TD, Brown RR, Monsell F. Slipped capital femoral epiphysis. *Hip Int.* 2007;17(4):185-193.
21. Loder RT, Dietz FR. What is the best evidence for the treatment of slipped capital femoral epiphysis? *J Pediatr Orthop.* 2012;32:S158-S165.
22. Castañeda P, Ponce C, Villareal G, Vidal C. The natural history of osteoarthritis after a slipped capital femoral epiphysis/the pistol grip deformity. *J Pediatr Orthop.* 2013;33:S76-S82.
23. Wensaas A, Gunderson RB, Svenningsen S, Terjesen T. Femoroacetabular impingement after slipped upper femoral epiphysis: the radiological diagnosis and clinical outcome at long-term follow-up. *J Bone Joint Surg Br.* 2012;94:1487-1493.
24. Ramachandran M, Azegami S, Hosalkar HS. Current concepts in the treatment of adolescent femoroacetabular impingement. *J Child Orthop.* 2013;7:79-90.
25. Kim HK. Pathophysiology and new strategies for the treatment of Legg-Calvé-Perthes disease. *J Bone Joint Surg Am.* 2012;94(7):659-669.
26. Wiig O, Terjesen T, Svenningsen S, Lie SA. The epidemiology and aetiology of Perthes' disease in Norway. A nationwide study of 425 patients. *J Bone Joint Surg Br.* 2006;88:1217-1222.
27. Wiig O, Terjesen T, Svenningsen S. Prognostic factors and outcome of treatment in Perthes' disease: a prospective study of 368 patients with five-year follow-up. *J Bone Joint Surg Br.* 2008;90:1364-1371.
28. Kim YJ, Novais EN. Diagnosis and treatment of femoroacetabular impingement in Legg–Calvé–Perthes disease. *J Pediatr Orthop.* 2011;31:S235-S240.
29. Lee CB, Mata-Rink A, Millis MB, et al. Demographic differences in adolescent-diagnosed and adult-diagnosed acetabular dysplasia compared with infantile developmental dysplasia of the hip. *J Pediatr Orthop.* 2013;33:107-111.
30. Murphy SH, Ganz R, Müller ME. The prognosis in untreated dysplasia of the hip. A study of radiographic factors that predict the outcome. *J Bone Joint Surg.* 1995;77:985-989.
31. Ziegler J, Thielemann F, Mayer-Athenstaedt C, et al. The natural history of developmental dysplasia of the hip. A meta-analysis of the published literature. *Orthopade.* 2008;37:515-516.
32. Wenger DR. Is there a role for acetabular dysplasia correction in an asymptomatic patient? *J Pediatr Orthop.* 2013;33:S8-S12.
33. Spence D, Kelly D, Mihalko M, Guyton J. Adolescent and young adult hip dysplasia. *Curr Orthop Prac.* 2013;24:567-575.
34. Ganz R, Klaue K, Vinh TS, et al. A new periacetabular osteotomy for the treatment of hip dysplasias. Technique and preliminary results. *Clin Orthop Relat Res.* 1988;232:26-36.
35. Kelly DM. Congenital and developmental anomalies of the hip and pelvis. In: Canale ST, Beaty JH, eds. *Campbell's Operative Orthopaedics.* Philadelphia, PA: Elsevier Mosby; 2013:1079-1118.
36. Heyworth BE, Voos JE, Metzl JD. Hip injuries in the adolescent athlete. *Pediatr Ann.* 2007;36(11):713-718.
37. Ferlic PW, Sadoghi P, Singer G, Kraus T, Eberl R. Treatment for ischial tuberosity avulsion fractures in adolescent athletes. *Knee Surg Sports Traumatol Arthrosc.* 2014;22:893-897.
38. Paletta GA Jr, Andrish JT. Injuries about the hip and pelvis in the young athlete. *Clin Sports Med.* 1995;14(3):591-628.
39. McKinney BI, Nelson C, Carrion W. Apophyseal avulsion fractures of the hip and pelvis. *Orthopedics.* 2009;32(1):42.
40. Smith TO, Hilton G, Toms AP, Donell ST, Hing CB. The diagnostic accuracy of acetabular labral tears using magnetic resonance imaging and magnetic resonance arthrography: a meta-analysis. *Eur Radiol.* 2011;21(4):863-874.

41. Haddad B, Konan S, Haddad FSH. Debridement versus re-attachment of acetabular labral tears: a review of the literature and quantitative analysis. *Bone Joint J*. 2014;96(1):24-30.
42. Anderson LA, Peters CL, Park BB, Stoddard GJ, Erickson JA, Crim JR. Acetabular cartilage delamination in femoroacetabular impingement: risk factors and magnetic resonance imaging diagnosis. *J Bone Joint Surg Am*. 2009;91(2):305-313.
43. Beaule PE, Zaragosa E, Motamedi K, Copelan N, Dorey FJ. Three-dimensional computed tomography of the hip in the assessment of femoroacetabular impingement. *J Orthop Res*. 2005;23(6):1286-1292.
44. Beck M, Kalhor M, Leunig M, Ganz R. Hip morphology influences the pattern of damage to the acetabular cartilage: femoroacetabular impingement as a cause of early osteoarthritis of the hip. *J Bone Joint Surg Br*. 2005;87(7):1012-1018.
45. Naal FD, Miozzari HH, Wyss TF, Notzli HP. Surgical hip dislocation for the treatment of femoroacetabular impingement in high-level athletes. *Am J Sports Med*. 2011;39(3):544-550.
46. Nwachukwu BU, McFeely ED, Nasreddine AY, Krcik JA, Frank J, Kocher MS. Complications of hip arthroscopy in children and adolescents. *J Pediatr Orthop*. 2011;31(3):227-231.
47. Ilizaliturri VM Jr, Martinez-Escalante FA, Chaidez PA, Camacho-Galindo J. Endoscopic iliotibial band release for external snapping hip syndrome. *Arthroscopy*. 2006;22(5):505-510.
48. Hoskins JS, Burd TA, Allen WC. Surgical correction of internal coxa saltans: a 20-year consecutive study. *Am J Sports Med*. 2004;32(4):998-1001.
49. Yamamoto Y, Hamada Y, Ide T, Usui I. Arthroscopic surgery to treat intra-articular type snapping hip. *Arthroscopy*. 2005;21(9):1120-1125.
50. Ruggieri P, Angelini A, Montalti M, et al. Tumours and tumour-like lesions of the hip in the paediatric age: a review of the Rizzoli experience. *Hip Int*. 2009;19(suppl 6):S35-S45.

26

hip arthroscopy
frontiers and limitations

ANIL S. RANAWAT, MD
BRIAN J. REBOLLEDO, MD
JACQUELINE M. BRADY, MD

Editor's Note: *Noted hip surgeon Anil Ranawat seems the right person to state where hip arthroscopy is headed over the next 2 to 3 years. From the Ranawat first family of hip surgery, Anil was born to do this. It is not surprising he chose his dad for the opening quote. Rumor has it that all the Ranawat middle names translate to mean "hip." In this chapter, Anil and his 2 younger colleagues make some bold statements about the direction of hip arthroscopy.*

The eye sees only what the mind knows.

—Chitranjan Ranawat, MD.

WHY ME?

After all, he was only 20 years old.

The strapping mid-fielder never envisioned that hip pain would be the ailment to slow him down so early in his career. After last year's playoff run, his team was supposed to be a serious contender. At first, the pain was manageable, but now in the crunch time of the season, the pain was a lot worse and medications were not doing the trick.

Finally, at the insistence of his mother, he called his team physician and came in right away for an evaluation. From all the off-season conditioning he felt strong, but certain maneuvers agonizingly aggravated the same darn groin pain. As the doctor pressed down on his flexed and internally rotated hip, he winced. "That's it, doc! That's the pain," he exclaimed.

The doctor held up the X-ray and waved his finger over an image of his hip. A "bump," he called it, along the neck of his femur was the likely culprit. What was apparent on X-ray was better defined by an MRI. He also had a labral tear. "It is a good thing," said the doctor. "We can fix this for you."

This story about a young athlete is becoming commonplace. As we understand better the causes for these pains, we have been devising more specific solutions. The emergence of hip arthroscopy set the stage for our new understandings and new-fangled managements of so many ailing young athletes. Since the whole field is still new and growing, the indications and techniques continue to evolve. In this chapter, we shall highlight some of the frontiers of hip arthroscopy and its expanding role in management of hip injuries. We shall also draw attention to some of the obvious limitations of hip arthroscopy, as we see it, and what the future holds.

Frontiers in Hip Arthroscopy

As our understanding of hip pathology develops, so does our capacity to treat the disorders, which are quickly becoming numerous. As Tom Byrd pointed out in a previous chapter, hip arthroscopy developed before we really knew what we could do with it. Now, through this less invasive technique, hip arthroscopy has become a powerful "change" tool. It has allowed us to recognize and more effectively treat more and more hip disorders. We must still appreciate that hip arthroscopy continues to evolve, and that we are finding new roles for it and also learning where we should not be applying this technique. Suffice it to say that this new technology is paving the way. Indications are expanding, and patient outcomes are improving.

We shall talk about 4 hip arthroscopic frontiers.

COMPUTERIZED NAVIGATION AND ROBOTICS FOR CAM RESECTIONS (FIGURE 26-1)

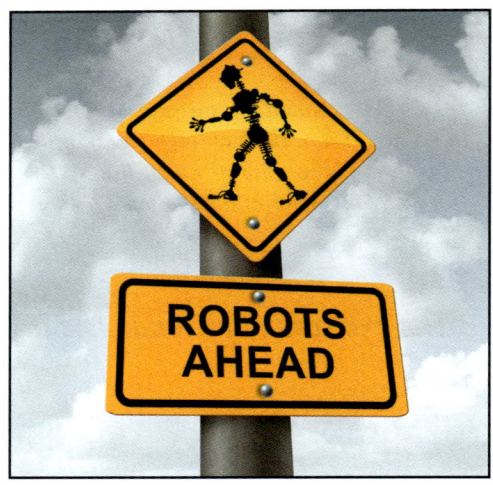

Figure 26-1.

A common reason for failure of hip arthroscopy is incomplete resection of a cam lesion[1,2] or sometimes resecting too much. A previous chapter talked about the importance of sphericity of the femoral head, and how loss of that causes injury to the acetabular labrum during the hip's range of motion.[3] Artful removal of the "bump" of a cam lesion, with restoration of sphericity, is the key to success for that type of impingement.

During femoral neck osteochondroplasty of a cam resection, the surgeon uses the combination of an arthroscopic shaver and burr to re-contour the femoral head and neck so that hip motion has minimal impingement on the chondrolabral junction. Direct intraoperative assessment of cam impingement is tricky, particularly while the lower extremity is captured in a traction device and the whole operative field is captured by just a 2-dimensional screen. Preoperative planning has also been limited by the absence of tools to understand how much of the cam bump to resect and how much not to. The 2-dimensional representation of a 3-dimensional problem doesn't quite do it. For instance, the "alpha angle" gives us a point where the femoral head loses its sphericity. However, it does not indicate the proximal and distal extent of the lesion on the femoral neck, nor quantify in any way the overall size or volume of the culprit bony lesion. Clohisy et al shouted this frustration when they called the utility of that same "angle" into question. They found basically the same range of values in patients with and without symptoms of impingement.[4] The relationships between the femoral heads and acetabula are affected in numerous ways, certainly by the shapes of the ball and the socket and, more importantly, by a combination of the 2 surfaces.

Three-dimensional CT scanning provides surgeons a means of visualizing clearly the location and extent of the cam lesion (Figure 26-2). Surface renderings help evaluate osseous impingements caused by either the proximal femur or pelvis side.[5] The location and size of each cam lesion are generally defined according to the clock face of the roughly spherical femoral head. The overall volume of the bony prominence area is actually very calculable.

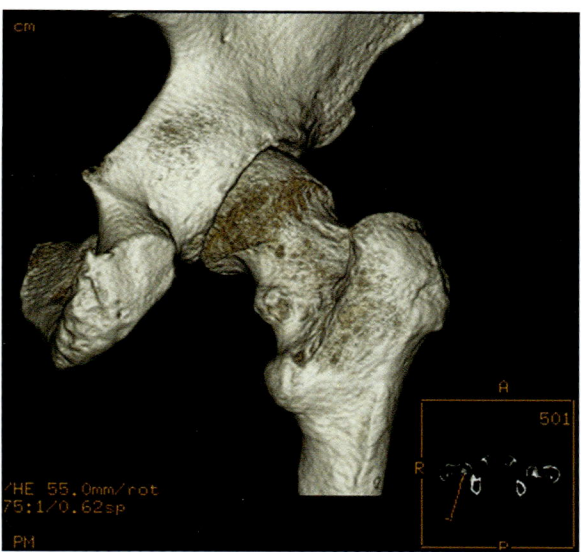

Figure 26-2. Imaging frontier for hip arthroscopy. Three-dimensional CT reconstruction. This technique is being used to visualize preoperatively a lesion along the femoral neck and to plan its removal.

Computerized navigation and robotics utilize the 3-dimensional imaging of the hip and acetabulum to provide the surgeon with an opportunity to characterize completely the 3-dimensional size and location of a femoral cam lesion and then accurately resect it. The area of planned resection can be identified 3-dimensionally preoperatively via a patient-specific reconstruction of the particular osseous anatomy. Depending on the software, virtual surgery may then be done digitally right in the laboratory. A proposed area can be resected and the resultant range of motion assessed again in the laboratory prior to the actual surgery. Navigation allows visualization of the surgical instruments in relation to the prior virtual reconstruction. So, in theory at least, the surgeon's "hands" can be guided magnificently during the actual surgery. Robotic-assisted surgery provides even more accuracy, combining both preoperative and navigation tools with a "guided" intraoperative cutting device automated according to a preoperatively drawn up "cut map."

This technology introduces several promising opportunities. The learning curve of hip arthroscopy, and particularly cam lesion resection, is known to be very "gradual." That means the surgeon must do many cases before he/she can perform consistently and confidently.[6] Therefore, a navigation system makes great sense. It seems a great stride toward the standardization of cam resection, both for the individual surgeon as well as for reducing the variability between surgeons.

In addition, trainees striving to master the surgical techniques in hip arthroscopy can do it with the 3-dimensional navigation device both in the laboratory during practice and on the operating suite "playing field" and live patients. A recent review by Nawabi et al argues for it. In that paper, navigation and robotic-assisted hip arthroscopy seemed to allow for more accurate osseous resection than did free-handed technqiues.[7] Cartiaux et al showed in a sawbones model that navigation and robot-assisted cutting devices were superior in accuracy than free-hand cuts.[8] We still don't know the costs of all this nor the overall cost-effectiveness. And we still certainly don't know how much, if any, it will bring with respect to overall clinical success.

But we will know these things soon.

HIP ARTHROSCOPY FOR EVALUATING THE PAINFUL TOTAL HIP

Another frontier for hip arthroscopy is the periprosthetic setting. Knee arthroscopy has long been used in the treatment of painful knee arthroplasty, and for the same reasons that Dr. Byrd points out, indications for periprosthetic hip arthroscopy have evolved more slowly. The new arthroscopic techniques actually allow us to see areas near the total hip better. Think of what can be done with these tiny scopes. We can inspect for signs of infection, to obtain a biopsy, or to assess wear or bone resorption. Then we can do procedures such as resect scar or symptom-causing adhesions.[9,10]

Early and proper diagnosis and treatment of infection associated with total hip arthroplasty can be life-saving. Removal of the prosthesis or any of the parts can be morbid. In the past, precise assessment has been difficult. One essentially had to guess based on clinical signs and symptoms. Now, suspected septic arthritis of both the native and prosthetic hip have become excellent indications for hip arthroscopy, culture, irrigation, and even synovectomy.[11,12] Some surgeons have particularly low thresholds to arthroscope the hip for suspected infection following total hip arthroplasty.[9,13] In some cases the decision to remove the prosthesis may be clear, based on a draining wound, elevated inflammatory markers, and positive aspirate cultures.[14-20] However, in most cases that decision is not so clear, and both the physician and patient don't want to remove it without the firmest evidence possible. Most of the time, patients have borderline serum markers, some redness around the wound, no drainage, and negative cultures. Plus, the patients usually don't feel or look too bad.

Hip arthroscopy is just plain simpler than the old open way of going into the hip. The surgeon has the ability to visualize the hip joint and obtain tissue cultures for analysis without subjecting patients to the risks of dislocation, secondary infection, and poor wound healing. The minimally invasive approach reduces the overall risk of medical complications.[21-23] Tissue histology and cultures are key in the ultimate decision and are now necessary components of the work-up for suspected periprosthetic infection. The tools used in hip arthroscopy permit so much more to be done with much less risk.[24,25] The arthroscopic setting, of course, does not afford the surgeon to exchange any prosthetic components. That can be done as a second stage if necessary.

ARTHROSCOPY FOR SYMPTOMATIC HIP DYSPLASIA

Hip preservation remains the main goal in developmental dysplasia of the hip (DDH). The methods to achieve this are somewhat challenging and controversial. Hip arthroscopy has several promising and seemingly appropriate roles. It is proving promising for the treatment of selected patients with pain. During periacetabular osteotomy, hip arthroscopy can help visualize the acetabular cartilage to be rotated into weightbearing positions. That can be quite helpful to maximize the chance of reducing pain after the osteotomy.[26] Arthroscopy can also help with labral fixation and capsular closure.

There is uncertainty with regard to the potential benefit of the latter procedures. As our indications for hip arthroscopy expand, it becomes increasingly important to analyze our outcomes critically. Perhaps nowhere else is this more important than in these patients with DDH.

There are a huge number of patients with painful hips but who don't quite fit the criteria for periacetabular osteotomy, such as those on the inner part of the spectrum of hip dysplasia (eg, lateral center-edge angle 20 to 25 degrees). The treatment remains controversial. Periacetabular osteotomy might seem too invasive, while hip arthroscopists worry about the potential for worsening symptoms, by exacerbating the dysplasia with their labral debridement or acetabular rim decompression. Despite the worry about causing hip instability, some hip arthroscopy techniques are showing promise for treating "microinstability" in selected settings of both traditional, global dysplasia and focal acetabular undercoverage.

One should not necessarily underplay the likelihood that the ligamentum teres contributes to stabilization of the native adult hip, especially during flexion, adduction, and external rotation. In addition to its known contribution to the blood supply of the pediatric hip, the ligament both contributes to the blood supply of the pediatric hip and has mechanoreceptors and nociceptors, which likely contribute to mechanical and proprioceptive factors involved in hip stability.[27] When there is both dysplasia and gross instability, the ligamentum teres is often torn. The ligament is traditionally sacrificed in open hip surgery. In contrast, arthroscopic reconstruction of the ligamentum teres may well aid with hip stabilization in any patient with deficient acetabular coverage.[28-30]

ARTHRO-ENDOSCOPIC PROCEDURES AROUND THE HIP

Don't forget that there is a large musculoskeletal world around the ball-and-socket hip joint that seems amenable to endoscopic procedures. The hip arthroscope can be utilized, and it seems we could design better scopes for that purpose. The hip arthroscope has already been used to assist in such things as proximal hamstring repair, psoas release, and nerve decompression. Such endoscopic procedures have the benefits of image magnification and limited exposure[31] and avoid such structures as the gluteus maximus and the sciatic nerve. Indications for hip endoscopy within the peritrochanteric space have expanded (eg, for refractory trochanteric bursitis and abductor tendon repair). The early results seem promising.[32-34] The hip arthroscope has shown promise for sciatic nerve decompression and piriformis syndrome.[35,36] Other extra-articular hip disease has also been attacked that way,[37] such as deep gluteal syndrome, another kind of sciatic nerve entrapment, involving the gluteus maximus, ischial tunnel syndrome, and pudendal nerve entrapment. The results are not all in.

The iliopsoas muscle/tendon deserves special mention in this section. It can compress the chondrolabral complex as it crosses over the acetabulum and create unusual labral pathology, leading to degeneration, inflammation, and tears. Domb et al described results addressing iliopsoas impingement by arthroscopic tenotomy, which resulted in improved postoperative clinical outcomes.[38] The labral injury is distinct from dysplasia and femoroacetabular impingement (FAI), in that the position of labral insult is located at the 3 o'clock position, where the tendon traverses. This is in contrast to FAI and dysplasia, where the neck impinges usually at the 1 o'clock position.

Young patients with chondral lesions have also benefited from recent advances with hip arthroscopy. Success has been shown with microfracture,[39] mosaicplasty,[40,41] osteochondral allograft transplantation,[42] and autologous chondrocyte implantation in the hip.[43] The early reports show promise, but these are mostly case series with limited long-term follow-up. Many of these techniques derive from articular cartilage-saving techniques of the knee. Some show great promise in stopping ongoing chondral degeneration.

Limitations of Hip Arthroscopy

Montgomery et al report a 365% increase in hip arthroscopic procedures in the United States since 2004.[44] This is due to a combination of increased number of trainees and a proliferation of innovative technical advances.[45] The advances and improving outcomes have called for expanded indications. Now many patients severely afflicted with hip pain can live better lives and hopefully avoid hip replacements.

However, hip arthroscopy continues to evolve and certain limitations remain. Certain complex hip disorders and patient populations pose particular risk. The procedure is not for everybody. Now let's highlight specific hip disorders that pose special challenges to us hip arthroscopists.

FEMOROACETABULAR IMPINGEMENT MORPHOLOGIC CHALLENGES

Osteochondral Defects

Hip arthroscopy effectively addresses various morphologies, including cam, pincer, and mixed-type FAI. By its nature, FAI may abnormally contact other areas of the hip not so easily addressed. The altered relationship between the head and acetabulum links to early osteoarthritic changes.[46] While not exclusive to FAI, one such problem is the osteochondral defect. This is thought to be a relative instability, resulting in shearing of the cartilage covering the femoral head. This poses a significant problem for the young patient not yet a candidate for arthroplasty.

Hip arthroscopy has provided a number of options to address the management of this difficult problem, but none of them are totally satisfactory. The limited blood supply and poor capacity for healing of the osteochondrum ensures a complex problem. Preventing further degenerative disease is difficult. Targeted strategies using hip arthroscopy include osteochondral allograft transplantation (OAT),[42,47,48] autologous chondrocyte implantation (ACI),[43,49] mosaicplasty,[41,50] and microfracture of the affected area[39,51,52] (Figure 26-3). Stafford et al reported 43 patients who underwent the use of fibrin adhesive for treatment of delaminated articular chondral damage to the femoral head.[53] They reported significant clinical and functional improvement in these patients up to 3 years after treatment. While relative success has been reported with these strategies, case reports and small case series still dominate the literature.

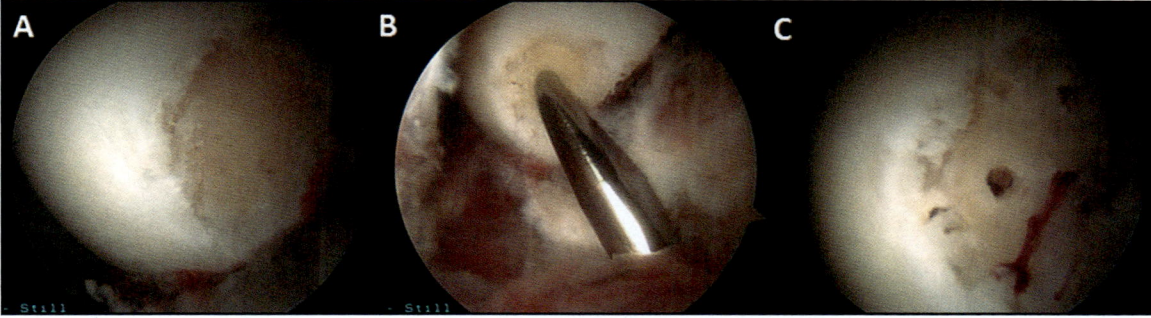

Figure 26-3. Arthroscopic photographs of "microfracture," in this case for a chondral lesion in the femoral head. (A) The bare area of the femoral head represents an articular surface void of cartilage. (B) An awl is used to perforate subchondral bone at the chondral defect. (C) Perforations stimulate fibrocartilage growth and allow for marrow contents to fill the defect.

It remains difficult to assess the viability and efficacy of these modalities without controlled trials or long-term data. El Bitar et al proposed a treatment algorithm based on the size of the full-thickness lesions of the femoral head and acetabulum.[54] For lesions less than 6 to 8 cm^2, the most viable options for hip preservation were OAT, microfracture, and mosaicplasty procedures, whereas lesions 8 cm^2 or greater should be referred for hip arthroplasty. They recommended only microfracture and suture repair on the acetabular side and only for nominal chondral lesions; lesions greater than 6 cm^2 should go to hip arthroplasty.

Coxa Profunda

Another difficult FAI condition to manage is an extreme form of pincer type, known as *coxa profunda* or *protrusio of the hip*. This occurs when there is essentially global acetabular overcoverage. The acetabular fossa can come in line with the ilioischial line or the femoral head may have migrated medial as far as the ilioischial line. Correction of the deformity requires a redirectional periacetabular osteotomy. The negative acetabular roof inclination may complicate things. In a small case series of 3 patients, arthroscopic acetabuloplasty showed improved function and decreased pain at 2.5 years of follow-up.[55] Tannast and Leunig have proposed that only mild global pincer FAI could be safely and effectively managed by arthroscopic means, because entering a deep socket and performing posterior rim resection is technically difficult.[56] As a result, open surgical techniques remain the mainstay of treatment for extreme forms of pincer FAI or global overcoverage.

Cam-Associated Asphericity

Cam-type FAI is associated with femoral head asphericity with a bulge often at the anterosuperior femoral head that eliminates the head-neck offset.[57] In order to address the anterolateral quadrant of the femoral head-neck, osteochondroplasty can be used to decrease the anteromedial abutment in order to improve deficits in internal rotation during hip flexion (Figure 26-4).

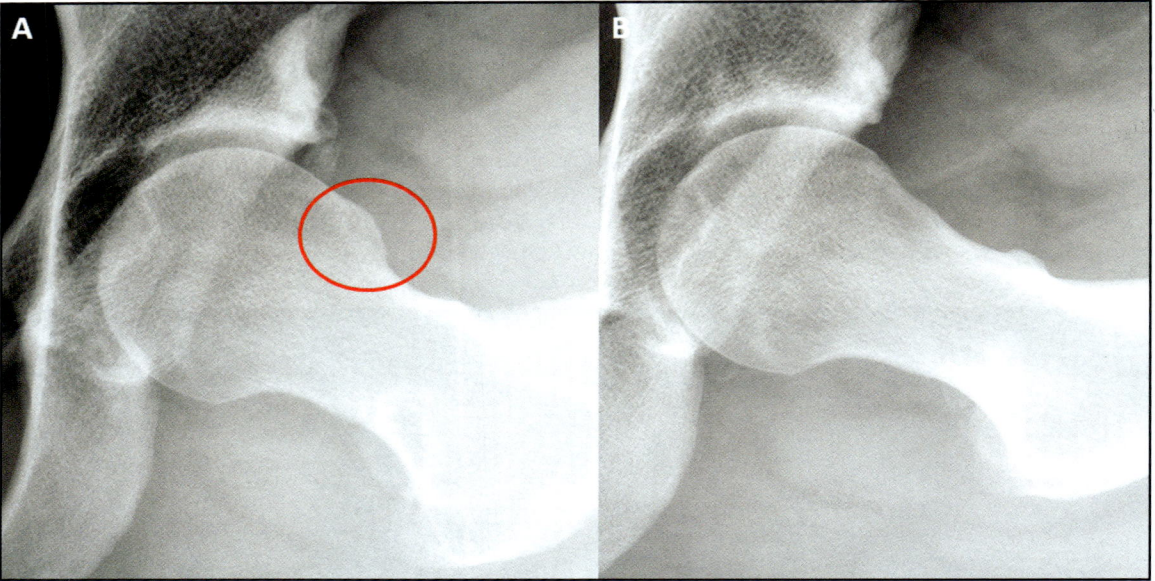

Figure 26-4. Osteochondroplasty for FAI. (A) A cam "bump" along the femoral neck that causes impingement (red circle). (B) X-ray image showing the femoral neck contour after bump removal, which alleviated the patient's impingement symptoms.

However, more severe forms of cam deformity may require posterior cam decompression or repair of the posterior labrum. In this scenario, access past the mid-coronal plane of the hip can pose certain limitations. One such obstacle is access for visualization of the posterior structures, which may require greater hip distraction, thus placing the patient at higher risk for traction injury. Another concern has been the vascular supply to the hip when venturing posteriorly. McCormick et al has suggested that cam osteochondroplasty on the anterior femoral neck is safe in not disrupting femoral head perfusion.[58] However, when osteochondroplasty is to be performed on the posterior superior aspect of the femoral neck, retinacular vessels likely to course within this region can be placed at risk. They recommend using the tip of the greater trochanter or the lateral synovial fold as an intraoperative landmark, or "safe zone," for preserving the blood supply. While not only technically challenging, such anatomic constraints place caution on using hip arthroscopy in more extreme forms of FAI.

Labral Deficiency

Labral deficiency that requires reconstruction can also be a challenging dilemma for surgeons. In this situation where repair would be futile, reconstructive options still remain limited. While open procedures have been used, arthroscopic reconstruction with autologous iliotibial band graft has shown promise. Boykin et al demonstrated in a retrospective review that elite athletes have benefited from arthroscopic reconstruction, with 85.7% returning to play.[59]

Femoral Head Fractures

Another controversial use of hip arthroscopy is the management of femoral head fractures. While historically managed by an open procedure, Park et al has suggested the use of hip arthroscopy as a less invasive means to address femoral head fractures.[60] They report treatment of a patient with a Pipkin Type IV femoral head fracture (femoral head fracture with associated acetabular fracture) by removal of loose osteochondral fracture fragments and posterior labral repair subsequent to internal fixation of the posterior wall of the acetabulum. Additional reports have also shown that femoral head fractures have been effectively treated by use of hip arthroscopy.[61,62] Recently, 2 cases were described using arthroscopic reduction and internal fixation of acetabular wall fractures.[63] Despite these examples, only case reports exist on such rare situations where arthroscopy can be used to manage fractures of the femoral head and acetabulum. Given the scenario where fixation of a large femoral head fragment or associated acetabular fracture exists, open treatment is still necessitated to address this complex injury.

COMPLEX PEDIATRIC DEFORMITIES

Complex disorders of the hip and pelvis in pediatric patients pose particular challenges for selecting who would benefit from hip arthroscopy. Being able to address the patho-anatomy adequately, and choosing the proper intervention to alter the natural history, is needed to give the best outcomes in this population. Still many of these complex hip disorders in the pediatric population have a limited role for hip arthroscopy at this point with further research needed to evaluate outcomes.

The etiology of FAI has been suggested to be initiated during childhood, with some authors having proposed that the deformity occurs in response to subclinical injury during childhood.[64,65] Still others have suggested that athletic activity during childhood can cause subsequent development of FAI.[66,67] Recently, Carsen et al has shown that cam deformity exclusively occurs in childhood during the period of physeal closure and is associated with increased levels of activity.[68] While the etiology of FAI in the pediatric population continues to be delineated, the determined role of hip arthroscopy may also follow suit with strategies to affect the disease course and prevent early degenerative changes.

Slipped capital femoral epiphysis (SCFE) represents the disorder of the epiphysis displacing posterior to the femoral neck during childhood development. Linked to mechanical and often endocrine factors that lead to SCFE, the cause is often multifactorial. Common practice for treatment of SCFE includes in situ pinning, which halts progression of the disease and relies on remodeling of the proximal femur. However, arthritic changes can still occur with an injury to the labrum and peripheral cartilage in SCFE patients.[69-71] Redirectional osteotomy, especially in cases of a severe slip, has been utilized to address the deformity that ensues. Still, without specific indications, the role of hip arthroscopy continues to evolve in SCFE patients. In early-onset or mild SCFE patients with an impingement deformity, previous literature has implicated that arthroscopic decompression may have a role.[72] It has also been advocated that in situ pinning, coupled with arthroscopic femoral osteochondroplasty is an effective means to treat SCFE patients concomitantly.[73] The limitations of hip arthroscopy arise when the disorder represents advanced disease that can involve femoral retroversion, dysplastic acetabular features, and significant epiphyseal displacement. Iatrogenic femoral neck fracture is a catastrophic occurrence associated with aggressive osteochondroplasty of the femoral neck in both arthroscopic and open procedures.[74,75] Mardones et al have suggested that up to 30% of the femoral neck can be resected without significant increase in risk of postoperative femoral neck fracture.[76] Further recommendations have included that femoral neck osteochondroplasty in SCFE patients can be particularly difficult and should be reserved for only mild deformities with slip angles less than 30 degrees.[77] Still the role of hip arthroscopy in early correction of symptomatic FAI in SCFE patients continues to be elucidated. Future studies and long-term follow-up will help to better define the role of early arthroscopic management in this population.

Legg-Calvé-Perthes disease (LCPD) is the process by which idiopathic avascular necrosis of the femoral head can lead to morphologic changes in the head with secondary changes of the pediatric acetabulum. Due to these changes, subsequent chondral damage, labral pathology, coxa breva and vara deformities along with mechanical dysfunction can exist following healed LCPD. Because of the complexity of the pathology, the treatment of LCPD and acetabular dysplasia in pediatric patients has also provided a limited role for hip arthroscopy. While not able to alter the natural history of the disease, it has been reported that selective cases of LCPD patients can experience decreased pain after hip arthroscopy.[78] Still, little data exist on follow-up in these patients, and whether the efficacy of arthroscopy in these affected patients can show long-term benefit.

THE ARTHRITIC HIP

Hip arthroscopy has shown promise in being able to address early degenerative changes of the hip in young patients; however, outcomes in the older patient with osteoarthritis (OA) have been less favorable.[79-81] Often affected by more severe cartilage wear and progression of OA, correction of deformity may not be able to address or alter the damage already incurred. While surgery for FAI has been associated with early pain relief and improved function, Clohisy et al showed that these patients can be at risk for persistent pain and be more likely to need arthroplasty.[82] It continues to be shown that hip arthroscopy in the setting of advanced OA are at risk for poorer clinical outcomes. That would seem obvious anyway, considering that these patients are heading downhill already, and the hip arthroscopy would be for salvage and a year or two of quality of life before putting a big foreign body into the body. Despite the aim of preventing the progression of OA in numerous conditions, there still remains a role for hip arthroscopy for those with progressive degenerative joint disease of the hip.

A long-term study by Byrd and Jones evaluated 50 patients at mean age of 38 years who underwent hip arthroscopy.[79] Remarkably, at 10-year follow-up, 79% of the patients with severe OA had progressed and required total hip arthroplasty. They concluded that older age and advanced OA were significant risk factors for failure of hip arthroscopy. Another large cohort of 106 patients with a mean age of 39 years who underwent hip arthroscopy with debridement and microfracture were evaluated up to 13 years after their index hip arthroscopy.[80] Based on multivariate analysis performed, those with less severe chondral damage, Outerbridge Grade I or II, had a 20% progression to hip arthroplasty, while those with Grade III or IV changes had 78% progression to hip arthroplasty.

In addition, short-term outcomes are affected by evidence of OA. In 28 patients with radiographic evidence of OA at a mean age of 41 years who underwent hip arthroscopy and debridement, only 21% had reported good-to-excellent outcomes, with 42% needing total hip arthroplasty at an average of 14 months after surgery.[81]

The recognition of patients who are at particular risk for having a poorer outcome is important. Patients shown to have longer duration of symptoms may signify chronic disease that would indicate more advanced OA. Still, not all patients with evidenced OA have been shown to have an inferior outcome. The young patient with FAI and nominal joint space narrowing has been shown to have a reduction of pain and improved function following hip arthroscopy.[83] Despite these findings, the dilemma arises as to when these patients would be better served by hip arthroscopy or arthroplasty referral. Consideration should take into account the degree of OA and preoperative symptoms in order to predict who may be best served by hip arthroscopy. There remain limited data, and further investigation is still needed to elucidate when OA can limit the success of hip arthroscopy.

THE LEARNING CURVE

One common critique of hip arthroscopy has been the technical difficulty and learning curve associated with the procedure.[84] Mastery of the procedure is often relegated to surgeons who have had specialty training in this area. As such, the Orthopaedic Residency Review Committee of the Accreditation Council for Graduate Medical Education has not recognized hip arthroscopy as a required competency, especially in light of relatively few academic centers that can provide such training. Still, hip arthroscopy remains technically demanding with outcomes inevitably affected by the level of training and experience of the surgeon. (See Figure 26-5.)

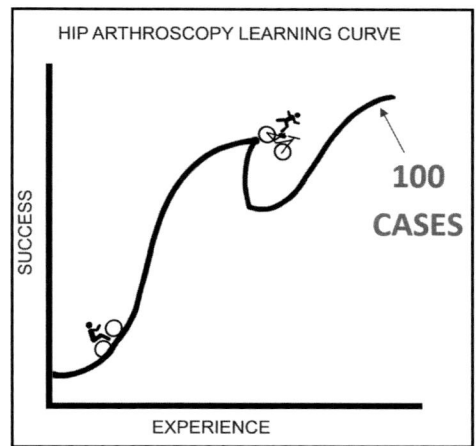

Figure 26-5.

A surgeon's experience has been linked to outcomes following hip arthroscopy.[6,85] Konan et al evaluated the first 100 hip arthroscopies performed by a single surgeon.[6] In subgroup analysis it was shown that there was an increase in complications of the first 30 patients compared to subsequent procedures, with the suggestion the learning curve was approximately 30 cases. Similarly, Lee et al showed that operation time and failure rates decreased significantly after the first 21 patients.[86] As such, it has been advocated that training should require a designated hip preservation fellowship, with exposure to high volumes of diverse hip pathology.[85] These reports mark decreased complications as part of the learning curve but do not address improved clinical outcomes as a measure of the learning process. We subscribe to the Malcom Gladwell notion of the "10,000 hour rule," which specifies that mastery of any subject requires extensive experience. This type of experience would allow for a better understanding of the utility and shortcomings of hip arthroscopy for individual patients.

The traditional model of education remains based upon the master-apprentice model in which trainees are given instruction by a senior surgeon.[87] In response, various alternative methods have been developed to improve the surgical skills of orthopedic trainees. Recent evidence has supported the use of surgical simulation in training orthopedic surgeons.[88] Various studies have shown the simulator model to be successful in skill development using arthroscopy models of the shoulder,[89] knee,[90] and wrist.[91] However, no study to date has evaluated a hip model for surgical simulation and whether this may be a viable option to training orthopedic surgeons outside the operating room. This can point to the need for further focus and research in providing high-quality training of hip arthroscopy to the next generation of orthopedic surgeons. As training experiences improve, highly skilled surgeons in hip arthroscopy may help to reduce these technical limitations associated with this procedure.

SUMMARY

The goal of treating hip disease in the young patient is to stave off the development of degenerative joint disease. As shown, hip arthroscopy has proven that it is a powerful tool to accomplish these means. The advent of navigation and robotics to improve outcomes and advances in chondral preservation are on the horizon. In addition, extra-articular causes of hip pain can also be addressed endoscopically, which may allow for less morbidity and faster recovery for the patient. Recognizing what the future holds also means identifying where the limitations currently lie. While problematic anatomic morphologies and progressive joint disease have shown limited success with arthroscopy, only limited data remain available. Nonetheless, the dynamic of hip preservation surgery has markedly evolved due to hip arthroscopy. The prospect of being involved in this rapidly growing field is enticing as we learn more on how best to optimize our results with hip arthroscopy.

SELECTED READINGS

Nawabi DH, Nam D, Park C, Ranawat AS. Hip arthroscopy: the use of computer assistance. *HSS J.* 2013;9(1):70-78.
  This review addresses the current status of navigation and robotic-assisted surgery within hip arthroscopy.
Bedi A, Chen N, Robertson W, Kelly BT. The management of labral tears and femoroacetabular impingement of the hip in the young, active patient. *Arthroscopy.* 2008;24(10):1135-1145.
  This systematic review addresses study outcomes related to hip arthroscopy in the young patient, focusing on clinical scores that show equivalence to historical to open procedures.

Montgomery SR, Ngo SS, Hobson T, et al. Trends and demographics in hip arthroscopy in the united states. *Arthroscopy.* 2013;29(4):661-665.
An epidemiological study that shows evidence of the recent surge of hip arthroscopy procedures being performed in the United States.

Byrd JWT, Jones KS. Prospective analysis of hip arthroscopy with 10-year followup. *Clin Orthop Relat Res.* 2010;468(3):741-746.
While few reports in the literature exist on long-term outcomes, this study substantiates the long-term effectiveness of hip arthroscopy at 10-year follow-up.

REFERENCES

1. Philippon MJ, Schenker ML, Briggs KK, Kuppersmith DA, Maxwell RB, Stubbs AJ. Revision hip arthroscopy. *Am J Sports Med.* 2007;35(11):1918-1921.
2. Heyworth BE, Shindle MK, Voos JE, Rudzki JR, Kelly BT. Radiologic and intraoperative findings in revision hip arthroscopy. *Arthroscopy.* 2007;23(12):1295-1302.
3. Leunig M, Beaule PE, Ganz R. The concept of femoroacetabular impingement: current status and future perspectives. *Clin Orthop Relat Res.* 2009;467(3):616-622.
4. Clohisy JC, Nunley RM, Otto RJ, Schoenecker PL. The frog-leg lateral radiograph accurately visualized hip cam impingement abnormalities. *Clin Orthop Relat Res.* 2007;462:115-121.
5. Kang RW, Yanke AB, Espinoza Orias AA, Inoue N, Nho SJ. Emerging ideas: novel 3-D quantification and classification of cam lesions in patients with femoroacetabular impingement. *Clin Orthop Relat Res.* 2013;471(2):358-362.
6. Konan S, Rhee SJ, Haddad FS. Hip arthroscopy: analysis of a single surgeon's learning experience. *J Bone Joint Surg Am.* 2011;93(suppl 2):52-56.
7. Nawabi DH, Nam D, Park C, Ranawat AS. Hip arthroscopy: the use of computer assistance. *HSS J.* 2013;9(1):70-78.
8. Cartiaux O, Paul L, Docquier PL, Raucent B, Dombre E, Banse X. Computer-assisted and robot-assisted technologies to improve bone-cutting accuracy when integrated with a freehand process using an oscillating saw. *J Bone Joint Surg Am.* 2010;92(11):2076-2082.
9. McCarthy JC, Jibodh SR, Lee JA. The role of arthroscopy in evaluation of painful hip arthroplasty. *Clin Orthop Relat Res.* 2009;467(1):174-180.
10. Lahner M, von Schulze Pellengahr C, Lichtinger TK, et al. The role of arthroscopy in patients with persistent hip pain after total hip arthroplasty. *Technol Health Care.* 2013;21(6):599-606.
11. Blitzer CM. Arthroscopic management of septic arthritis of the hip. *Arthroscopy.* 1993;9(4):414-416.
12. Yamamoto Y, Ide T, Hachisuka N, Maekawa S, Akamatsu N. Arthroscopic surgery for septic arthritis of the hip joint in 4 adults. *Arthroscopy.* 2001;17(3) 290-297.
13. Hyman JL, Salvati EA, Laurencin CT, Rogers DE, Maynard M, Brause DB. The arthroscopic drainage, irrigation, and debridement of late, acute total hip arthroplasty infections: average 6-year follow-up. *J Arthroplasty.* 1999;14(8):903-910.
14. Barrack RL, Harris WH. The value of aspiration of the hip joint before revision total hip arthroplasty. *J Bone Joint Surg Am.* 1993;75(1):66-76.
15. Mulcahy DM, Fenelon GC, McInerney DP. Aspiration arthrography of the hip joint. its uses and limitations in revision hip surgery. *J Arthroplasty.* 1996;11(1):64-68.
16. Muller M, Morawietz L, Hasart O, Strube P, Perka C, Tohtz S. Diagnosis of periprosthetic infection following total hip arthroplasty—evaluation of the diagnostic values of pre- and intraoperative parameters and the associated strategy to preoperatively select patients with a high probability of joint infection. *J Orthop Surg Res.* 2008;3:31.
17. Parvizi J, Adeli B, Zmistowski B, Restrepo C, Greenwald AS. Management of periprosthetic joint infection: The current knowledge: AAOS exhibit selection. *J Bone Joint Surg Am.* 2012;94(14):e104.
18. Shih LY, Wu JJ, Yang DJ. Erythrocyte sedimentation rate and C-reactive protein values in patients with total hip arthroplasty. *Clin Orthop Relat Res.* 1987;Dec(225):238-246.
19. Spangehl MJ, Masri BA, O'Connell JX, Duncan CP. Prospective analysis of preoperative and intraoperative investigations for the diagnosis of infection at the sites of two hundred and two revision total hip arthroplasties. *J Bone Joint Surg Am.* 1999;81(5):672-683.
20. Squire MW, Della Valle CJ, Parvizi J. Preoperative diagnosis of periprosthetic joint infection: role of aspiration. *AJR Am J Roentgenol.* 2011;196(4):875-879.
21. Berend KR, Lombardi AV Jr, Morris MJ, Bergeson AG, Adams JB, Sneller MA. Two-stage treatment of hip periprosthetic joint infection is associated with a high rate of infection control but high mortality. *Clin Orthop Relat Res.* 2013;471(2):510-518.
22. Alberton GM, High WA, Morrey BF. Dislocation after revision total hip arthroplasty: an analysis of risk factors and treatment options. *J Bone Joint Surg Am.* 2002;84-A(10):1788-1792.
23. van Diemen MP, Colen S, Dalemans AA, Stuyck J, Mulier M. Two-stage revision of an infected total hip arthroplasty: a follow-up of 136 patients. *Hip Int.* 2013;23(5):445-450.
24. Pandey R, Drakoulakis E, Athanasou NA. An assessment of the histological criteria used to diagnose infection in hip revision arthroplasty tissues. *J Clin Pathol.* 1999;52(2):118-123.
25. Pandey R, Berendt AR, Athanasou NA. Histological and microbiological findings in non-infected and infected revision arthroplasty tissues: the OSIRIS collaborative study group: Oxford Skeletal Infection Research and Intervention Service. *Arch Orthop Trauma Surg.* 2000;120(10):570-574.
26. Ross JR, Zaltz I, Nepple JJ, Schoenecker PL, Clohisy JC. Arthroscopic disease classification and interventions as an adjunct in the treatment of acetabular dysplasia. *Am J Sports Med.* 2011;39(suppl):72S-78S.
27. Sarban S, Baba F, Kocabey Y, Cengiz M, Isikan UE. Free nerve endings and morphological features of the ligamentum capitis femoris in developmental dysplasia of the hip. *J Pediatr Orthop B.* 2007;16(5):351-356.
28. Lindner D, Sharp KG, Trenga AP, Stone J, Stake CE, Domb BG. Arthroscopic ligamentum teres reconstruction. *Arthrosc Tech.* 2012;2(1):e21-e25.

29. Simpson JM, Field RE, Villar RN. Arthroscopic reconstruction of the ligamentum teres. *Arthroscopy.* 2011;27(3):436-441.
30. Philippon MJ, Pennock A, Gaskill TR. Arthroscopic reconstruction of the ligamentum teres: technique and early outcomes. *J Bone Joint Surg Br.* 2012;94(11):1494-1498.
31. Dierckman BD, Guanche CA. Endoscopic proximal hamstring repair and ischial bursectomy. *Arthrosc Tech.* 2012;1(2):e201-e207.
32. Voos JE, Rudzki JR, Shindle MK, Martin H, Kelly BT. Arthroscopic anatomy and surgical techniques for peritrochanteric space disorders in the hip. *Arthroscopy.* 2007;23(11):1246.e1-1246.e5.
33. McCormick F, Alpaugh K, Nwachukwu BU, Yanke AB, Martin SD. Endoscopic repair of full-thickness abductor tendon tears: surgical technique and outcome at minimum of 1-year follow-up. *Arthroscopy.* 2013;29(12):1941-1947.
34. Voos JE, Shindle MK, Pruett A, Asnis PD, Kelly BT. Endoscopic repair of gluteus medius tendon tears of the hip. *Am J Sports Med.* 2009;37(4):743-747.
35. Martin HD, Shears SA, Johnson JC, Smathers AM, Palmer IJ. The endoscopic treatment of sciatic nerve entrapment/deep gluteal syndrome. *Arthroscopy.* 2011;27(2):172-181.
36. Dezawa A, Kusano S, Miki H. Arthroscopic release of the piriformis muscle under local anesthesia for piriformis syndrome. *Arthroscopy.* 2003;19(5):554-557.
37. Reich MS, Shannon C, Tsai E, Salata MJ. Hip arthroscopy for extra-articular hip disease. *Curr Rev Musculoskelet Med.* 2013;6(3):250-257.
38. Domb BG, Shindle MK, McArthur B, Voos JE, Magennis EM, Kelly BT. Iliopsoas impingement: a newly identified cause of labral pathology in the hip. *HSS J.* 2011;7(2):145-150.
39. Philippon MJ, Schenker ML, Briggs KK, Maxwell RB. Can microfracture produce repair tissue in acetabular chondral defects? *Arthroscopy.* 2008;24(1):46-50.
40. Hart R, Janecek M, Visna P, Bucek P, Kocis J. Mosaicplasty for the treatment of femoral head defect after incorrect resorbable screw insertion. *Arthroscopy.* 2003;19(10):E1-E5.
41. Girard J, Roumazeille T, Sakr M, Migaud H. Osteochondral mosaicplasty of the femoral head. *Hip Int.* 2011;21(5):542-548.
42. Krych AJ, Lorich DG, Kelly BT. Treatment of focal osteochondral defects of the acetabulum with osteochondral allograft transplantation. *Orthopedics.* 2011;34(7):e307-e311.
43. Fontana A, Bistolfi A, Crova M, Rosso F, Massazza G. Arthroscopic treatment of hip chondral defects: autologous chondrocyte transplantation versus simple debridement—a pilot study. *Arthroscopy.* 2012;28(3):322-329.
44. Montgomery SR, Ngo SS, Hobson T, et al. Trends and demographics in hip arthroscopy in the United States. *Arthroscopy.* 2013;29(4):661-665.
45. Bedi A, Chen N, Robertson W, Kelly BT. The management of labral tears and femoroacetabular impingement of the hip in the young, active patient. *Arthroscopy.* 2008;24(10):1135-1145.
46. Ito K, Leunig M, Ganz R. Histopathologic features of the acetabular labrum in femoroacetabular impingement. *Clin Orthop Relat Res.* 2004;(429):262-271.
47. Meyers MH. Resurfacing of the femoral head with fresh osteochondral allografts: long-term results. *Clin Orthop Relat Res.* 1985;(197)(197):111-114.
48. Evans KN, Providence BC. Case report: fresh-stored osteochondral allograft for treatment of osteochondritis dissecans the femoral head. *Clin Orthop Relat Res.* 2010;468(2):613-618.
49. Akimau P, Bhosale A, Harrison PE, et al. Autologous chondrocyte implantation with bone grafting for osteochondral defect due to posttraumatic osteonecrosis of the hip—a case report. *Acta Orthop.* 2006;77(2):333-336.
50. Nam D, Shindle MK, Buly RL, Kelly BT, Lorich DG. Traumatic osteochondral injury of the femoral head treated by mosaicplasty: a report of two cases. *HSS J.* 2010;6(2):228-234.
51. Haviv B, Singh PJ, Takla A, O'Donnell J. Arthroscopic femoral osteochondroplasty for cam lesions with isolated acetabular chondral damage. *J Bone Joint Surg Br.* 2010;92(5):629-633.
52. Karthikeyan S, Roberts S, Griffin D. Microfracture for acetabular chondral defects in patients with femoroacetabular impingement: results at second-look arthroscopic surgery. *Am J Sports Med.* 2012;40(12):2725-2730.
53. Stafford GH, Bunn JR, Villar RN. Arthroscopic repair of delaminated acetabular articular cartilage using fibrin adhesive: results at one to three years. *Hip Int.* 2011;21(6):744-750.
54. El Bitar YF, Lindner D, Jackson TJ, Domb BG. Joint-preserving surgical options for management of chondral injuries of the hip. *J Am Acad Orthop Surg.* 2014;22(1):46-56.
55. Safran MR, Epstein NP. Arthroscopic management of protrusio acetabuli. *Arthroscopy.* 2013;29(11):1777-1782.
56. Tannast M, Leunig M, Session Participants. Report of breakout session: coxa profunda/protrusio management. *Clin Orthop Relat Res.* 2012;470(12):3459-3461.
57. Siebenrock KA, Wahab KH, Werlen S, Kalhor M, Leunig M, Ganz R. Abnormal extension of the femoral head epiphysis as a cause of cam impingement. *Clin Orthop Relat Res.* 2004;(418):54-60.
58. McCormick F, Kleweno CP, Kim YJ, Martin SD. Vascular safe zones in hip arthroscopy. *Am J Sports Med.* 2011;39(suppl):64S-71S.
59. Boykin RE, Patterson D, Briggs KK, Dee A, Philippon MJ. Results of arthroscopic labral reconstruction of the hip in elite athletes. *Am J Sports Med.* 2013;41(10):2296-2301.
60. Park MS, Yoon SJ, Choi SM. Hip arthroscopic management for femoral head fractures and posterior acetabular wall fractures (Pipkin type IV). *Arthrosc Tech.* 2013;2(3):e221-e225.
61. Lansford T, Munns SW. Arthroscopic treatment of pipkin type I femoral head fractures: a report of 2 cases. *J Orthop Trauma.* 2012;26(7):e94-e96.
62. Matsuda DK. A rare fracture, an even rarer treatment: the arthroscopic reduction and internal fixation of an isolated femoral head fracture. *Arthroscopy.* 2009;25(4):408-412.
63. Kim H, Baek JH, Park SM, Ha YC. Arthroscopic reduction and internal fixation of acetabular fractures. *Knee Surg Sports Traumatol Arthrosc.* 2014;22(4):867-870.
64. Fraitzl CR, Kafer W, Nelitz M, Reichel H. Radiological evidence of femoroacetabular impingement in mild slipped capital femoral epiphysis: a mean follow-up of 14.4 years after pinning in situ. *J Bone Joint Surg Br.* 2007;89(12):1592-1596.
65. Goodman DA, Feighan JE, Smith AD, Latimer B, Buly RL, Cooperman DR. Subclinical slipped capital femoral epiphysis: relationship to osteoarthrosis of the hip. *J Bone Joint Surg Am.* 1997;79(10):1489-1497.
66. Murray RO, Duncan C. Athletic activity in adolescence as an etiological factor in degenerative hip disease. *J Bone Joint Surg Br.* 1971;53(3):406-419.

67. Siebenrock KA, Ferner F, Noble PC, Santore RF, Werlen S, Mamisch TC. The cam-type deformity of the proximal femur arises in childhood in response to vigorous sporting activity. *Clin Orthop Relat Res*. 2011;469(11):3229-3240.
68. Carsen S, Moroz PJ, Rakhra K, et al. The Otto Aufranc award on the etiology of the cam deformity: a cross-sectional pediatric MRI study. *Clin Orthop Relat Res*. 2014;472(2):430-436.
69. Abraham E, Gonzalez MH, Pratap S, Amirouche F, Atluri P, Simon P. Clinical implications of anatomical wear characteristics in slipped capital femoral epiphysis and primary osteoarthritis. *J Pediatr Orthop*. 2007;27(7):788-795.
70. Leunig M, Casillas MM, Hamlet M, et al. Slipped capital femoral epiphysis: early mechanical damage to the acetabular cartilage by a prominent femoral metaphysis. *Acta Orthop Scand*. 2000;71(4):370-375.
71. Sink EL, Zaltz I, Heare T, Dayton M. Acetabular cartilage and labral damage observed during surgical hip dislocation for stable slipped capital femoral epiphysis. *J Pediatr Orthop*. 2010;30(1):26-30.
72. Larson CM, Giveans MR. Arthroscopic management of femoroacetabular impingement: early outcomes measures. *Arthroscopy*. 2008;24(5):540-546.
73. Leunig M, Horowitz K, Manner H, Ganz R. In situ pinning with arthroscopic osteoplasty for mild SCFE: a preliminary technical report. *Clin Orthop Relat Res*. 2010;468(12):3160-3167.
74. Laude F, Sariali E, Nogier A. Femoroacetabular impingement treatment using arthroscopy and anterior approach. *Clin Orthop Relat Res*. 2009;467(3):747-752.
75. Ayeni OR, Bedi A, Lorich DG, Kelly BT. Femoral neck fracture after arthroscopic management of femoroacetabular impingement: a case report. *J Bone Joint Surg Am*. 2011;93(9):e47.
76. Mardones RM, Gonzalez C, Chen Q, Zobitz M, Kaufman KR, Trousdale RT. Surgical treatment of femoroacetabular impingement: evaluation of the effect of the size of the resection. *J Bone Joint Surg Am*. 2005;87(2):273-279.
77. Azegami S, Kosuge D, Ramachandran M. Surgical treatment of femoroacetabular impingement in patients with slipped capital femoral epiphysis: a review of current surgical techniques. *Bone Joint J*. 2013;95-B(4):445-451.
78. Freeman CR, Jones K, Byrd JW. Hip arthroscopy for Legg-Calvé-Perthes disease: minimum 2-year follow-up. *Arthroscopy*. 2013;29(4):666-674.
79. Byrd JWT, Jones KS. Prospective analysis of hip arthroscopy with 10-year followup. *Clin Orthop Relat Res*. 2010;468(3):741-746.
80. McCarthy JC, Jarrett BT, Ojeifo O, Lee JA, Bragdon CR. What factors influence long-term survivorship after hip arthroscopy? *Clin Orthop Relat Res*. 2011;469(2):362-371.
81. Farjo LA, Glick JM, Sampson TG. Hip arthroscopy for acetabular labral tears. *Arthroscopy*. 1999;15(2):132-137.
82. Clohisy JC, St John LC, Schutz AL. Surgical treatment of femoroacetabular impingement: a systematic review of the literature. *Clin Orthop Relat Res*. 2010;468(2):555-564.
83. Larson CM, Giveans MR, Taylor M. Does arthroscopic FAI correction improve function with radiographic arthritis? *Clin Orthop Relat Res*. 2011;469(6):1667-1676.
84. Zaltz I, Kelly BT, Larson CM, Leunig M, Bedi A. Surgical treatment of femoroacetabular impingement: what are the limits of hip arthroscopy? *Arthroscopy*. 2014;30(1):99-110.
85. Mei-Dan O. Hip preservation: reality check on training. *Orthopedics*. 2013;36(4):244-245.
86. Lee YK, Ha YC, Hwang DS, Koo KH. Learning curve of basic hip arthroscopy technique: CUSUM analysis. *Knee Surg Sports Traumatol Arthrosc*. 2013;21(8):1940-1944.
87. Engels PT, de Gara C. Learning styles of medical students, general surgery residents, and general surgeons: implications for surgical education. *BMC Med Educ*. 2010;10:51.
88. Atesok K, Mabrey JD, Jazrawi LM, Egol KA. Surgical simulation in orthopaedic skills training. *J Am Acad Orthop Surg*. 2012;20(7):410-422.
89. Gomoll AH, Pappas G, Forsythe B, Warner JJ. Individual skill progression on a virtual reality simulator for shoulder arthroscopy: a 3-year follow-up study. *Am J Sports Med*. 2008;36(6):1139-1142.
90. Martin KD, Belmont PJ, Schoenfeld AJ, Todd M, Cameron KL, Owens BD. Arthroscopic basic task performance in shoulder simulator model correlates with similar task performance in cadavers. *J Bone Joint Surg Am*. 2011;93(21):e1271-e1275.
91. Obdeijn MC, Bavinck N, Mathoulin C, van der Horst CM, Schijven MP, Tuijthof GJ. Education in wrist arthroscopy: past, present and future. *Knee Surg Sports Traumatol Arthrosc*. 2015;23(5):1337-1345.

27

complex **core-hip** considerations in the athlete

from "lighting the lamp" to "getting your face washed"

MARC J. PHILIPPON, MD
WILLIAM R. MOOK, MD
KAREN K. BRIGGS, MPH

Editor's Note: *It seems fair to say that co-editor Marc Philippon has long been regarded as the most important innovator in hip arthroscopy. Marc sits high on top of this specialty's mountain and sees many things before others. As a result, he has operated on many high-level athletes and other famous people. I asked Marc to write about the intricacies of hip arthroscopy. Marc's research director and fellow join him as co-authors.*

There is no such thing as a routine diagnosis.

—Marc J. Philippon, MD.

Please forgive all the ice hockey parallels in this section. I can't help it. I love the sport, and I love taking care of many of the sport's players. Their lingo has become part of my nature.

In that vein, the main goal in this chapter is to avoid bumps, fights, and distractions and to score more goals than our opponents. Our opponents in the hip joint are all the factors that contribute to the symptoms of femoroacetabular impingement (FAI). We need to do whatever it takes to score goals against that bad anatomy.

Making an accurate diagnosis of FAI may sometimes seem easy, and treating it through the scope is as straightforward as lighting the lamp (Figure 27-1). That phrase refers to a red light flashing, whenever the siren sounds, to indicate that someone has scored a goal. In the eyes of young professional ice hockey players, all goals are "easy."

The same thing basically holds for new hip arthroscopists. Once one has developed the tools and training to arthroscope hips, correcting hip impingement usually seems easy. Both the young professional hockey players and young arthroscopists are wrong. Rarely are things as straightforward as they seem.

Just as Tom Byrd pointed out in an earlier chapter, the improved understanding of the pathophysiology, anatomy, and natural history of FAI is all a recent phenomenon. Our new understanding has led already to improved outcomes and novel arthroscopic techniques. Yet, we remain still very much within a learning phase with respect to our knowledge base. Therefore, unavoidable surgical pitfalls still leave many patients in need for revision surgery.

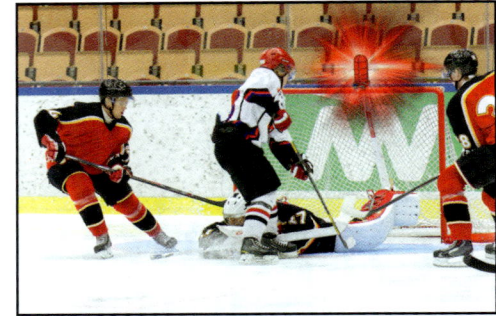

Figure 27-1. Lighting the lamp.

The second ice hockey idiom—getting your face washed (Figure 27-2)—refers both to ice hockey and hip arthroscopy. In hockey, the expression means being taken into the boards by an opponent and having that player's sweaty, smelly hockey glove rubbed all over your face. The same holds for hip arthroscopy, only the opponent is the player's seemingly straightforward bad hip anatomy.

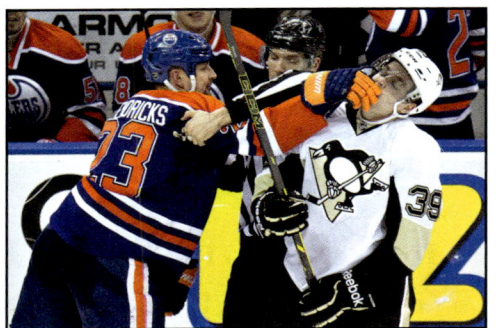

Figure 27-2. Getting your face washed. (Reprinted with permission from AP Photo/Canadian Press, Jason Franson.)

This chapter will do 3 things:
1. Expand on Dr. Reinhold Ganz's initial description of FAI
2. Review the diagnosis and treatment of FAI as we understand it today
3. Connect some of this current understanding to other parts of the core and its potential muscular imbalances

We will try to keep this chapter as simple and straightforward as possible. We shall share some illustrative clinical examples from the world of sports. We shall also provide what we think is a pretty reasonable treatment algorithm for the evaluation and treatment of patients with continued pain and/or dysfunction following hip arthroscopy. Finally, we shall hone in on what may be an important target for FAI prevention.

A good hockey player plays where the puck is.
A great hockey player plays where the puck is going to be.

—Wayne Gretzky. Nicknamed "The Great One," Gretzky had more goals and assists than any other player in NHL history.

HIP INJURY DURING SPRING TRAINING

In parallel with Dr. Meyers's experience with core muscle injuries and his prior description of a prominent quarterback, we have been dealing with many elite professional athletes suffering from un- or misdiagnosed injuries in the region of the hip. Let us tell you about one baseball star who came to us in the middle of spring training (Figure 27-3).

This elite slugger was referred for evaluation of his groin pain that prevented him from turning effectively on pitches. He could not hit the ball with full strength and described "hip weakness and tightness." The pain was hurting his performance. Such vague but real complaints are all too common in today's competitive athlete. In years past, without high-resolution diagnostic imaging and the option of predictable success with minimally invasive treatment, the radiographic findings of FAI and a labral tear usually went unnoticed and untreated.

Fortunately, this elite athlete's all-star team of coaches, trainers, and doctors recognized the reason for his declining performance. The team had the foresight to recognize "where the puck was going to be," prior to irreversible damage to his joint, and referred him for treatment.

Complex Core-Hip Considerations in the Athlete—From "Lighting the Lamp" to "Getting Your Face Washed"

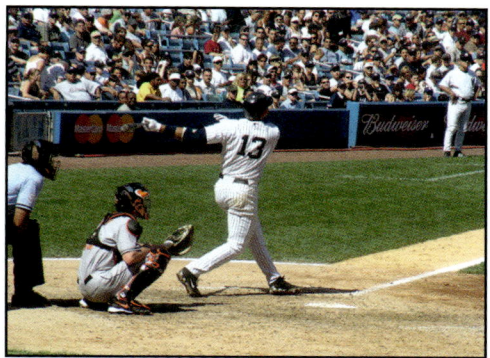

Figure 27-3. New York Yankee Alex Rodriguez hitting a home run during spring training.

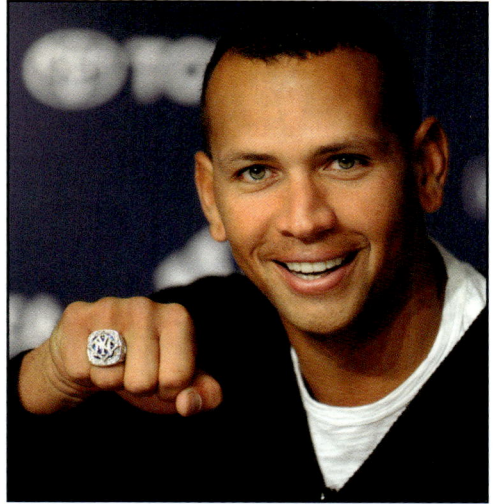

Figure 27-4. Alex Rodriguez with his 2009 World Series ring. (Reprinted with permission from AP Photo/Bill Kostroun.)

Often, it takes 5 to 6 months to recover from such surgery. This future Hall-of-Famer lit the lamp. With the bony impingement and labral tear addressed, he made a full recovery and returned the same season and helped lead his team to a World Series championship (Figure 27-4).[1-3]

The most common sports hip problem is FAI, which comes, literally, in all shapes and forms. We see athletes, and nonathletes, from all over the world, and I remain amazed at how much we continue to learn and how much we still need to learn. FAI remains in its infancy with respect to our understanding of its pathophysiology and natural history. We know much more about short- and medium-term consequences.

SEEING WHERE THE PUCK WAS GOING

Wayne Gretzky's famous quotation describes my friend and colleague, Reinhold Ganz, the world's top expert in hip preservation. Reinhold, still Professor Emeritus at the University of Bern, had eyes that no one else had. Dr. Ganz watched from behind the net, just like Gretzky, and recognized "where the puck was going to be." He saw the various femoral and acetabular shapes most likely associated with soft tissue labral tears and subsequent arthritis.[4,5] Dr. Ganz went even further and described FAI as a distinct clinical syndrome that was determined by the bony architecture of the hip.

He asserted, basically, that action at a certain anatomic site placed individuals at great risk for arthritis: the abutment of the acetabular rim (ie, hip socket) against the femoral head-neck junction.[4-6] He described several distinct subtypes of FAI. He referred to abnormalities of the acetabulum as *pincer* deformities, and those of the femoral head or neck as *cam* deformities. Then, of course, there were deformities at both the acetabulum and femur, which he called the *mixed-type* FAI (Figure 27-5).

With the cam deformity, there is a bony prominence or "bump" of the proximal femoral head-neck junction. The bump prematurely engages the acetabulum during hip flexion. This contact is what leads to shearing there between the articular cartilage of the femur and the fibrocartilaginous labrum. Damage occurs to either the articular cartilage or the labrum or both. Both cam-type and pincer-type impingements may cause groin pain and disability in young adults, and particularly those who participate in athletic activities. Unquestionably, the deformities combined with the bony contact may predispose patients to osteoarthritis.[7,8]

In addition to my personal experience, several authors have also noted that a large percentage of patients with cam, pincer, and mixed-type FAI bony abnormalities also tend to develop changes of global joint degeneration at a relatively young age.[9-11] Dr. Ganz's appreciation of these bony abnormalities as a definite source of articular cartilage and labral damage, and possible cause of hip osteoarthritis, have paved the way for the development of the diagnostic and treatment technologies that have led to our current understanding of FAI.

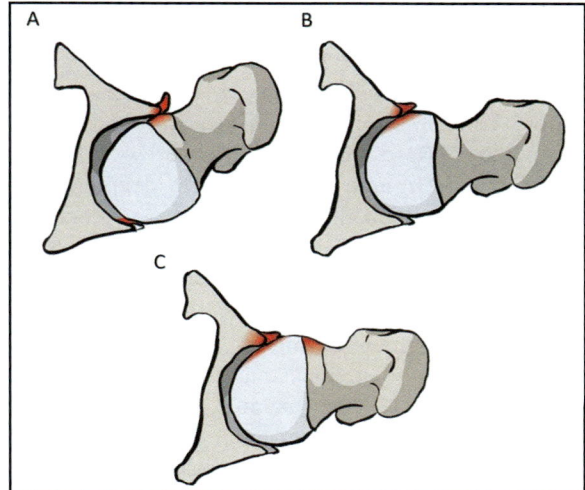

Figure 27-5. Types of FAI. (A) Pincer: Overhang of the acetabulum pinches against the femur. (B) Cam: Femoral head-neck bump pinches against the acetabulum. (C) Mixed-type. (Adapted from Leunig M, Ganz R. FAI—concept and etiology. *Orthopade*. 2009;38[5]:394-401.)

I am going to be ambitious with this chapter and try to accomplish 6 things:
1. Expand on Dr. Ganz's initial description of FAI
2. Correlate the pathology of FAI to other parts of the core, particularly the core muscles and back
3. Kibitz on our current concepts about the diagnosis and management of FAI
4. Share several cases that illustrate particular diagnostic and/or treatment challenges
5. Propose an algorithm for evaluation and treatment of patients with continued or new dysfunction following hip arthroscopy
6. Theorize about where we want "the puck to be" (ie, I will present a hypothesis aimed at preventing FAI, ideally the ultimate goal for all well-meaning arthroscopic scientists)

Wow, I am exhausted already. That was the longest sentence I've ever written!

THE WAY IT WAS

The concept of FAI dates back to 1936,[12] not long after Burman first introduced arthroscopic surgery in the hip.[13] Abnormal bony features of the hip were not associated with cartilage injury and the early onset of osteoarthritis until the 1960s and 1970s. Murray and Stulberg were the first to describe an abnormal relationship between the femoral head-neck junction in patients with unexplained early arthritis of the hip.[14,15] They coined the terms *head tilt* and *pistol grip* deformities of the proximal femur. Although forward thinking, they did not offer an explanation as to how the abnormal radiographic bony features of the hip led to cartilage injury and later joint degeneration.

It wasn't until the 1990s when Dr. Ganz and his colleagues theorized that decreased clearance of the femoral head-neck at the bony socket led to pathologic contact of the 2 surfaces. Repetitive abutment of the neck against the acetabular rim, in turn, led to labral and articular cartilage shearing, ending up in joint degeneration. Ganz's group also was the first to act preemptively on the proposed abnormal anatomic relationship. They attempted to correct it surgically.

Consider the hip joint a highly congruent ball-and-socket joint buried deep within an environment of muscular, ligamentous, capsular, and neurovascular structures where complex dynamic interactions allow for amazing athletic feats. Historically, this complex anatomy struck fear with respect to accessing the hip joint surgically. Traditional open surgical approaches appeared invasive and associated with potential complications. Additionally, the proximal femur has a complex vascular anatomy that might be disrupted. So, even though surgeons, like Murray and Stulberg, were able to see the bony impingement abnormalities associated with cartilage injuries, surgical correction of the abnormalities was another matter. Safe surgical repair seemed a pipe dream. Native hip anatomy posed a substantial obstacle.

Then Ganz and his colleagues fastidiously characterized the vessels that maintained the integrity of the femoral head and neck.[16] For example, the lateral epiphyseal vessels of the medial femoral circumflex artery were important. In the setting of a traumatic hip dislocation or fracture, damage to those vessels would starve the articular surface of the nutrients it needs, and the hip would undergo the dreaded degenerative process called *avascular necrosis*.

An open surgical technique then emerged, based on the vascular anatomy described by Ganz. The technique involved exposure of the hip joint by dislocating the ball and socket. This allowed anterior exposure of the hip joint by cutting through bone (ie, osteotomy), so as to preserve the medial femoral circumflex artery, the main blood supply of the femoral head.[17] The technique permitted a 360-degree view of the femoral head and neck and acetabular socket. With this exposure, surgeons could eliminate the bony or other abnormalities causing impingement and also create freer motion. With his excellent results, Ganz convinced others that the pain and other symptoms of hip impingement could be relieved. Possibly, they could even prevent further joint space narrowing, particularly if the problem was recognized early and addressed prior to the development of severe hip joint osteoarthritis.[18]

The development of minimally invasive arthroscopic techniques in the hip lagged behind the developments in other joints due to these obvious anatomic limitations. Although the first report of a clinical application for hip arthroscopy was presented in 1939 by Takagi,[19] it wasn't until the late 1970s and 1980s that the technique re-emerged as a viable option for the treatment of intra-articular disorders. Dr. James Glick, in San Francisco, should be credited with popularizing hip arthroscopy and providing the foundation in the late 1980s. He paved the way for modern hip arthroscopists and the techniques developed in North America.[20,21] Thomas Byrd then essentially redefined how hip surgeons should approach the hip arthroscopically and popularized the supine approach, which is the one most utilized.[22] Technological advancements and techniques of hip arthroscopy have swiftly accelerated since the early 1990s.

The minimally invasive nature of hip arthroscopy delivers valuable advantages, such as minimal morbidity, fast recovery, and quicker return to sport or other normal activities. It affords the same 360-degree access to the femoral head, neck, and acetabular socket as surgical hip dislocation. Modern hip arthroscopy greatly expanded the practical applications of a whole new therapy envisioned by Dr. Ganz, who had the new eyes and set the foundation. Modern surgeons now help numerous young people, and some older ones, who have the condition we call FAI. Recovery from surgery is probably faster than Ganz initially conceived, and elite athletes can return to their pre-injury levels of play after numerous nonoperative measures have been tried.

THE WAY IT IS

The ball-in-socket hip joint does not exist in isolation. It is part of the core—the whole region of the body from the mid-chest to the mid-thighs. The core, as we define it, includes everything in this region of the body. For convenience, we divide it into the 4 parts outlined in an earlier chapter: the back, the core muscles and rest of the pelvic bones, the hip, and then everything else—all the organ systems, nerves, blood vessels, etc.

The advances in our arthroscopic technology and techniques for treating disorders of the hip joint over the past decade are remarkable, and it is amazing how much we can do now within that narrow space called the hip. But we should also recognize that our understanding of the relationship between the dynamic and static stabilizers of the core, hip, and lower extremity is expanding and that this is critical to the evaluation and treatment of the athlete with pain about the pelvis and the pelvis's many articulations. The primary point is to remember that as we focus more on the pathology in the ball-in-socket hip joint, hip injuries rarely occur only there, in isolation. To understand fully why many hip injuries occur, the relationship between the hip and rest of the core must be more fully appreciated.

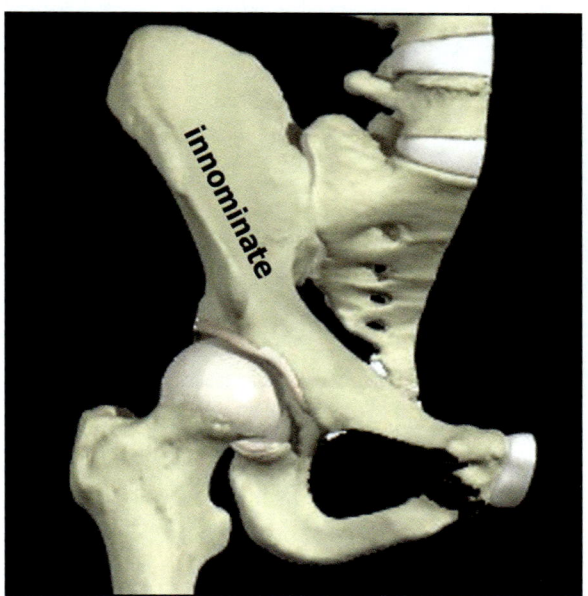

Figure 27-6. The hemi-pelvis or innominate bone provides the physical connection between the spine and the lower extremities.

For starters, think about this. Each bony hemipelvis, or innominate bone, provides the physical connection between the spine and both lower extremities, via the sacroiliac joints and the pubic symphysis, respectively. Each innominate bone of the pelvis also contains the acetabulum (ie, hip socket), which provides the proximal bony articulation for each hip joint (Figure 27-6). The position of the pelvis relative to the lower extremities is a result of the interplay between its inherent bony architecture and the forces that act on it in the form of muscular attachments.

Pelvic Tilt

The position of the pelvis relative to the lower extremity is often objectively quantified radiographically by a measurement referred to as *pelvic tilt*. Pelvic tilt is my (MJP) pet venture into understanding how the hip interacts with the rest of the core. As I see it, in his chapter, Thomas Byrd identified 4 likely important, contributing extra-articular anatomic factors involved in FAI: the core muscles, lumbar lordosis/kyphosis, femoral version, and pelvic orientation. Based on my biases, I have chosen a specific type of pelvic orientation, pelvic tilt, on which to focus a fair amount of my attention.

Basically, I see 2 different ways to understand pelvic tilt. One way is to think of the pelvic bones tilting forward or backward compared to the spine (Figure 27-7A). An angle is created between a horizontal line connecting the anterior superior iliac spine (ASIS) and the sacrum, and a line connecting the ASIS with the PSIS (posterior superior iliac spine). Consequently, the hip gets involved via the acetabulum, which is part of the pelvis. The second way is to get the hip more "actively" involved in the definition (Figure 27-7B). Pelvic tilt then becomes essentially a radiographic parameter defined as the angle between a line extending from the middle of the first sacral endplate to the center of the femoral head and a vertical plumb line on a lateral view of the pelvis.[23,24]

Emerging evidence seems to demonstrate that pelvic tilt can be dynamically altered by the activity of surrounding core musculature and by the lower extremity.[25-28] Associated factors likely play significant roles in the predispositions of the hip joint for the bony impingement of FAI. Ross and colleagues studied the effect of pelvic tilt on hip range of motion. The location of bony contact changes when the pelvic orientation (ie, tilt) is made to alter, either anteriorly or posteriorly.

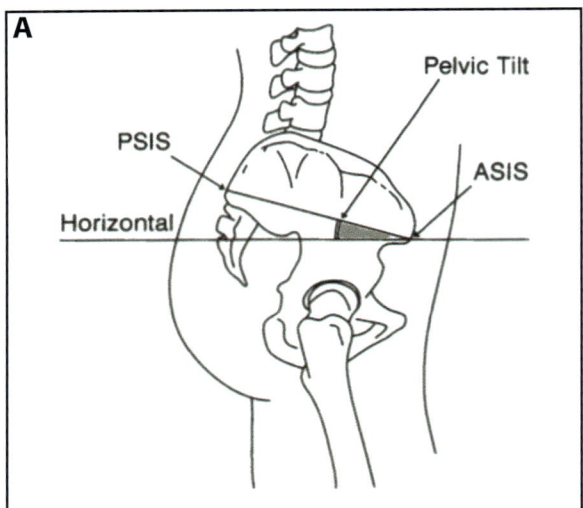 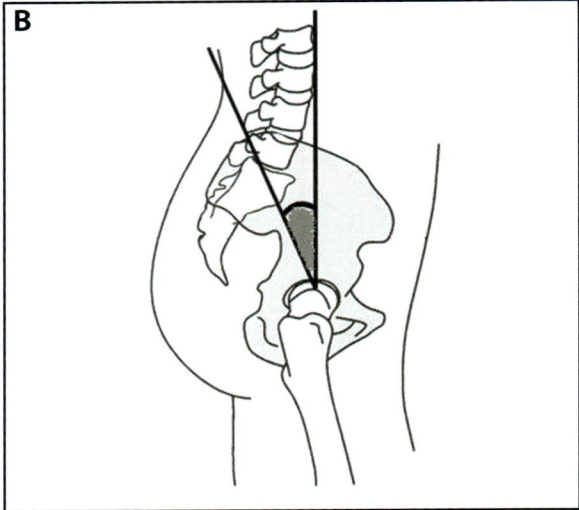

Figure 27-7. Two ways to think about pelvic tilt. (A) An angle between a horizontal line through the ASIS and sacrum compared to one between the ASIS and PSIS. (Adapted from Levine D, Whittle MW. The effects of pelvic movement on lumbar lordosis in the standing position. *J Orthop Sports Phys Ther.* 1996;243:130-135.) (B) Angle between a line through the femoral head and the middle of the first sacral endplate and a vertical plumb line in front of the lumbar vertebrae.

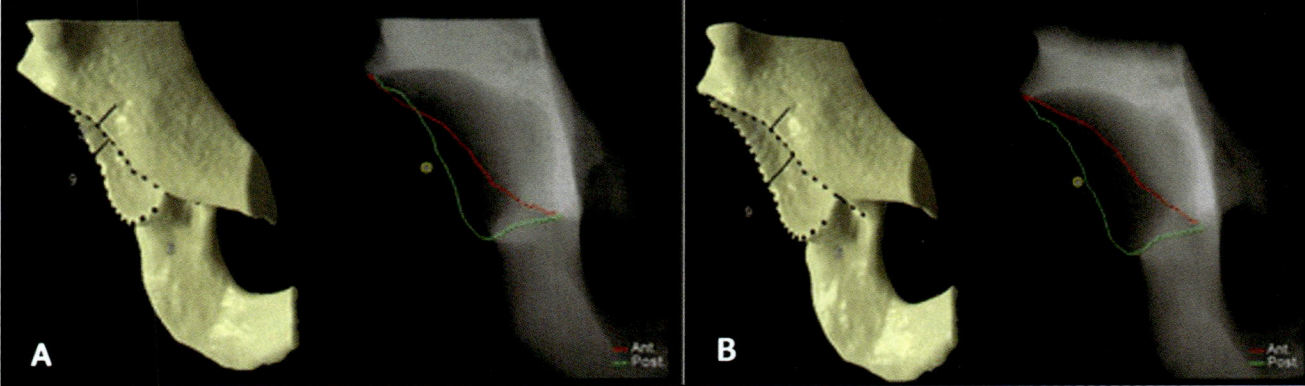

Figure 27-8. It is important to realize that the subject of pelvic tilt is complicated and needs more study. Anterior tilt exacerbates FAI. In this experimental model, a slight (10-degree) anterior change in pelvic tilt (A) resulted in a significant increase in the retroversion (ie, posterior orientation) of the acetabulum vs neutral alignment (B). In turn, this alteration resulted in an earlier occurrence of bony impingement during femoral flexion and internal rotation. Look at the red and green lines and how they cross or not. These changes are subtle but real. Certainly, these effects are important. We need to know more about them.

They utilized a 3-dimensional computer simulation based on preoperative radiographs in patients with FAI anatomy.[29] A 10-degree anterior change in pelvic tilt (Figure 27-8) resulted in a significant increase in the retroversion (ie, posterior orientation) of the acetabulum. In turn, this alteration resulted in an earlier occurrence of bony impingement during femoral flexion and internal rotation. Conversely, with 10 degrees of posterior tilt change, impingement between the acetabulum and femoral neck occurred later in "arc susceptible motion" of the hip (Figure 27-9).

Ross's findings have profound implications in terms of the potential for nonsurgical intervention to improve impingement-free range of motion of the hip. For example, normal running involves 15 to 20 degrees of anterior pelvic tilt. The normal range can vary by as much as 5 to 7 degrees between asymptomatic individuals.[30,31] Most people become more anteriorly tilted as their running speeds increase.[31] Ross's data imply that small dynamic changes in posterior pelvic tilt during that activity, by altering the neuromuscular control of the pelvis, should, theoretically, target less bony impingement even when the bony anatomy of FAI deformities is present.[32] If the theory holds, deleterious effects on impingement-free motion must be caused by imbalances in the core muscle groups responsible for both anterior pelvic tilt, such as the iliopsoas, erector spinae, and rectus femoris muscles, **and** posterior pelvic tilt, such as the rectus abdominis, abdominal obliques, gluteus maximus, and hamstrings.

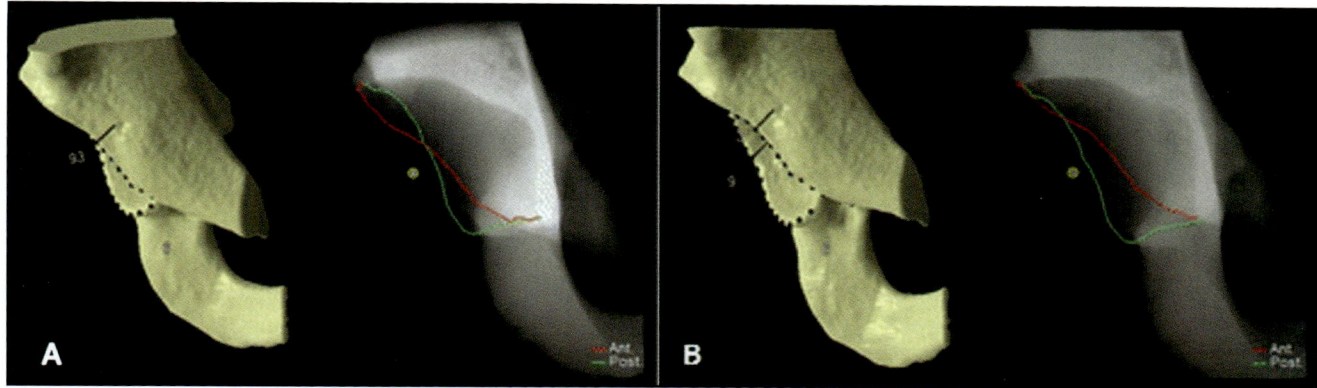

Figure 27-9. Again, be ready for subtle differences. Posterior tilt lessens FAI. In this experimental model, a slight (10-degree) posterior tilt change (A), impingement between the acetabulum and femoral neck occurred later in "arc susceptible motion" of the hip vs neutral alignment (B). Look at the red and green lines and how they cross or not. Again, these changes are subtle but real.

To carry the theory even further, such imbalances can become manifest in the form of muscle contractures, iliopsoas dysorientations,[33] the acute or chronic core muscle harness (see Chapter 8) injuries of the syndromes formerly called *athletic pubalgia*,[34] or simply sport-specific adaptations favorable for optimal performance. While those adaptations favor performance, they also place FAI anatomically susceptible individuals at risk for repetitive abutment.[35] Therefore, it might be critical to evaluate fully and possibly train the lumbar spine muscles and pubic attachment muscles in certain ways depending on the specific FAI anatomy. These conceptual issues have got to be real. The pathologic entities involving the hip and core muscles are so clinically interrelated. As our understanding these complex dynamic relationships evolve, nonsurgical pelvic tilt strategies have got to form the basis for nonsurgical treatment of FAI.

Current Concepts About Femoroacetabular Impingement

No doubt, muscular injuries or imbalances predispose an athlete to FAI symptoms. The underlying bony anatomy is what ultimately leads to limitations in motion and subsequent labral and articular cartilage injuries. Therefore, let's go through, in some more detail, the various bony abnormalities that lead to FAI. (See Table 27-1.)

Table 27-1
The Morphologic Variations of the Femur and Acetabulum That Lead to Femoroacetabular Impingement

Morphologic Variations of the Femur	Morphologic Variations of the Acetabulum
• Cam • Femoral version	• Pincer • Acetabular version • Pelvic tilt • Dysplasia

No one has elucidated the reasons for these bony abnormalities. Likely they occur primarily as either a developmental disorder **or** as secondary responses to abnormal stresses during or after adolescence **or** as a combination of those 2 factors. Regardless of the primary etiology, impingement anatomy does lead to injury to the acetabular labrum[36] and articular cartilage,[6] as well as changes of the head-neck shape.[37]

Our clinical experience over the past 2 decades with arthroscopic management of FAI includes both young[38] and mature athletes,[39,40] as well as recreational[41] and elite professional athletes.[42,43] We have found that when the patients' histories and physical findings correlate with their radiographic abnormalities, then arthroscopic corrections of their bony abnormalities, combined with labral repair, lead to a predictable improvements in their symptoms and return to preinjury activity or sports participation levels.

Clinical Presentation and Exam

The symptoms of a patient with FAI may be acute or chronic. Notwithstanding the duration of symptoms, the most common complaint is anterior groin pain exacerbated by hip flexion, internal rotation, and/or abduction. Sitting for long periods of time and steep inclines often aggravate the symptoms of FAI.

Physical examination begins with evaluation of the patient's gait, and subsequently includes palpation, assessment of his/her range of motion, isometric strength, neurovascular structures, and concludes with special, provocative tests. Over recent years, we have learned to be especially cognizant of coexisting core muscle problems and lumbar pathology that may occur in association with the intra-articular causes of pain that are our focus. Patients with FAI often have restricted internal rotation, external rotation, flexion, extension, and abduction.[44] Our special provocative tests include the following.

- **Anterior impingement test (Figure 27-10):** The hip is placed in a position of 90-degree passive hip flexion and maximally internally rotated. This test is positive if the patient's pain symptoms are reproduced.[45]
- **Posterior impingement test (Figure 27-11):** With the pelvis stabilized, the femur is brought into a position of extension and external rotation. This test is positive if pain is reproduced or range of motion is decreased.[45]
- **FABER distance test (Figure 27-12):** The hip is placed in a position of flexion-abduction-external rotation, and the distance from the knee to the table is measured and compared to the other extremity. Patients with restricted motion are at higher risk of symptoms from cam impingement.

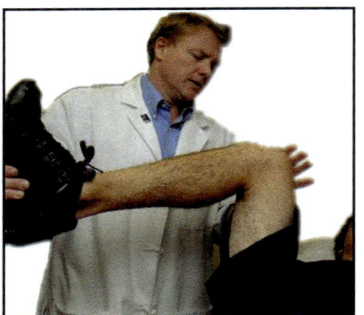

Figure 27-10. Anterior impingement test.

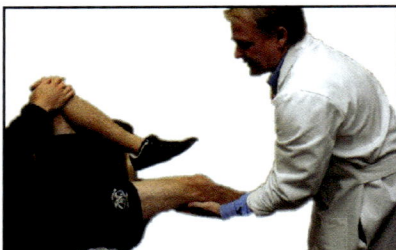

Figure 27-11. Posterior impingement test.

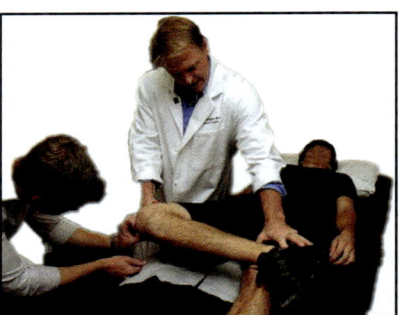

Figure 27-12. FABER distance test.

- **Imaging:** We routinely obtain 2 plain radiographic views as part of our initial assessment: a neutral pelvic tilt AP radiograph of the pelvis and a Dunn lateral view of the affected hip.[46] The plain radiographs help in the evaluation of osteoarthritis, dysplasia, and the various types of FAI. MRI can help in the evaluation of articular cartilage and labrum in cross section. Three-dimensional CT also occasionally helps determine bony detail not visualized well with MRI, particularly in the assessment of dysplasia.
- **Hip arthroscopy:** Like Dr. Byrd, our preferred arthroscopic approach is with the supine position and a standard fracture table. Patients are anesthetized with a combined spinal and epidural anesthetic. Fluoroscopy is utilized to confirm adequate distraction of the limb prior to introduction of a 70-degree arthroscope. An anterolateral portal is established with a needle and guidewire, and a direct anterior portal is established under direct arthroscopic visualization. Once access to the hip joint is established, the hip can be dynamically examined for impingement, as well as for articular and labral pathology. Treatment of the acetabular socket and labrum is performed with the leg in traction. Treatment of peripheral injuries is performed with traction relaxed.

Let's go through our standard arthroscopic treatment of 7 types of hip pathology:

1. **Cam impingement:** A cam lesion is confirmed with dynamic arthroscopic examination at the beginning of the case.[47] The area of impingement is typically found at the anterior head-neck junction as an area of abnormal convexity. The lesion is then removed by performing an osteoplasty that restores the femoral head-neck offset with an arthroscopic burr, changing the convex surface to a concave surface. We resect just enough bone to relieve the FAI. This is determined by periodically dynamically examining the hip by flexing and internally rotating the femur. Indirectly, this will restore the alpha angle to less than 55 degrees[48] (Figure 27-13).

2. **Pincer impingement:** The labrum is initially assessed to determine if repair is possible or debridement/reconstruction is necessary. Overhanging bony acetabular rim is then resected with a burr or arthroscopic osteotome and adequate resection is confirmed with dynamic exam (Figure 27-14). Care should be taken not to remove too much of the acetabular rim in hips with limited coverage or borderline dysplasia.

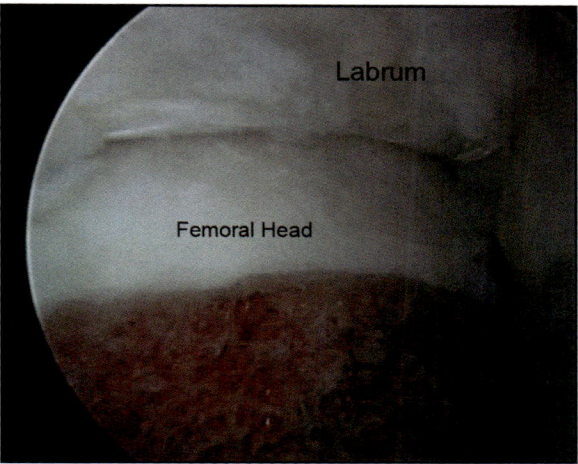

Figure 27-13. Arthroscopic photo demonstrating the femoral head following resection of a cam lesion.

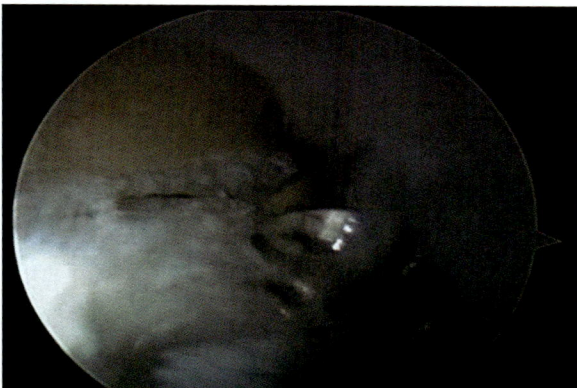

Figure 27-14. Arthroscopic photo demonstrating a cut above the labrum and shaving of the overhanging bony acetabular rim (pincer).

3. **Labral tear/detachment:** Following acetabular rim trimming, if tissue quality of the labrum is adequate, repair is undertaken by reattaching the labrum with suture anchors (Figure 27-15).

4. **Labral reconstruction:** Outcomes for labral preservation are superior to those of debridement.[49,50] Therefore, if tissue quality of the labrum is poor, the remaining labrum is resected and reconstruction is performed with an iliotibial band auto- or allograft. The graft is secured to the acetabulum with suture anchors similar to labral repair (Figure 27-16).

5. **Articular cartilage defects:** When defects in the articular cartilage are encountered, we perform chondroplasty, or smoothing of the cartilage, with a shaver that removes unstable cartilage surfaces. Once unstable cartilage has been removed, injuries that burrow to the underlying bone (ie, full thickness) are treated with microfracture. Microfracture is a technique by which small perforations are made in the underlying bone and allow for the release of marrow pluripotent stem cells (Figure 27-17). These stem cells differentiate into fibrocartilage with morphological features of healthy chondrocytes.[51] Our experience has demonstrated that return to high-level athletics, including professional hockey, is predictable utilizing this technique.[52,53]

6. **Labral tears in dysplastic hips:** Careful selection for surgery is necessary for patients with the combination of labral tears and underyling dysplasia (ie, extra-shallow acetabular sockets). Arthroscopic surgery is indicated only in mild cases. Labral refixation is performed as previously described, followed by capsular plication, at which time the capsule of the hip is closed slightly tighter than its original state. In our experience, excellent outcomes can be expected.

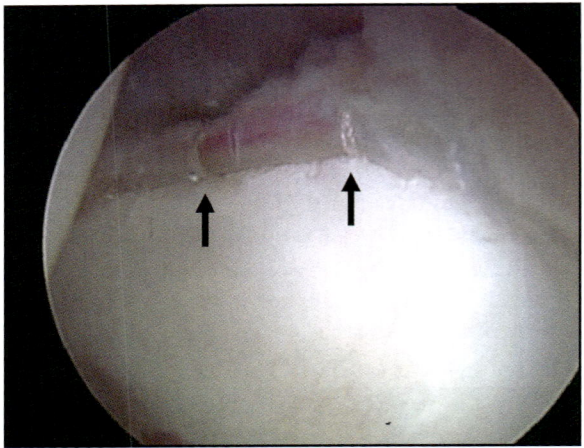

Figure 27-15. Arthroscopic photo of a repaired labrum with suture anchors (arrows).

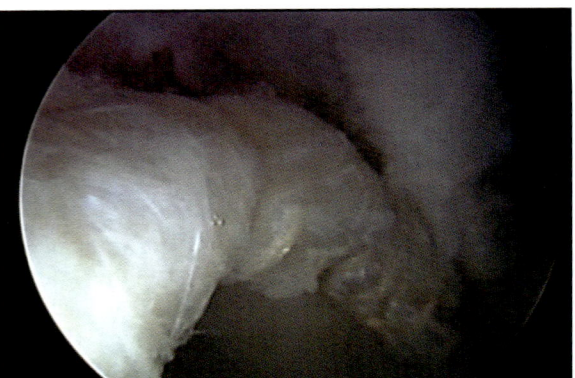

Figure 27-16. Arthroscopic photo of labral reconstruction with an iliotibial band graft.

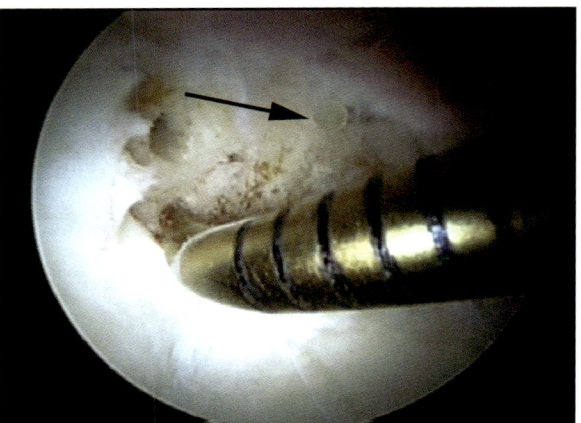

Figure 27-17. Arthroscopic photo of microfracture for full-thickness chondral defects.

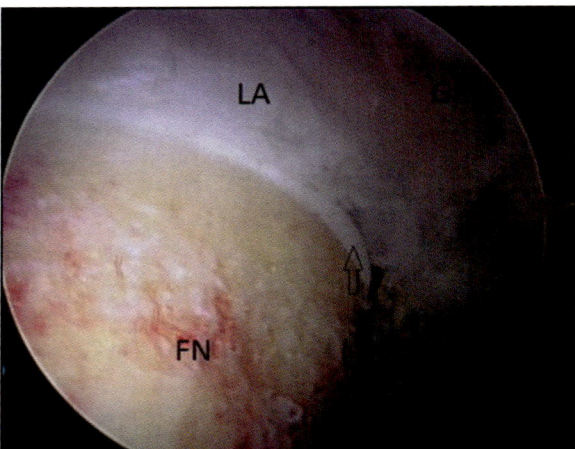

Figure 27-18. An arthroscopic photo demonstrating placement of a capsulolabral allograft spacer (arrow) to treat adhesions between the labrum and the capsule following hip arthroscopy. FN = femoral neck, GR = graft, LA = labrum. (Reprinted with permission from Philippon MJ, Ferro FP, Nepple JJ. Hip capsulolabral spacer placement for the treatment of severe capsulolabral adhesions after hip arthroscopy. *Arthrosc Tech.* 2014;3[2]:e289-e292.)

7. **Capsular adhesions and stiffness following previous arthroscopy:** Occasionally, capsulolabral adhesions develop in patients prone to excessive scarring following hip arthroscopy. When conservative measures fail, revision arthroscopy with lysis of adhesions and placement of a capsulolabral allograft spacer should be considered. The plane between the labrum and capsule is recreated, and an iliotibial band allograft spacer fixed between the 2 structures, in order to both prevent recurrent adhesion and maintain the suction seal of the previously repaired labrum (Figure 27-18).[54]

Hypothesis and a Plea to Search for Prevention

Analogous to what Dr. James Andrews and his colleagues have done for adolescent baseball pitchers throwing curve balls and sliders in excessive amounts, placing their elbows and shoulders at risk for injury,[55] we have observed that pee wee ice hockey players are likely subjecting their hips to undue risk. Kinematic study of pee wee hockey players have shown that the commonly endorsed sprint start of their skating regimens places the hip repeatedly into a high-risk impingement position of flexion and internal rotation.[56] Furthermore, the radiographic alpha angles of asymptomatic adolescent hockey players compared to an asymptomatic cohort of skiers shows significantly increased alpha angles in the skaters.[8] In other words, routine motions of skating may place youth hockey players at risk for repeated injury even if there is no pre-existent impingement anatomy. Repetitive trauma then may cause callus and other morphological changes of the proximal femur that can result in cam-type FAI (Figure 27-19).

Could youth hockey players be placing themselves at risk for symptomatic FAI later in life? Could this be worse when competitive hockey begins at a young age, when the femoral growth plates are particularly susceptible to remodeling? We are not sure of the answers to either of those questions. If we think that either is true, then we should be asking more questions, such as could the pathology be prevented by limiting ice hours prior to skeletal maturity? We are not sure of the answer to that one either. However, these associations have peaked our interest. We are actively investigating such questions as possible avenues for prevention of FAI. Stay tuned.

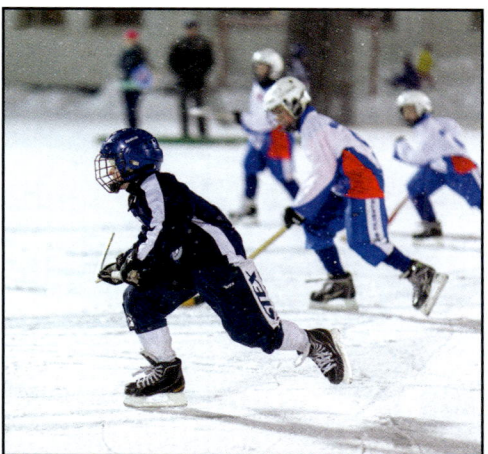

Figure 27-19. Youth hockey players. Repetitive hip trauma associated with the warm-up routine of stop-and-starts may cause morphological changes and lead to subsequent injury.

MANAGEMENT FOR FAILED ARTHROSCOPY

When hip arthroscopy is unsuccessful, there are several potential causes. A systematic approach based on the signs and symptoms allows for successful navigation of these often-murky waters. Residual cam or pincer (ie, not shaving enough bone) is a culprit. Instability is another, and it can arise from shaving too much bone, in addition to unrecognized dysplasia, capsular insufficiency, and a ligamentum teres injury. Figure 27-20 outlines a systematic approach to patients following failed hip arthroscopy.

SUMMARY

Our understanding of the causes for FAI and implications of FAI with respect to development of degenerative joint disease is evolving. The outcomes of arthroscopic treatment continue to improve as we understand more. In general, arthroscopic approaches allow for minimal perioperative morbidity and a return to high levels of function for the appropriately selected surgical candidates. But we are nowhere near perfect. Not all the patients get all the way better, and it is possible to make them worse. We still have a lot to learn.

The increased usage of arthroscopy for FAI, on the other hand, is a double-edged sword. With more readily available surgeons, more patients can be cured. This has also led to numerous patients in need of revision surgery. The pitfalls that lead to the need for revision are sometimes unavoidable. Usually, but not always, redo surgery is successful. The treatment options within this revision scenario are growing and merit further investigation. Short- and mid-term results of the arthroscopic treatment of FAI, in general, remain promising. But, as mentioned before, longer term follow-up remains crucial. We must see that we are truly preserving hips over the long term before we proclaim that Dr. Ganz's predictions have truly lit the lamp.

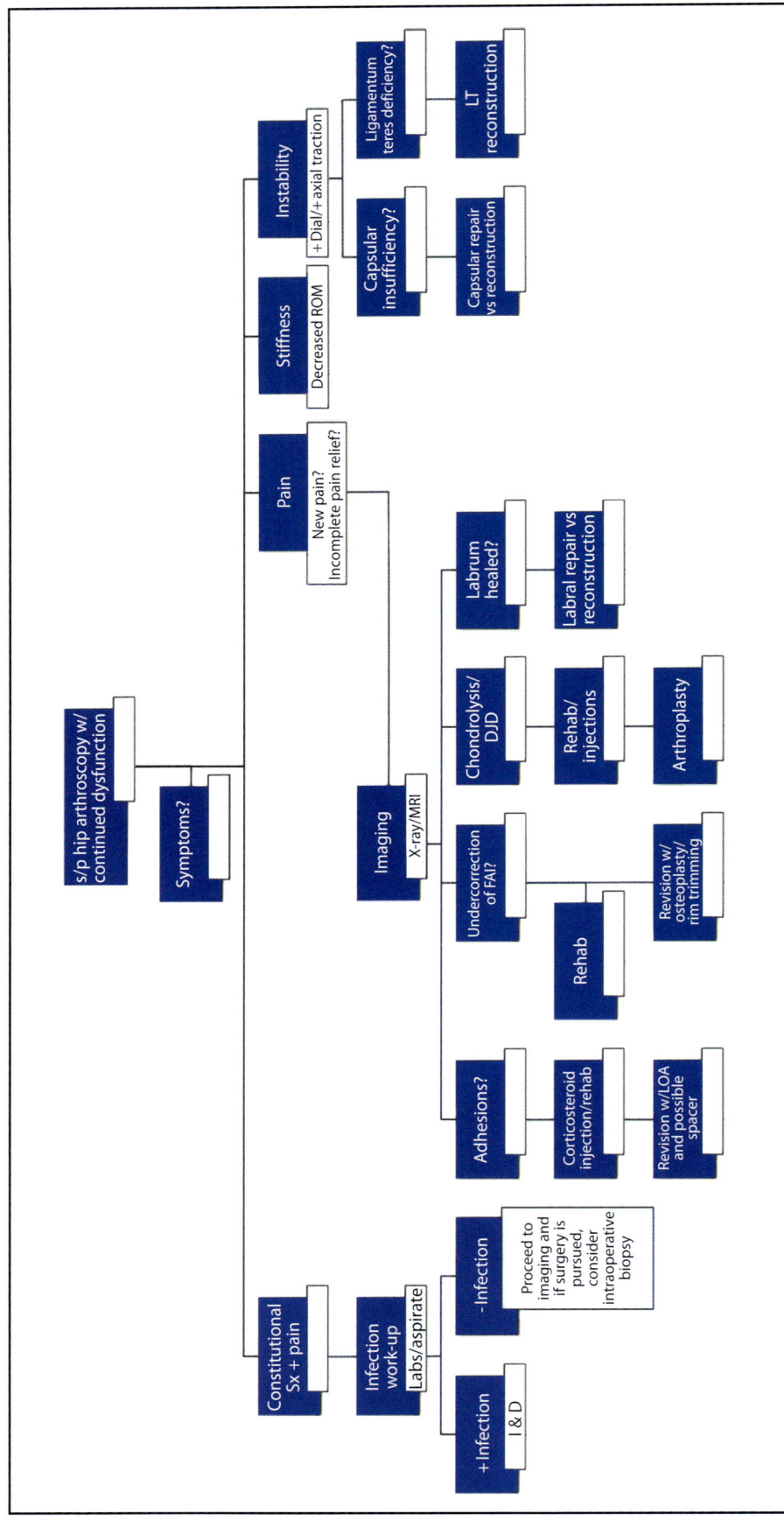

Figure 27-20. Management algorithm for failed hip arthroscopy.

Selected Reading

Philippon MJ, Ho CP, Briggs KK, Stull J, LaPrade RF. Prevalence of increased alpha angles as a measure of cam-type femoroacetabular impingement in youth ice hockey players. *Am J Sports Med.* 2013;41(6):1357-1362.
Our research suggests that routine motions of skating may place youth hockey players at risk for hip injury and that we should propose changes to the way we train young hockey players.

References

1. Doctors: A-Rod hip surgery "went exactly as planned." Fox News. http://www.foxnews.com/story/2009/03/09/doctors-rod-hip-surgery-went-exactly-as-planned.html. Published March 9, 2009. Accessed September 10, 2018.
2. LaPointe J. Alex Rodriguez to begin rehab after hip surgery. *The New York Times.* https://www.nytimes.com/2009/03/10/sports/baseball/10arod.html. Published March 9, 2009. Accessed September 10, 2018.
3. A-Rod committed to "hard road back" after hip surgery set for mid-Jan. *New York Post.* https://nypost.com/2012/12/08/a-rod-committed-to-hard-road-back-after-hip-surgery-set-for-mid-jan/. Published December 8, 2012. Accessed September 10, 2018.
4. Ito K, Minka MA 2nd, Leunig M, Werlen S, Ganz R. Femoroacetabular impingement and the cam-effect. A MRI-based quantitative anatomical study of the femoral head-neck offset. *J Bone Joint Surg Br.* 2001;83(2):171-176.
5. Lavigne M, Parvizi J, Beck M, Siebenrock KA, Ganz R, Leunig M. Anterior femoroacetabular impingement: part I. Techniques of joint preserving surgery. *Clin Orthop Relat Res.* 2004;(418):61-66.
6. Notzli HP, Wyss TF, Stoecklin CH, Schmid MR, Treiber K, Hodler J. The contour of the femoral head-neck junction as a predictor for the risk of anterior impingement. *J Bone Joint Surg Br.* 2002;84(4):556-560.
7. Johnson AC, Shaman MA, Ryan TG. Femoroacetabular impingement in former high-level youth soccer players. *Am J Sports Med.* 2012;40(6):1342-1346.
8. Philippon MJ, Ho CP, Briggs KK, Stull J, LaPrade RF. Prevalence of increased alpha angles as a measure of cam-type femoroacetabular impingement in youth ice hockey players. *Am J Sports Med.* 2013;41(6):1357-1362.
9. Clohisy JC, Dobson MA, Robison JF, et al. Radiographic structural abnormalities associated with premature, natural hip-joint failure. *J Bone Joint Surg Am.* 2011;93(suppl 2):3-9.
10. Ecker TM, Tannast M, Puls M, Siebenrock KA, Murphy SB. Pathomorphologic alterations predict presence or absence of hip osteoarthrosis. *Clin Orthop Relat Res.* 2007;465:46-52.
11. Nicholls AS, Kiran A, Pollard TC, et al. The association between hip morphology parameters and nineteen-year risk of end-stage osteoarthritis of the hip: a nested case-control study. *Arthritis Rheum.* 2011;63(11):3392-3400.
12. Smith-Petersen MN. Treatment of malum coxae senilis, old slipped upper femoral epiphysis, intrapelvic protrusion of the acetabulum, and coxa plana by means of acetabuloplasty. *J Bone Joint Surg.* 1936;18:869-880.
13. Burman MS. Arthroscopy or the direct visualisation of joints. An experimental cadaver study. *J Bone Joint Surgery.* 1931;13A:669-695.
14. Murray RO. The aetiology of primary osteoarthritis of the hip. *Br J Radiol.* 1965;38(455):810-824.
15. Stulberg SD. Unrecognized childhood hip disease: a major cause of idiopathic osteoarthritis of the hip. In: Cordell LD, Harris WH, Ramsey PL, MacEwen GD, eds. *The Hip: Proceedings of the Third Open Scientific Meeting of the Hip Society.* St. Louis, MO: CV Mosby; 1975:212-228.
16. Ganz R, Gill TJ, Gautier E, Ganz K, Krugel N, Berlemann U. Surgical dislocation of the adult hip a technique with full access to the femoral head and acetabulum without the risk of avascular necrosis. *J Bone Joint Surg Br.* 2001;83(8):1119-1124.
17. Gautier E, Ganz K, Krugel N, Gill T, Ganz R. Anatomy of the medial femoral circumflex artery and its surgical implications. *J Bone Joint Surg Br.* 2000;82(5):679-683.
18. Beck M, Leunig M, Parvizi J, Boutier V, Wyss D, Ganz R. Anterior femoroacetabular impingement: part II. Midterm results of surgical treatment. *Clin Orthop Relat Res.* 2004;(418):67-73.
19. Takagi K. The classic. Arthroscope. Kenji Takagi. J Jap Orthop Assoc, 1939. *Clin Orthop Relat Res.* 1982;(167):6-8.
20. Glick JM. Hip arthroscopy using the lateral approach. *Instr Course Lect.* 1988;37:223-231.
21. Glick JM, Sampson TG, Gordon RB, Behr JT, Schmidt E. Hip arthroscopy by the lateral approach. *Arthroscopy.* 1987;3(1):4-12.
22. Byrd JWT. Hip arthroscopy utilizing the supine position. *Arthroscopy.* 1994;10(3):275-280.
23. Legaye J, Duval-Beaupere G, Barrau A, et al. Relationship between sacral pelvic incidence and acetabular orientation. *Hip Int.* 2011;21(1):87-97.
24. Legaye J, Duval-Beaupere G, Hecquet J, Marty C. Pelvic incidence: a fundamental pelvic parameter for three-dimensional regulation of spinal sagittal curves. *Eur Spine J.* 1998;7(2):99-103.
25. Stevens VK, Vleeming A, Bouche KG, Mahieu NN, Vanderstraeten GG, Danneels LA. Electromyographic activity of trunk and hip muscles during stabilization exercises in four-point kneeling in healthy volunteers. *Eur Spine J.* 2007;16(5):711-718.
26. Tateuchi H, Taniguchi M, Mori N, Ichihashi N. Balance of hip and trunk muscle activity is associated with increased anterior pelvic tilt during prone hip extension. *J Electromyogr Kinesiol.* 2012;22(3):391-397.
27. Yoo WG. Effect of individual strengthening exercises for anterior pelvic tilt muscles on back pain, pelvic angle, and lumbar ROMs of a LBP patient with flat back. *J Phys Ther Sci.* 2013;25(10):1357-1358.
28. Yoo WG. Effect of the individual strengthening exercises for posterior pelvic tilt muscles on back pain, pelvic angle, and lumbar ROM of a LBP patient with excessive lordosis: a case study. *J Phys Ther Sci.* 2014;26(2):319-320.
29. Ross JR, Nepple JJ, Philippon MJ, Kelly BT, Larson CM, Bedi A. Effect of changes in pelvic tilt on range of motion to impingement and radiographic parameters of acetabular morphologic characteristics. *Am J Sports Med.* 2014;42(10):2402-2409.
30. Cairns MA, Burdett RG, Pisciotta JC, Simon SR. A biomechanical analysis of racewalking gait. *Med Sci Sports Exerc.* 1986;18(4):446-453.
31. Novacheck TF. The biomechanics of running. *Gait Posture.* 1998;7(1):77-95.

32. Oh JS, Cynn HS, Won JH, Kwon OY, Yi CH. Effects of performing an abdominal drawing-in maneuver during prone hip extension exercises on hip and back extensor muscle activity and amount of anterior pelvic tilt. *J Orthop Sports Phys Ther*. 2007;37(6):320-324.
33. Domb BG, Shindle MK, McArthur B, Voos JE, Magennis EM, Kelly BT. Iliopsoas impingement: a newly identified cause of labral pathology in the hip. *HSS J*. 2011;7(2):145-150.
34. Meyers WC, McKechnie A, Philippon MJ, Horner MA, Zoga AC, Devon ON. Experience with "sports hernia" spanning two decades. *Ann Surg*. 2008;248(4):656-665.
35. Tyler T, Zook L, Brittis D, Gleim G. A new pelvic tilt detection device: roentgenographic validation and application to assessment of hip motion in professional ice hockey players. *J Orthop Sports Phys Ther*. 1996;24(5):303-308.
36. Leunig M, Werlen S, Ungersbock A, Ito K, Ganz R. Evaluation of the acetabular labrum by MR arthrography. *J Bone Joint Surg Br*. 1997;79(2):230-234.
37. Beall DP, Sweet CF, Martin HD, et al. Imaging findings of femoroacetabular impingement syndrome. *Skeletal Radiol*. 2005;34(11):691-701.
38. Philippon MJ, Ejnisman L, Ellis HB, Briggs KK. Outcomes 2 to 5 years following hip arthroscopy for femoroacetabular impingement in the patient aged 11 to 16 years. *Arthroscopy*. 2012;28(9):1255-1261.
39. Philippon MJ, Briggs KK, Carlisle JC, Patterson DC. Joint space predicts THA after hip arthroscopy in patients 50 years and older. *Clin Orthop Relat Res*. 2013;471(8):2492-2496.
40. Philippon MJ, Schroder ESBG, Briggs KK. Hip arthroscopy for femoroacetabular impingement in patients aged 50 years or older. *Arthroscopy*. 2012;28(1):59-65.
41. Philippon MJ, Briggs KK, Yen YM, Kuppersmith DA. Outcomes following hip arthroscopy for femoroacetabular impingement with associated chondrolabral dysfunction: minimum two-year follow-up. *J Bone Joint Surg Br*. 2009;91(1):16-23.
42. Philippon M, Schenker M, Briggs K, Kuppersmith D. Femoroacetabular impingement in 45 professional athletes: associated pathologies and return to sport following arthroscopic decompression. *Knee Surg Sports Traumatol Arthrosc*. 2007;15(7):908-914.
43. Byrd JW. Femoroacetabular impingement in athletes, part 1: cause and assessment. *Sports Health*. 2010;2(4):321-333.
44. Ito K, Leunig M, Ganz R. Histopathologic features of the acetabular labrum in femoroacetabular impingement. *Clin Orthop Relat Res*. 2004;(429):262-271.
45. Leunig M, Beaule PE, Ganz R. The concept of femoroacetabular impingement: current status and future perspectives. *Clin Orthop Relat Res*. 2009;467(3):616-622.
46. Clohisy JC, Carlisle JC, Beaule PE, et al. A systematic approach to the plain radiographic evaluation of the young adult hip. *J Bone Joint Surg Am*. 2008;90(suppl 4):47-66.
47. Philippon MJ, Stubbs AJ, Schenker ML, Maxwell RB, Ganz R, Leunig M. Arthroscopic management of femoroacetabular impingement: osteoplasty technique and literature review. *Am J Sports Med*. 2007;35(9):1571-1580.
48. de Sa D, Urquhart N, Philippon M, Ye JE, Simunovic N, Ayeni OR. Alpha angle correction in femoroacetabular impingement. *Knee Surg Sports Traumatol Arthrosc*. 2014;22(4):812-821.
49. Ayeni OR, Alradwan H, de Sa D, Philippon MJ. The hip labrum reconstruction: indications and outcomes—a systematic review. *Knee Surg Sports Traumatol Arthrosc*. 2014;22(4):737-743.
50. Philippon MJ, Briggs KK, Hay CJ, Kuppersmith DA, Dewing CB, Huang MJ. Arthroscopic labral reconstruction in the hip using iliotibial band autograft: technique and early outcomes. *Arthroscopy*. 2010;26(6):750-756.
51. Steadman JR, Rodkey WG, Rodrigo JJ. Microfracture: surgical technique and rehabilitation to treat chondral defects. *Clin Orthop Relat Res*. 2001;(391):S362-S369.
52. McDonald JE, Herzog MM, Philippon MJ. Performance outcomes in professional hockey players following arthroscopic treatment of FAI and microfracture of the hip. *Knee Surg Sports Traumatol Arthrosc*. 2014;22(4):915-919.
53. McDonald JE, Herzog MM, Philippon MJ. Return to play after hip arthroscopy with microfracture in elite athletes. *Arthroscopy*. 2013;29(2):330-335.
54. Philippon MJ, Ferro FP, Nepple JJ. Hip capsulolabral spacer placement for the treatment of severe capsulolabral adhesions after hip arthroscopy. *Arthrosc Tech*. 2014;3(2):e289-e292.
55. Lyman S, Fleisig GS, Andrews JR, Osinski ED. Effect of pitch type, pitch count, and pitching mechanics on risk of elbow and shoulder pain in youth baseball pitchers. *Am J Sports Med*. 2002;30(4):463-468.
56. Stull JD, Philippon MJ, LaPrade RF. "At-risk" positioning and hip biomechanics of the Peewee ice hockey sprint start. *Am J Sports Med*. 2011;39(suppl):29S-35S.

28

biomechanics

(A) tilt and version

ERIC J. KROPF, MD
STRUAN H. COLEMAN, MD, PHD
ALEXANDER E. POOR, MD

Editor's Note: *Eric Kropf is a trusted colleague and Chairman of Orthopedic Surgery at Temple University. An excellent hip arthroscopist, Eric talks a lot about the importance of the different orientations of the hip and rest of the pelvis. Eric joins Struan and co-editor Alexander Poor in expanding upon the theme of pelvic geometry playing an important role in human performance and the surgery that we do. They present the basic concepts in a fun way. Keep in mind that very little basic research exists on this subject.*

Come on, let's twist again, like we did last summer.
Let's twist again, like we did last year!
—Lyrics from the music of Chubby Checker (born Ernest Evans). Chubby may now be known also for propagating the roles of pelvic tilt and version. Popularizer of The Twist, The Limbo Rock, The Fly, and The Pony, Checker changed the way we dance to music. Before The Twist, grown-ups never danced to teenage music. Raised in the projects of Philadelphia, Checker tops Billboard's list of the most popular singles ever and holds the record for placing 5 albums in the Top 12 at once.

Chubby's New Eyes

Think about Chubby and The Twist. How many twists, turns and contortions does your pelvis go through when you do The Twist? "Justin Timberlake, Britney Spears, all the rappers, they're doing my dances and they're making billions doing my dances. When they do that little thing they do with their hands? That's The Fly and The Pony!"

Those were Chubby's words. Chubby saw what's going on; he saw the movements. Chubby lived all the different variations of pelvic tilt and version. No doubt, he also knows about all the other orientations of the bones and muscles of the pelvis and hips.

In the last chapter, Dr. Philippon traveled quickly through some clinical implications of the various anatomies of the hip. In the next chapter, Marc Safran digs deeper into the biomechanics. Let's pause here for a moment, go up 30,000 feet, with Chubby, and place a few biomechanical definitions on what Chubby, Justin, Beyoncé, and Eminem are doing when they dance.

"Three" Orientations

No, we are not talking about sex again. We are talking about 3 different orientations that factor into movements that we create when we use our pelvis.

We will keep this simple. Think of the pelvis as having 3 important orientations. The pelvis, of course, has way more than 3 orientations. But just think about 3: tilt and version. Wait a minute, that's just 2, isn't it? We said 3. Before you designate us not-mathematical whiz kids, understand that when it comes to the hip, there are 2 types of version. That makes 3: tilt plus 2 types of version.

Now, think of the entire set of pelvic bones as one entity. Think of it as a planting pot holding a tree. Tilt refers to the orientation of that pot. The planting pot can tilt in any direction. The direction and degree of tilt will, obviously, affect the tree and whatever supports the pot (Figure 28A-1).

Version refers to each of the supporting posts of the pot. In the case of the human being, we have 2 supporting posts holding up that pot, or pelvis. Perhaps aliens have 3 or more. On Earth, we call these 2 supporting posts the lower extremities, and we call the connecting apparatus for each of those 2 posts the ball-in-socket hip joint. Therefore, now understand that we now have 3 types of orientation: one for the whole pelvis (tilt), and the second and third for each of the 2 hips jointly with their posts (versions). See, we have made this simple as promised. Thanky Panky, we only have to think about 2 types of orientation. What holds for one hip likely holds for the other.

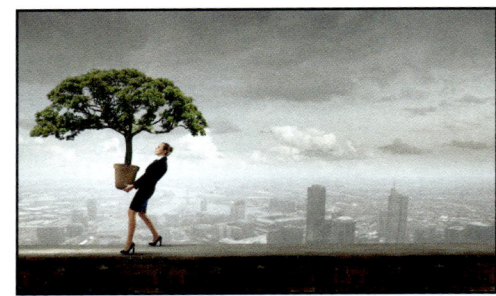
Figure 28A-1.

Wait again. Two posts do not provide stability. Won't it fall over? Doesn't it take a triad of posts to stabilize the pelvis or a pot otherwise hanging in the air? Yes, that would be true if there were no movement, and all we did was stand still. Then we would usually simply fall over.

But we have movement here, and a lot of it. Our body has to stay dynamic to keep its balance. That is how we maintain our 2-leggedness and our superiority in the species hierarchy. Balance and stability occur via dynamic interplays of opposing forces. Tilt and version are big parts of normal body dynamism. To quote Coach Belichick, "It is what it is." These orientations keep us doing what we are doing. Belichick probably said that, too.

The pelvis tree-pot can tip in any direction. It can tip in 3 ways, from (1) what is going on in the tree, (2) something within the pot itself, or (3) an issue involving either (or both) of its post connectors.

TILT TYPES

Anterior pelvic tilt occurs when the pelvis (or "pot") tips forward. The anterior pubis drops, and the sacrum and rest of the posterior pelvis rise. Consequently, anterior soft tissue structures—such as the rectus abdominis, adductors, iliopsoas, rectus femoris, and sartorious—shorten, and posterior soft tissue structures—such as the erector spinae, hamstrings, and glutes—lengthen. Lengthening past normal tensile parameters causes weakness, and the whole process may lead to instability owing to inability of the shortened muscles to generate force enough to correct imbalances and restore neutrality.

Posterior pelvic tilt refers to the opposite situation. The pelvis tips backward; the flexors, adductors, and rectus abdominis lengthen; and the posterior muscles shorten. Instability may occur via a process complementary to anterior pelvic tilt (ie, weakened anterior muscles and/or ineffective posterior muscles). (See Figures 28A-2 and 28A-3.)

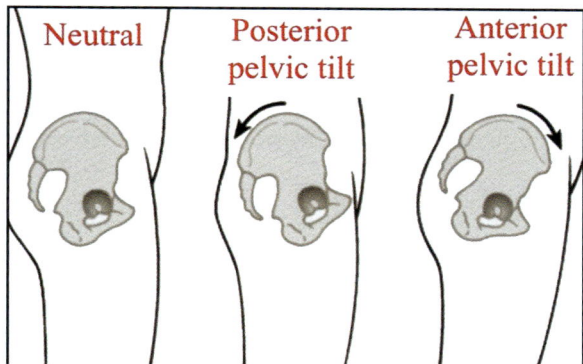

Figure 28A-2. Anterior and posterior pelvic tilt. (Reprinted with permission from Joel Kouyoumjian [admin@iseecrookedpeople.com] of Manchester-Bedford Myoskeletal [www.mbmyoskeletal.com] in Bedford, New Hampshire.)

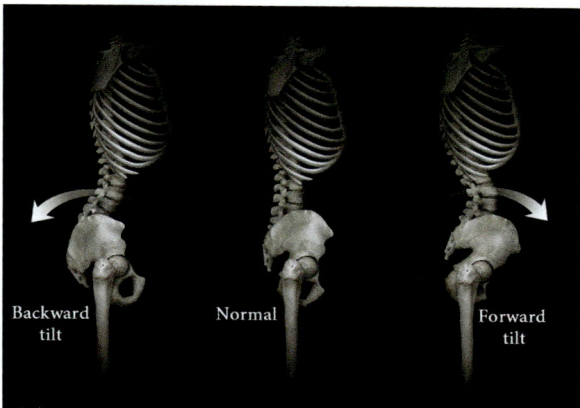

Figure 28A-3. The bony arrangement of anterior and posterior pelvic tilt. Basically, think of tilt as the relationship between the entire bony pelvis and (1) the femur and rest of the bony lower extremity and (2) the spine. Note that both the lower extremity and spine must make adjustments.

Lateral pelvic tilt, as you might surmise, occurs when the pelvis tips to either side (Figure 28A-4). This most commonly ensues from structural abnormalities such as limb length discrepancies or spinal scoliosis. Left vs right pelvic tilt refers to the side tipped down. In other words, with left tilt, the right iliac wing appears elevated, and with right tilt, the left iliac wing is higher.

When pelvic tilt matters, the designations permanent or variable hold importance with respect to designing treatment. *Permanent* refers to the inability to correct the actual tilt itself. This may be related either to inherent anatomical structure or the consequence of injury or an otherwise nonfunctional part (eg, after a stroke). Treatment then focuses on palliation via influencing the consequences of the permanent deficit. *Variable* refers to just that, the tilt is fixable either through physical therapy, more invasive intervention, alternative therapies, or a combination of treatments.

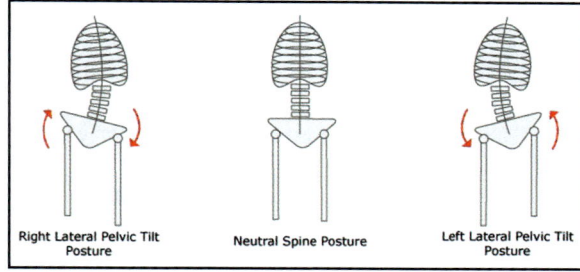

Figure 28A-4. Schematic of lateral pelvic tilt. (Reprinted with permission from Dr. Jason Gray of My Rehab Connection [www.myrehabconnection.com].)

WHEN TILT MATTERS

Size and shape of the pelvis comes into this big time. Let's start out with the horse, and then go to the monkey and human. Review Chapter 20 and some of the evolutionary/developmental/comparative anatomic factors.

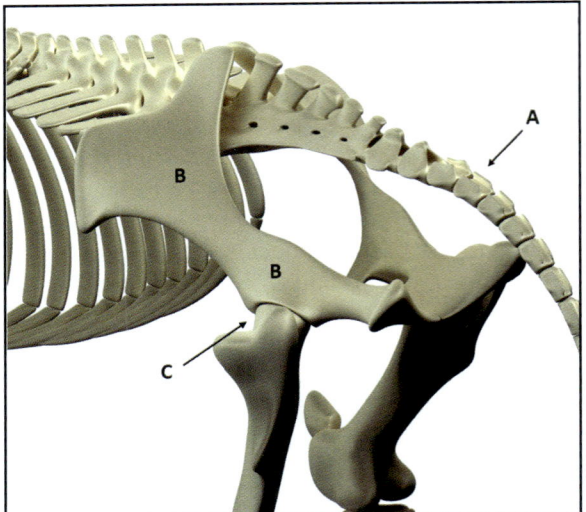

Figure 28A-5. The horse's pelvis. (A) The tail. (B) The long iliac bone. (C) The "tight" hip (ie, the acetabular socket completely enveloping the femoral ball).

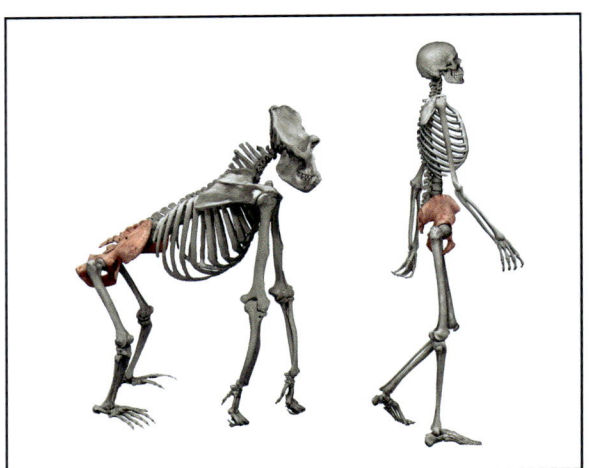

Figure 28A-6. Chimp and human pelves have different structures. The most obvious difference is the chimp's longer pelvis, probably important for locomotion.

Look at the horse's pelvis (Figure 28A-5). Consider the anatomical factors that distinguish this 4-legged animal. There are, basically, 3 things: (1) the extension of the sacrum as a tail (okay, we don't have that); (2) a long, vertical iliac bone; and (3) tight hips.

Now look at a gorilla or chimp and compare it to upright us (Figure 28A-6). First, look at the iliac bone. It is also much longer and more vertical in the gorilla. This anatomical feature distinguishes the 4-legged creatures from us upright hierarchal leaders. The height and size of the iliac bone helps fixate those creatures into 4-legged postures. The overall size and shape of the pelvis help determine acetabular depth and shape.

Think of the 4-legged posture as the extreme of anterior pelvic tilt (Figure 28A-7). We, as humans, normally vary in the size and shape of our pelvis. We can think of ourselves as all having some degree of "gorilla" in our posture. Could this be why the "set position" in most sports (see Chapter 7) involves just a little bit of anterior pelvic tilt?

Also see how much more limited anteriorly within the socket our hips appear to be. The monkey's hips are more limited in their anterior range of motion. The horse and other 4-leggeders have grossly limited ranges of hip motion. In general, all 4-legged postures compellingly fixate both posture and hip motion; the exception indeed being the human baby.

In humans, alterations of tilt and version limit anterior hip range of motion.[1] In the extreme, we become more like 4-legged animals. Considering the species comparisons, doesn't it seem best to think of this fixation as creating both an advantage and a disadvantage?

The advantage is that limitation of movement can also serve as a fulcrum, by its very nature of decreasing range of motion. If our muscles are fit, we can "fly" in a multitude of ways. But, of course, we can't jump as high as many of the 4-leggeders. The ability to jump high seems obviously related to the vertical length of the pelvic bones, glutes, psoases, and other muscles. Think about it, think about all the parallels of comparative anatomy and how we might apply them in sports.

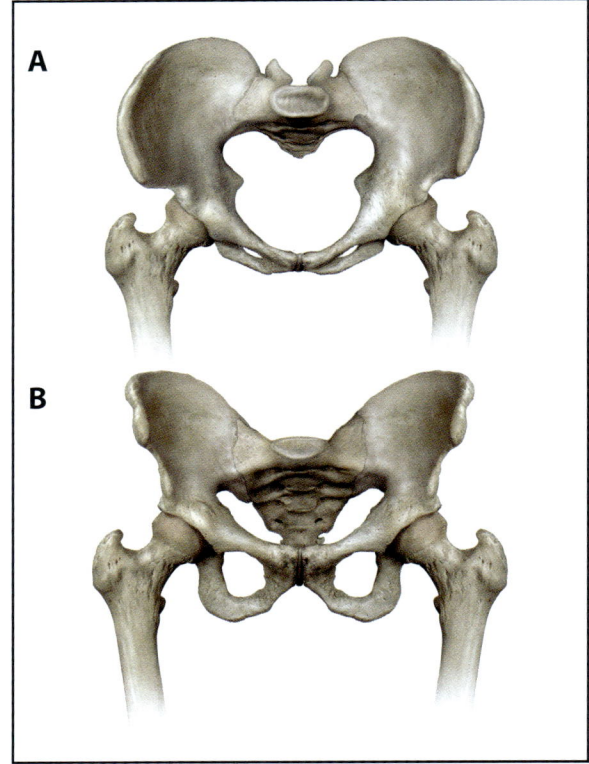

Figure 28A-7. Extremes of pelvic tilt shown by comparing (A) gorilla and (B) man. Think about where the third baseman's baseball set position fits in.

How Variable Tilt Becomes Bad

The earlier discussion pertained mostly to the permanent type of pelvic tilt—something we are born with, either as a species or just individual variability. Alterations in resting pelvic tilt generally involve muscle weakness or contracture or joint or ligamentous instability or contracture. When one form of variable pelvic tilt stays for long, compensatory muscle activation patterns occur. The result may be chronic pain or even acute muscle injury. Sometimes, injuries occur in predictable patterns.

For example, with continuous anterior pelvic tilt, the spine must assume a relatively hyperextended position in order to maintain balance and strength. This results in paradoxical lengthening of the rectus abdominis and shortening or contracture of the erector spinae musculature. In this scenario, the spine may demonstrate increased lordosis or the athlete may compensate by bringing the hips into a flexed position. This further amplifies anterior muscular contracture of the hip flexors or even of the adductor compartment.

Conversely, to maintain balance in the setting of posterior pelvic tilt, the spine will roll forward and "round," resulting in contracture of the erector spinae. The lumbar spine then assumes a kyphotic position. With excessive lateral tilt, the hip abductors will need to increase their forces during single-leg stances. The glute medius and minimus exert maximal effort in order to elevate the pelvis in the single-leg stance so that the pelvis on the elevated side does not fall to the floor.

Standing and Sitting in the Office All Day Are Both Bad

Pelvic tilt issues occur for a variety of reasons. The most common clinical scenario is excessive anterior pelvic tilt. Most people remain unaware that their daily routine may be dangerous and result in the chronic muscle imbalances that create anterior pelvic tilt. Either standing or sitting throughout the day contribute to pelvic tilt issues. The best position for standing in neutral pelvic tilt involves mild knee flexion. Then the hip flexors and extensors become relatively balanced. However, this requires considerable muscular effort to maintain this position. Work creates fatigue.

Then it becomes more energy efficient to stand with the knees extended or hyperextended. In this position, the pelvis tips slightly anteriorly. The muscle groups in the anterior hip muscles contract and gradually tighten more and more. The muscles include the rectus femoris and iliopsoas. A repetitive cycle turns a mild muscular imbalance into a fixed contracture. A fixed anterior hip contracture then balances with increased lumbar lordosis. One ends up with a lot of stress across intervertebral discs and low back pain.

Our world has evolved into one in which people spend tremendous amounts of time sitting in front of a computer or television screen.[2] Sitting turns out to be the worst way to spend our lives, from the standpoint of pelvic tilt problems. In our new cyberworld, jobs regularly require preposterously extended sitting. In the normal sitting posture, we usually lean forward for large amounts of time. Consequently, our trunks drift anteriorly. Of course, the position minimizes energy expenditure. And at the same time, it rocks the pelvis forward and forces the lumbar spine into lordosis, creating the condition for an anterior muscular contracture.

Let's digress for a moment from the topic of sitting or standing all day and talk in general terms about muscular injury. Usually, muscular "pulls" occur when muscle fibers are stretched beyond their normal working length. All fitness instructors know that a lack of flexibility contributes to and increases the risk of injury. So, in layperson's terms, the greater the tightness (resting contracture of a muscle unit), the less force (or excursion) it takes to stretch that muscle beyond acceptable length. In short, this is why pelvic tilt abnormalities result in muscle injury.

We often see patients reinjuring the same muscle groups over and over again. Plus, we see athletes with similar injury patterns year in and year out. Many of these recurrences likely come from tilt habits of daily living. Therefore, increasing our understanding of pelvic tilt shall likely yield new insights into correct rehabilitation protocols. One can guess that varying our postures during routine daily activity shall remain a component of the protocols. For now, we should study our job's daily requirements and come up with basic biomechanical alterations to prevent injuries.

Affecting Impingement

In cam impingement, the misshapen, femoral ball does not fit perfectly into the spherical acetabular socket. This anatomical incompatibility creates shear that damages articular cartilage or labrum. In pincer impingement, the socket, rather than the ball, is the culprit. We should not underestimate the role of pelvic tilt as a cause or aggravator of either process. The exact position derives originally from the overall position of the pelvic bones. In extreme cases, clinical impingement may occur even without discernible ball-or-socket incongruities. For example, the anterior lip of the acetabulum may tip forward and down and abut the femur during hip flexion positions.

The previous observations emphasize the importance of recognizing pelvic tilt or other more regional anatomical imbalances for optimal treatment of clinical FAI. We see many patients with functional impingement and pain and no obviously significant cartilage or labral injury. We also see patients with miniscule or no apparent bony incongruity. Developing appropriate physical therapy regimens for these patients remains another matter in need of more thought and research. Some of these patients improve using only present-day knowledge about correcting pelvic tilt issues.

Aversions to Version

Version

Remember that we stated that we will discuss 3 orientations of the pelvis? That means we still have 2 left to cover. Think back to the planting pot holding a tree, and recall that version refers to the orientation of the 2 posts that hold up the pot. Version, like tilt, has a big impact on how well the ball and socket fit together. Think about version like the way a submarine periscope spins around. The femur even looks kind of like a periscope (Figure 28A-8). There are 2 types of version: femoral and acetabular.

Femoral Version

The orientation of the femur in the hip joint is femoral version. If the ball of the femur pushes toward the front of the hip joint, this is femoral anteversion. Folks with a lot of femoral anteversion walk around pigeon-toed. Subconsciously, they rotate their legs inward to keep their balls within their sockets. Femoral retroversion is just the opposite. The ball tucks deep into the back of the socket and makes the grinding of hip impingement more dramatic (Figure 28A-9).

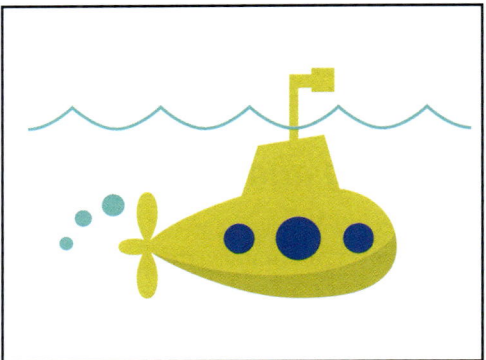

Figure 28A-8. Think of version like a submarine and its periscope. Both the submarine and the periscope can rotate in various ways.

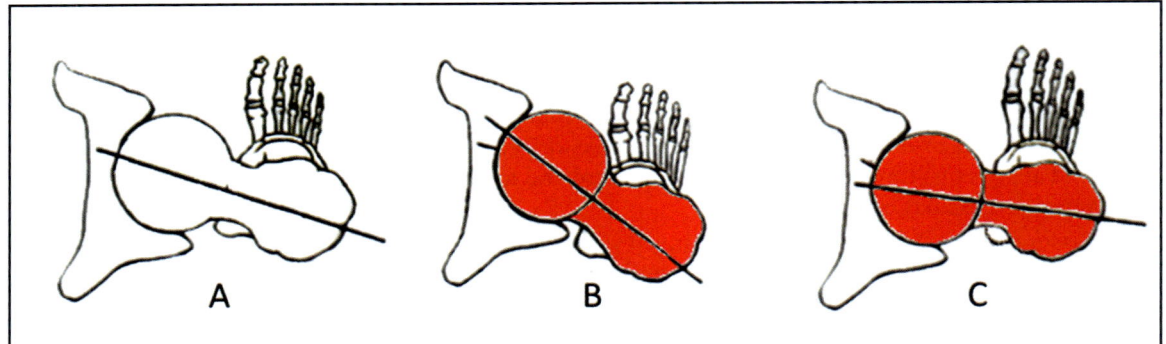

Figure 28A-9. Femoral version refers to the rotation of the femoral head (in red) relative to the rest of the femur and is independent of the acetabulum. By our definition, (A) normal femoral version is slightly anteverted. (B) Abnormal (excessive) femoral anteversion is more than that. (C) Femoral retroversion is less than normal anteversion. Don't let this be too confusing.

Acetabular Version

The other type of version, acetabular version, refers to the orientation of the socket (Figure 28A-10). Again, think of a periscope rotating toward the front or back of the body. Normally, the hip socket orients about 20 degrees toward the front. We call this *normal acetabular anteversion*. If the socket rotates too much toward the front, this gives rise to instability and predisposes the joint to sublux or dislocate, which, logically, puts more stress on surrounding muscles, ligaments, and other structures. When the socket is rotated toward the back (retroverted), it can, like femoral retroversion, create more impingement and cause pain. It also makes FAI harder to treat surgically, probably because these folks are more likely to have some instability after surgery. They may also have grinding in funny locations within the hip, but all we really know is that they tend not to do as well after hip surgery.[3]

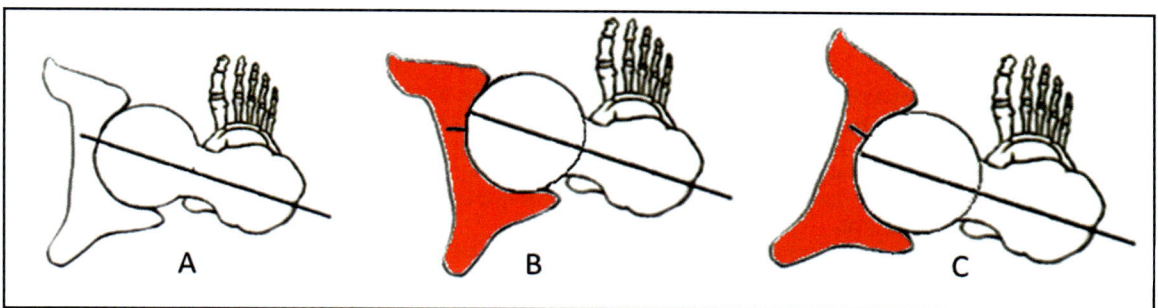

Figure 28A-10. Acetabular version refers to the orientation of the acetabulum (in red) relative to the femoral head. Note that the acetabular alignment changes in all 3 examples while the femoral head stays the same. (A) Normal acetabular anteversion. (B) Abnormal (excessive) acetabular anteversion. (C) Acetabular retroversion.

Many Versions of Version

If your head is spinning trying to keep track of the spinning bones, you are not the only one! In fact, someone was kind enough to create a composite scoring system that summarizes the overall picture of version. It is called the McKibbin instability index, and it is basically a combination of how much the socket is rotated forward or backward plus the rotation of the femur. A normal McKibbin index is 30 to 60 degrees. Higher than that tends to lead to an unstable joint and may even need surgery to break the bones of the socket and remodel the shape. People with lower than normal McKibbin indices tend to have pain from grinding within the joint. Reportedly, they develop arthritis more quickly.[4]

TWISTING NEXT SUMMER

Let's consider Chubby Checker's lyrics. If we twist again like we did last summer, how about next summer? Or the summers after that? What will all that twisting do to us? To come up with the right answers, we must shrewdly observe our dancing moves, plus determine which specific postures are best to sit or stand while watching the others on the dance floor. We need new dances, along with perhaps fresh styles for activities of daily living. Pelvic tilt and version abnormalities are real and cause various muscular and bony imbalances. These factors stand (like the pun?) as key components to understanding the core and preventing injury. We also must know more about how daily routine affects our dancing.

SELECTED READINGS

Healy GN, Dunstan DW, Salmon J, et al. Breaks in sedentary time: beneficial associations with metabolic risk. *Diabetes Care*. 2008;31(4):661-666.
   An early article that helped trigger the popular phrase: "Sitting is the new smoking."

Vernikos J. *Sitting Kills, Moving Heals: How Simple Everyday Movement Will Prevent Pain, Illness, and Early Death—and Exercise Alone Won't*. Fresno, CA: Quill Driver Books; 2011.
   A former NASA director, Dr. Vernikos applies anti-gravity lessons learned from space to terrestrial health problems. Operative terms relate to body alignment rather than tilt and version, but the gist is similar.

Ross JR, Nepple JJ, Philippon MJ, Kelly BT, Larson CM, Bedi A. Effect of changes in pelvic tilt on range of motion to impingement and radiographic parameters of acetabular morphologic characteristics. *Am J Sports Med*. 2014;42(10):2402-2409.
   This article highlights how subtle changes in pelvic orientation may have pronounced effects on our quality of life. Its complexity also demonstrates that we still have a lot to learn about the whole subject.

REFERENCES

1. Ross JR, Nepple JJ, Philippon MJ, Kelly BT, Larson CM, Bedi A. Effect of changes in pelvic tilt on range of motion to impingement and radiographic parameters of acetabular morphologic characteristics. *Am J Sports Med.* 2014;42(10):2402-2409.
2. Schwartz B, Kapellusch JM, Schrempf A, et al. Effect of a novel two-desk sit-to-stand workplace (active office) on sitting time, performance and physiological parameters: protocol for a randomized control trial. *BMC Public Health.* 2016;16:578.
3. Hartigan DE, Perets I, Walsh JP, Close MR, Domb BG. Clinical outcomes of hip arthroscopy in radiographically diagnosed retroverted acetabula. *Am J Sports Med.* 2016;44(10):2531-2536.
4. Tönnis D, Heinecke A. Current concepts review: acetabular and femoral anteversion: relationship with osteoarthritis of the hip. *J Bone Joint Surg Am.* 1999;81:1747-1770.

(B) altered hip **biomechanics** and the **muscles**

Marc R. Safran, MD
Joshua Sampson, MD

Editor's Note: *About 20 years ago, we observed that hip and core muscle pathologies often manifest simultaneously. This was not a "shocker" at all to us at the time. The observation seemed natural considering the close anatomic proximity of the ball and socket to other core structures. To our surprise, the observation created consternation, way more than we thought it would. The consternation probably came from hip surgeons living within their proverbial "box"; or perhaps we should call it "socket." Whatever the case, many people now have validated the observation. Past bewilderment probably relates to the primary topic of Chapter 2.*

I asked Marc Safran, one of the smartest young hip surgeons on the planet, with incredible vision, to tell us what his eyes see as possible answers. Keep in mind that while Marc's eyes connect to the brain and heart of a hip surgeon, he no longer sees the hip as the center of the universe. He grasps the importance of the pubic bone and surrounding muscles.

Marc's fellow Joshua Sampson joins him as a co-author. Joshua is the son of Tom Sampson, one of the original pioneers in hip arthroscopy.

Hip hop has always been braggin' and boasting and "I'm better at you than this" and "I'm better at you than that."

—Eminem.

304 Chapter 28

ILLUSTRATIVE CASE

A young professional ATP (Association of Tennis Professionals) tennis player was fighting his way up the world rankings in 2012 when his play started to decline from a nagging injury. He had been suffering from groin pain for nearly a year but had continued playing given the high pressure to perform on the international circuit. Like many high-level athletes, he believed he had to work through the pain, but after his level of play started to drop, he realized that the injury needed to be addressed. He was referred to a hip specialist for further work-up.

The patient's physical exam included pain with adduction, internal rotation, and resisted sit-up. He underwent a CT scan showing bilateral cam lesions and os acetabuli fragments near the acetabular rim (Figure 28B-1). The surgeon diagnosed the patient with femoroacetabular impingement (FAI) and suggested he undergo hip arthroscopy to relieve his symptoms.

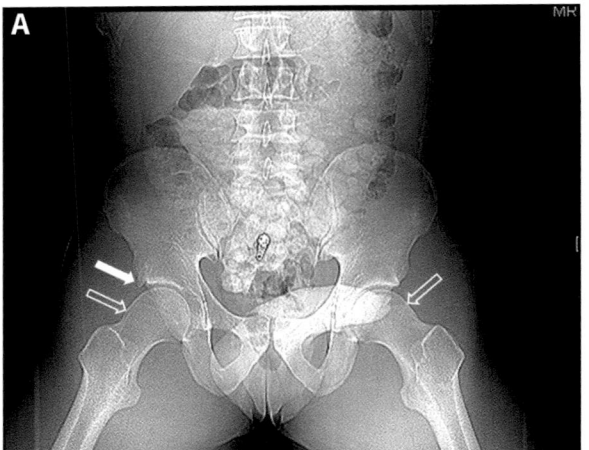 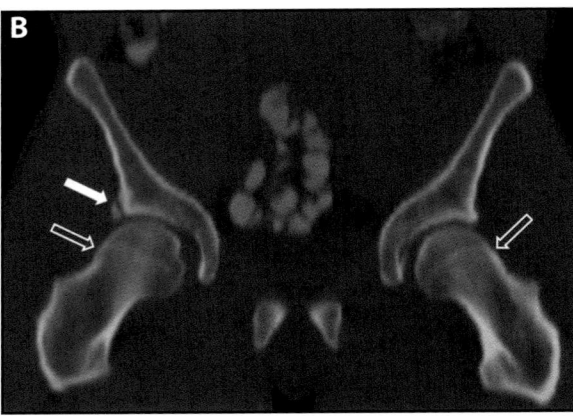

Figure 28B-1. (A) Plain X-ray and (B) CT scan, each showing both bilateral cam lesions (open arrows) and an os acetabuli fragment (closed arrows) near the acetabular rim of the right hip.

Being a high-level athlete, the patient sought a second opinion from another hip sports specialist and tennis medicine provider who agreed with the physical exam findings. However, more detailed evaluation revealed that the patient's pain was located deep in the groin, lower abdomen, and upper/inner thigh and no pain was emanating from the joint. Further, the pain elicited with flexion, adduction, and internal rotation did not recreate the patient's pain, but resisted adduction and resisted sit-up did reproduce the pain that was limiting his pain. As such, another MRI scan was obtained to evaluate for core muscle injury. The results of the MRI were said to be consistent with a *core muscle injury*, which we should all know by now is the right term. The surgeon recommended the patient undergo muscular repair. (See Figure 28B-2.)

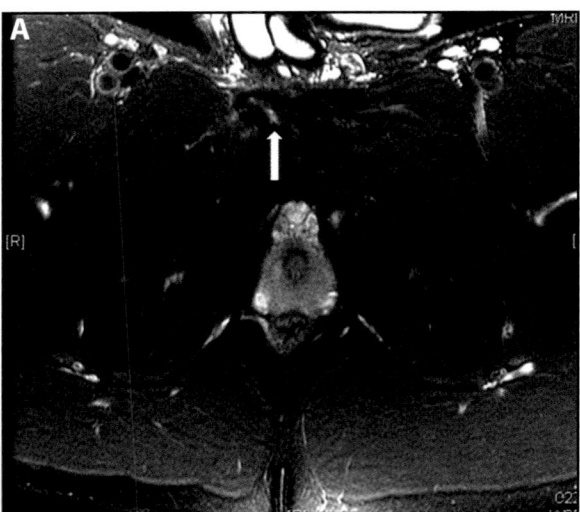 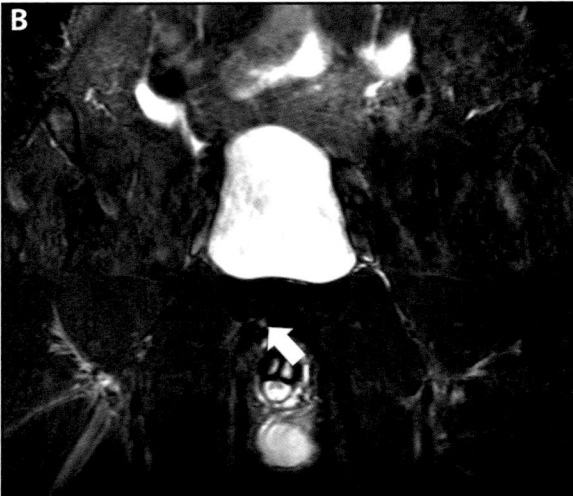

Figure 28B-2. Core muscle/pubic plate injury. Arrows show fluid between the fibrocartilage plate and right pubic body. (A) Axial image shows the right-sided plate separation. (B) Magnified coronal view.

Within 6 weeks of the core muscle surgery, the young tennis player was pain free. He underwent rehabilitation and went on to reach his highest ranking in professional tennis within the year following the surgery. Three years later, the player has had no recurrence of groin pain, nor has he had any hip pain, or needed any injections or surgery for either hip, while he remains on the ATP tour.

THE ASSOCIATION BETWEEN CORE MUSCLE INJURIES AND FEMOROACETABULAR IMPINGEMENT

FAI and core muscles injury have been observed in similar athletic populations, and concurrently in the same athletes. The sports include soccer, ice hockey, and football, which require cutting, pivoting, and acceleration. The coexistence of FAI and core muscle injury pertains to many patients with chronic groin or hip pain.

Focusing on high-level athletes, Larson et al studied a subset of patients with both symptomatic intra-articular hip pathology and athletic pubalgia. Management of the muscle injuries alone led to only a 25% return to pre-injury level of play. Treating both intra- and extra-articular symptoms concurrently led to an 85% return to pre-injury level of play. Treating both sets of problems in a stepwise manner yielded a 93% return to pre-injury level of play.[1]

A recent study conducted by Economopoulos et al found radiographic evidence of FAI in 86% of patients who were treated surgically for athletic pubalgia.[2] The evidence seems to be mounting that a relationship exists between limited range of motion ("tight hips") and chronic groin injuries.[3]

Advancements in the role of arthroscopic hip surgery have also allowed us to focus more on the overall effects of bony morphology of the hip and, in particular, the role of FAI on the rest of the pelvis. FAI describes a physical abutment of the proximal femur and the acetabulum secondary to overgrowth of bone at the proximal femur and/or acetabular rim. The result is usually a reduction of hip range of motion. Impingement may result in labral tears and articular damage.[4] Studies comparing patients with FAI to healthy controls have strongly suggested an association with alterations in gait in 3 planes of hip motion. Kinematic differences occurred in extension, adduction, and internal rotation during otherwise the stance phase of the gait cycle.[5,6]

To maintain stride length and/or hip range of motion (ROM) with sporting activities, the body must somehow compensate for FAI impingement. ROM must increase somewhere else in the pelvis. Birmingham et al studied the dynamics of FAI on pubic symphyseal joint motion.[7] The study revealed obvious motion at the pubic symphysis in all 3 planes of motion, with the majority (~60%) occurring in the transverse plane. With bony impingement about the hip joint, important rotation at the pubic symphysis seemed to occur. Cam impingements seemed to cause as much as 35% more symphyseal rotation at every level of torque. It is safe to say that at least some patients with FAI have increased motion at the pubic symphysis joint. (See Figure 28B-3.)

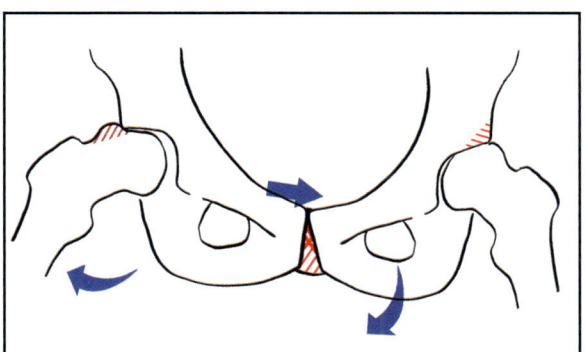

Figure 28B-3. Artist's sketch of a right-sided cam lesion forcing rotation at the pubic symphysis, resulting in alteration in left-sided forces.

The muscles attaching at or near the pubic symphysis may not be designed to stabilize effectively the symphyseal joint. The attachments are oriented to let the muscles function as abdominal flexors (rectus abdominis) or thigh adductors (eg, the adductor longus, pectineus, adductor brevis, and gracilis). Excess symphyseal motion "stresses" those muscles. Repeated excess motion at the symphysis compels those muscles to contract and help stabilize that joint. However, because these muscles are not designed biomechanically to do so, repetitive loading of the fibrocartilage (formerly thought of as the musculotendinous) sleeve around the pubis may separate this "plate" from the pubic periosteum and lead to "osteitis pubis." Formerly, it was thought that a pubic symphyseal disc played a role in this process,[8,9] but as mentioned in Chapter 7, recent evidence challenges the existence of such a disc.

Basic Biomechanics of the Hip

Understanding the biomechanics provides a better understanding of hip joint function as well as the relative importance of the anatomic structures in and around the hip joint. Think of the hip joint as connecting the trunk to the lower extremities. The 2 hips represent the main articulation between the pelvis and the femurs. Think of each hip as classically described—a ball-and-socket joint, with the head of the femur acting as the ball and the acetabulum as the socket.

The hip also supports much of the weight of the body both while standing (static) as well as moving (dynamic). The entire hip region is much more complex with more than 20 muscles crossing over the joint. Plus, the muscles and bones have wide variations in morphologies.[10]

The hip exists in at least 3 planes of motion: flexion-extension, abduction-adduction, and internal-external rotation. In addition, there are 3 "translation" planes called anterior-posterior, medial-lateral, and proximal-distal. The movement that occurs between the femoral head and the acetabulum "translates" in all 3 of those planes.[11,12]

Limitation of hip motion commonly arises from the bony structure, forcing the capsuloligamentous structures, muscular, and other soft tissue structures around the hip to stretch. In addition, flexion-extension at the knee impacts hip movement. For example, hip flexion decreases whenever the knee extends. This reduction comes from the increased tension in the muscles crossing posteriorly across both joints. Hip extension has multiple influences (eg, on the iliofemoral ligament, anterior capsule, and hip flexors).[13]

ROM is greatest in the sagittal plane. A normal hip can undergo anywhere from 120 to 140 degrees of flexion while the knee is flexed, but only 90 degrees when the knee is fully extended. The hip can undergo 10 to 20 degrees of active extension with up to 30 degrees of passive extension.[13-15]

While in flexion, the hip can undergo 0 to 70 degrees of internal rotation and 0 to 90 degrees of external rotation. The short external rotator muscles and ischiofemoral ligament limit internal rotation. The lateral band of the iliofemoral ligament, the pubofemoral ligament, the internal rotator muscles, and femoral neck anteversion all limit external rotation. Internal and external rotation is more limited in extension due to soft tissue tension.[15,16]

A normal hip abducts to 50 degrees and adducts to 30 degrees.[15] Johnston and Smidt examined the range of motion of the hip during daily activities. They observed that a basic activity such as shoe tying requires abduction and external rotation of 20 degrees and hip flexion of 120 degrees.[17] As the hip ages, it loses ranges of motion, especially flexion and extension, which makes daily activities more challenging.[18]

Bony morphology and the degree of ligamentous or muscular suppleness play important roles in hip range of motion. The former factor may be best shown by the extremes of acetabular coverage (eg, dysplastic acetabulum vs the deep pocket of coxa profunda). The wide range of motion of an ice hockey goalie may come from some degree of hip dysplasia, whereas it is doubtful someone with coxa profunda would ever be able to play that position very well. Do not discount the roles, however, of ligamentous or muscular laxity alone; either may lead to an apparent hip hypermobility.[15]

The Gait Cycle

The hip plays a large role in the gait cycle. Think of the cycle as having 2 phases: the stance phase, when the foot is planted on the ground, and the swing phase, when the foot is off the ground. The durations of the 2 phases vary on a spectrum that depends on the activity being performed. For example, walking engages the stance phase roughly 60% of the cycle. As a result, both feet remain planted on the ground about 20% of the time. We define walking by this "double support" phase, and running by the relative absence of the double support phase. Less than 50% of the gait cycle comprises the stance phase during running. The stance phase percentage decreases as running velocity increases. That gets us into the float phase when both legs lift off the ground, and at no point both feet plant at the same time.[19-21]

The role of the hip during the gait cycle occurs mainly with flexion and extension in the sagittal plane. In the swing phase, the hip goes through flexion, abduction, and external rotation. The stance phase begins following the final part of the swing phase when the hip is maximally flexed. The stance phase takes the hip through extension, adduction, and internal rotation and brings our center of gravity closer in line with the joint. The gait cycle produces a continuous spectrum for the hip, which assumes various positions combining abduction/adduction with flexion/extension.[15,20,22] Normal walking involves roughly 30 degrees of flexion and roughly 10 degrees of extension.[15,22] Flexion increases with even casual running and then much more with sprinting, as opposed to extension, which differs slightly and actually decreases with sprinting.[19,23]

The hip maximally extends when the heel comes off the ground, and maximally flexes at the end of the swing phase.[24] Maximal hip flexion increases during the swing phase as we walk faster and transition into running. Maximal flexion is greater than 55 degrees during sprinting and is less than 50 degrees during walking or jogging. The amount of adduction and abduction at the hip also varies during the walking to running transition. Adduction peaks at 15 to 20 degrees. That takes place just prior to the heel striking the ground. In contrast, abduction peaks after the toe comes off the ground during the swing phase.[15]

The muscles around the hip work in a coordinated fashion during the gait cycle. The hip flexors get involved mainly during the swing phase and the extensors during the stance phase. The gluteus maximus and hamstrings become more active during thigh deceleration in the swing phase.[19,25] The adductors work throughout the gait cycle of running, but only in the swing to mid stance portion of walking.[20] The gluteus medius and tensor fascia lata factor prominently in pelvic stabilization during ambulation and running.[25]

Now consider what happens with FAI. The results should be pretty obvious. Patients with FAI, or other processes that limit the range of motion, may not achieve a full stride. That may be most apparent in athletes, who achieve exaggerated motions during competition. Resultantly, the body compensates and creates motion in locations not designed for such forces. The compensation leads to increased motion in such places as the lumbosacral spine, other parts of the hemipelvis, sacroiliac joint, or pubic symphysis. We previously mentioned the core muscle and osteitis problems that happen. Think also about the sacroiliac joint dysfunction and the "back" pain that occurs at that location. The latter problem occurs very frequently with FAI.

SUMMARY

Increasing evidence shows that patients with FAI are more likely to develop core muscle injuries and other problems in the pelvis. Depending on the situation, one should be careful about doing surgery on the muscle problem alone.[2] The best way to treat many of these patients may be to consider addressing both problems in a coordinated fashion.[1] As we learn more about the hip and regional pelvic biomechanics, there is no doubt we will treat these conditions better.

SELECTED READINGS

Birmingham PM, Kelly BT, Jacobs R, McGrady L, Wang M. The effect of dynamic femoroacetabular impingement on pubic symphysis motion: a cadaveric study. *Am J Sports Med.* 2012;40(5):1113-1118.
   This article was the first biomechanical study to demonstrate that FAI can lead to compensatory motion at the pubic symphysis. This article confirmed the hypothesis that FAI may biomechanically cause osteitis pubis and/or core muscle injury.

Verrall GM, Slavotinek JP, Barnes PG, Esterman A, Oakeshott RD, Spriggins AJ. Hip joint range of motion restriction precedes athletic chronic groin injury. *J Sci Med Sport.* 2007;10(6):463-466.
   This article was one of the first to confirm that limited hip range of motion, as with FAI, is associated with chronic groin pain and core muscle injury.

Larson CM, Pierce BR, Giveans MR. Treatment of athletes with symptomatic intra-articular hip pathology and athletic pubalgia/sports hernia: a case series. *Arthroscopy.* 2011;27(6):768-775.
   This landmark article demonstrated the association of FAI and core muscle injury, and the need to treat both the symptoms and underlying cause. More explicitly, this study showed that surgical treatment of the core muscle injury alone may not resolve the patient's problem. Combined surgical management of the muscle and hip yielded the most satisfactory returns to sport.

REFERENCES

1. Larson CM, Pierce BR, Giveans MR. Treatment of athletes with symptomatic intra-articular hip pathology and athletic pubalgia/ sports hernia: a case series. *Arthroscopy.* 2011;27(6):768-775.
2. Economopoulos KJ, Milewski MD, Hanks JB, et al. Radiographic evidence of femoroacetabular impingement in athletes with athletic pubalgia. *Sports Health.* 2014;6(2):171-177.

3. Verrall GM, Slavotinek JP, Barnes PG, et al. Hip joint range of motion restriction precedes athletic chronic groin injury. *J Sci Med Sport*. 2007;10(6):463-466.
4. Ganz R, Parvizi J, Beck M, et al. Femoroacetabular impingement. A cause for osteoarthritis of the hip. *Clin Orthoped*. 2003;417:112-120.
5. Hunt MA, Guenther JR, Gilbart MK. Kinematic and kinetic differences during walking in patients with and without symptomatic femoroacetabular impingement. *Clin Biomech (Bristol, Avon)*. 2013;28(5):519-523.
6. Kennedy M, Lamontagne M, Beaule P. Femoroacetabular impingement alters hip and pelvic biomechanics during gait: walking biomechanics of FAI. *Gait Posture*. 2009;30(1):41-44.
7. Birmingham PM, Kelly BT, Jacobs R, McGrady L, Wang M. The effect of dynamic femoroacetabular impingement on pubic symphysis motion: a cadaveric study. *Am J Sports Med*. 2012;40(5):1113-1118.
8. Garvey JF, Read JW, Turner A. Sportsman hernia: what can we do? *Hernia*. 2010;14(1):17-25.
9. Williams PR, Thomas DP, Downes EM. Osteitis pubis and instability of the pubic symphysis: when nonoperative measures fail. *Am J Sports Med*. 2000;28(3):350-355.
10. Botser IB, Safran MR. *Delee & Drez's Orthopaedic Sports Medicine: Principles and Practice*. 4th ed. Philadelphia, PA: Elsevier; 2014:917-932.
11. Charbonnier C, Kolo FC, Duthon VB, et al. Assessment of congruence and impingement of the hip joint in professional ballet dancers: a motion capture study. *Am J Sports Med*. 2010;39(3):557-566.
12. Safran MR, Lopomo N, Zaffagnini S, et al. In vitro analysis of periarticular soft tissues constraining effect on hip kinematics and joint stability. *Knee Surg Sports Traumatol Arthrosc*. 2013;21(7):1655-1663.
13. Hamill J, Knutzen K. *Biomechanical Basis of Human Movement*. 3rd ed. Baltimore, MD: Lippincott Williams & Wilkins; 2009:187-254.
14. Dewberry MJ, Bohannon RW, Tiberio D, et al. Pelvic and femoral contributions to bilateral hip flexion by subjects suspended from a bar. *Clin Biomech*. 2003;18:494-499.
15. Hughes PE, Hsu JC, Matava MJ. Hip anatomy and biomechanics in the athlete. *Sports Med Arthrosc*. 2002;10(2):103-114.
16. Nordin M, Frankel VH. *Basic Biomechanics of the Musculoskeletal System*. 3rd ed. Baltimore, MD: Lippincott Williams & Wilkins; 2001:203-221.
17. Johnston RC, Smidt GL. Hip motion measurements for selected activities of daily living. *Clin Orthop*. 1970;72:205.
18. Murray R, Bohannon R, Tiberio D, et al. Pelvifemoral rhythm during unilateral hip flexion in standing. *Clin Biomech*. 2002;17:147-151.
19. Mann RA, Hagy J. Biomechanics of walking, running, and sprinting. *Am J Sports Med*. 1980;8(5):345-350.
20. Nicola TL, Jewison DJ. The anatomy and biomechanics of running. *Clin Sports Med*. 2012;31(2):187-201.
21. Novacheck TF. The biomechanics of running. *Gait Posture*. 1998;7(1):77-95.
22. Polkowski GG, Clohisy JC. Hip biomechanics. *Sports Med Arthrosc*. 2010;18(2):56-62.
23. Franz JR, Paylo KW, Dicharry J, et al. Changes in the coordination of hip and pelvis kinematics with mode of locomotion. *Gait Posture*. 2009;29(3):494-498.
24. Murray MP, Kory RC, Clarkson BH. Walking patterns in healthy old men. *J Gerontol*. 1969;24:169-178.
25. Cappellini G, Ivanenko YP, Poppele RE, et al. Motor patterns in human walking and running. *J Neurophysiol*. 2006;95(6):3426-3437.

29

what lies **behind** the hip
the **deep derrière**

Hal David Martin, DO

Editor's Note: *Hal Martin has been leading the way into the deepest, darkest aspects of the core—what has been regarded as the "black hole" of our anatomy, a place where many pains seem to originate and stay. It seemed appropriate to ask Hal to write this chapter on the anatomy posterior and otherwise immediately adjacent to the hip.*

Pain in the front can also be a pain in the butt.

—The chapter author.

JOE THE PLUMBER (FIGURE 29-1)

Joe has his own plumbing business and comes into the clinic with aching groin pain and "fat wallet" syndrome. The latter occurs not because he makes a lot of money—Joe does okay—but because he can't sit for more than 10 minutes on one side of his butt without pain. And when he does sit, he leans onto the unaffected side as though he has a fat wallet. Joe needs to be able to sit. Otherwise, he has to do all his plumbing work squatting, which isn't so bad, except squatting for so long, eventually, tires him out. He grades the pain an 8 on a 10-point scale, and completes our modified Harris Hip Score form, which catalogs him as an F (with 55 out of 100 points).

To investigate the issue, we go through our evaluation routine. This begins with a comprehensive history and physical examination. We then confirm our clinical impression with several tests. The pain radiates down the backside of the affected leg and worsens with activity. We rule out the lumbar spine with a back examination and magnetic resonance imaging (MRI). We do a bunch of other physical examination maneuvers. Palpation suggests the culprit to be the piriformis muscle. The pain increases with the seated piriformis stretch test (ie, we move one straight leg over the other and rotate it inward). This maneuver stretches the piriformis muscle, which sometimes compresses the sciatic nerve and does not allow normal nerve motion.

Then we do the active piriformis test. Joe lies on his unaffected side, bends his knee, drives his heel into the table, and rotates his knee away from his body against resistance. This activity makes the piriformis contract. This, again, increases the pain. We know the sensitivity and specificity of doing both these tests together to be 0.91 and 0.80, respectively. We become convinced that the problem is entrapment of the sciatic nerve. We follow with diagnostic/therapeutic injections, MRI, and nerve conduction studies.

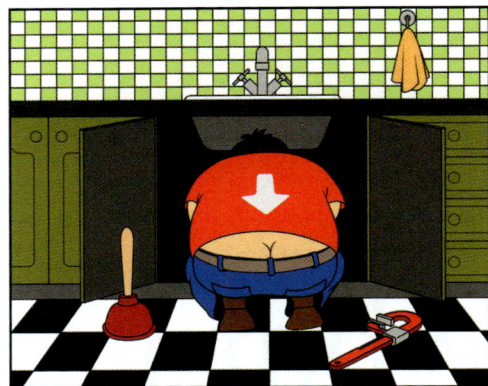

Figure 29-1.

Joe wants nonoperative treatment, and we put him on a physical therapy program. He achieves more mobility of the piriformis muscle and hip external rotators with focused piriformis stretch exercises. Joe sits with both legs flat to the ground. He bends the affected side knee and places his foot on the lateral aspect of the opposite knee. He initiates the stretch by pulling his knee inward, as far has he can, toward his chest. This set of exercises greatly alleviates the pain for several months. After 6 months, it comes back, even more piercingly than it had ever been. Our surgical treatment options include open or endoscopic sciatic nerve decompression. He chooses the minimally invasive approach and gets piriformis partial tenotomy. The procedure restores normal sciatic nerve motion and cures him.

Now, 1 year after definitive therapy, Joe's pain is 0 and his modified Harris Hip score A+, with a 100 out of 100 total. He is back full time to work, sitting and squatting without pain, and making a good living.

The effort invested in "getting it right" should be commensurate with the importance of the decision.

—Daniel Kahneman, 2002 Nobel Prize winner in Economics and author of the best-selling book *Thinking, Fast and Slow.*

Getting It Right

Professor Daniel Kahneman's beautiful prose tells us that we arrive on a decision by either thinking fast or thinking slowly. A huge distinction exists between fast intuitive thought and slow deliberate thought processes. Solving the mystery of a perplexing problem in this region of our body comes only by thinking slowly—piecing together a puzzle of anatomy, biomechanics, clinical diagnostics, and treatment outcomes.

The first piece of the puzzle is hip pain that does not fit the usual clinical profile. Then arrives the search for the anatomical and biomechanical pieces. We have learned to recognize those pieces from our research in the laboratory. The puzzle begins to take shape when we complete the diagnostics and make the decisions. By carefully observing the outcome, hopefully, we complete the puzzle. The final answer comes after recycling the same pieces and puzzle-solving methods over and over again, and seeing if the same methods and pieces continue to solve similar puzzles.

The Formerly Mysterious Region

The hip, the way we have defined it, is just the ball and socket. The anatomical territory behind the hip has remained a "black hole" (Figure 29-2) for too long. We are talking about the region deep to the glutes, where so much pain in so many people seems to originate. The anatomy, it turns out, is readily identifiable. Most problems that reside here can be unearthed via a comprehensive history and physical examination.

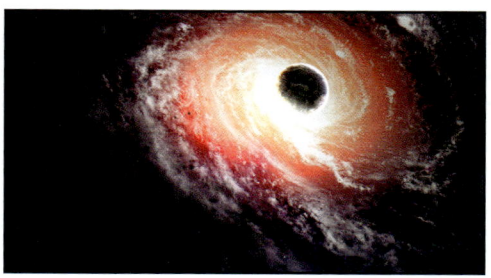

Figure 29-2. Aerospace experts talk about a mysterious black hole in the middle of galaxies where stars, debris, and other materials enter and disappear. The analogy here is to the anatomy posterior to the hip, where so many pains dwell, and diagnoses fleetingly exist and then disappear.

The realization that one can diagnose the problems in this region requires a thorough understanding of the anatomy and biomechanics of the hip and this surrounding territory. Close anatomic and kinematic relationships exist among the lumbar spine, pelvis, and hip, so, of course, to determine what exactly is going on entails a structured approach. Failure to identify a cause of pain in this region, especially in a timely manner, can have devastating effects. In fact, delay in diagnosis can increase the perception of pain, and thereby diminish the quality of life and take away hope.

We think of the region as having 5 different anatomic levels: osseous, capsulolabral, musculotendinous, neurovascular, and kinematic (ie, adjacent anatomy relating to motion or directly to the kinematic chain). Imaging tools and other ancillary tests are usually confirmatory. Physical therapy and guided injections may provide good initial treatment options. Open or endoscopic surgical techniques show promise in selected patients.

The bottom line is that pinpointing the involved anatomy remains essential. The skill to see this spectrum of afflictions necessitates seeing what we see now in terms of functional anatomy, and also learning the knowledge that is rapidly evolving about ways that intra-articular anatomy connect to structures outside the hip joint. Much of this important dynamic occurs behind the hip.

The Crucial Concept

The number of causes and consequent treatment options for posterior core pain grow as our understanding of clinical anatomy and biomechanics in this region expand.[1] Think of the hip as the center axis of the largest lever-arm of the human body. These biomechanics entail a balance of interactions between the osseous and soft tissue structures that exist there, the natural ranges of motion of the contained joints and superimposed neuromuscular activity.[2] Any alteration in the balance might produce pain due to disturbances of the kinematic chain in any direction from the hip joint.

That means that deep derrière pain can occur from any number of causes that emanate from intra- or extra-articular sources. The main diagnoses are intra-articular hip pathologies, spine issues, intrapelvic abnormalities, pudendal nerve entrapment, something we call *ischiofemoral impingement* (IFI), hamstring origin tendinopathy, deep gluteal syndrome (DGS), and secondary lumbar spine influences (SLSI). Often, DGS and SLSI come from abnormal kinematics arising from primary hip joint pathology.

Abutments in the Butt

Much of the book thus far has focused on different types of bony impingements inside the hip joint (ie, cam, pincer, or mixed). That's not the only place where abnormal abutments may occur. Many impingements also happen outside the hip joint, and, in particular, behind it. For example, subtle abnormalities in the orientation of the femoral neck or lesser trochanter may lead to extra-articular hip impingement, and then kinematic chain disturbances and posterior pain.[3]

Table 29-1 lists the anatomical landmarks relevant to posterior hip pain. These include different structures at each level (bone, capsulolabral and ligamentous, musculotendinous, neurovascular, and kinematic). As we have stated, intra-articular and extra-articular sources of posterior hip pain can usually be identified through a comprehensive history and physical examination.

Table 29-1
The Five Anatomic Considerations in the Deep Derrière

Bone	Capsulolabral and Ligamentous
- Sacroiliac joint - Posterior acetabulum - Greater trochanter (posterior aspect and tip) - Lesser trochanter (size and version) - Femoral neck (torsion and femoral neck-shaft angle) - Ischium - Ischiofemoral space - Greater trochanter/ischial space	- Sacrotuberous ligament - Posterior labrum - Posterior capsule - Ischiofemoral ligament
Musculotendinous	**Neurovascular**
- Gluteus maximus muscle - Gluteus medius muscle - Piriformis muscle and tendon - Hamstring origin tendons - Adductor magnus origin - Obturator internus muscle and tendon - Quadratus femoris muscle	- Sciatic nerve - Posterior femorocutaneous nerve - Pudendal nerve - Fibrovascular bands - Inferior gluteal artery
	Kinematic
	- Sagittal and coronal spinal axes - Pelvic tilt and rotation - Triplanar lower leg mechanical axis

Version, the Trochanters, and Ischiofemoral Impingement

A recent study assessed the relationship between the femoral neck "version" and lesser trochanter "version" with IFI using a standardized MRI protocol. Femoral neck version and lesser trochanter angle were significantly increased in patients with symptomatic IFI.[4] A cadaveric study by Martin et al showed that even the greater trochanter can impinge on the ischium during a combination of hip flexion, abduction, and external rotation.[5] This phenomenon is also called *greater trochanteric pelvic impingement*. While IFI is a common problem often left unrecognized, the occurrence of such greater trochanter impingement demonstrates the importance of considering each person's anatomy individually.

Relationships Between the Back and the Posterior

Limitations in range of motion due to femoroacetabular or any other type of impingement lead to adaptations in lumbopelvic kinematics. One provisional biomechanical study suggested that "pelvic inclination" may help increase loads on the lumbar spine.[6] Another cadaveric study proved a relationship between simulated IFI and lumbar facet load changes during terminal hip extension.[7] Problems such as flexor contracture, posterior acetabular overcoverage, and femoral retroversion can also limit terminal hip extension and have similar effects on the lumbar spine. Secondary pelvic rotation, hyperlordosis, and facet joint overload may explain lower back symptoms in patients with hip pathologies. Limitation of terminal hip extension can increase hyperlordosis, and also narrow foramina thereby compressing adjacent lumbar nerve roots.[8] One take-away from all these analyses—Every hip exam should include a back exam and every back exam should include a hip exam.

The Sciatic Nerve

The sciatic nerve plays a huge role in many of these pains (Figure 29-3). Sciatic nerve kinematic adaptation (and irritation) occurs within a dynamic narrowing of the ischial tunnel in posterior hip impingement.[5,8] The sciatic nerve enters the pelvis via the sciatic notch and moves considerably with hip movement. In fact, Coppieters et al[9] found that the sciatic nerve has 28 mm of excursion during hip flexion. Sciatic motion may also be greatly affected by "penetration" of the piriformis muscle. That muscle actually pierces portions of the sciatic nerve in 16.2% of the population.[10]

In normal situations, the sciatic nerve glides across the posterior border of the greater trochanter as the hip moves into deep flexion, abduction, and external rotation. Greater trochanteric impingement occurs when the sciatic glide is absent. These observations about the sciatic nerve also turn out to be important with respect to understanding the principles of many types of rehabilitation. In the fully flexed, abducted, and externally rotated state, the semimembranosus muscle origin and the posterior edge of the greater trochanter can come into contact.[5] During hip flexion with knee extension, a spiraling phenomenon of the sciatic nerve has been observed, and then the tension gets better with hip abduction and knee flexion.[11] Study of the kinematics of the sciatic nerve within the ischial tunnel continues to bear fruit.

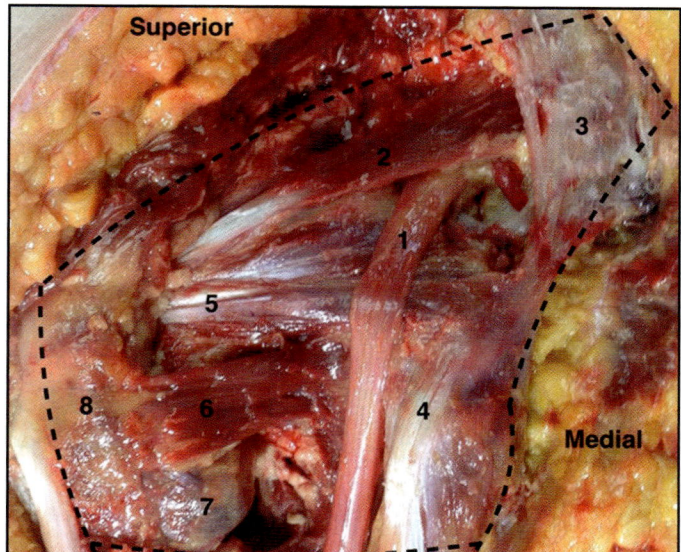

Figure 29-3. Deep gluteal space. A cadaveric left hip with the gluteus maximus reflected. The course of the sciatic nerve (1) as it enters the pelvis at the sciatic notch anterior to the piriformis muscle (2) and sacrotuberous ligament (3). As the nerve courses distally toward the ischium and hamstring origin (4), it passes posterior to the gemelli-obturator internus complex (5) and quadratus femoris (6) with the inferior portion removed to expose the lesser trochanter. Lateral structures include the lesser trochanter (7) and greater trochanter (8). (© Hal David Martin, Manoj Reddy, Juan Gomez-Hoyos 2015. *J Hip Preserv Surg*. Published by Oxford University Press.)

The Hamstrings

Chronic hamstring origin abnormalities can occur in patients with posterior impingements.[12] Therefore, these mechanisms should also be considered in the evaluation of posterior pain. Most hamstring injuries are from indirect trauma (ie, overuse injuries from excessive stretching or repeated forceful contractions), which leads to muscle strains, tears, or even avulsions.[13]

Hamstring tears, regardless of cause, lead to sciatic nerve irritation and lower buttock pain due to inflammation and scar. We call this problem *ischial tunnel syndrome* or *hamstring syndrome*. This is an important diagnosis to consider in most patients with posterior hip pain.[14]

Several studies demonstrate, beyond a doubt, the close relationship among the sciatic nerve, hamstring origin, and ischium (Figure 29-4). A cadaveric study by Miller and Webb[15] emphasizes the intimate anatomic relationship the sciatic nerve has with the ischium and hamstring origin. The sciatic nerve lies an average of 1.2 ± 0.2 cm from the most lateral aspect of the ischial tuberosity. The branches situated there are likely to be irritated. Branches to the long head of the biceps femoris and semitendinosus muscle emerge at a close distance to the ischial tuberosity (6.9 and 7.1 cm, respectively), although this area is highly variable.[16]

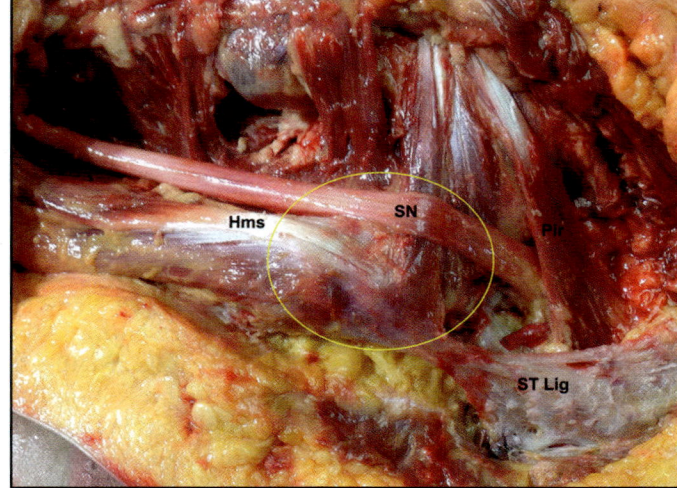

Figure 29-4. Hamstring (Hms) and sciatic nerve (SN) anatomy. Pir = piriformis muscle, ST Lig = sacrotuberous ligament. (© Hal David Martin, Manoj Reddy, Juan Gomez-Hoyos 2015. *J Hip Preserv Surg*. Published by Oxford University Press.)

Deep Gluteal Syndrome

DGS describes the entrapment of the sciatic nerve in the deep gluteal space. A number of structures may entrap the sciatic nerve: fibrous bands containing blood vessels, gluteal muscles, hamstring muscles, the gemelli-obturator internus complex, bone structures, vascular abnormalities, and space-occupying lesions.[1] One should also remember that abutments of the sciatic nerve may also occur in locations above or below the deep gluteal space, such as by intrapelvic vascular and gynecologic abnormalities.[17]

Pudendal Nerve Issues

One should also remember that the pudendal nerve may a play a role in some of the mysterious pains. Pudendal nerve entrapment and/or irritation can occur at various locations, such as the intrapelvic region, near the piriformis muscle or at the sciatic notch, or involving the sacrospinous ligament or sacrotuberous ligament.[18]

It's all about location, location, location.

—Numerous real estate moguls lay claim to this declaration.
The statement probably originated in Chicago in the early 1900s.

LOCATING THE PAIN (TABLE 29-2)

The exact location of the pain, plus the elicitation of that pain on examination, often leads to the right answers. As discussed in Chapter 18, the site of pain or tenderness can fool you, but don't start out with that negative attitude. Probably, nothing is more instructive than identifying where the pain is and what causes and relieves it, and then finding the exact site of tenderness and reproducing the pain with various physical examination maneuvers. So, take off your modesty hat, get a chaperone, and ask the daring questions during your history; then track down the correct diagnosis with your physical examination.

Use the ischial tuberosity as a reference point (Figure 29-5). Hamstring tendon pathologies lie lateral or posterior to the ischial tuberosity. IFI (or ischial tunnel syndrome) also occurs lateral to the ischial tuberosity, but not so lateral. DGS pain (ie, sciatic nerve impingement) manifests superiorly and laterally; that means at the sciatic notch or beyond that along the course of the sciatic nerve. Pudendal nerve entrapment signs and symptoms occur medial to the ischial tuberosity.

History

Sitting aggravates pudendal-origin and other pain manifesting medial to the ischial tuberosity. A toilet seat or sitting donut usually alleviates these pains, as does standing or a good night's rest off one's butt. The pudendal nerve entrapment patient often awakens in the morning feeling good. Then the pain progresses and gets worse and worse during the day. Pudendal nerve entrapment generates pain often described as burning, tearing, stabbing, lightning-like, electrical, sharp, or shooting. Patients often describe foreign body sensations and changes in skin sensation.[18,19]

Patients with sciatic nerve entrapment often have a history of trauma and sit-pain (the inability to sit for more than 30 minutes). They also often have radicular pain emanating from the low back or "hip," with paresthesias of the affected leg.[9] Patients with hamstring syndrome or IFI present similarly, so either syndrome, or the coexistence of the two, must come to mind when you observe such descriptions in lateral (to the ischial tuberosity) locations.[20]

Patients with distal sciatic nerve impingement have different complaints than those with more proximal causes. Take, for example, hamstring vs IFI. The hamstring patient often exacerbates the pain by sitting (eg, driving), whereas, in general, patients with IFI are more comfortable sitting. Conversely, IFI patients have more pain during the terminal hip extension part of walking. In the driving position,[10,21] the hip rests in a 30-degree flexion position. Therefore, the semimembranosus of the hamstring has a different (and worse from the standpoint of pain) force vector angle. Holding the hip in 30 degrees flexion with the hamstring activated, no matter the mechanism, can reproduce sciatic nerve complaints. The

Table 29-2
The Main Posterior Disorders and Their Anatomic Associations

Diagnosis	Osseous	Capsulolabral and Ligamentous	Musculotendinous	Neurovascular	Kinematic
Sacroiliac joint dysfunction	X	X			X
Deep gluteal syndrome/sciatic nerve entrapment	X		X	X	X
Ischiofemoral impingement	X		X	X	X
Greater trochanter/pelvic impingement	X			X	
Hamstring origin tendon avulsion/ischial tunnel syndrome	X		X		
Pudendal nerve entrapment		X	X	X	
Hip-spine syndrome	X	X	X	X	X
Sacrotuberous ligament avulsion		X			
Ischiofemoral ligament strain		X			
Buttock claudication			X	X	
Adductor magnus origin avulsions			X		
Posterior femoroacetabular impingement and labral tears	X	X			X
Intrapelvic nerve entrapment	X		X	X	X
Spinal disorders	X		X	X	X

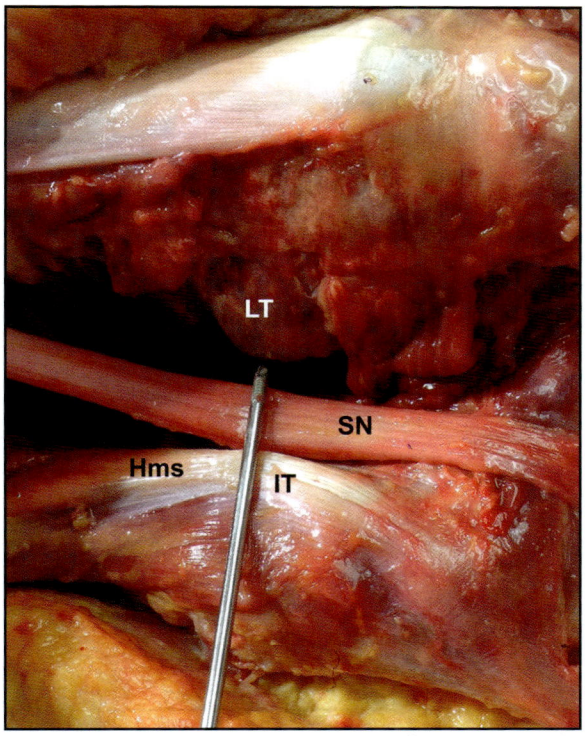

Figure 29-5. Ischial tuberosity (IT) is a reference point. The right side of the figure is superior, top lateral, and bottom medial. Hms = hamstrings, LT = lesser trochanter, SN = sciatic nerve. (© Hal David Martin, Manoj Reddy, Juan Gomez-Hoyos 2015. *J Hip Preserv Surg*. Published by Oxford University Press.)

terminal hip extension of walking diminishes the space between the ischium and the lesser trochanter and squeezes the sciatic nerve in IFI.

Any sort of posterior abutment can also cause low back pain, which makes the separation of spinal and posterior core issues even trickier. Limited hip range of motion has long been known to affect spine mobility and function.[22-26] Patients with IFI have those symptoms due to the limited hip extension. Gomez-Hoyos confirmed that direct relationship in a cadaveric study by artificially decreasing the ischiofemoral space and seeing lumbar intrafacet joint pressure increase.

Distinguishing between sacroiliac joint disorders and hip or other posterior core disorders can be thorny, particularly considering how often hip and sacroiliac joint problems occur together. We use the rule that pain inferior and medial to the posterior superior iliac spine points to sacroiliac joint disorders. However, we must rule out gluteus maximus tendinitis. Ask whether the pain is "on" or "in" the sacroiliac joint? Only 4% of patients with sacroiliac joint pain mark that they have pain above the L5 vertebra on pain drawings,[27] so the rule does has practical applicability. Sacroiliac tenderness, combined with that location of pain, has the highest sensitivity. One must remember, still, the lack of specificity. Beware that any pathology that produces loss of hip extension can cause sacroiliac joint pain and tenderness.

Table 29-3
Physical Examination Tests for Posterior Pain

Test	Maneuver	Positive if...
Standing position		
Long-stride walking test[8]	The patient is asked to walk with long strides and then short strides.	Pain is reproducible lateral to the ischium during hip extension with long strides while pain is alleviated when walking with short strides.
Seated position		
Hamstring active test[13]	The patient tries to flex the knee against resistance in seated position at 30 degrees of knee flexion and then at 90 degrees of knee flexion.	Weakness and pain at 30 degrees and pain is improved at 90 degrees.
Passive seated piriformis test[27]	The patient is seated over the edge of an examination table with the hip flexed to approximately 90 degrees and the knee extended. The examiner palpates the sciatic notch and adducts and internally rotates the limb.	Provokes pain at piriformis.
Supine position		
FABER test[19]	The patient lies supine as the examiner crosses the same-side foot over the opposite-side thigh. The pelvis is stabilized at the opposite ASIS by the hand of the examiner. A gentle force is steadily increased on the same-side knee of the patient, exaggerating the motion of hip flexion, abduction, and external rotation.	Provokes pain at a specific location. The test is useful for problems such as sacroiliac joint dysfunction and greater trochanteric/ischial impingement.
Thigh thrust test[19]	The patient lies supine with one hip flexed to 90 degrees. The pelvis is stabilized at the opposite ASIS with the hand of the examiner. The examiner stands on the same side as the flexed leg. The examiner provides steady and increasing pressure through the axis of the femur.	Provokes pain at the sacroiliac joint.
Sacroiliac distraction test[19]	The patient lies supine and is asked to place his/her forearm behind lumbar spine to support the natural lordosis. A pillow is placed under the patient's knees. The examiner places hands on the anterior and medial aspects of the patient's left and right ASIS with arms crossed and elbows straight. A slow and steady pressure is applied by leaning toward the patient.	Provokes pain at the sacroiliac joint.
Gaenslen test[20]	The patient lies supine near the edge of the table and is asked to flex the opposite hip grasping his/her knee. This action "locks" the sacroiliac joint in position prior to the next step. The examiner then slides the near-side leg (typically starting with the painful side) off the table and applies a steady extension force while simultaneously applying a flexion force through the opposite leg. The patient assists with the opposite-side hip flexion.	Provokes pain at the sacroiliac joint.

(continued)

Table 29-3 (continued) Physical Examination Tests for Posterior Pain

Test	Maneuver	Positive if...
Lateral position		
Sacroiliac joints lateral compression test[19]	The patient is placed in a side-lying position, facing away from the examiner, with a pillow between the knees. The examiner places a steady downward pressure through the anterior aspect of the lateral ilium, between the greater trochanter and iliac crest.	Provokes pain at the sacroiliac joint.
Active piriformis test[27]	The examiner palpates the piriformis as the patient is instructed to drive heel into the examination table, initiating active hip abduction and external rotation against the resistance by the examiner.	Provokes pain at piriformis.
Posterior rim impingement test	Patient lies supine, and the examiner places the patient's hip in extension and external rotation.	Provokes posterior pain or apprehension.
Ischiofemoral impingement test[8]	The examiner extends the hip in neutral or mild adduction and then extends it again in hip abduction.	Pain is present in hip extension with a neutral or adducted hip, and is absent or very mild in hip extension with an abducted hip. A clinically evident increase of the lumbar lordosis during hip extension is considered a "positive hip-spine test."
Prone position		
There are no specific tests for posterior hip pain in prone position. However, Craig test for femoral version and Ely's test for rectus femoris contracture add information to the therapeutic decision-making process.		

Physical Examination (Table 29-3)

Since the various posterior entrapments/impingements occur with movement or in different positions, we perform our examinations during 5 different postures. The most efficient order of examinations turns out to be: (1) standing, (2) seated, (3) supine, (4) lateral, and finally (5) prone.[28] At the same time, we look for alterations in normal biomechanical postures or axes, such as gait patterns, pelvic tilt, rotation, foot progression, comparative leg lengths, global laxity, spinal or hip ranges of motion, femoral neck version, muscular contractures, laxities, or asymmetrical strength. Concurrently, we try to exclude such diagnoses as tumors and inflammatory spondyloarthropathies.[29] That sounds like a lot of labor and thinking. It is. We warn you: a careful diagnostic examination for posterior core pain takes a while.

There are many things to consider.

Biomechanical axis alignment is one of them. It provides information of pelvic positioning. Abnormal pelvic positioning contributes to weakness or, as the patient says, "stiffness" of the core muscles surrounding the hip. Normally, there is a balance between hip flexors and extensors. A bad balance creates an uncomfortable feeling. The opposite is true too: injury to the muscles or hip creates a bad balance and messes up pelvic positioning. It is easiest to think of the posterior core in the sagittal axis. There is no doubt that sagittal axis misalignment contributes to the development of both DGS and IFI.[30-33] That being said, we spend a lot of time trying to distinguish between DGS and IFI.

Another factor is gait. Gait analysis can reveal important information that leads to the diagnosis. The long-stride walking test can differentiate hamstring syndrome from IFI. As mentioned, IFI occurs more frequently with increased femoral version.[21,34] The long-stride walking test is positive when the patient refers pain lateral to the ischium during terminal extension that is relieved with short steps[3,4] (Figure 29-6). The internal foot progression angle during gait can uncover the increased femoral version of IFI.[34]

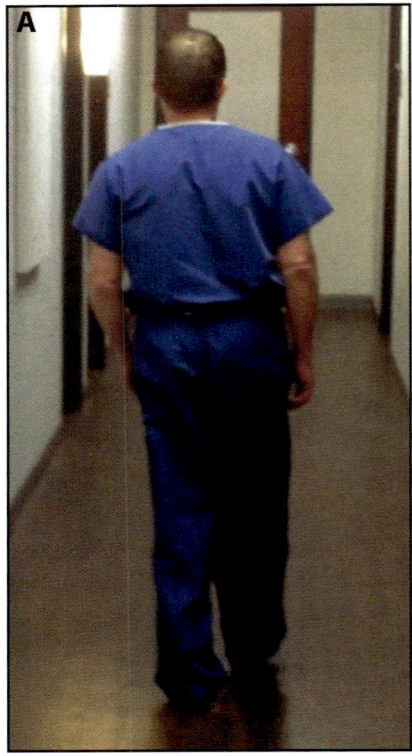

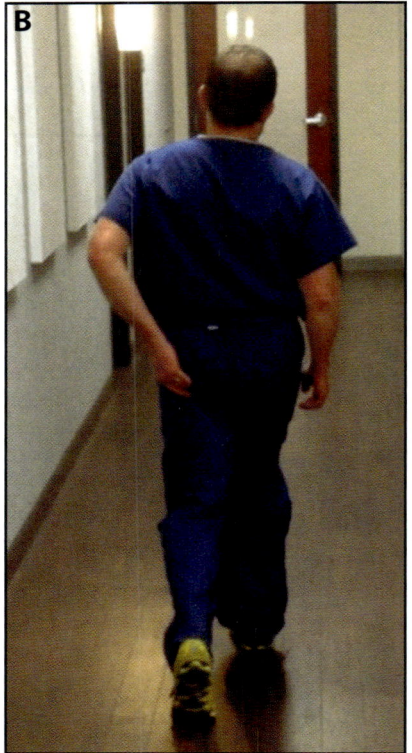

Figure 29-6. Long-stride walking test. (A) Weight on left leg. (B) Weight on right leg. (© Hal David Martin, Manoj Reddy, Juan Gomez-Hoyos 2015. *J Hip Preserv Surg.* Published by Oxford University Press.)

A positive Trendelenburg sign usually indicates weakness of the gluteus medius muscle. The analysis may reveal adduction and pelvic tilt abnormalities associated with the rotational motion and axial load of the lesser trochanter rubbing against the ischium (ie, IFI).[10,21,34] Specific pain patterns during gait deliver important clues. For example, one may see during the initial heel strike that the hamstring muscles activate eccentrically and decelerate the leg. The subject may be guarding against pain lateral to the ischial tuberosity. This is a positive sign for proximal acute or chronic hamstring tears. This contrasts with the long-stride walking test mentioned, which serves as a critical diagnosis tool for IFI.[3,4] For that diagnosis, Gomez-Hoyos et al showed that the latter test had a sensitivity of 0.94 and specificity of 0.85.

What we said, in general, about location holds in spades for the physical examination. Palpation of the gluteal structures in the seated position using the ischial tuberosity as a reference point guides the diagnosis.[10] The sitting position facilitates activation of the hamstring test. The patient is asked to actively flex the knee at 30 or 90 degrees against the resistance of the examiner (Figure 29-7). Reproduction of the pain identical to the complaint usually means a proximal hamstring tendon injury. Then one thinks of the hamstring syndrome and sciatic nerve subluxation into the ischial tunnel.[10] Proximal vs distal entrapment then follows simply by noting the precise location of the accordingly provoked pain.

DGS describes the presence of pain in the buttock caused from nondiscogenic and extrapelvic entrapment of the sciatic nerve. Several structures can be involved in sciatic nerve entrapment within the gluteal space. Usually, we think in terms of identifying the precise location where the sciatic nerve is trapped (ie, from proximal to distal). Two tests in seated position are particularly helpful. The piriformis stretch test (sensitivity 0.52; specificity 0.90) is performed with the hip in flexion, adduction, and internal rotation. The examiner extends the knee (ie, engaging the sciatic nerve) and passively moves the flexed hip into more adduction and internal rotation while palpating the piriformis muscle, which lies lateral to the ischium and external rotators, or, more proximally, at the sciatic notch. A positive test recreates the pain at the piriformis.[5]

Two more sets of tests help differentiate IFI from DGS. We move the patient into the lateral decubitus position. First, we have the active and passive piriformis tests. These tests have a sensitivity of 0.78 and specificity of 0.80. The patient drives his/her heel into the examination table, initiating active hip abduction and external rotation against resistance from the examiner. Like the piriformis stretch test, elicitation of pain at the level of the piriformis or external rotators constitutes a positive test.[5] Then we perform the second test, which we call the *IFI test*. The patient stays in the lateral decubitus position, and the examiner extends the hip in a neutral position. The production of pain lateral to the ischium means IFI. This impression gets confirmed by a "control" test, which means the examiner then extends the hip again while abducting it. The absence of pain during the latter maneuver functionally clinches the presence of IFI. In our studies, the IFI test has a sensitivity of 0.82 and specificity of 0.85, when done in combination with the long-stride walking test[3] (Figure 29-8).

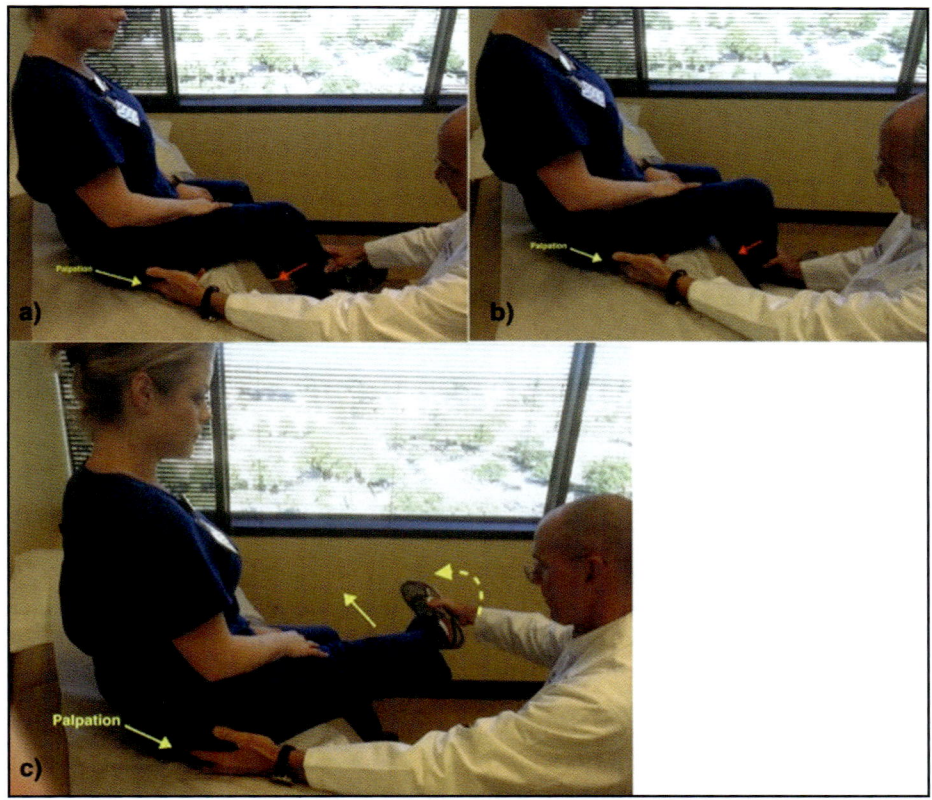

Figure 29-7. Hamstring active test and piriformis stretch test. (A) Active hamstring test at 45 degrees knee flexion. (B) Active hamstring test at 90 degrees knee flexion. (C) Piriformis stretch test. (© Hal David Martin, Manoj Reddy, Juan Gomez-Hoyos 2015. *J Hip Preserv Surg*. Published by Oxford University Press.)

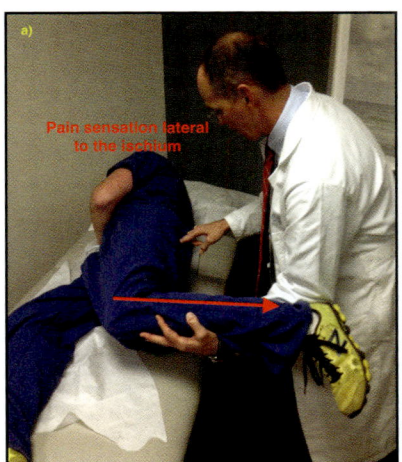 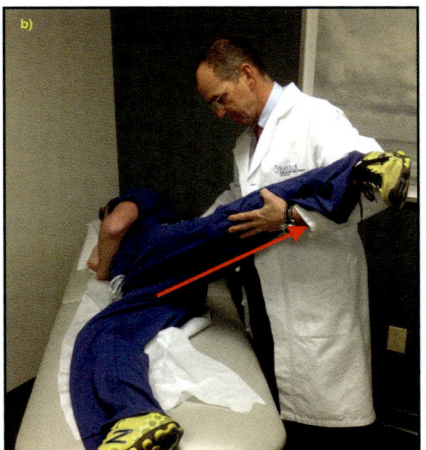 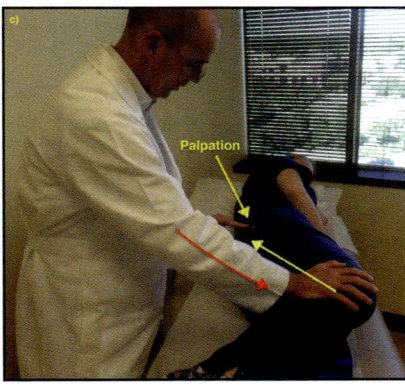

Figure 29-8. Lateral position tests that help differentiate between the "distal" causes of DGS. (A) IFI test (ie, attempt to recreate pain lateral to the ischium). (B) Attempt to alleviate symptoms with leg abduction and extension. (C) Piriformis muscle test (ie, attempt to recreate pain lateral to the piriformis muscle). This test helps distinguish proximal from distal etiologies. (© Hal David Martin, Manoj Reddy, Juan Gomez-Hoyos 2015. *J Hip Preserv Surg*. Published by Oxford University Press.)

Traps

Of course, as you might imagine, not only are there many anatomic entrapments in this region, but there are also many diagnostic traps for the clinician. This book talks about the 4 different parts of the core, and *le derrière* incorporates all 4 parts. Some of the more common traps that we encounter are urogynecologic (eg, endometriosis, bladder or bowel issues, and dysmenorrhea)[10,16,17] and neural (ie, entrapment of nerves in unusual locations). Think of all the nerves that coalesce here, spinal nerve roots, peripheral nerves, etc. The pudendal nerve is complex by itself, and the sciatic nerve can be entrapped in more than one location (eg, at the piriformis or obturator internus muscle, by the sacrotuberous or sacrospinous ligaments, or at the falciform process). Sometimes, a pelvic floor manual test performed by a physical therapist with the right anatomic experience, assists this differentiation between these different diagnoses.[17,35,36]

Imaging and Other Ancillary Tests (Table 29-4)

Standard plain roentgenograms include the standing AP pelvis, false profile, and lateral images. MRI helps rule out intrapelvic sources of sciatic nerve entrapment vs extrapelvic sciatic nerve entrapment. A T3 MRI and patient positioning turn out to be important. The feet are secured in a neutral walking position, in order to best recreate the ischiofemoral space during this dynamic phase. Otherwise, a false positive decreased ischiofemoral space may occur.

The T2 axial or T2 coronal series best visualizes the semimembranosus and its orientation to the lateral ischium. This view also allows best detects partial or undersurface musculotendinous tears. Dynamic MRI or ultrasound may be useful for detecting subluxation. For the dynamic ultrasound, the patient lies prone and performs a bicycling motion activating the hamstring. If the latter pathology is present, the semimembranosus then subluxes into the ischial tunnel recreating sciatic nerve radicular pain. Scarring is best assessed with the T1 and T2 axial and coronal series. T3 MRI best assesses intrapelvic gynecologic or vascular sciatic nerve entrapments.

Other testing may include dynamic EMG, which we have found tricky to interpret. Injections of precise anatomical sites may sometimes localize important pathology. A double injection technique of anesthetic and corticosteroid in the region of the piriformis muscle relieved the pain in 41 out of 45 patients. Certainly, ultrasound may help in the critical assessment of IFI vs hamstring causes of posterior pain. Fluoroscopy can be helpful in the recreation of pain under direct bony observation, such as in the diagnosis of greater trochanteric sciatic nerve impingement. Also, sometime overall kinematic study of the hip may be helpful in localizing exact locations of impingement in difficult-to-diagnose patients. The latter makes more sense than fluoroscopy when soft tissue, rather than bony, impingements are suspected culprits.

Treatment

Nonoperative

This usually means a combination of physical therapy, steroidal or nonsteroidal injections,[10,37,38] and neuropsychological evaluation/treatment.[10,36] Educational strategies addressing activities of daily living and handouts containing home exercise programs may also have merit for some patients.

The physical therapy treatment for hamstring syndrome, IFI, or DGS includes lumbosacral spine alignment and stabilization, pelvic floor and/or intra-articular structures. The aim is to rebalance the muscle-articular functioning of the hip/pelvis and spine through soft tissue mobilization, stretching, strengthening, and aerobic conditioning. Depending on the suspected degree of pelvic floor involvement, pelvic floor massage and other internal therapy may apply.

For Joe the Plumber, we mentioned one exercise aimed at increasing sciatic nerve mobility within the deep gluteal space. This exercise combines the piriformis stretch with sciatic nerve-greater trochanter mobilization (Figure 29-9).[36]

Sometimes, IFI may be resolved by simple solutions such as a shoe lift to moderate leg length inequality or gait therapy (eg, addressing a hyperpronated hind foot by bringing the extremity into less internal rotation during midfoot stance phase). At the same time, one must beware of the presence of concurrent pathologies, such as genu valgum or coxa valga, which may narrow the ischiofemoral space, which may result in more exaggerated pain during implementation of these therapeutic attempts.

Table 29-4
Main Clinical and Imaging Features of the Most Important Differential Diagnosis in Patients With Posterior Hip Pain

Diagnosis	History Highlights	Physical Exam	Main Diagnostic Tools
Deep gluteal syndrome/sciatic nerve entrapment	Aching, burning, or cramping sensation Sitting pain with square sitting avoidance	Production of pain by palpation at the sciatic notch Could have abnormal reflexes or weakness Active piriformis tests Passive seated piriformis test	T1 MRI showing fibrovascular bands reaching the sciatic nerve and/or tendinous structures crossing the nerve T2-weighted MRI showing perineural hyperintensity and/or vascular engorgement Imaging-guided injection to the periphery of the nerve and/or the suspected source of entrapment (more commonly piriformis muscle) Electromyography and nerve conduction
Pudendal nerve irritation	Pain medial to the ischium Sitting pain Pain relief when standing and absent upon awakening Foreign body sensation Cyclic variations in pain Painful intercourse Bladder and bowel issues Numbness	Production of pain by palpation medial to the ischium	Perineural hyperintensity on 3T MRI T2-weighted axial sequences Imaging-guided injections at the sciatic notch, sacrospinous ligament, sacrotuberous ligament, and obturator internus muscle Intrapelvic examination
Ischiofemoral impingement	Pain lateral to the ischium during terminal hip extension Lower back pain (hip-spine effect)	Production of pain by palpation lateral to the ischium Long-stride walking test Ischiofemoral impingement test	Dynamic CT scan or MRI T2-weighted MRI showing narrow ischiofemoral (< 17 mm) and quadratus femoris spaces (< 8 mm) with or without quadratus femoris edema Hamstring tendinosis in 50% of the cases
Greater trochanteric ischial/sciatic nerve impingement	Pain lateral to the ischium or at the posterior aspect of the greater trochanter during flexion-abduction-external rotation of the hip Radiating pain Hyperlaxity	Production of pain by palpation lateral to the ischium and/or posterior to the greater trochanter Patrick/FABER test	Dynamic CT scan or MRI Dynamic ultrasonography showing abnormal sciatic nerve kinematics into the ischial tunnel T2-weighted MRI showing greater trochanteric bursitis associated to hamstring tendonitis or tear Imaging-guided injection at the posterior greater trochanter and/or lateral ischium

(continued)

Table 29-4 (continued)
Main Clinical and Imaging Features of the Most Important Differential Diagnosis in Patients With Posterior Hip Pain

Diagnosis	History Highlights	Physical Exam	Main Diagnostic Tools
Hamstring origin avulsion	Pain lateral or posterior to the ischium during heel strike Increasing pain with hip flexion plus knee extension Radiating pain (ischial tunnel syndrome)	Production of pain by palpation lateral and/or posterior to the ischium Hamstring active test	Dynamic ultrasonography showing avulsed hamstring tendons T2-weighted MRI showing hyperintensity between the hamstring tendons and the ischium Imaging-guided injection to the hamstring origin
Sacroiliac joint pain/dysfunction	Pain inferior to the posterior superior iliac spine	Production of pain by palpation medial at the sacroiliac joint Thigh thrust test Sacroiliac joint distraction test Gaenslen test Sacroiliac lateral compression test	T2-weighted MRI showing bone marrow and/or subchondral bone hyperintensity around the sacroiliac joint Fluid/inflammation at the sacroiliac joint can be observed in sacroiliitis Imaging-guided injection to the sacroiliac joint
Posterior femoroacetabular impingement/labral tear	Mechanical symptoms, including clicking, locking, catching, or giving way mainly during hip extension	Posterior femoroacetabular impingement test	X-ray showing prominent posterior wall T2-weighted MRI showing posterior labral tear
Gluteus maximus claudication	Fatigue after walking or muscle activation, and alleviated by rest	Production of fatigue or claudication by maintained gluteus maximus activation against resistance	T1 MRI showing gluteus maximus muscle atrophy Arteriography showing gluteal arteries stenosis
Hip-spine syndrome	Lower back pain Hip pain at a location according to the primary hip pathology Radiating pain due to nerve root compression	Limited terminal hip extension Hip-spine test Clinical evidence of any other hip problem related to the hip-spine effect	Lumbosacral X-ray showing lack of sagittal or coronal spine balance Imaging features of hip problems producing limitations on hip range of motion

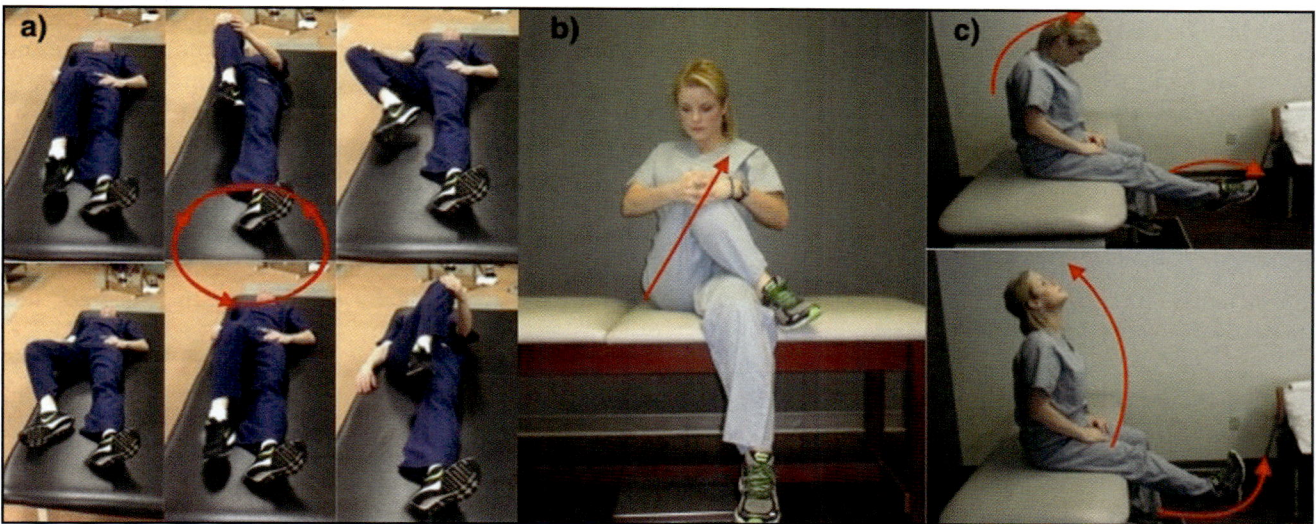

Figure 29-9. Rehabilitation exercises designed to mobilize the sciatic nerve and stretch the piriformis and external rotator muscles. (A) Hip circumduction (go counter-clockwise). (B) Piriformis stretch. (C) Neural mobilization. (© Hal David Martin, Manoj Reddy, Juan Gomez-Hoyos 2015. *J Hip Preserv Surg*. Published by Oxford University Press.)

Surgery

The precise surgical treatment, of course, depends on both the specificity of the clinical diagnoses, as well as the radiologic and targeted injection correlations. The surgery, obviously, must address the relevant pathology. The goal of surgery is to restore normal anatomy and neuromuscular function.

The correct surgical procedure for IFI must encompass consideration of the entire biomechanical axis. If femoral torsion is greater than 30 degrees of femoral anteversion, one must consider femoral de-rotational osteotomy. The latter decision depends on 3 planar osseous assessments, a McKibbin's index with precise acetabular and femoral version analyses, and sagittal plane and bimalleolar axis assessments.

With well-selected patients, the endoscopic techniques have proven successful using multiple functional hip and return to sport grading systems and 2-year follow-up.[4] The surgical options involve open, endoscopic, or combination open-closed techniques. The goal is a functionally normal ischiofemoral space (ie, between the ischium and lesser trochanter). This may involve either lesser trochanteroplasty or ischioplasty or both. The patient is placed supine on a traction table with 20 degrees contralateral tilt. The procedure involves 3 portals—anterolateral, posterolateral, and "auxiliary" (at level of lesser trochanter).

Traction ensues for less than 15 minutes for a complete examination of the intra-articular space, and the remainder of the procedure performed without traction. A 70-degree high-definition arthroscope is introduced initially through the anterolateral portal, while the other ports are used mainly for other instrumentation. A window of resected quadratus femoris is necessary to access the lesser trochanter between the medial circumflex femoral artery and first perforating femoral artery. After the surgical trochanteric remodeling, one verifies the decompression by moving around the hip under fluoroscopy.[4]

The cases of proximal hamstring injury plus IFI require a combination of ischioplasty and hamstring repair, with or without lesser trochanteroplasty. The goal here is basically the same (ie, to recreate the space for normal terminal hip extension, plus to avoid any kinematic lumbar consequences). Decompression of the sciatic nerve, of course, remains critical for optimal results. Hamstring avulsions are repaired at the same time using, again, either an open or endoscopic approach. Fully endoscopic repairs are becoming more popular,[2,39] but those closed repairs limit how much the hamstring can be mobilized. The closed repairs become very difficult for retractions greater than 5 cm.[39]

As so nicely illustrated by Drs. Dodson and Woods in Chapter 31, the open approach for hamstrings avulsion is generally preferred when a large amount of scar is predicted.[40] We have found that Achilles allografts may be necessary for tears older than 3 months. For anyone intending to do such hamstring repairs, we strongly recommend to first do a thorough review of the literature.[40-45]

An alternative surgical approach within the deep derrière is a "mini-open" surgical technique, which means by dry endoscopy combined with neuromonitoring. The goal of neuromonitoring is to reduce the intraoperative risk of nerve damage.[46-48]

The mini-open, transgluteal approach is performed with the patient in a prone position. The ischial tuberosity and ischiofemoral space are identified under fluoroscopy. Hamstrings are accessed through the gluteus maximus. The size and severity of hamstring avulsion are identified through an 8-cm incision, and once the degenerated tendon fibers and bursa are removed, the footprint of the torn tendon is decorticated with a 4.0-mm burr. The hamstrings are reattached to the anatomic footprint using 4.5-mm sutures and direct fluoroscopic visualization.

One must take into account the ischial angle, which reflects the degree of ischioplasty resection. The overall goal is to create a flat surface by which the semimembranosus can be repaired at the same time as recreation of a proper ischiofemoral space. Should the space remain narrow after the maximally achieved ischial resection, one can still internally rotate the femur and approach the lesser trochanter via the central portion of the quadratus femoris, like before. All potentially culprit adhesions are divided, and nerve mobility is assessed prior to closure. We usually lock the knee in 45 degrees flexion for 3 to 4 weeks postoperatively, depending on the degree of tension.

Effective open and endoscopic techniques have been described for hamstring origin repair,[13,14,47] ischiofemoral decompression,[8,14,48] piriformis release/sciatic nerve decompression,[23,40] and posterior labral tears with or without rim fractures.[49,50]

Optimistic people play a disproportionate role in shaping our lives. Their decisions make a difference; they are inventors, entrepreneurs, political and military leaders—not average people. They got to where they are by seeking challenges and taking risks.

—Daniel Kahneman.

THE BOTTOM LINE

With regard to the deep derrière, the posterior, what lies behind the hip, whatever you want to call this region, the bottom line reverberates in Daniel Kahneman's above quote. For so many years, this region has remained mysterious. It has maintained the status, perhaps, of the black hole and frightened orthopedists and so many others away. Diagnoses, such as piriformis syndrome, have come and gone. Certainly, there is a lot going on here. There is a lot more going on than just the piriformis muscle.

The bottom line is to stay optimistic and recognize that the anatomy here is identifiable and the pathology very diagnosable. With this recognition, we can make the right decisions in terms of doing something good, doing something to cure the various pains that reside here. In short, there are just 5 aspects of the anatomy to consider. And only 8 main sets of diagnoses to contemplate: hip, spine, intrapelvic, pudendal, IFI, hamstring, sciatic, and secondary lumbosacral. Of course, more than one diagnostic category can occur at the same time, and that may make things seem more complicated.

But, do not let things in this anatomic region get complicated. KISS…Keep it simple (stupid). For any given patient, we must, as Kahneman says, "think slowly." We have to think deliberately and comprehensively. Each patient's affliction then becomes a solvable puzzle. We can solve that puzzle by fitting together the right pieces of anatomy, biomechanics, kinematics, and clinical expertise. We already have most of the right diagnostic tools. We have, or are developing, the right therapeutic approaches.

SELECTED READINGS

Martin HD, Khoury A, Schroder R, Palmer IJ. Ischiofemoral impingement and hamstring syndrome as causes of posterior hip pain: where do we go next? *Clin Sports Med.* 2016;35:469-486.
An excellent (of course, we wrote it!) recent review of the anatomy, biomechanics, clinical, and diagnostics of posterior hip pain.

Martin HD. Mini symposium: evolving concepts in extra-articular hip pathology. *J Hip Pres Surg.* 2015;2(2):91-122.

This report comes from a fun symposium, featuring hot topics and cutting-edge techniques, such as cavernous laparoscopic approaches; subtleties of the deep gluteal syndrome; entirely endoscopic periacetabular, femoral, and pubic symphyseal osteotomies and fusions; and much-less-invasive hamstring approaches. Discussion contains details of the surgical practices of such pioneers as Lemos, Possover, Martin, Reddy, Gomez-Hoyos, Matsuda, and Guanche.

REFERENCES

1. Martin HD, Reddy M, Gomez-Hoyos J. Deep gluteal syndrome. *J Hip Preserv Surg.* 2015;2(2):99-107.
2. Chambers HG, Sutherland DH. A practical guide to gait analysis. *J Am Acad Orthop Surg.* 2002;10(3):222-231.
3. Bardakos N V. Hip impingement: beyond femoroacetabular. *J Hip Preserv Surg.* 2015;2(3):206-223.
4. Gomez-Hoyos J, Schroder R, Reddy M, Palmer I, Martin H. Femoral neck anteversion and lesser trochanteric retroversion in patients with ischiofemoral impingement. *Arthroscopy.* 2016;32(1):13-18.
5. Kivlan B, Martin RL, Martin HD. Defining the greater trochanter-ischial space: a potential source of extra-articular impingement in the posterior hip region. *J Hip Preserv Surg.* 2016;3(4):352-357.
6. Popovich JM, Welcher JB, Hedman TP, et al. Lumbar facet joint and intervertebral disc loading during simulated pelvic obliquity. *Spine J.* 2013;13(11):1581-1589.
7. Gomez-Hoyos J, Khoury A, Schroder R, Johnson E, Palmer I, Martin H. The hip-spine effect: a cadaveric study of simulated ischiofemoral impingement in hip extension effecting loads in lumbar facet joints. XVI Congresso Brasileiro de Quadril, Fortaleza, Brazil; 2015.
8. Hatem MA, Palmer IJ, Martin HD. Diagnosis and 2-year outcomes of endoscopic treatment for ischiofemoral impingement. *Arthroscopy.* 2015;31(2):239-246.
9. Coppieters MW, Alshami AM, Babri AS, Souvlis T, Kippers V, Hodges PW. Strain and excursion of the sciatic, tibial, and plantar nerves during a modified straight leg raising test. *J Orthop Res.* 2006;24(9):1883-1889.
10. Smoll NR. Variations of the piriformis and sciatic nerve with clinical consequence: a review. *Clin Anat.* 2010;23(1):8-17.
11. Khoury A, Schroder R, Gomez-Hoyos J, Reddy M, Palmer I, Martin H. The effects of hip abduction on sciatic nerve during terminal hip flexion. ISHA Annual Meeting, Cambridge, United Kingdom; 2014.
12. Torriani M, Souto SCL, Thomas BJ, Ouellette H, Bredella MA. Ischiofemoral impingement syndrome: an entity with hip pain and abnormalities of the quadratus femoris muscle. *Am J Roentgenol.* 2009;193:186-190.
13. Guanche CA. Hamstring injuries. *J Hip Preserv Surg.* 2015;2(2):116-122.
14. Gomez-Hoyos J, Reddy M, Martin HD. Dry endoscopic-assisted mini-open approach with neuromonitoring for chronic hamstring avulsions and ischial tunnel syndrome. *Arthrosc Tech.* 2015;4(3):e193-e199.
15. Miller SL, Webb GR. The proximal origin of the hamstrings and surrounding anatomy encountered during repair. Surgical technique. *J Bone Joint Surg Am.* 2008;90(suppl 2):108-116.
16. Seidel PM, Seidel GK, Gans BM, Dijkers M. Precise localization of the motor nerve branches to the hamstring muscles: an aid to the conduct of neurolytic procedures. *Arch Phys Med Rehabil.* 1996;77(11):157-160.
17. Lemos N, Possover M. Laparoscopic approach to intrapelvic nerve entrapments. *J Hip Preserv Surg.* 2015;2(2):92-98.
18. Filler AG. Diagnosis and treatment of pudendal nerve entrapment syndrome subtypes: imaging, injections, and minimal access surgery. *Neurosurg Focus.* 2009;26(2):E9.
19. Dreyfuss P, Michaelsen M, Pauza K, McLarty J, Bogduk N. The value of medical history and physical examination in diagnosing sacroiliac joint pain. *Spine.* 1996;21(22):2594-2602.
20. Dreyfuss P, Dreyer SJ, Cole A, Mayo K. Sacroiliac joint pain. *J Am Acad Orthop Surg.* 2004;12(4):255-265.
21. Cibulka MT, Sinacore DR, Cromer GS, Delitto A. Unilateral hip rotation range of motion asymmetry in patients with sacroiliac joint regional pain. *Spine J.* 1998;23(9):1009-1015.
22. Halbertsma JP, Göeken LN, Hof a L, Groothoff JW, Eisma WH. Extensibility and stiffness of the hamstrings in patients with nonspecific low back pain. *Arch Phys Med Rehabil.* 2001;82(2):232-238.
23. Neumann DA. Kinesiology of the hip: a focus on muscular actions. *J Orthop Sports Phys Ther.* 2010;40(2):82-94.
24. Ekstrom RA, Donatelli RA, Carp KC. Electromyographic analysis of core trunk, hip, and thigh muscles during 9 rehabilitation exercises. *J Orthop Sports Phys Ther.* 2007;37(12):754-762.
25. Sullivan MK, Dejulia JJ, Worrell TW. Effect of pelvic position and stretching method on hamstring muscle flexibility. *Med Sci Sports Exerc.* 1992;24(12):1383-1389.
26. Gomez-Hoyos J, Martin R, Schroder R, Palmer I, Martin H. Accuracy of two clinical tests for ischiofemoral impingement in patients with posterior hip pain and endoscopically confirmed diagnosis. *Arthroscopy.* 2016;32(7):1279-1284.
27. Martin HD, Kivlan BR, Palmer IJ, Martin RL. Diagnostic accuracy of clinical tests for sciatic nerve entrapment in the gluteal region. *Knee Surg Sports Traumatol Arthrosc.* 2014;22(4):882-888.
28. Van Dillen LR, Gombatto SP, Collins DR, Engsberg JR, Sahrmann SA. Symmetry of timing of hip and lumbopelvic rotation motion in 2 different subgroups of people with low back pain. *Arch Phys Med Rehabil.* 2007;88(3):351-360.
29. Van Dillen LR, Bloom NJ, Gombatto SP, Susco TM. Hip rotation range of motion in people with and without low back pain who participate in rotation-related sports. *Phys Ther Sport.* 2008;9(2):72-81.
30. Hibner M, Desai N, Robertson LJ, Nour M. Pudendal neuralgia. *J Minim Invasive Gynecol.* 2010;17(2):148-153.
31. FitzGerald MP, Kotarinos R. Rehabilitation of the short pelvic floor. II: treatment of the patient with the short pelvic floor. *Int Urogynecol J Pelvic Floor Dysfunct.* 2003;14(4):269-275.
32. Schröder RG, Martin RRL, Bobb VL, et al. Outcomes of non-operative management of deep gluteal syndrome: a case series of six patients. *J Musculoskelet Disord Treat.* 2016;2:012.

33. Michel F, Decavel P, Toussirot E, et al. Piriformis muscle syndrome: diagnostic criteria and treatment of a monocentric series of 250 patients. *Ann Phys Rehabil Med.* 2013;56(5):371-383.
34. Ellison JB, Rose SJ, Sahrmann S. Patterns of hip rotation range of motion: a comparison between healthy subjects and patients with low back pain. *Phys Ther.* 1990;70(9):537-541.
35. Fishman LM, Dombi GW, Michaelsen C, et al. Piriformis syndrome: diagnosis, treatment, and outcome: a 10-year study. *Arch Phys Med Rehabil.* 2002;83(3):295-301.
36. Fetzer GB, Fischer DA. Hamstrings injuries. In: Guanche C, ed. *Hip and Pelvis Injuries in Sports Medicine.* Philadelphia, PA: Lippincott Williams & Wilkins; 2010:181-192.
37. Mica L, Schwaller A, Stoupis C, Penka I, Vomela J, Vollenweider A. Avulsion of the hamstring muscle group: a follow-up of 6 adult non-athletes with early operative treatment: a brief report. *World J Surg.* 2009;33(8):1605-1610.
38. Sallay P, Ballard G, Hamersly S, Schrader M. The effect of collar on aseptic loosening and proximal femoral bone resorption in hybrid total hip arthroplasty. *Orthopedics.* 2008;31(3):227.
39. Lempainen L, Sarimo J, Mattila K, Vaittinen S, Orava S. Proximal hamstring tendinopathy: results of surgical management and histopathologic findings. *Am J Sports Med.* 2009;37(4):727-734.
40. Chakravarthy J, Ramisetty N, Pimpalnerkar A, Mohtadi N. Surgical repair of complete proximal hamstring tendon ruptures in water skiers and bull riders: a report of four cases and review of the literature. *Br J Sports Med.* 2005;39(8):569-572.
41. Cross M, Vandersluis R, Wood D, Banff M. Surgical repair of chronic complete hamstring rupture in the adult patient. *Am J Sports Med.* 1998;26(6):785-788.
42. Porat M, Orozco F, Goyal N, Post Z, Ong A. Neurophysiologic monitoring can predict iatrogenic injury during acetabular and pelvic fracture fixation. *HSS J.* 2013;9(3):218-222.
43. Calder HB, Mast J, Johnstone C. Intraoperative evoked potential monitoring in acetabular surgery. *Clin Orthop Relat Res.* 1994;305:160-167.
44. Baumgaertner MR, Wegner D, Booke J. SSEP monitoring during pelvic and acetabular fracture surgery. *J Orthop Trauma.* 1994;8:127-133.
45. Rust D, Giveans MR, Stone RM, Samuelson KM, Larson CM. Functional outcomes and return to sports after acute repair, chronic repair, and allograft reconstruction for proximal hamstring ruptures. *Am J Sports Med.* 2014;42(6):1377-1383.
46. Truong WH, Murnaghan L, Hopyan S. Ischioplasty for femoroischial impingement. *JBJS Case Connect.* 2012;2(3):e51.
47. Martin HD, Shears SA, Johnson JC, Smathers AM, Palmer IJ. The endoscopic treatment of sciatic nerve entrapment/deep gluteal syndrome. *Arthroscopy.* 2011;27(2):172-181.
48. Filler AG, Haynes J, Jordan SE, et al. Sciatica of nondisc origin and piriformis syndrome: diagnosis by magnetic resonance neurography and interventional magnetic resonance imaging with outcome study of resulting treatment. *J Neurosurg Spine.* 2005;2:99-115.
49. Yoon SJ. Arthroscopic treatment in acetabular posterior wall fractures. ISHA Annual Meeting, Cambridge, United Kingdom; 2014.
50. Cross MB, Shindle MK, Kelly BT. Arthroscopic anterior and posterior labral repair after traumatic hip dislocation: case report and review of the literature. *HSS J.* 2010;6(2):223-227.

section four

shared responsibility*

*from both Democratic and Republican Presidential platforms

30

fixing everything
putting the **core universe** into perspective

Editor's Note: *Section Four covers both generally accepted and alternative perspectives on the core. The main point is that no particular specialist "owns" the core. We should pay attention to all who work within this region of the body: physical therapists, osteopaths, yogi, nonoperative sports physicians, the list is long. An important theme is that everything in the core is connected. One fixes one part of the body only to find out that something else is broken! Osteopathy, chiropractic, and yoga, for example, offer explanations for this corporal connectivity. As we realize that the core defines a scientific discipline, those "alternative" disciplines may no longer seem quite so alternative.*

As we explore this new world in the next chapters, recognize 3 dangers that lurk in the shadows. (1) Beware of the impostors, people who profess they already know all about the core. They are out there, big time, in all the disciplines. With your antennae up, they are easy to recognize. (2) Resist our own natural tendencies, as therapists, to try to cure everything. Instead, identify the specific goals of each patient or client. For each patient, chart, unambiguously, that person's right course. And (3) look out for the "Twilight Zone." For example, in this first chapter, we shall travel through the fourth dimension and then into the fifth. We know we can get you into the fifth dimension. The problem is getting you back from there.

In this, let's say, "capsule" of a chapter, we shall travel up high again, way past 30,000 feet this time, so that we visualize the entire universe of core anatomy and diagnoses depicted in the Venn diagram of Figure 19-3. While we sit gazing in space, we catch glimpses of an unidentified planet darting between and behind the other core planets. We wonder if this is real. Is it a high-speed meteorite? As we look closer, it looks more like a planet. A neon sign flashes from this furtive spheroid. The sign says: "Perfect Core Health and Maximal Performance Planet." This is definitely not a comet. This is the Perfect Core Planet. This is our Holy Grail! Is it for real? (See Figure 30-1.)

We ask others sitting on nearby space mobiles, "Have you ever seen this Perfect Planet?"

All say no, except one pompous bonehead, who crows, "I live there. I can tell you all of its secrets."

This is BB, the bloviating blowhard. He is obviously BS-ing. The Perfect Planet, in actuality, remains elusive. No one has actually landed there. If, by chance, a wandering soul has ever arrived there, certainly that soul would not have recognized the place, nor would he/she have stayed there stay for long.

Just for a moment now, in the yet-unboggled part of your brain, imagine you have a desire to fix or optimize everything that might possibly ail in somebody's core, and then to deliver that perfect physical specimen, decorated with a bow, to the Perfect Planet. How do you do that? Where do you begin?

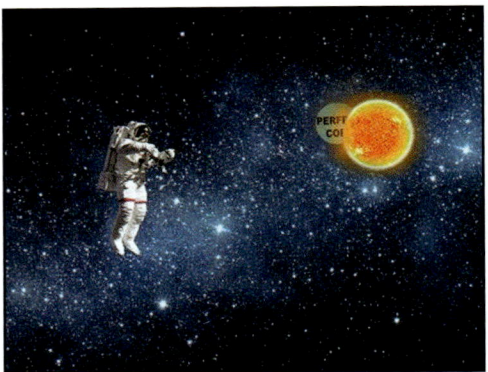

Figure 30-1.

THE MAGIC ITINERARY

What is the magic formula for optimizing our engine room, this region of the body we call the core? First, ask the question that gets us closer to reality: What is our best strategy to do that? Now ask the even simpler question: What's the best way to begin to think about the best strategy to optimize the core?

Okay, here's the formula. There are 5 legs to our journey (Table 30-1).

- Leg 1: We must recognize our limitations. In space parlance, we allude to this leg by the expression: Don't travel too close to the sun.
- Leg 2: We set practical goals. This usually means cooling our jets, and sometimes shooting for the moon. In space parlance, we say: See all the planets, but don't necessarily travel there.
- Leg 3: We need to know what we know; plus, the corollary to that statement: We need to know when we don't know. In space parlance, that means: Know our own planet.
- Leg 4: We must catalog the varieties of therapy that might help and determine how to apply them. In other words, we make a list of what we can do, and add to that list the therapies we don't know how to do, and then highlight in yellow or green whether or not we can find out how to do those other therapeutic modalities or have to find someone to do them for us. In space parlance, this means: Know our travel options.
- Leg 5: The final leg of the journey is the decision-making (ie, determining what actually to do and also when and how to apply techniques or seek consultants). Optimal strategy figures in cost, likelihood of success, individual biases, efficiencies, and other practicalities like the need to find an expert with more experience. Then and only then, we execute the strategy. This last leg of the core journey goes by the parlance: We have lift off.

Now let's go through the sights we see during each of the 5 legs of this magical mystery voyage toward perfection.

LEG 1: DON'T TRAVEL TOO CLOSE TO THE SUN
(IE, KNOWING OUR LIMITATIONS)

From the journey's beginning, we must be aware of 3 limitations. The first limitation is knowing we don't know everything about the core. There are just too many systems that reside there for anyone to know it all in depth. Plus, we have way too much still to learn about it. The core belongs to us all, not any one individual or individual specialty. We may know a lot about parts of the core, but no one knows it all. This limitation insinuates 2 things.

The first insinuation is that we should respect all specialties that deal with the core in any fashion. That means chiropractors, osteopaths, yoga and Pilates instructors, fitness fanatics…everybody. They all have something to offer. We may not agree with what they say or do, but we must watch and listen. Experience means a lot in this field right now.

It is not too late for new paradigms to appear. Many specialists are looking at the core from dramatically different perspectives. Even though we may not "get it" right away, this may be on account of that "unsee phenomenon" that we talked about in Chapter 4. Therefore, in Section Four, we have included several chapters written by such specialists. From the outset, we, the editors, admit that we do not agree about everything they say. But we do recognize these specialists still might be right, at least about certain things. As we said earlier, everybody has partial ownership of the core. Nobody owns it all.

The second insinuation is that we also must watch out for the charlatans in this field. While we all strive for the perfect core, we should not let our gusto fool us. We must learn to identify the bloviating blowhard, whom we shall call BB. As we have said before, this developing field of study provides many opportunities, especially for scam artists. BB usually lays claim to total ownership. BB talks but does not listen. We go more into the recognition of BB in the rehabilitation and performance chapter. BB prospers in all specialties within the core, not just those.

Table 30-1
The Five-Legged Trip to the Perfect Core

1. Don't Travel Too Close to the Sun
2. See All the Planets
3. Know Your Own Planet
4. Know Your Travel Options
5. Lift-Off

The second limitation is the built-in oxymoron of any fitness specialty: Getting fit means traumatizing our tissues. We talked about this in Chapters 20 and 21. Growth and development are body-molding processes, just like lifting weights. Cam impingement may come from exercising too much the wrong way during adolescence. Exercise and microtrauma go together. Some cardiologists even argue that anything more than minimal exercise is bad for us.

Certainly, we should not ignore any of those arguments. Face it. Life should be a process of becoming more fit, and, at the same time, minimizing trauma to ourselves. Perhaps that is why we call it survival of the fittest. So, we must think of life and fitness as a series of graphic curves. Yes, charts (Figures 30-2 and 30-3). Each of us has our own life curves. The trick is recognizing which curve we should be on. Our inability to be sure about the right curve for any one individual is our second inherent limitation. It's like that old analogy: If one glass of wine allows us to live longer, how about two? What about more?

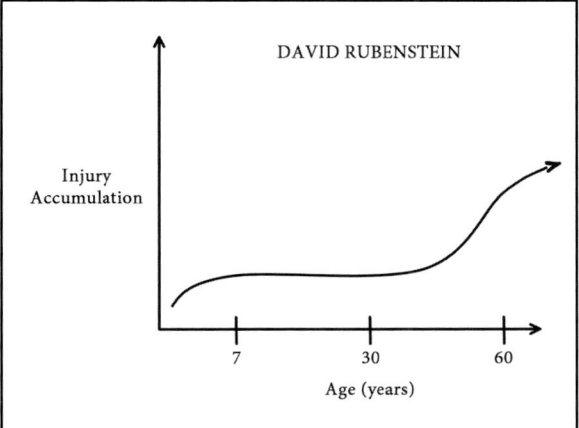

Figure 30-2. Remember the quote, from Chapter 21, by David Rubenstein, CEO of the Carlisle Group: "I was a great athlete until I was 7. Then I took time off. Now I can beat most of my friends in tennis because they have artificial hips and knees." This graph would be his "life injury accumulation curve" and shows how David might defeat his tennis opponents as he gets older. Contrast this with Figure 30-3.

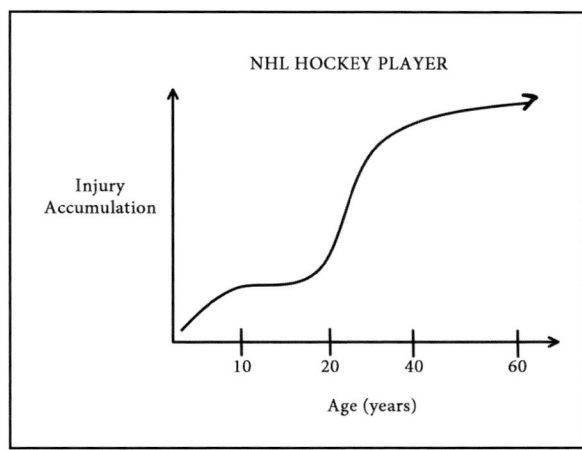

Figure 30-3. Life injury accumulation curve for an NHL hockey player, whom David Rubenstein might beat in tennis.

The third limitation is experience, or lack of it. Like any developing field, experience matters. Not size…experience! No matter how wide our eyes may open, we can't see everything just by just looking. We may say, or convince ourselves, that we can see everything, but we can't. When we blind ourselves to that reality, we become just like BB, the know-it-all, bloviating blowhard mentioned above. When it comes to diagnosing someone correctly, or prescribing the right exercises, or deciding pushing forward rather than resting…true experience matters. The learning curves are steep within this still-developing field. It is easy to harm someone in this field.

Leg 2: See All the Planets but Don't Necessarily Travel There (ie, Setting Practical Goals)

You aren't trying to make everyone into an Adrian Peterson or a Mia Hamm. Fitness and repair strategies depend on goals of the individual patients or clients. Goals get more complicated the more accomplished the person or athlete. As we said in Chapter 21, proper goals derive from proper teamwork between the patient/client and the therapist. Here are some goal categories that are frequently requested:
- Simple optimization of the core, no apparent injury
- To improve a generally poor quality of life due to pain or weakness
- To "get back" right away after acute pain or injury
- To get back without pain as soon as possible
- To restore pre-injury performance level before the start of the "next season" while no time pressure looms
- To achieve the unachievable

We phrased the above examples of goals so they might apply to any person, not just high-performance athletes. Athletes, and we common folks, seek help for many reasons and from an assortment of perspectives. And to make matters even more complicated, some people have particular treatment methods etched already in their minds before they come to see us therapists, and seek only endorsement of their preprogrammed viewpoints. Our job as therapists is to understand, implement wisely, maintain the passion, and, at the same time, create a team. Our job is not necessarily to modify the goals.

Leg 3: Know Our Own Planet (ie, Knowing What We Know and What We Don't Know)

There's not too much more to say here. Either we have this ability to know our limitations or we do not. That skill or innate ability is a hard one to develop. Yet, this ability is what separates excellence from run of the mill. We must quote Bill Belichick again, "It is what it is." And no, Bill is not BB to whom we were referred before. Bill Belichick is Bloviating Blowhard's antithesis.

Leg 4: Know Our Travel Options (ie, Cataloging the Therapies)

This important leg of the journey goes along with the previous one. You have to travel through Leg 3 in order to get to Leg 4 of the journey. If we don't know what we know and don't know, how the heck are we supposed to recognize what resides on other planets?

Think in terms of the various types of injuries, surgical options, or rehabilitation options. If we do make it to Leg 4, then all we do is list the options. Multiple types of lists may apply here—pure performance enhancement techniques, operative vs nonoperative approaches, physical therapy options, alternative therapies…

Here, we consider one more gigantic factor: temporizing vs definitive therapy. For high-performing athletes, there are 3 categories of thought here. And think in parallel ways for recreational or nonathletes. The 3 categories are:
1. Purely temporizing, definitive fix after the season
2. Temporizing, no need or plan for fix
3. Definitive fix

This list leads to additional lists such as future plans for the athlete (eg, retirement, lifestyle modification, desire to continue high-level play) or specific injury type (eg, will it get better on its own, does it need surgical fix, will temporizing hurt the chances of definitive surgical fix)? Remember that these injuries, these core injuries, can rear their ugly heads even years later. Take offensive lineman Brian Baldinger, for example, who had successful core muscle surgery during his NFL career and then, after 20 years of successful broadcasting, he developed a problem on the other side kicking a soccer ball on the beach. And no, Brian is not BB, to whom we referred earlier.

After listing the options, we begin our way toward the fifth and final stage. For each option, we consider such things as success rates, duration of therapy to achieve success, the time pressures... Again, the lists go on. At some point, we have to stop. The latter reality, however, should not diminish the importance of the thought and effort that goes into developing the catalogs.

Leg 5: The Final Stage—We Have Lift-Off (ie, the Decisions)

Keep in mind that all decisions should take into account the totality of the patient. For example, if we fix a specific problem, what does that mean with respect to overall fitness and prevention of nuisance or severe issues in the future? So, in this fifth and final leg of our journey, we need, again, to go up way past 30,000 feet, and predict the life curves that we talked about in the second limitation of Leg 1.

No matter the decisions (eg, temporizing solution, surgical vs nonoperative approach), we must consider how each intervention impacts those life curves. For example, Jakoi et al's article in the *American Journal of Sports Medicine* (see Selected Readings) showed a generally deteriorating career after "sports hernia repairs" for NHL hockey players when they had their surgery after 7 full seasons. This paper brings up big questions about the normal life curves of NHL hockey players or what happens to them after other injuries (eg, ACL repair, concussion). On top of that, consider that many of these NHL hockey players with problems had their mesh hernia repairs!

Our decision-making about what to do for a specific injury must take into account these bigger questions. Not only must we ask what can we fix? We should also ask about the impact of that fix upon future problems or injury. If it is not possible to fix everything, then how much can we really fix and how much should we try to fix? Certainly, fixing the core, as mentioned before, likely prevents other injuries. How impactful that reduction in risk really is, we still don't know. Certainly once one has fixed a portion of the core, we should attempt to prevent future injury by instituting the best performance regimens that we can, both to enhance future performance and to minimize future injuries.

The same life-curve question comes up with respect to the co-occurrence of hip and core muscle injuries. We ruminated, in several earlier chapters, on the reasons for this central theme in our understanding of the core. No doubt, the pathophysiology for this combination injury is a 2-way street. It can be a primary hip issue, with the muscles subject to tearing because they are contracting so much in attempts to limit range of motion. Or it can be a primary core muscle issue because severe tears increase in hip ranges of motion and allow hips with femoroacetabular impingement (FAI) anatomy to rub their bones more.

Let's transport this theme to a practical issue concerning fixing combination core injuries (ie, relating to combined FAI and core muscle injuries). And let's say the patient needs repairs for both parts of the anatomy. Why not fix them both at the same time? That certainly would reduce anaesthesia risk, and save rehab time provided the postoperative rehabilitation protocols are compatible.

Over the past few years, we have found, in fact, that this is the best way to approach selected combination hip/core muscle injury patients. The results have been tremendously satisfactory in our first 300 patients.

Clinical Correlation

Apply the 5 legs of this journey to any kind of treatment or other goal for the core. This could mean preparing an aspiring NFL player for the combine or designing a physical therapy plan for a specific hamstring injury.

The surgical example mentioned previously is a good one. Say, for example, you encounter a male soccer player with an injury of the adductor longus seemingly at its attachment onto the pubic bone. Here are possible considerations:
- Leg 1—Do we know how to handle this? What is our experience with this? Have we defined the injury enough by imaging?
- Leg 2—What are our goals here? Is it to get the player through the season? Is it to prevent the injury from extending and becoming a career-threatening problem? Where is the player in his/her contract? If we get him/her back out playing, how good will he/she be if we do get him/her back out playing soon? Will he/she look good to prospective teams if he/she is to become a free agent?
- Leg 3—What are all the possible therapies out there? Which ones are we capable of?

- Leg 4—We catalog the therapies out there, and which ones might make a difference? Do we need to send him/her somewhere else? Is this core muscle injury in isolation? Is there an associated hip injury? What caused the injury in the first place? Was it related to the foot injury that has never healed perfectly?
- Leg 5—So, the patient looks like he/she needs surgery. Do we fix the core muscle and underlying hip problem at the same time? Do we fix the muscle and see if he/she can perform well the rest of the season and then decide about the hip? Do we suggest, instead, a long-term core therapy program for the off-season? If so, which one?

Do you get it? We shall never achieve the Perfect Planet. Therefore, we should set our goals unambiguously and do what's right.

THE VOYAGE HOME—WHAT'S NEXT?

Okay, we have gotten you way out into space. The problem now is getting you back home. Since we are not sure we can, you might as well stay out here and enjoy it a while. Perhaps, you will get more glimpses of the Perfect Planet.

The next chapters bring you deeper into the fifth dimension. They go from a rising superstar in sports medicine talking about how how he fixes hamstring ruptures, to the basics of rehabilitation and performance, and then to interesting perspectives about the core from other health care specialists. Remember the theme of this section is that the core belongs to everyone who ventures into this space. Some of this fifth dimension shall boggle your mind. To maintain sanity, remember that you do not have to agree with these perspectives.

In Section Five, we shall bring you back home. We promise.

SELECTED READINGS

Knapik DM, Gebhart JJ, Nho SJ, Tanenbaum JE, Voos JE, Salata MJ. Prevalence of surgical repair for athletic pubalgia and impact on NFL performance in football athletes participating in the NFL combine. *Arthroscopy.* 2017;33(5):1044-1049.
   This delightful article is from the standpoint of these players having received optimal early results from their core muscle surgeries. Certainly, the docs and athletic trainers must have gone through the "5 legs of the journey" mentioned in this chapter. Undoubtedly, the health professionals made excellent decisions for the short term. Will these decisions hold up for the long term? We do not know, owing to the infancy of this field.

Meyers WC. Core muscle injuries or athletic pubalgia: finally the real sausage, not just the same ole baloney. *Arthroscopy.* 2017;33(5):1050-1052.
   This flattering commentary on the Knapik et al above-listed Selected Reading emphasizes the importance of understanding the injuries, performing the right imaging, and monitoring the right end-points. The critique demonstrates how a case control series such as this can extract tremendously beneficial information about this new field that we call "the core," for sports physicians, athletic trainers, management, agents, players, and all of us Sunday afternoon, TV-watching football experts.

Jakoi AJ, O'Neill C, Damsgaard C, et al. Sports hernia in National Hockey League players: does surgery affect performance? *Am J Sports Med.* 2013;41(1):107-110.
   This article, written by one of Dr. Meyers's surgical residents, is worth reading from the perspective of pondering life's natural "injury accumulation curves." Certainly, many factors, such as age, contract status, and variability in diagnosis and treatment, enter into how NHL players perform as they get older. A valid comparison for this article might have included anterior cruciate repairs.

31

managing the **ruptured** proximal hamstring

Christopher C. Dodson, MD
Daniel P. Woods, MD

Editor's Note: *Okay, a quick reminder...as we go into this chapter on the hamstrings, remember we are talking about "the core." We are not talking about just the hamstrings. Instead, we are talking about the whole thing—mid-chest to mid-thigh— our center that controls our whole body. Do not veer off this concept. Look at the balancing elephant in Figure 31-1, and ask what allows him (her?) to use its hamstrings and balance like this. It's about the whole kit and caboodle, and how the caboodle interacts with the brain. The top works so effortlessly with the bottom; the sides work so naturally with each together. It's remarkable. It's not just the hamstrings, which do provide most of the strength of the posterior thigh. It's also about how the strength works with the other cylinders in the engine room of this enormous creature.*

Now consider the hamstrings. These are obviously important muscles. They are big. They take up much of the posterior thigh mass of humans and many creatures. So, they must provide much strength. But they also provide much more than that; for example, they contribute a huge part of our balancing and the elephant's.

The hamstrings are hugely important in sport and in everyday life. To emphasize their importance in sports, all one has to do is look at the FIFA and other sports' injury lists. Hamstring injuries usually lead the lists. Sports injury prevention protocols often segregate out the hamstrings and provide them with loads of, actually too much, attention. We will get to the latter point soon.

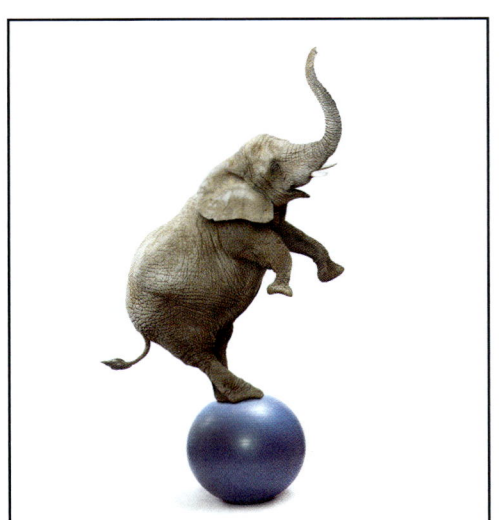

Figure 31-1.

These are the hamstrings (Figure 31-2).

There are 3, the ones highlighted in red. In athletes, they get a lot bigger and take up most of the space of the posterior thigh. This is the traditional way to think about these muscles. It is necessary to think about the hamstrings' attachments, their muscle mass and their importance in thigh extension. It is important to understand their anatomy, particularly if they are broken and you have to repair them.

But don't think about the hamstrings in isolation. They are a big part of the core; as we said, almost all of the posterior thigh (Figure 31-3).

For rehabilitation or performance purposes, don't think about the hamstrings as a segregated set of muscles. Like the rectus abdominis and other muscles, too much strengthening of the hamstrings sets up people for injury. Too many isolated hamstring exercises is one problem with the presently constructed FIFA injury prevention program. Think about all the recent hamstring injuries in prominent soccer players and ask if that program is working well. Don't think a hamstring workout should be all about this (Figure 31-4)…

Think about the hamstrings as an enormous part of the bottom and posterior part of the core, a valuable part of our power. They attach to the butt muscles and, in turn, to the back muscles. The power does no good unless it attaches to the rest of our body. Think balance. Think about the elephant. We can abuse any muscle in our body by exercising them too much in isolation. We need to be particularly careful about that with the hamstring.

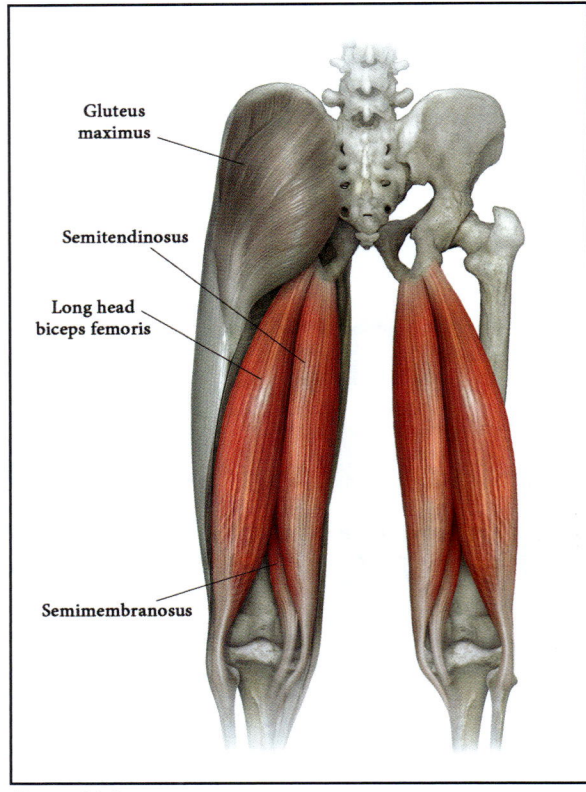

Figure 31-2.

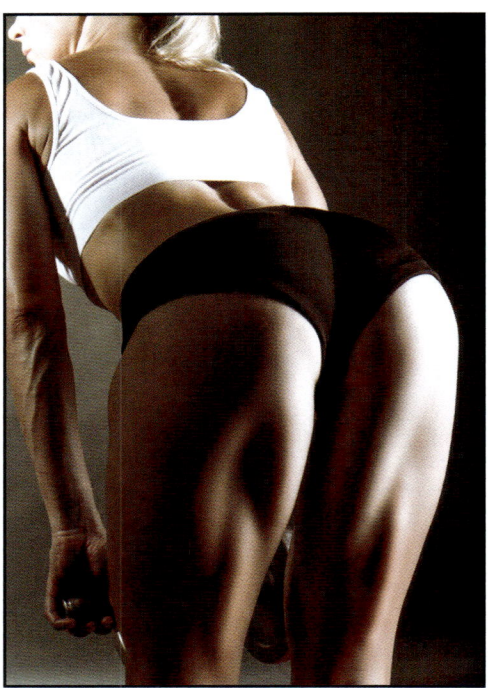

Figure 31-3.

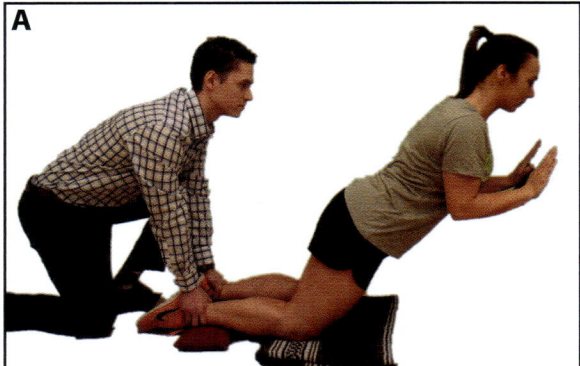

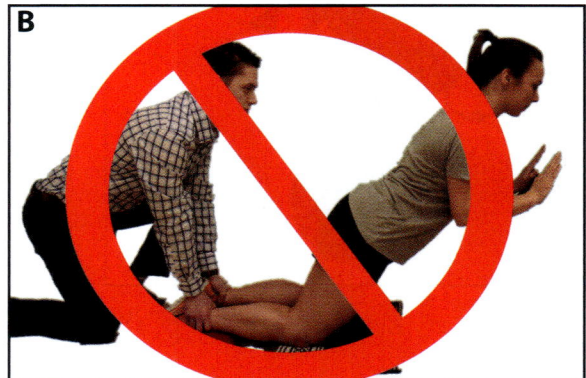

Figure 31-4. (A) This exercise isolates the hamstrings. (B) Too many of these place these muscles at risk.

A good hamstring workout incorporates planks and multiple other exercises that include the butt, the back, the front thigh, and abdomen. With any workout, it is fine to focus somewhat on a particular muscle group, but not too much and not in total isolation.

Consider workouts like Rob King's.[VID 1] *With these, be careful still. The videos show people using a lot of weight. In reality you don't need much, and you certainly have to work your way up.*

Okay, time to get back to business. With respect to the core, we should not ignore the old, traditional ways to do things. Hamstring avulsions cause enormous problems. For an athlete, laborer, or anyone like ourselves who wants to stay somewhat fit, hamstring integrity is a large part of good core function. When that muscle group rips off, we should be aggressive about fixing it. I have asked one of my young colleagues, superstar sports medicine orthopedist Chris Dodson, to update us on this. Chris is now both the Sixers' and the Eagles' doc and asked his sports medicine fellow to join him in writing this chapter.

Not all hamstring injuries are created equal.

—The chapter authors.

JOE THE TRUCK DRIVER

Joe, a 56-year-old male truck driver, loads his truck and slips on a patch of ice. His right thigh springs forward into a kind of forced hip flexion with his knee extended. He just did the "splits" for the first time in his life. At the same time, he felt a "pop" and a "ripping" in his posterior thigh. Immediately, he couldn't sit without excruciating pain. Unable to walk or put any pressure whatsoever on his injured leg, he goes to the worker's compensation physician. The doctor diagnoses a severe hamstring sprain. He starts on anti-inflammatories and rest.

Two months pass. He sees several more physicians and therapists who all advise time and physical therapy. He feels relatively okay, has much less pain, but still can't sit without lots of pain and feels "real weak" in his lower extremity. Physical therapy focuses on strengthening the hamstrings, and during this he develops lots of new aches and pains in his back, flank, and abdomen. More time passes and the pain gets worse, and he begins to feel an electric sensation going down the injured leg, and then numbness and now pain from the thigh to below his knee. Frustration grows and he finally gets an MRI. He has a 3-tendon proximal hamstring avulsion and tremendous inflammation around the sciatic nerve associated with the retracted tendons. He sees an operative orthopedist.

After the initial evaluation, surgical intervention was planned to reattach the proximal hamstring. He and the surgeon discussed the possibility of utilizing an Achilles allograft if the tendons had retracted too far away. At surgery, the sciatic nerve was freed from impenetrable inflammatory strictures, and an Achilles allograft came into play. Overall, the surgery went well and the hamstrings fit back to their appropriate positions on the ischial tuberosity.

Postoperatively, Joe does well and has no pain with sitting at 2 months. His strength returns completely, and he is back at work after 6 months, able to perform just like he did before. Joe is finally happy.

Not all hamstring injuries are created equal. This patient had a severe central injury. It involved the central part of his core. It was disabling. Early recognition of this injury pattern would have avoided significant down time, pain and frustration.

THE WAY IT WAS

"It's just a hamstring strain." How many times have we heard that in our athletic careers? Rest, anti-inflammatories, physical therapy, and gradual return to play are all that's necessary to return to action. It's a very simplistic algorithm for treatment that does indeed lead to excellent outcomes in the vast majority of patients. But it does not always work. And you can usually recognize the ones that won't get better with our simple, long-standing formula. There is a huge difference between a simple hamstring strain and a proximal hamstring tendinous avulsion.

Hamstring injuries in the athletic population are extremely common with the overwhelming majority treated successfully nonoperatively.[1] In the early 1900s, the evaluation of strains and sprains was thought to be very simple as "only a cursory examination"[2] was felt to be necessary in the diagnosis.[3] As scientific and clinical evaluations became more sophisticated, the specifics of a muscular strain vs an actual avulsion became more clearly delineated. The advent of MRI brought about a clear understanding of the fact that a simple cursory evaluation is not always able to demonstrate clearly the extent of actual injury as often those strains diagnosed by the clinician can be over- or underrecognized in terms of severity.[4] In the past 20 years, the evidence supports examining the specific location and pathoanatomical nature of the hamstring injury to determine the appropriate treatment regimen rather than symptom severity.[3,5]

Some of the early management at the turn of the 20th century of such injuries included "holding the affected limb under cold water as long as you can bear it, and as often as possible,"[6] plaster immobilization in the muscle fiber direction,[7] which was popular until the 1950s[6] with rest for 3 to 6 days followed by active work and massage creams.[3] In the early 1900s, musculotendinous bone avulsions were first noted to be an injury that required a much longer period of immobilization,[4] and as early as 1902, these injuries were treated with surgical intervention in the form of primary suture repair of avulsions.[2] As these injuries became recognized as responding better to operative intervention, newer techniques were developed including drill holes and primary suture repair, suturing of the ruptured portion of the hamstring tendon to surrounding tendons, and utilizing a fascia lata and carbon fiber graft to recreate the hamstring insertion on the ischial tuberosity.[8,9] With the advent of suture anchors and improved understanding of the particular injury patterns, the surgical indications and refined technique have allowed up to a 98% satisfaction rate and greater than 75% return of strength.[10] Despite the advances in diagnostic and surgical capabilities, many of these injuries continue to be misdiagnosed and can lead to sciatic nerve irritation and prolonged hamstring weakness.[10]

THE WAY IT IS

Nomenclature

The concept of a *proximal hamstring avulsion* entails the detachment of the confluence of the 3 tendons: *semitendinosus, semimembranosus,* and *long head of the biceps femoris* from its insertion on the *ischial tuberosity*. This injury is the result of a forceful hip flexion with an extended knee. Various degrees of this injury include avulsion of one tendon, 2 tendons both with and without retraction, and avulsion of all 3 tendons. The degree of injury dictates conservative vs surgical treatment. An *acute* injury is defined as an avulsion surgically treated within the initial 4 weeks after the injury, whereas a *chronic* injury is greater than 4 weeks until surgical treatment is initiated. This injury occurs in both the athletic population and in middle-aged adults. It should be differentiated from a distal hamstring avulsion, which is treated conservatively very successfully, and an apophyseal injury in an adolescent, which is treated based on the degree of separation of the avulsed fragment. A *chronic proximal hamstring tendinopathy* is also a separate entity, which is caused by repeated stress on the hamstring insertion and is often encountered in endurance athletes. If separation of the proximal hamstring tendons occurs, it can be treated operatively.

Clinical Experience

Introduction

Advanced imaging techniques and recognition of this specific injury pattern have allowed appropriate identification of proximal hamstring avulsions. Despite the newer knowledge and diagnostic tools, still a large number of these injuries are overlooked as a recent case series noted the average time from injury to surgical intervention was 2.4 months.[11] Although surgical management of chronic hamstring avulsions has been nearly as successful as acute primary repair,[12] it increases the surgical difficulty as the avulsed tendons may have developed adhesions to the sciatic nerve and the loss of tendon length may require the addition of an allograft to reach its origin on the ischial tuberosity.[10]

History and Physical Examination

The initial evaluation of a patient with a suspected proximal hamstring avulsion should consist of a detailed history of the inciting event. The most common mechanism of injury consists of a forceful flexion of the hip with the knee in an extended position.[11,13,14] These injuries may occur in the younger athletic population while doing sporting activities, including running, jumping, kicking, and winter sports, or may occur in the middle-aged sedentary population often due to a fall or slip on ice with a similar mechanism.[13-15] The patient may report the sensation of a shot in his/her posterior thigh with subsequent pain near the ischial tuberosity and difficulty with ambulation. A stiff-legged gait that avoids hip flexion or knee extension is a common presentation.[13] The patient often reports a significant amount of pain with sitting in the area of the avulsed tendon.

Managing the Ruptured Proximal Hamstring 339

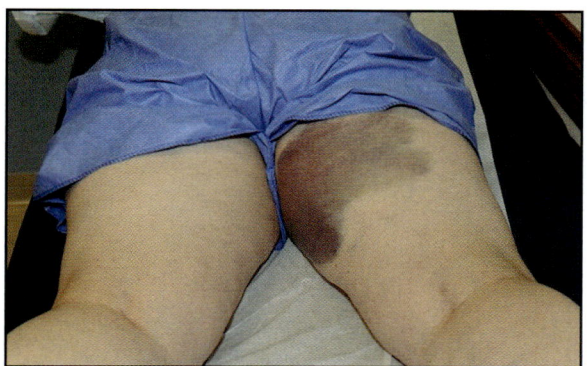

Figure 31-5. Acute proximal hamstring rupture. Note the tremendous amount of bruising, which is common.

A thorough physical examination of the patient is paramount to determining the degree of hamstring injury, as well as recognizing which patients need additional imaging to determine the appropriate treatment. Initially the posterior thigh should be closely inspected, as the presence of a diffuse ecchymosis (Figure 31-5) may represent a significant myotendinous injury, vs a proximal or distal avulsion of the hamstring tendons.[14] Next, the thigh should be palpated along the extent of the hamstring as with a proximal or distal avulsion there may be a palpable gap and thickened subcutaneous tissue near the area of injury.[16] The range of motion should be assessed, and an increased popliteal angle in the affected extremity compared to the contralateral limb may indicate hamstring injury.[17] The strength should be assessed with the patient prone with the knee in 90 degrees of flexion and an eccentric contraction with the knee in 30 degrees of flexion may recreate the mechanism of injury and aid in injury pattern recognition.[14]

Imaging

In those patients whose presentation appears suggestive of significant avulsion-style injury, imaging of the affected extremity should be undertaken. Plain radiographs may reveal a bony avulsion of the proximal hamstrings from the ischial tuberosity. However, the majority of radiographs are negative.[13,18] Although ultrasound has been utilized successfully,[19] MRI is the diagnostic study of choice for evaluating proximal hamstring avulsions. If a proximal avulsion is suspected, the image should include bilateral ischial tuberosities and extend through the proximal to mid thigh. The image will clearly demonstrate both the extent of the bony avulsion as well as the distance of distal retraction of the tendons (Figures 31-6 and 31-7).[20] The MRI characteristics are utilized for surgical decision-making.

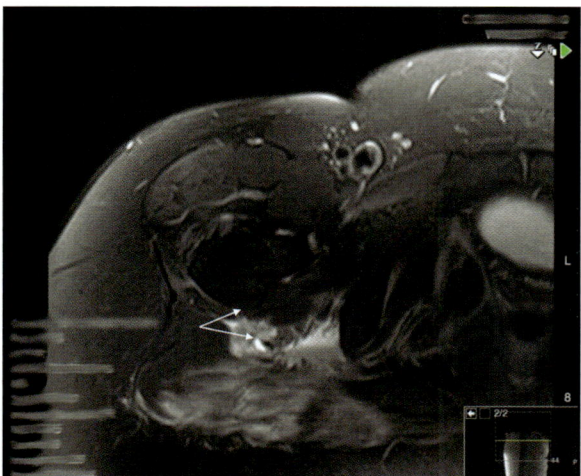

Figure 31-6. MRI (axial T2 image) of an acute 3-tendon proximal hamstring avulsion. Arrows point to gap between the bare ischial tuberosity and the hamstring tendon.

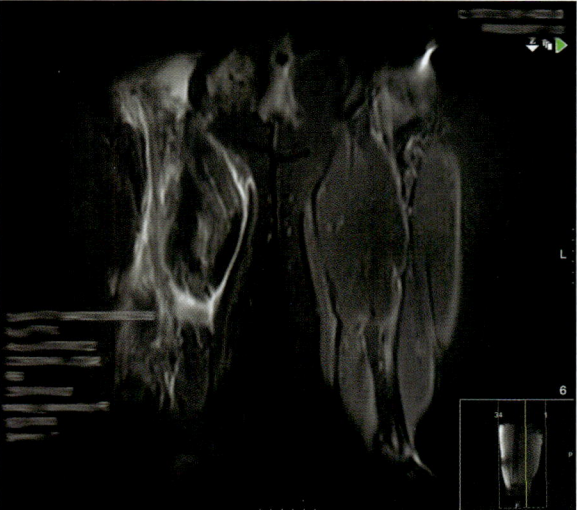

Figure 31-7. Coronal T2 MRI of the same avulsion as Figure 31-6, showing the extent of the hematoma.

Indications for nonsurgical management of proximal hamstring ruptures include single-tendon injuries and 2-tendon injuries with minimal retraction.[10] Surgical reattachment should be undertaken in 2 tendon tears when it is retracted more than 2 cm and in all 3 tendon tears regardless of retraction.[13,14] Additionally, in a chronic tendinopathy picture, if the MRI reveals a crescent-shaped "sickle sign" signifying the tendon separating from the ischial tuberosity (Figure 31-8), this is also an indication for debridement and reattachment of the proximal hamstring tendon.[21]

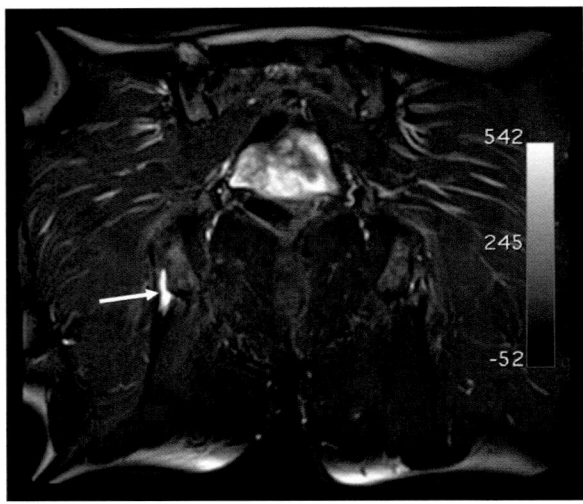

Figure 31-8. An MRI "crescent sign" that occurs with a "chronic proximal hamstring tendinopathy." Note the partial gap (arrow pointing to fluid that appears white) between the tendon and the right ischial tuberosity.

Management

Nonoperative management of a proximal hamstring avulsion consists of activity modification, nonsteroidal anti-inflammatory drugs (NSAIDs), and image-guided corticosteroid injection.[13,21] In addition, shock wave therapy, edema control, and electrical stimulation have been used concurrently with a physical therapy program.[22] If these measures are not successful, platelet-rich plasma injections have been utilized with varying success.[23] These injuries can take up to 6 to 8 weeks to improve, and return to play is only considered when the patient is asymptomatic and the strength is within one grade of the uninjured extremity.[14,24] Failure of nonoperative management, due to continued pain or inability of the athlete to return to sport, should result in further evaluation and consideration of operative management, which has been successful in this patient population.[21]

Authors' Preferred Surgical Management

Operative management of a proximal hamstring injury consists of reattachment of the proximal hamstring to its insertion on the ischial tuberosity. The patient is placed prone on an operating table with all bony prominences appropriately padded. The area around the affected proximal hamstring is then prepped and draped in normal sterile fashion, carefully separating the perineal area from the surgical field. The authors' preferred surgical technique initially consists of a transverse incision at the level of the gluteal crease.[13] Dissection is taken down through the subcutaneous fascia avoiding the posterior femoral cutaneous nerve until the gluteal fascia is encountered, and a subsequent transverse incision is made in the gluteal fascia.[13,14] The gluteus maximus muscle belly is retracted superiorly, uncovering the hamstring fascia, which is incised longitudinally. There may be additional fibrous tissue that has formed around this area, which makes it appear that the tendons are still intact.[13] This must also be incised in a longitudinal fashion to encounter the ruptured tendons, and it is usually accompanied by a large hematoma in cases of acute fixation.[13] The tendons are then mobilized and tagged with a heavy suture. After the sciatic nerve is identified lateral to the tendon, a Deaver retractor is utilized to protect it.

Next, the insertion of the tendons on the ischial tuberosity is identified, and a Cobb, curet, and/or periosteal elevator is used to denude the soft tissue from the bone and obtain a bleeding base for healing of the tendon to its insertion.[13,14] It is pertinent to recreate the anatomy of the hamstring insertion as closely as possible to allow for optimal functional outcome. The proximal hamstring insertion consists of a 2.7 x 1.8 cm oval area on the medial aspect of the tuberosity that composes the most medial long head of the biceps femoris and more lateral semitendinosus tendons.[25] The semimembranosus tendon insertion is more crescent-shaped and is the most lateral portion of the insertion.[25] The sciatic nerve is palpated, identified, and retracted laterally away from the operative field.[13,14] With these portions of the tendons identified, 2 or 3 double-loaded suture anchors are placed on the ischial tuberosity. Three limbs of the double-loaded suture anchor are passed through the tendon in Krackow fashion, while the fourth is placed as a simple stitch acting as a post. The sutures from the 2 or 3 anchors are all passed. Then the simple sutures from each are all pulled simultaneously to "parachute" the tendon snugly to the bone. These limbs are tied down with the knee held in approximately 30 degrees of flexion (Figure 31-9). Multiple muscle belly episiotomies/fasciotomies may help bring the muscles up without tension.

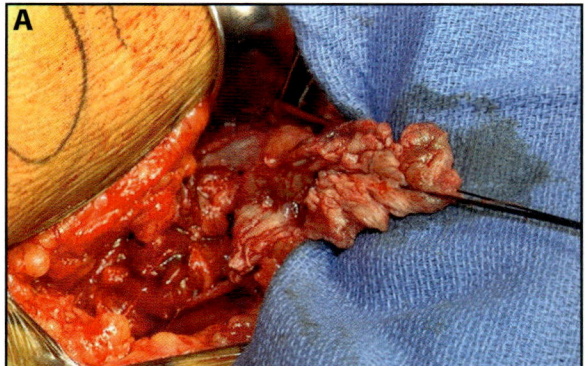
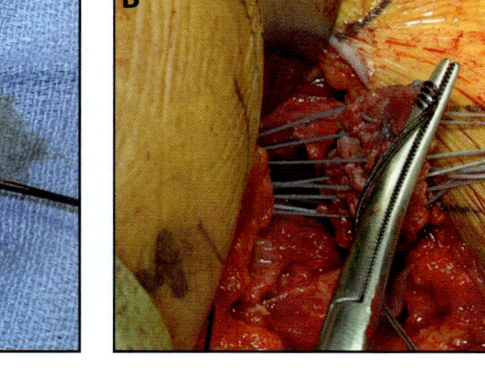
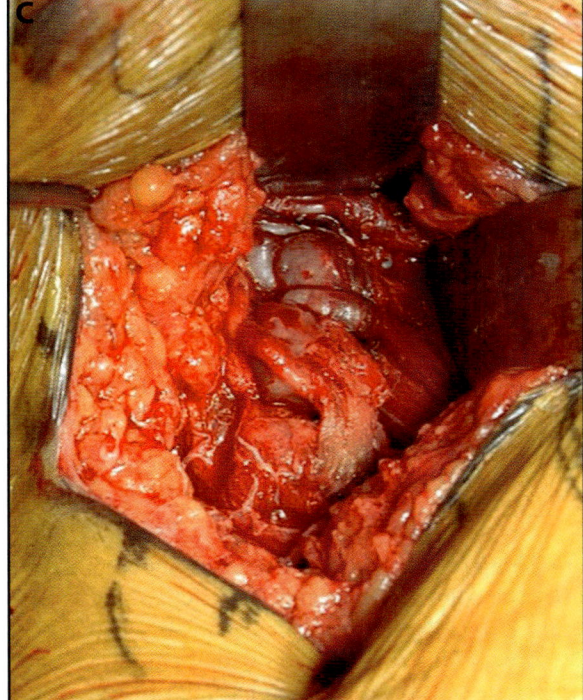

Figure 31-9. Operative photographs of a hamstring repair. (A) Mobilized tendon. (B) Suture anchors bringing tendon back to ischial tuberosity. (C) Completed repair. Note retractors protecting the sciatic nerve (not clearly shown).

In cases of a chronic hamstring rupture with a long retraction gap, an Achilles allograft can be utilized to allow the tendon to reach its appropriate insertion.[12] With the tendon reinserted, the gluteal fascia is closed with absorbable sutures and the skin and subcutaneous tissues reapproximated. The dressing is carefully placed avoiding any contamination from the perineal area, and the patient is placed in a prefabricated custom hip orthosis that limits hip flexion from 15 to 30 degrees before being awoken from anesthesia.

The postoperative rehab protocol initially consists of 2 weeks of toe touch weightbearing in the operative extremity, with the patient using crutches. A gradual increase in weightbearing is undertaken until the patient reaches full weight-bearing by 6 weeks.[13] Passive range of motion of the hip and knee is initiated at 2 weeks and active range of motion at 4 weeks.[14] The second phase of rehabilitation begins at 6 weeks with the removal of the brace and includes continued range of motion, initiation of aqua therapy, and isotonic strengthening exercises.[13,14] When the patient is 12 weeks from the operation, the final phase is initiated, which includes running and sport-specific activities. The athlete is allowed to return to competition when isokinetic testing at 60°/s, 120°/s, and 180°/s shows the involved side to be 80% of the uninvolved limb.[13] Typically, return to sport occurs 6 to 10 months postoperatively.[26]

Outcomes

The outcomes of proximal hamstring repair have been good to excellent in the majority of cases. Initial surgical outcomes, which included drill holes in the bone and suture repair reported 62% good outcomes at an average follow-up of over 5 years.[9] Outcomes in patients who underwent a longitudinal incision with 2 to 3 suture anchors reported a 91% success rate with patients achieving an average of 85% strength.[27] Subsequent studies evaluated the usage of metal anchors, and at 20 months postoperatively with an average of 3.5 suture anchors used per repair, 75% of athletes had returned to sport with a 10% deficit in isokinetic strength.[28] The functional results of the surgical technique utilizing a 5-suture anchor repair report 98% satisfaction rate, with 67% return to strenuous/sporting activities, but did document statistically significant improvement in outcomes in those patients who underwent acute hamstring repair vs those with a chronic repair.[10]

Illustrative Cases

Case 1

A 50-year-old female tri-athlete reported chronic right buttock pain. The pain initially began during an ultra-marathon approximately 6 months ago, and was not associated with any particular traumatic injury. The pain was localized to the right ischial tuberosity, and she reported significant pain with sitting. She had sought medical treatment, but physical therapy and anti-inflammatories did not relieve her pain. She did continue to attempt to run, swim, and bike, but this had become more and more difficult. An ultrasound-guided corticosteroid injection improved her pain significantly for a few weeks, but she was still unable to compete due to weakness. An MRI revealed significant right- and left-sided proximal hamstring tendinopathy, but the right side displayed a "crescent" sign at the proximal insertion. Surgical intervention was recommended, and the tendon was noted to have chronic degenerative changes. Fortunately, enough tendon was available to debride the degenerative portion, release the adhesions to the sciatic nerve, and primarily repair the proximal hamstring insertion utilizing the previously noted 5-suture anchor repair. The patient had immediate pain relief in the region of the right ischial tuberosity and returned to triathlon training and competition 6 months after fixation.

Case 2

A 46-year-old woman fell on the ice with the injured extremity outstretched. She felt a significant pop in the posterior thigh at the time of injury. She presented to the office 1 week after the fall with an antalgic gait and a significant amount of ecchymosis on the posterior thigh. Exam demonstrated tenderness to palpation at the hamstring insertion and notable weakness compared to the contralateral side. MRI revealed a 3-tendon hamstring avulsion with 4 cm retraction distally. Surgical reattachment was recommended and undertaken in the acute setting, allowing for primary repair with suture anchor fixation as described previously.

Case 3

A 33-year-old professional football player injured his left lower extremity when a player fell on him, forcing his knee into extension and his hip into hyperflexion. He had immediate pain in the posterior thigh and was unable to continue playing. The majority of his pain was localized to the region around the ischial tuberosity, and exam did reveal some mild ecchymosis around the area. A subsequent MRI revealed a semimembranosus tear only with no retraction of the torn tendons. Nonsurgical management was initiated (one tendon avulsion with no retraction) including NSAIDs, physical therapy, and localized platelet-rich plasma injection. He continued to improve, and his strength reached 90% of the uninjured limb by 7 weeks post-injury. He was able to return to play 8 weeks following the injury with no subsequent injuries.

Algorithm

The simplified algorithm for treatment of a proximal hamstring injury is shown in Figure 31-10.

Summary

A proximal hamstring avulsion injury, which is caused by forced hip flexion accompanied by knee extension, is one that necessitates further evaluation. An MRI should be ordered in all cases in which this injury is suspected. The treatment plan is based on the extent of injury to the tendons. Surgical reattachment of the avulsed tendons utilizing suture anchors has been associated with good-to-excellent outcomes and a high satisfaction rate in patients undergoing the procedure. A return to full athletic activity or occupational activity takes 6 to 10 months. Anatomic repair continues to be the treatment of choice in patients with surgical indications.

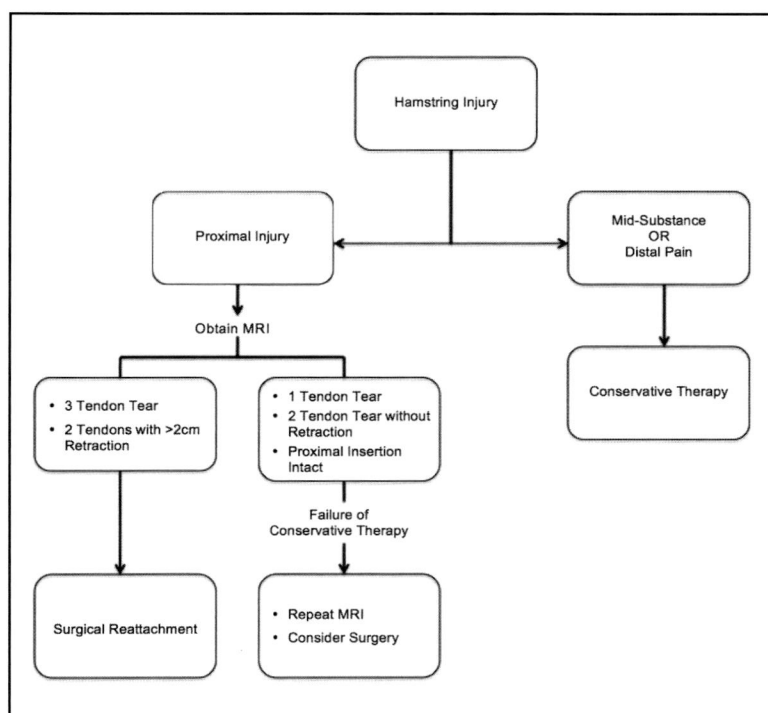

Figure 31-10. Simplified algorithm for diagnosis and treatment of hamstring injuries.

Selected Readings

Ahmad CS, Redler LH, Ciccotti MG, Maffulli N, Longo UG, Bradley JP. Evaluation and management of hamstring injuries. *Am J Sports Med.* 2013;41(12):2933-2947.
   An excellent and up-to-date review of the treatment of the gamut of hamstring injuries including proximal hamstring avulsion.

Cohen SB, Bradley JP. Acute proximal hamstring rupture. *J Am Acad Orthop Surg.* 2007;15(6):350-355.
   A review of proximal hamstring injury from evaluation to repair.

Cohen S, Rangavajjula A, Vyas D, Bradley JP. Functional results and outcomes after repair of proximal hamstring avulsions. *Am J Sports Med.* 2012;40(9):2092-2098.
   An outcomes article that examines differences between acute and chronic injuries.

References

1. Clanton TO, Coupe TJ. Hamstring strains in athletes: diagnosis and treatment. *J Am Acad Orthop Surg.* 1998;6:237-248.
2. Crowley, DD. Suturing of muscles and tendons. *Cal State J Med.* 1902;1(2):48-54.
3. Hamilton B. Hamstring muscle strain injuries: what can we learn from history? *Br J Sports Med.* 2012;46:900-903.
4. Verrall GM, Slavotinek JP, Barnes PG, Fon GT, Esterman A. Assessment of physical examination and magnetic resonance imaging findings of hamstring injury as predictors for recurrent injury. *J Orthop Sports Phys Ther.* 2006;36(4):215-224.
5. Askling C, Saartok T, Thorstensson A. Type of acute hamstring strain affects flexibility, strength, and time to return to pre-injury level. *Br J Sports Med.* 2006;40(1):40-44.
6. Andrews H. *Training for Athletics and General Health.* London, United Kingdom: C. Arthur Pearson Limited; 1904.
7. Wilbur RL. Football injuries. *Cal State J Med.* 1906;4(6):170-172.
8. Delarue NC. The treatment of athletic injuries. *Can Med Assoc J.* 1954;70(4):408-416.
9. Orava S, Kujala UM. Rupture of the ischial origin of the hamstring muscles. *Am J Sports Med.* 1995;23:702-705.
10. Cohen S, Rangavajjula A, Vyas D, Bradley JP. Functional results and outcomes after repair of proximal hamstring avulsions. *Am J Sports Med.* 2012;40(9):2092-2098.

11. Sarimo J, Laimpainen L, Matilla K, Sakari O. Complete proximal hamstring avulsions: a series of 41 patients with operative treatment. *Am J Sports Med.* 2008;36(6):1110-1115.
12. Folsom GJ, Larson CM. Surgical treatment of acute vs chronic proximal hamstring avulsions: results of a new allograft technique for chronic reconstructions. *Am J Sports Med.* 2007;36(1):104-109.
13. Cohen SB, Bradley JP. Acute proximal hamstring rupture. *J Am Acad Orthop Surg.* 2007;15(6):350-355.
14. Ahmad CS, Redler LH, Ciccotti MG, Maffulli N, Longo UG, Bradley JP. Evaluation and management of hamstring injuries. *Am J Sports Med.* 2013;41(12):2933-2947.
15. Ali K, Leland JM. Hamstring sprains and tears in the athlete. *Clin Sports Med.* 2012;31(2):263-272.
16. Cooper DE, Conway JE. Distal semitendinosis injuries in elite level athletes: low success rates of non-operative management. *Am J Sports Med.* 2010;38(6):1174-1178.
17. Bradley PS, Portas MD. The relationship between preseason range of motion and muscle strain injury in elite soccer players. *J Strength Cond Res.* 2007;21(4):1155-1159.
18. Clanton TO, Coupe KJ. Hamstring strains in athletes: diagnosis and treatment. *J Am Acad Orthop Surg.* 1998;6(4):237-248.
19. Mariani C, Caldera FE, Kim W. Ultrasound versus magnetic resonance imaging in the diagnosis of an acute hamstring tear. *PM R.* 2012;4(2):154-155.
20. Bresler M, Mar W, Toman J. Diagnostic imaging in the evaluation of leg pain in athletes. *Clin Sports Med.* 2012;31(2):217-245.
21. Bowman KF, Cohen SB, Bradley JP. Operative management of partial thickness tears of the proximal hamstring muscles in athletes. *Am J Sports Med.* 2013;41(6):1363-1371.
22. Standaert CJ. Shockwave therapy for chronic proximal hamstring tendinopathy. *Clin J Sport Med.* 2012;22(2):170-171.
23. Finnoff JT, Fowler SP, Lai JK, et al. Treatment of chronic tendinopathy with ultrasound-guided needle tenotomy and platelet-rich plasma injection. *PM R.* 2011;3(10):900-911.
24. Mendiguchia J, Brughelli M. A return-to-sport algorithm for acute hamstring injuries. *Phys Ther Sport.* 2011;12(1):2-14.
25. Miller SL, Gill J, Webb GR. The proximal origin of the hamstrings and surrounding anatomy encountered during repair: a cadaveric study. *J Bone Joint Surg Am.* 2007;89(1):44-48.
26. Askling CM, Tengvar M, Saartok T, Thorstensson A. Acute first-time hamstring strains during slow-speed stretching: clinical, magnetic resonance imaging, and recovery characteristics. *Am J Sports Med.* 2007;35(10):1716-1724.
27. Klingele KE, Sallay PI. Surgical repair of complete proximal hamstring tendon rupture. *Am J Sports Med.* 2002;30:742-747.
28. Brucker PU, Imhoff AB. Functional assessment after acute and chronic complete ruptures of the proximal hamstring tendons. *Knee Surg Sports Traumatol Arthrosc.* 2005;13:411-418.

VIDEO

1. http://www.robkingfitness.com/strength-training-2/4-hamstring-exercises/

32

rehabilitation and performance
from **snake oil** salespeople to **well-oiled** machines

ALEXANDER E. POOR, MD
JIM McCROSSIN, MS, ATC, CSCS, PES, CES, CKTP
ALEX McKECHNIE, PT, MCSP

Editor's Note: *I asked Jim McCrossin and Alex McKechnie, two of the world's leaders in core physical therapy and performance training, to help write this chapter. Both are partners in the Vincera Institute. Jimmy, the Philadelphia Flyers' head athletic trainer, runs the Vincera Rehab Center. Alex, Director of Sports Science for the Toronto Raptors, was one of the conceptualizers of the Institute. Alex originated some of the core performance and rehab fundamentals employed there. He also created the device called Core-X. Another Alex, co-editor Alex Poor, brings together Jim's and Alex's thoughts, and adds some of his own.*

THE IMPORTANCE OF ATHLETIC TRAINERS AND MANY OTHERS IN THE FITNESS WORLD

Athletic trainers, physical therapists, strength coaches, and some alternative therapists—not necessarily docs—presently command the core. These therapists deal with the core all the time and see the problems with it. I got into this field via the heartfelt convictions of certified athletic trainers. In the mid-1980s, two of them from a professional football team approached me saying, "Doc, this player has a real injury. The coach thinks he's faking, and our team docs are stumped. No one can diagnose him. We have staked our reputations that he has a real injury, and that you can fix it. Make us look good, Doc."

Athletic trainers may be the most dedicated group of health professionals right now in the United States. With essentially the same educational background as registered nurses, they have the dedication and tirelessness of physicians of the old day. Often underappreciated, they spend countless hours with their athletes, looking out for them, making house calls, hospital and pharmacy visits—whatever it takes to get their athletes into the best health and mental and physical conditions. Athletic trainers have also become the primary health communicators for many teams, often more than the team doctors, coaches, agents, or administrative staffs.

With that dedication, athletic trainers sometimes even identify these core injuries precisely. More than the rest of us, they know when a player really hurts, and when the injury seems important. Athletic trainers are always "there"—on the field, in the training rooms, and by the players' sides. They notice the grimaces. They see the impact of these injuries more than any other group of health professionals. They became convinced about the concept of the core way before docs.

Through the insistence of athletic trainers that there were a variety of injuries in this region, I got interested in the core despite a large liver practice, and performed the initial laboratory experiments described in Chapters 3 through 5. At the same time, I cannot minimize the influence of my colleagues, Duke doctors Frank Bassett and Bill Garrett. Frank and Bill encouraged me to listen to the athletic trainers. Frank and Bill saw the core as an undiscovered scientific field, and its study would likely yield the fundamentals of physical performance and optimal use of our muscles, bones, and brain. The bases of this field turn out to be basic anatomy, physiology, pathology, and pharmacology.

Athletic trainers, physical therapists, strength coaches, docs, and so many others turn out to be so important with respect to the core; not only for prevention of injuries, but also for achieving maximal performance in general as well as after surgery. Having said that, we must mention a few words of caution…

WATCH OUT FOR THE SNAKE OIL SALESPERSON (FIGURE 32-1)

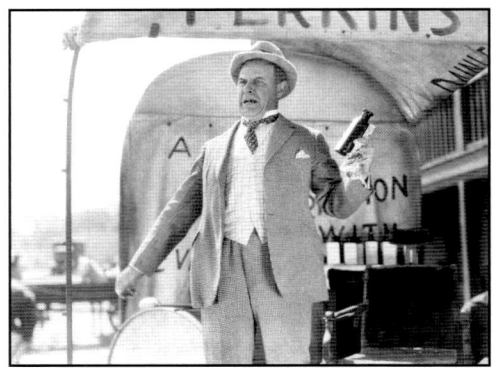

Figure 32-1. A snake oil salesperson.

Right now, in this complex world with so much commercialism and so little established scientific data, the lay public logically will have difficulty picking out good therapists from the snake oil salespeople. As we have mentioned multiple times previously, it is easy to injure someone with the wrong training regimens and/or the wrong devices. We have previously talked about the oft-sexy, 2 AM television ads that promote the latest products that may be dangerous. On the other hand, particularly in this developing scientific field, we must keep our minds. Some people who seem like snake oil salesmen or -women may, in fact, be onto something. Let's be wary, but also not be too quick to label their wares as snake oil.

One tell-tale sign of a snake-oil salesperson is the supposed therapist who says: "I know all about the core; I know exactly what to do." Whether or not that therapist has a great background, be cautious. Nobody knows all about the core, not yet. In the least, that therapist reflects a closed mind about learning more.

You, sir, are the scion of an ancestral procession of idiots stretching back to the Missing Link.

—Samuel Langhorne Clemens, aka Mark Twain, the author of *Tom Sawyer* and *Huckleberry Finn*. The quote comes from a letter from Clemens to a snake oil peddler on November 20, 1905.

MOVING FORWARD

Certainly, we all have a lot more still to learn. Several principles for core training have emerged. Not everyone knows these. One reason may be that the principles have never been expressed clearly in a textbook. Alas, that excuse should hold true no longer…

We certainly recognize that enumerating "basic principles" may trigger debate. Plus, what gives us the right to do this? The answer to this is we don't know. We had the opportunity to write this book, so we figured we have been helping drive this field, so why not? Someone had to start somewhere. We welcome debate and alternative hypotheses about the fundamentals. In the next few chapters, we have assembled some megastars in core physical therapy and athletic training. We already mentioned Alex and Jimmy. We also have Andrew Small, a young Australian physical therapist, and then Tracey Vincel and Andrew Barr, therapists in New York City in whom I have a lot of confidence.

Success is never final, failure is never fatal. It's courage that counts.

—John Wooden, the "Wizard of Westwood,"
who won 10 NCAA basketball titles with UCLA in a 12-year time frame.

We divide this chapter into 2 parts: how to recognize the right therapist from the snake oil salesperson and the right principles.

IDENTIFYING THE RIGHT THERAPIST

Ask yourself any of the following 3 questions.
1. I want to get back into shape, who do I get to help me?
2. I pulled a big muscle in my thigh, who knows what to do?
3. How do I get an athlete from the operating table all the way back to stardom?

For all 3, you start out by trying to identify the right therapist.

The third question may seem the easiest to answer because of the abundant resources often available to a potential star athlete. The reality is that the answer to Question 3 may be the most difficult, even considering the optimal settings. Getting the player "all the way back" shall be addressed further in the following chapter.

So, where does one start? How does one find the "right therapist"? Look at the choices: physical therapist, strength coach, personal trainer, athletic trainer, physiatrist…the list goes on. For a patient, or even a referring doc, it can be mind-boggling trying to decipher where to go. Consider all the specialties, the special credentialing, and the many initials that follow each specialist's name. Lines of distinction between fitness specialties remain obscure, at least to most people out there. Know that that the fitness world is now second to the financial world in terms of number of workers within it. Inability to discriminate causes frustration. No wonder so many people go out and buy the latest fitness video, and give up the quest to find the right therapist.

Let's say you are not a therapist. You are just anybody and either have an injury that you deem not serious or have simply decided you want to get back into shape. What do you do? Where do you go? If you have no background whatsoever in any of the fitness fields, you undoubtedly will feel lost. Probably, you would latch onto the first person whom a friend suggests, or who sounds good, or who talks a good game and acts like he/she knows something. In reality, figuring out the right therapist, without some direction, may be like finding the "eighth" wonder of the world.

Many experienced therapists get frustrated thinking about the above scenario. So many people, it seems, claim to be fitness experts nowadays. Then frustration can turn to exasperation when a therapist compares the educational backgrounds. Consider reading an article written in *Men's Health* written by Bryan Krahn.[1] Krahn articulates, with unpleasant language, that exasperation. The world is, certainly, not as bad as Krahn portrays it, but he does make a valid point about the huge amount of deception that lurks within the fitness industry.

Eight Tips for Finding the Right Therapist

In the spirit of Krahn's blog (without the crassness) and the "eighth" wonder, we have come up with 8 tips for patients/clients/athletes for deciphering a good therapist:

1. Look at the therapist's training. The initials ("credentials") after the therapist's name may, or may not, mean something. In general, the longer the list…the more you should question. Watch out for quantity (eg, number of credentials or number of spoken words) substituting for quality. Find out specifically where the therapist trained, did internships, etc. Ask how long those internships lasted (eg, a few weeks or a month vs a full year or two). Make sure they were not online courses. Look up the reputation of the schools and ask directly or research the meaning of those initials.

2. See if the therapist is currently working with legitimate colleagues. Many therapists list well-known people as colleagues. Watch out; there are lots of ways to fudge those data. Ask specifically about the schools, institutions, doctors, etc, with whom he/she affiliates. Look up the institutions and doctors if you don't recognize them. Challenge the therapist with respect to the specific ways that therapist works with the colleagues or institution listed.

3. Find current clients of the therapists and quiz them. Don't be swooned by the names of big-name athletes, performers, etc. Some of the best and worst therapists drop names like you wouldn't believe. Be wary of the "nutritional" side. You have seen the scams chronicled in newspapers involving anabolic steroids. Some of those scams grew out of legitimate clinics. On the other hand, recognize that sometimes there is a real rationale for anabolic steroids, and that their acceptance is actually evolving. Right now, most anabolic steroid usage is inappropriate. You do have to pay attention to criminal conviction or eviction of a therapist from a legitimate organization. Currently, the best therapy locales often make special points to differentiate themselves from such activities. On the other hand, keep your mind open here.

4. Find a therapist who is flexible in his/her thinking. A good therapist should truly read through an existent protocol from an outside doc and be willing to call directly and work with previous therapists or treating physicians. The refusal to do that is an absolute indicator of someone with whom you don't want to work. For example, the right kind of early, aggressive, postsurgical physical therapy is very important at Vincera with respect to rehabilitation after core muscle repairs, in order to prevent certain types of scar build-up; so much so that the patient begins therapy the day after surgery. When we get a report that an outside therapist has looked at our postop protocol and pronounced impulsively, "This is way too aggressive—you need to wait a while before you start this," we tell the patient to switch therapists. We actually coach our patients on comments of a potentially bad therapist.

    In general, therapists should be willing to, in the least, pick up the phone and call, and go through a referrer's protocol with the referrer, particularly when that has been requested. Without that, critical statements serve only to undermine the confidence in everybody.

5. Watch out for big words and ultra-aggressive people. The therapist should also be able to talk to you so that you can understand. When you hear big words or phrases that you do not understand, know there are only 2 possible explanations for that. The therapist may be sincere and innocently overlooking your lack of training; or the therapist is, indeed, double-talking. As implied previously, lots of double-talking scammers live in this field. Absolutely, you should ask them to explain things so that you understand them. If they cannot, politely say "Adios, Amigo."

    Think the same way for the ultra-aggressive people. Distrust the therapist who insists on interventional therapy that just plain seems wrong (eg, active release therapy within a few days after surgical repair, or, for that matter, dry-needling or extreme stretching). The therapist may even legitimize the offer by citing the initials after his/her name to show that he/she is well-credentialed in a particular therapy. Keep in mind, however, that many of those therapies do have roles. The point is that they must be used wisely.

6. Krahn says, "Beware of the liars and scammers." The top 3 clues that you are dealing with a scammer are (1) goofy qualifications, (2) evasiveness about the qualifications, and (3) "buzzword wizardry." The last refers to a form of double-talking, using seeming catchwords or phrases with the explanations just not making perfect sense. Trust your instincts: If you don't totally understand the rationale for a therapy, believe yourself not the therapist. Other things to watch out include the big promises (eg, you will become the next superhero), the overly talkative therapist, and the terribly out-of-shape therapist. If the therapist can't keep in reasonable shape, don't trust the person's ethic. Also, watch out for the scam artist, who tells you, ad nauseam, about his/her superhero background, or the one who prioritizes entertainment over exercise, or therapists who try to convince you to also take pills or buy a club membership.

7. Trust a well-known athlete who has gone through something similar, if you can get access to one of them. The chances are that the athlete, or one of his/her agents, has gone through the research. Of course, make sure the athlete has done well. Know, however, that this recommended process is, by no means, failsafe.

8. And finally, look at the soft stuff. Pay attention to your general feelings about the therapist. Consider the therapist's flexibility and modesty. Do you like him/her? Do you think you will be able to trust the prospective therapist? Trust, good vibes, and convenience (travel time, etc) mean a lot. Don't be fooled by the well-publicized reputation. The therapist with the great name may also be set in his/her ways (ie, to a fault).

THE RIGHT PRINCIPLES

When one says "the right principles," one may mean a lot of things. Let's narrow that down for this chapter. We are talking about the right principles that athletic trainers should have when they take care of their players. We are talking about the total care of the player—physical, psychological, nutritional, and whatever else it takes to make the player as great as he/she can. We shall provide a case example, and then list what we think are the right core rehabilitation and performance principles. Like all other aspects of this book, you may argue with any of these. These principles merely open the discussion.

Let us begin with Kyle Lowry. His story was written up as a "Medical Mystery" for the Sunday *Philadelphia Inquirer* newspaper.[2] Consider this case from the perspective of what the athletic trainers and physical therapists did for Kyle. They watched him like hawks and figured out a really bad thing that what was going on with him. They corrected the problem and subsequently provided first-class core care that helped Kyle to become a mega-star in the NBA.

Diagnosing and Managing a Tricky Core Injury

As we said, Kyle's story appeared in the Sunday *Philadelphia Inquirer* within a series called "Medical Mysteries." We present it here, in a modified form, from the same perspective.

The Mystery

Kyle was in his sixth year of the NBA. The Villanova University standout was drafted in 2006, after his sophomore year. He finally had the chance to play regularly. It was now March 2012, and he was a point guard with the Houston Rockets. Kyle knew he could be a star (Figure 32-2). But that darn pain in his belly was such a distraction.

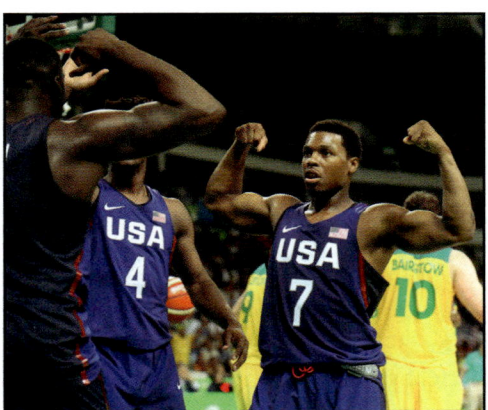

Figure 32-2. NBA basketball star Kyle Lowry.

For 6 months, the tormenting pain below his belly button had shifted from one side to the other. Like many professional athletes, he played through it. Somehow, he could no longer keep the nagging pain out his mind. It had begun to hurt his performance. Spending more time than ever in the gym and training room no longer seemed to be getting him anywhere. Simply working harder wasn't working. The pain kept getting worse. The athletic trainers paid attention to everything—his nutrition, his mindset, his overall health. They knew something was wrong. They couldn't put their finger on it. They just knew Kyle was not right.

The night before, Lowry had pushed himself nearly to the brink against Toronto—the team he would eventually join. He thought he had the flu, except he had never heard of the flu feeling like a knife stabbing him in the guts. He remembered Michael Jordan once performing well in the playoffs with a fever and severe congestion. He was determined to do the same. And he did. Lowry led his team in assists that night, although Houston lost to Toronto. He remembers being exhausted at the end of the game. Once the adrenaline rush was over, the pain became unbearable.

Lowry remembers being in New Jersey, preparing for the next game against the Nets at the Prudential Center in Newark. The athletic trainers saw that he did not look right. They asked for him to be taken out of the game. He was sweating too much and seemed to be experiencing chills. Kyle denied there was a problem. This was how he felt during every game, he told them.

After that, the details became vague. At one point, one of the athletic trainers took his temperature: 101°F. An hour later, it was 105°F.

Kyle next remembers lying in a hospital bed at a top institution in New York. The doctors were talking about appendicitis or a kidney infection. No one was paying attention to the fact that he had been hurting for months. They started antibiotics and ordered CAT scans, MRIs, and ultrasounds of every part of his body. The tests produced no other diagnosis, though. Everything came back normal. Antibiotics would take care of it.

But antibiotics did not work. The pain and the fever continued. Doctors decided to take him to the operating room and look inside his abdomen with a scope. Again, everything appeared normal.

Eventually, after the surgery, one test came back positive. A bug was growing in his blood. No one explained why he had this blood infection, known as sepsis. Two weeks of intravenous antibiotics made the fever go away, but they had no effect on the pain in his belly.

The pain had been going on for 6 months. Then he had become septic. His athletic trainers decided it was time for Lowry to see somebody else.

The Solution

By the time Kyle Lowry reached Philadelphia, he was no longer overtly septic. Most of the excitement from his life-threatening scare had subsided. There was mostly frustration and pain. He could no longer play.

The clinic specialized in core injuries—everything in the body region from nipples to knees.

Three things were considered. (1) It was extremely unusual for a young, elite athlete to have a life-threatening episode of sepsis, and even more unusual for there to be no known diagnosis. (2) This lower abdominal pain had to have a cause. And (3), as the famous doctor Sir William Osler once said: Two simultaneously occurring unusual events in medicine must be connected.

Sure enough, Lowry still had a subtle sign of sepsis, although he had no fever and had been off antibiotics for a week. His pulse rate was in the 80s, which may be normal for most people but way too fast for Kyle, whose was documented at 50 in his preseason physical. Lowry's pubic bone also was exquisitely tender, and when he pulled in his thighs against resistance, he triggered the same pain.

A specialized MRI showed significant fluid where some time ago he had obviously pulled several core muscles completely off his pubic bone. Osler, a cofounder of Johns Hopkins Hospital in 1889, would have agreed that, in the absence of any other abnormality, such a fluid collection likely was the source of sepsis.

The way to explain all this is by the following. For 6 months, Lowry had been stoically playing with, and continuously extending, the core muscle injury. Bacteria seeded a resulting collection of fluid, called a *hematoma*, and eventually entered his bloodstream.

Fixing his 2 problems turned out to be simple: Drain the fluid and repair the muscles.

Lowry was back on the court in 5 weeks. He ended the season with a personal record of 14.3 points per game.

Houston athletic trainers Keith Jones and Jason Biles deserve tremendous credit for Kyle's overall health care and for observing him so closely and then finally recognizing that somehow things "were not right." Kyle had a truly life-threatening core muscle injury. The athletic trainers remained convinced that Lowry's pain and sepsis were intimately linked. That turned out to be the key factor in solving his mystery.

Alex McKechnie took charge of his rehab and performance training in Toronto after Houston traded Kyle in 2012. Kyle has become a perennial All-Star; in 2016-17, he sported career bests in minutes played (37.7 mpg), scoring (22.8 ppg), and field goal percentage (46.3) and a second best in assists (6.9 apg).

One cannot credit Lowry enough, and his athletic trainers. Five years earlier, he had played through incredible pain and a big-time illness. His character, will, and determination enabled him to get by these huge obstacles. Kyle also humanizes the importance of athletic trainers and physical therapists standing by the right principles.

The Core Rehab Principles

The story in the Philadelphia paper understates an important factor in Kyle's return to play and his emergence as a star in the NBA—his rehabilitation. In fact, that was critical. Jimmy McCrossin, then his Houston athletic trainers, and finally Alex all participated vigorously in that. Over the months prior to diagnosis, Kyle had lost tremendous muscle mass. He had to build these things back up the right way.

For simplicity, let's go through 5 core principles.

1. **Early activation:** It turns out that early activation of the core muscles following repair is essential. Immediately following repair the 2 processes that are most likely to cause problems with return to play (scarring and loss of muscle tone) have already kicked in. Understandably, folks are nervous about re-injury and intuitively want to off-load and rest the repaired muscles. But this is simply wrong. The body rapidly applies inelastic scar tissue to the area and, unopposed, results in constriction of the muscle compartment (akin to a compartment syndrome in the lower leg) and decreased flexibility to passive stretch. Couple the scarring with the loss of strength that comes with disuse and you will have frustration and pain when you finally try to get back to training. Not every case is as exciting as Kyle Lowry's (thankfully), but rehabilitating any core injury requires a detailed understanding of the core anatomy, a good foundation of training, a willingness to be aggressive and adapt to changes as they arise, and persistence to push through setbacks and find the right help when things aren't working.

2. **Sequential activation:** The sequence of muscle activation has been mapped for most athletic movements. In many, such as pitching, kicking, and swinging, there are 3 phases to the movement: an initiation phase, an acceleration phase, and a follow-through. The initiation phase involves creating potential energy through activation of 29-plus opposed muscle groups. This sets the timing pattern and tone for the remainder of the motion and ends at a point where all of the forces are in balance. As illustrated in Figure 32-1, which describes the muscle firing sequence for hip extension, there are opposing forces involved in all movement. The acceleration phase is when the coiled up energy is released and, most importantly, the speed of the arm or leg or club head is generated by the large, proximal muscles. Once again, one half of the body is moving in opposition to the other, and these forces are transferred between the legs and torso via one point. Think about the muscle slings and the patterns of muscle activation, at the center of those forces in opposition is the pubic bone. The final phase, the follow-through, allows a controlled and balanced deceleration (Figure 32-3).

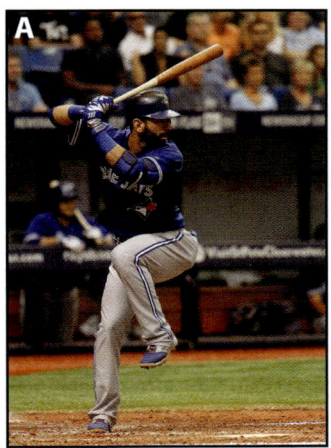
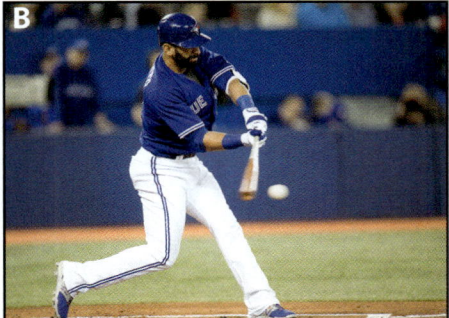
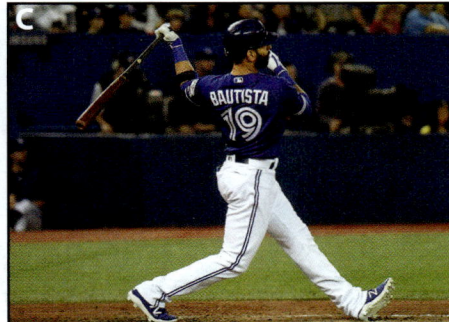

Figure 32-3. The 3 phases of movement for most sports. Power, balance, and the ability to hit the ball is generated by sequential movements known as 3 phases: (A) initiation, (B) acceleration, and (C) follow-through. The core governs these movements in conjunction with the brain. Note the vertical left leg of José Bautista in the initiation phase. The acceleration phase channels the power, as the bat drives into the ball. An ideal follow-through exhibits balance and satisfaction, which José's swing so well demonstrates. Sometimes, the swing is so well executed, it concludes with a bat flip that resembles taunting. (Reprinted with permission from *USA Today Sports,* with permission from José Bautista.)

3. **Harnessing power:** Myofascial slings and what additional training and therapy?! Assuming one has the right physical therapist in his/her corner, there are some principles to follow while coming back from a core muscle injury: strengthen muscles together in functional groups (rather than in isolation) pay attention to the sequence of muscle activation, understand the harness that attaches to the pubic bone, and protect the harness. These principles apply to everyone and are important in preventing core injuries. Some of this stuff is not new, but armed with your new perspective—seeing all of the core—you'll have a new appreciation of why it makes sense.

   The pubic bone sits in the center of an array of myofascial slings that stabilize the pelvis and balance the torso on the legs (Figure 32-4). These slings make up the outer unit of the core. The inner unit consists of the pelvic diaphragm, multifidus, transverse abdominus, and diaphragm.[3-6] There are 3 or 4 slings (depending on whom you believe) made up by the muscles: on the front of the torso (the anterior sling), on the back of the torso (the posterior oblique sling), and deep in your back and butt (the deep longitudinal sling). The anterior sling is made up of the external oblique, internal oblique, and the adductor of the opposite side. The posterior oblique sling is made up from the latissimus dorsi, thoracolumbar fascia, and gluteus maximus of the opposite side. Deep longitudinal sling comprises of erector spinae, sacrotuberous ligament, and the biceps femoris (hamstring) of the opposite side.[7,8] Training a single muscle in isolation creates imbalances, while working all of the components of a sling together creates functional strength. Imbalanced pulling across the pubic bone is a set-up for a core muscle injury.

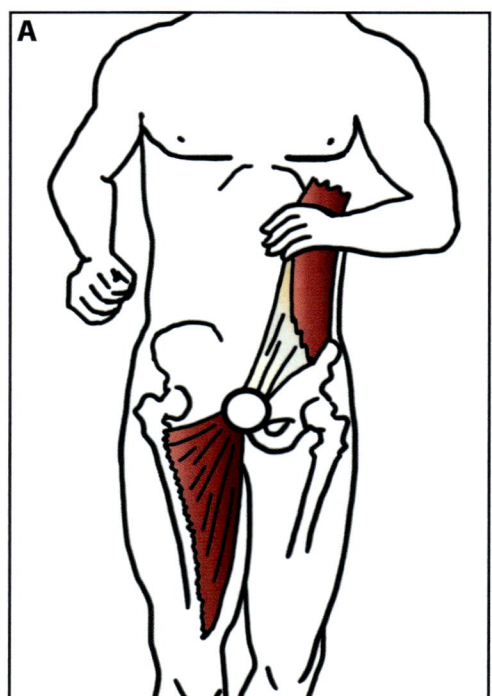
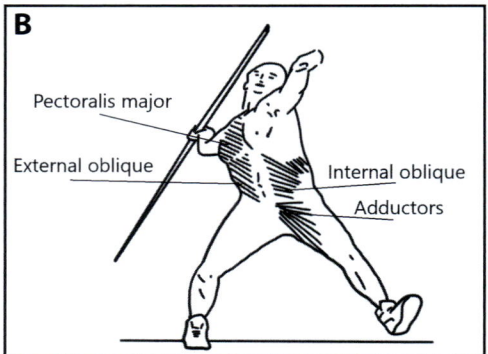

Figure 32-4. (A) A myofascial sling and (B) myofascial slings in action.

4. **Protecting the harness:** If you think about these slings and how they are arranged across the pubic bone, you can predict how these muscles should fire with a certain movement. It turns out that the sequence of muscles firing basically follows these slings. Muscle scripting follows the basic rule that the most proximal muscle groups contract first, giving a stable foundation on which the more distal muscles engage movement. Some refer to this as *stability before mobility*, which is much easier to say than to understand.[9] Pain and/or loss of strength in a muscle or loss of joint range will directly affect the efficiency of muscle contraction, therefore influencing the outcome of the fine movements. Contraction of the most proximal group of muscle (ie, the inner unit [pelvic diaphragm, transverse abdominus, multifidus, and diaphragm]) is important for strength, balance, and power. The sequence of contraction continues with firing of the outer unit or the myofascial slings. These muscles are slow-twitch, postural muscles and need to be trained differently than the more easily fatigable distal muscles. If the proximal muscles are fatigued or injured, the sequence of muscle contraction will be altered to compensate. Often this means distal, more easily fatigable muscles take on responsibility for maintaining posture, and this loss of proximal stability means more wobbles in the joints; slower, less-efficient movements; and more risk for subsequent injury.

5. **Thinking function, not isolation:** The principle of central/proximal stability serving as the foundation for peripheral movements is derived from relatively small muscles. The muscles that insert directly into the fibrocartilage covering of the pubic bone create the harness through which all of the power of the legs, butt, and back are transferred into purposeful upper body movements. The muscles of the harness (rectus abdominis, pectineus, adductor longus, and adductor brevis) insert on a relatively small area of the pubic bone. If you think about the size of these muscles and their attachment relative to the glutes, quads, and hamstrings, these attachments are a point of weakness. There are tremendous forces applied to this point during any athletic activity, and we should be training with protecting this relative weak spot in mind. So much training is focused on strengthening the rectus abdominis, but overemphasizing this muscle simply directs more force on a point of weakness. Go back to the muscles that make up the slings: these are the muscles to focus on for improving stability and efficiency of movement and at the same time protecting the harness from wear.$^{\text{VID 1}}$

Protecting the harness needs to be a primary concern during all phases of rehab: acute, return to sport, and maintenance. Unfortunately, the rehab market has been split into 2 independent universes: rehab and performance. This leaves folks who are coming back from an injury with a decision, do they seek out someone who understands their injury or do they throw their lot in with someone who will get them ready to play more quickly? Clearly the best answer is somewhere on the spectrum between the two, but taking someone through all phases of his/her rehab is not easy and, apparently, not good business either.

Sticking to the Protocol and Early Return to Previous Skill Sets

We have seen 2 main issues result from well-intended, but not fully informed, therapists unfamiliar with our postoperative rehabilitation core muscle repair protocols.

The first is not adhering to the protocol. This stems from a natural, though very wrong, instinct that rest must be required for a week or two at least after surgery. The reality is that scar tissue is our main enemy postoperatively. We emphasize the importance of early vigorous activity in certain controlled fashions. In the same vein, early gentle massage empirically reduces the possibility of formation of balls of scar, which can become problematic later; yet, early active release (eg, Graston techniques) cause harm through disruption of tissue, repair sites, and bruising. Athletic trainers and physical therapists love to do active release massage, but after surgery this can be dangerous.

The second is the fear of early return to skill sets. It turns out that gentle soft toss catch for a baseball player or quarterback or careful, controlled skating for an NHL hockey player is good when instituted very early in the rehab program. It helps both with respect to preventing scar in key areas as well as allowing the player not to avoid the feeling of having to start from "scratch" when resumption of play really begins.

Assessing Outcomes

This is tricky. As you might expect within a nascent field, there will be loads of confusion with regard to the best measurements for this. For example, how do we best measure when an athlete is truly "back"? What do we really mean by that? While we may all agree that returning to play is a primary goal, shouldn't we also be looking also at how the athlete feels he/she is performing? How do we establish precise scoring systems for the different types of injuries? Or, for that matter, what about the athlete who is not injured and who is training simply to get "fitter"? How do you measure that? We cannot always use the specific measures used in the NFL or MLS Combine.

The fact looms that we need better measurements. The established hip measurement outcome scores don't cut it for assessing high-level athletes. For example, when it comes to treatments of hip impingement, the modified Harris Hip Score (mHHS) and others like it[10,11] cover, rather extensively, issues like pain, function, range of motion, and deformity. Yet, they don't tell you whether athletes are truly happy with their overall sports performance. Those measurement sticks do not cover intimate feelings that athletes experience and use to assess whether he/she is truly back to pre-injury levels of play. We have found a simple 1 to 5 grading system, based solely on sequential athlete self-assessments, to be the most useful for differentiating subtle changes compared to the way he/she felt before injury.[12]

In actuality, Thorborg, Hölmich, and colleagues' Copenhagen Hip and Groin Outcome Score (HAGOS)[13] does pretty well with regard to answering the challenge of producing a scoring system analogous to the tools for measuring outcomes after hip surgery. Per Hölmich has been creating the forefront of nonoperative core treatment for several decades.

Alex McKechnie Performance Principles (in His Words)

I have 4 main performance principles:

1. **Make default postures the correct ones.** Every athletic body defaults into postures unique for the individual and the individual's sport or position with consideration to right or left dominance. Default postures come as a direct result of repetition. Performance evaluation requires the identification of 2 factors: (1) the repetitive natures of the sport and (2) the postural defaults peculiar to the individual. Maximizing performance requires the matching of the two, and ridding the individual of suboptimal defaults.

   Injuries or pre-existing conditions reduce joint range or weaken baseline strength or otherwise create dysfunctional movement patterns that have significant effects on default and movement dynamics.

   The practitioner/clinician must use skilled manual therapy, joint mobilization, and muscle activation techniques to address the identified deficiencies.

   Recognition and correction of default postures will greatly improve the chance of positive outcomes from core strength and functional movement strategies.

   Core muscle injuries without a history of acute trauma are almost always the result of training errors; hence, the importance of identifying and correcting default postures before the athlete enters the weight room.

2. **Have an exercise system designed to train and strengthen the core properly.** That is what I had in mind when I designed the Core X program (http://corexsystem.com/). The primary goal of Core X is to train through repetition and establish what I call the *core neutral* posture, then to be able to sustain that posture while training balance and central-to-peripheral sequential movement. We want the core neutral posture to endure and help to create a profound and smooth ground force reaction. The end result should reduce torsion, load, and shear forces to which gravity subjects us.

   The most important movement principles involve a combination of endurance of the core neutral posture and establishment of proximal to distal muscle firing patterns that ensures stability before mobility.

   The end result is proper core control that maximizes the athlete's efficiency of movement à la Baryshnikov, Beckenbauer, or Messi.

3. **It's all about VVT.** Reinforcing the correct posture takes constant correction and repetition. This means using 3 tools that we call:
   - Visual: Imaging (ie, both video and mirrors) to provide continuous feedback
   - Verbal: A skilled observer who provides constant correction and utilizes key commands
   - Tactile: Manual positioning (ie, touching)

4. **Get the patient/client/player all the way back.** One of the most daunting tasks the practitioner/clinician faces is the transition from the treatment room back to the performance venue.

   Rehabilitation must constantly challenge the patient to get closer to the activities of play or of his/her previous daily activities. For the athlete, that means getting closer and closer to the demands of the sport in terms of strength, mobility, and duration. That transition back to the performance venue and, hopefully, to the same pre-injury level of performance would be seamless, except for the erratic adrenaline rushes, which, by their nature, bring unpredictability and, moreover, new forces that the player may not have seen in a while.[VID 2]

THE NEXT STEP

Okay, we have listed some important principles for identifying the right therapist and then designing spot-on rehabilitation and performance protocols. Now we go into more detail about a particularly tricky part of rehab, the one Alex lists as Performance Principle 4 (ie, getting the athlete all the way back).

SELECTED READINGS

Bizzini M, Dvorak J. FIFA 11+: an effective programme to prevent football injuries in various player groups worldwide—a narrative review. *Br J Sports Med*. 2015;49:577-579.

This article represents what may be the largest and most successful injury prevention program in soccer. While people may quibble with some of the specific exercises, the concept of coaches using a standard routine, from several perspectives, makes a lot of sense.

Hölmich P, Uhrskou P, Ulnits L, et al. Effectiveness of active physical training as treatment for long-standing adductor-related groin pain in athletes: randomised trial. *Lancet*. 1999;353(9151):439-443.

Dr. Hölmich has refined the art of nonoperative approaches to core muscle injuries. Over decades, he has developed sound rehab principles that are used throughout the world.

McKechnie A. The Core X System. https://www.youtube.com/watch?v=w99aTmTFi0I.

The video advertises an exercise system developed by Alex after many years of experience. It features several patients jointly treated by Alex and Dr. Meyers. From simply watching the advertisement, one may get some insight into several principles mentioned by Alex in this chapter.

REFERENCES

1. Krahn B. 5 ways to spot a bad trainer. *Men's Health*. https://www.menshealth.com/fitness/a19537433/how-to-spot-a-bad-trainer/. Published February 15, 2014. Accessed February 13, 2017.
2. Meyers WC, Poor AE. He wanted to have game, got pain. *The Philadelphia Inquirer*. 2015;Jan 18:G02.
3. Hodges PW, Richardson CA. Contraction of the abdominal muscles associated with movement of the lower limb. *Phys Ther*. 1997;77:132-142.
4. Hodges P, Richardson C, Jull G. Evaluation of the relationship between laboratory and clinical tests of transversus abdominis function. *Physiother Res Int*. 1996;1(1):30-40.
5. Hodges PW, Sapsford R, Pengel LH. Postural and respiratory functions of the pelvic floor muscles. *Neurourol Urodyn*. 2007;26(3):362-371.
6. Willett GM, Hyde JE, Uhrlaub MB, Wendel CL, Karst GM. Relative activity of abdominal muscles during commonly prescribed strengthening exercises. *J Strength Cond Res*. 2001;15(4):480-485.
7. Macintosh JE, Bogduk N, Gracovetsky S. The biomechanics of the thoracolumbar fascia. *Clin Biomech*. 1987;2(2):78-83.
8. Vleeming A, Schuenke MD, Danneels L, Willard FH. The functional coupling of the deep abdominal and paraspinal muscles: the effects of simulated paraspinal muscle contraction on force transfer to the middle and posterior layer of the thoracolumbar fascia. *J Anat*. 2014;225(4):447-462.
9. Bliss LS, Teeple P. Core stability: the centerpiece of any training program. *Curr Sports Med Rep*. 2005;4(3):179-183.
10. Harris WH. Traumatic arthritis of the hip after dislocation and acetabular fractures: treatment by mold arthroplasty. An end-result study using a new method of result evaluation. *J Bone Joint Surg Am*. 1969;51:737-755.
11. Murray D. The hip. In: Pynsent D, Fairbank J, Carr A, eds. *Outcome Measurements in Orthopaedics*. Oxford, United Kingdom: Butterworth-Heinemann; 1993:198-227.
12. Meyers WC, Foley DP, Garrett WE, Lohnes JH, Mandlebaum BR, PAIN Study Group. Management of severe lower abdominal or inguinal pain in high-performance athletes. *Am J Sport Med*. 2000;28(1):2-8.
13. Thorborg K, Hölmich P, Christensen R, Petersen J, Roos EM. The Copenhagen Hip and Groin Outcome Score (HAGOS): development and validation according to the COSMIN checklist. *Br J Sports Med*. 2011;45(6):478-491.

VIDEOS

1. https://youtu.be/vuZZDAPOYUc
2. https://www.youtube.com/watch?v=w99aTmTFi0I

33

the **final** stage of rehab
getting **all the way** back

ANDREW SMALL, PT, CSCS, RSCC*D, MPHTYST, BSC (HMS-EXSCI)

Editor's Note: *The first parts of rehabilitation are relatively easy with respect to every athlete's psyche. You follow the right protocol, strength returns appropriately, scar is minimized, and the pain goes mostly away. Psychology comes into action in this final part of rehab—the stage of getting the player, or even the construction worker, all the way back to his/her sport or other activity. This is when the pressure begins. Expectations and the real timeline for return for participation begin to overlap. Pressure grows on everybody (eg, player, management, fans, agents, and doctors). Conflicting goals abruptly cloud the picture. Nonmedical factors enter into the scenario—contract status, team security, disability payments; the list is long.*

A number of years ago, during spring training, a star MLB centerfielder going into his free agency year gets hurt and has surgery for a simple rectus abdominis tear. The return-to-play time was predicted to be only 3 weeks. The player might have to do a minor league "rehab stint" after that, before rejoining the "big show" team. At the same time, an important person within the team management hierarchy decides he wants to see how well a promising minor league centerfielder might perform during this star's absence. The thinking is this: If the promising centerfielder plays well, then contract negotiations with the veteran star centerfielder's agent might go better. The team's management person tells the owner it might be "3 months" rather than 3 weeks before the star would return. Of course, it becomes difficult for that management person's agenda to stay private. The player finds out and gets upset. Things start to play out in the press.

This case exhibits the complexity of return to play. The contemplations go way beyond the medical aspects of the patient/player. They enter the world of psychology, politics, and sometimes into a spooky expanse—what Rod Serling used to call "The Twilight Zone."

I asked Andrew Small, an excellent young Australian sports physical therapist, to comment on this final stage of rehab.

The greatest accomplishment is not in never falling, but in rising again after you fall.

—Vince Lombardi, legendary NFL football coach.

I will never forget standing in the Great Court at the University of Queensland, speaking to my former mentor. Humble and always willing to talk though my issues, he threw me through for a loop this time.

"I want to study physical therapy and work with athletes."

I fully expected him to support this. He was my wisest advisor and strongest advocate, plus an internationally respected coach, researcher, and educator with over 30 years of experience working with elite athletes, including 12 Olympians. His words stunned me.

"Are you sure you want to do this?"

He went on, "It may seem glamorous traveling around the world, working with these stars. But there are so many, let's say, challenges. It's not glamorous. They want results way beyond realistic expectations."

I think, but am still not sure, that he was just testing me. As we talked more, he became convinced of my passion. He said athletes want results "yesterday" and that the return-to-sport phase was the trickiest part of the physio's job. "There are so many conflicts of interest that keep you from doing the job the way you want." Having let off his steam, he finally succumbed and congratulated me on my chosen career.

Since then, I have learned that the return-to-play part of rehab is actually the most rewarding. It remains tremendously gratifying to see an athlete overcome injury and return stronger and actually better than ever before. That's our aim in rehab of core injuries. We think that most athletes do not get the core training they should, and when they do after surgery, they often beat their previous personal bests.

RISING TO DIVE AGAIN

Okay, let me tell you about a specific case, a diver before the Olympics (Figure 33-1). Just 4 weeks prior to the big qualifying event, this athlete suffered a mid-muscle belly rectus abdominis strain. He couldn't dive at all. The medical team and I had just 7 days to wean the athlete back to full competition loads following 3 weeks off.

We immediately implemented corrective and strengthening exercises to improve the capacity of both involved and uninvolved structures. With the qualifiers only 4 weeks away, we had 3 things to accomplish: (1) allow injured tissue to heal, (2) continue to improve his overall physical condition, and (3) preserve his technical abilities. The immediacy of a situation sometimes necessitates extraordinary treatment. The old concept of rest simply does not usually apply to core muscle injury.

Don't get me wrong, we did some degree of modified rest. We used the combination of pain and performance as our guide, graded by some specific functional tests. Exercises were designed to protect as well as improve the capacity of that one specific area to load. He was allowed to work through some pain. Ranges of motion of the hips and lumbar spine and hip were maintained. We stepped up massage and other manual therapy, and monitored strength with a diving-specific 5-stage test. Our diver re-entered the pool after he completed the test without symptoms. He had just 1 week left before competition.

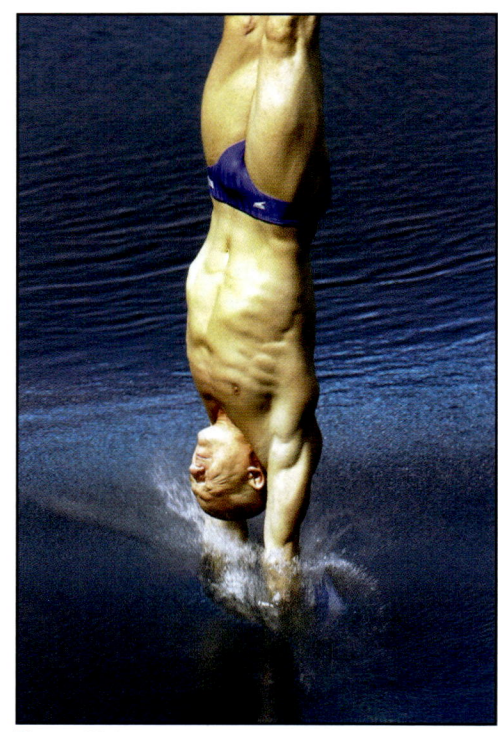

Figure 33-1.

The coaches kept in close contact, and technical training was planned jointly. The extra-swift training began with both dry land and pool sessions with modifications to reduce stress on injured tissue. We used how the symptoms reacted to the different types of sessions as measures of tolerance of the injured tissue to specific loads. The loads grew each day until our technical and physical goals of the demands of training reached the demands of competition. The coaches kept in close contact, and they planned the technical training.

We began with modified 1-m and 5-m drills. Then, fortunately, the day before competition, the athlete had earned the right to compete his full list from 10 m. The athlete competed successfully the next day and made the Olympic team and surpassed all expectations in the Olympics.

The diver shows that sometimes we physical therapists, athletic trainers, and other fitness people need to break from what we usually do. This is how I learned about these injuries. I developed a totally different attitude about return to play and changed all my protocols. Sometimes, we just have to cast away our old eyes and put on new specs.

A star on a movie set is like a time bomb.
That bomb has got to be defused so people can approach it without fear.

—Jack Nicholson, the famous Hollywood actor.

THE WAY IT WAS

A recent author referred to the area we in this book are calling the core as "the Bermuda Triangle of sports medicine."[1] That has been the prevailing thought. Defuse that bomb. Many specific injuries occur there. Learn what they are and how to identify them and then treat them appropriately. We certainly don't know everything yet about the core, but we know a lot, so at least know what we know. Don't fear this area of the body any more.

From our rehabilitation point of view, therapists still get nonspecific referral notes from docs prescribing things as vague as a teenager's description of what he/she did last night, scripts like "rehab for groin pain," nothing specific, no directions. The plan then develops according to whims of the therapist and nonspecific, existing rehab protocols. The program then progresses to disagreements between the different rehab people, because the patient does not get better or reaches a plateau from which there is no escape. Arguments ensue regarding diagnosis and subsequent management.[2-4] We therapists liken this situation to a ticking time bomb.

For estimating the best time for return to play, therapists generally have quantified loads and loosely used various monitoring devices. These approaches remain mostly guesswork.

Progress lies not in enhancing what is, but in advancing toward what will be.

—Khalil Gibran.

NEW EYES

Over a 20-year period, technology and awareness of core muscle injuries have increased significantly.[5-9] Paradigms[10-12] are evolving. The science has become much more straightforward, although no reliable formulas exist with regard to the precise timing for return to play. You still have to consider all kinds of factors. The best decisions demand a lot of experience. The factors include such things as precise identification of the injury, its severity and implications with respect to development of other injuries, many biomechanical considerations, current and necessary levels of strength, the playing season, and player contracts.

With a click of a button, we may come up with some technique. Beware, though, that the knowledge out there on the internet is usually wrong and often dangerous. On the other hand, we should embrace new technology, such as GPS accelerometers and cloud-based athlete management software.

As physical therapists, we also need to pay more attention to our performance and exercise colleagues. The 2 sets of professions actually complement each other. We need to adopt some of those traditional strength and conditioning principles. Recent research has demonstrated that the right amount of stress/load applied in a specific way can produce an adaptive cellular response in a number of tissues such as bone and tendon.[13-17]

Old Lessons Applied in New Ways

The concept of load is as simple as it sounds. With human movement, various tissues are placed under load or stress. Whether it is compressive, like a knee joint, or tensile, like an Achilles tendon, many structures undergo stress during human movement. Too much load causes tissue failure and too little leads to weakness and an inability to tolerate stress.[18-22] Believe it or not, we shall never find the Holy Grail. Finding the exact "right load" is similar. Various concepts have nonetheless emerged as part of that righteous search such as mechano-therapy and mechano-transduction.[23]

Load monitoring has improved with the GPS and accelerometer technology. It allows us to compare objective loads to objective measures of tissue tolerance such as pain, swelling, tightness, and muscle tone. Patterns can be tracked and provide therapists with more information. We can make therapy decisions based on this.

Performance and strength coaches talk in terms of "specific adaptations to imposed demands," or SAIDs. We as therapists must also understand those demands for specific tissues relative to the timelines for healing. If an athlete must run, we must figure out the tissue strength and what the muscles and bones need to withstand during running progression. The load and high-velocity movements shall be specific to the athlete and sport. Yes, we make a lot of judgments based on how the athlete feels. It is important to point out that we may easily correlate how the athlete feels to our objective parameters and make subsequent judgments based on multiple sets of data.

Streaming is the concept used extensively in sports performance education around the world.[24] It involves categorizing movements into sequential linear progressions involving multiple muscle groups. One stream may involve a series of exercises to develop single leg strength, another to develop horizontal push. Be familiar with the term. Use it. It conveys the right principles of involvement of multiple muscles in a sequential way. We use it a lot in our return-to-play lingo.

For the core, we choose streams that develop hip adductor/abductor strength, abdominal endurance, single-leg strength, single-leg hop abilities, as well as running progressions. These streams can be customized depending on the various deficits observed after physical examination, the type and extent of injury, as well as the movement goals of the patient. A structured approach allows us to set a plan that ensures that an athlete earns the right to progress to higher loads.

History and Physical Examination Factors

History and physical examination remains the backbone of the treatment plan. We must consider all aspects of the core: the hip, back, core muscles, and all those important viscera and systems that reside there. On top of that, we as physical or other therapists should identify previous training errors and load difficulties. We palpate a lot and use the elicitation of pain (ie, tenderness) as one of our important guideposts. We must be ready to communicate our findings when they differ with the referring doctor.

We should palpate the pubic bone, adductor, and rectus abdominis insertions and all the muscles that attach to or pass by the pubic bone. Specific strength tests may provide additional information such as adductor squeeze (Figure 33-2)[25,26] and pubic symphysis stress test (Figure 33-3).[27] Some recent work suggests hand-held dynamometry may help assess hip muscle strength in at-risk populations.[28-32] There is no question that strength imbalances are risk factors for core injuries.[32,33] Nobody yet is perfect with the use of these devices but they measure things objectively, which can be used as baselines for athletes who are injured or who just want to improve. We can devise our own protocols based on these data for return to play. We must recognize, however, that these are just tools. We really don't know much.

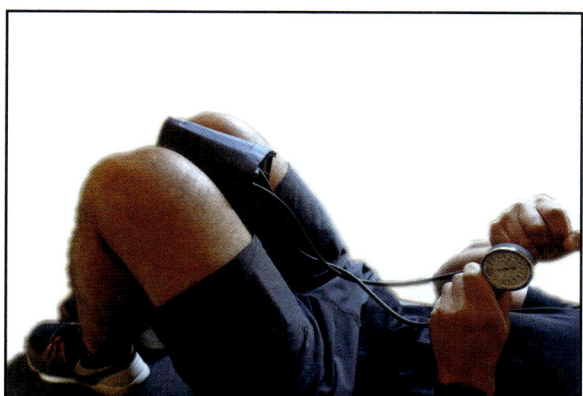

Figure 33-2. Pectineus squeeze test.

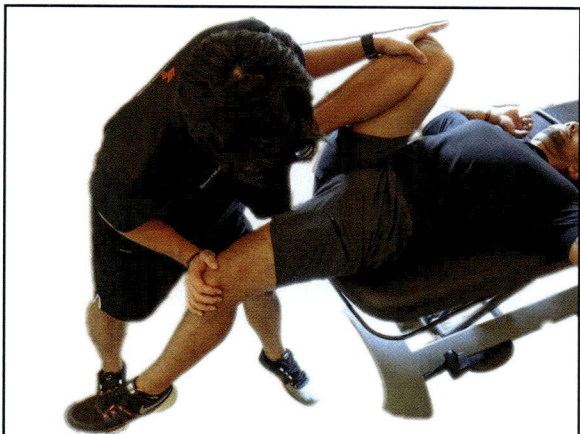

Figure 33-3. Pubic symphysis stress test. The therapist opposes flexion and extension.

Restricted ranges of motion may be risk factors for core muscle injury.[34-36] Therefore, it is important to measure as precisely as we can, hip internal and external rotation, abduction, flexion and extension, etc.

Functional performance measures are ones that relate to specific tasks that an athlete or worker commonly performs. One has to find or make up the applicable tests (eg, standardized lower limb tests)[37-40] or baseline GPS running data.

In summary, for return to play, we should first assess 6 things by history and physical exam:
1. Structure or structures causing pain and disability
2. The extent of injury to the respective injured tissues
3. Loads required to elicit pain and disability
4. Other areas that need to be addressed to reduce excess load on the injured structures (biomechanical, areas of uncontrolled movement)
5. Objective measures to monitor and assess change
6. External factors that could affect return to play (training errors, biomechanical, psychological, social, environment)

Management

Generally, the determination as to whether an athlete may return all the way to his/her sport is generally based on a number of criteria. These may include:
- No acute signs (eg, swelling, pain, heat, tenderness)
- Adequate tissue healing has occurred with respect to the relevant timelines
- Full range of motion
- Adequate strength and endurance with respect to the demands of the sport
- Appropriate level of coordination and balance
- Sport relevant skill/technique preserved
- Correction of biomechanical abnormalities
- Psychologically prepared to return to activity
- Clearance by coach and other support staff

With respect to core muscle injuries in particular, the return-to-play estimate in terms of timing is tricky based on the injury mainly and other factors mentioned previously. We think in terms of 3 phases of rehab: acute, subacute, and final (Figures 33-4 through 33-6).

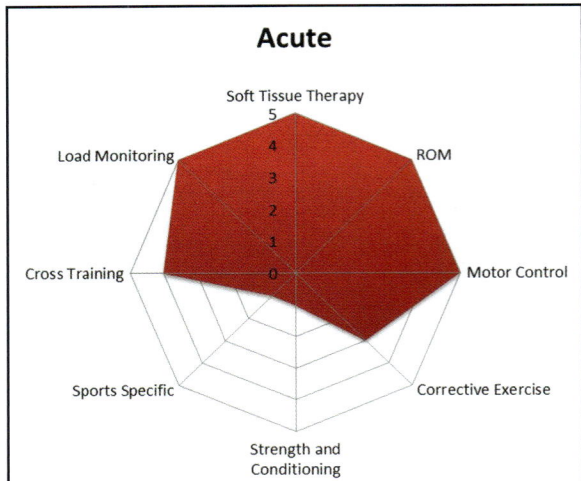

Figure 33-4. Acute phase rehabilitation multimodal therapy graphic for a core injury. In this initial stage, the emphasis is on manual therapy and decreasing pain and swelling.

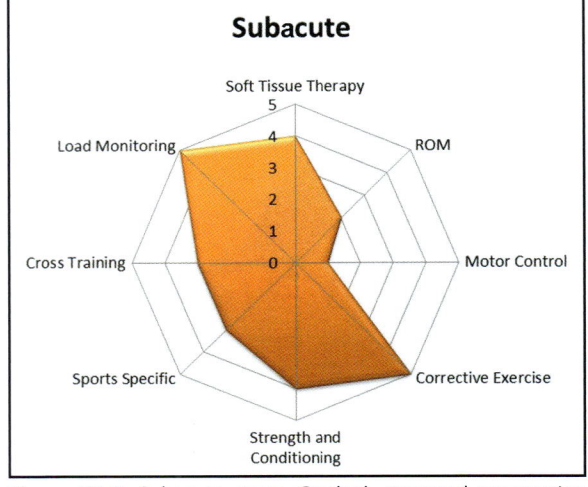

Figure 33-5. Subacute stage. Gradual, streamed progression into strength and conditioning.

Success in the first 2 phases does affect how we approach the third one. For this, the return-to-play phase, the physical condition must be at a level that can withstand the loads applied in the return-to-play phase of rehabilitation. The athlete must be able to withstand expected setbacks such as scar tissue break-up, no matter how severe. We need to have all the baseline data we can get when we formally begin this final stage. We usually use light jogging as the first step in the return-to-play phase, if this has not already begun. There is a whole science related to how we monitor and advance the running.

We should regard ourselves as both the interpreter and adviser for both the coach and doctor. Coaches and therapists may aim for at least 2 weeks of full practice, without aggravation, before graduating. During this phase, athlete-monitoring software and technology may be useful and provide objective data to guide practice intensity, frequency, and playing time when the player returns. There are all sorts of ways you can do this, so long as you pay attention to the player.

Professional sports teams and organizations around the world are currently using many of the mentioned concepts to manage their athletes. Although many of the mentioned concepts may seem simple in isolation, when put together they provide a powerful tool to guide the rehabilitation process. Think of this final phase of rehab like rowing at the Olympics. Consider the teams from all the different countries, their different methods of training, their quirky coaches and therapists and strength conditioners… and think how they all finish within a second of each other. In the end, they all did what worked, given all their different limitations.

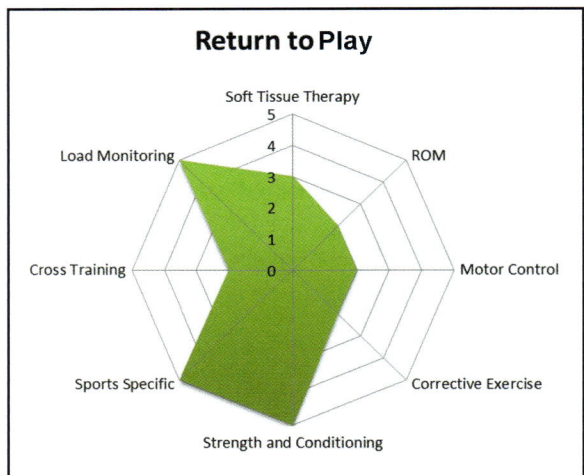

Figure 33-6. Return-to-play therapy. We can't emphasize enough the importance of the subacute and return-to-play stages (ie, robust strength and conditioning programs) to get patients all the way back to the demands of their sports. In the United States, physical therapists, in general, turn over this phase of rehab to the athletic trainers, strength coaches, etc. Other countries offer combined degrees in physical therapy and exercise science.

Still an Art

No doubt, the final-final stage of rehab—actual return to play—can be a tricky one. Picking the optimal take-off point for this final leap remains more of an art than a science. As we progress in understanding sports science, more objectivity and devices shall come into play. One unstudied area likely to prove useful for adjudging optimal return to play is cognitive function tests, similar to the tests described in Chapter 6.

It makes sense that injury causes diminution in sports cognition. If one could measure those decreases, and then see when, let's say, reaction times, balance, and visual fields correct, cognition might yield the ideal measures of healing and athlete confidence for determining optimal timing for return to play.

We believe that return to normal of cognitive tests after correction of a core injury shall likely equate to optimal timing for return to play. Perhaps then, maximal cognitive performance would equate to confidence.

The art is not in only working out what data points to collect, but also in the ability to use those measures to bring back the best for the individual performers, other interested parties, and perhaps also, the team. With continued advances in technology, our ability to assess the function, and perhaps even the confidence level of our athletes, shall continue to improve. The art of acting on these insights at the right time and with a maximal effect, in terms of meaningful change, shall remain in therapists' hands.

Selected Readings

Khan KM, Scott A. Mechanotherapy: how physical therapists' prescription of exercise promotes tissue repair. *Br J Sports Med.* 2009;43(4):247-252.
*Understanding how mechanical loads and "stress" promote physiological connective tissue responses leads to the development of new therapies. This article provides insight into the process called **mechanotransduction** and how we exercise therapists may apply some new, important principles to common musculoskeletal injuries.*

Blanch P, Gabbett TJ. Has the athlete trained enough to return-to-play safely? The acute:chronic workload ratio permits clinicians to quantify a player's risk of subsequent injury. *Br J Sports Med.* 2016;50(8):471-475.
Peter Blanch and Tim Gabbett address the subject of when the athlete has trained "enough" to return to full competition safely. The authors postulate that an acute:chronic workload ratio holds promise for the return-to-play decision-making.

Palisch A, Zoga AC, Meyers WC. Imaging of athletic pubalgia and core muscle injuries: clinical and therapeutic correlations. *Clin Sports Med.* 2013;32(3):427-447.
Correct imaging of the abdomen, pelvis, and thigh is essential for accurate diagnosis and rehabilitation of many athletic injuries of the core. This article discusses a specific protocol for imaging this region.

References

1. Bizzini M. The groin area: the Bermuda triangle of sports medicine? *Br J Sports Med.* 2010;45(1):1-1.
2. Orchard J, Read JW, Verral GM, Slavotinek JP. Pathophysiology of chronic groin pain in the athlete. *Intern J Sports Med.* 2000;1(1):134-147.
3. Minnich JM, Hanks JB, Muschaweck U, Brunt LM, Diduch DR. Sports hernia: diagnosis and treatment highlighting a minimal repair surgical technique. *Am J Sports Med.* 2011;39(6):1341-1349.
4. Robertson IJ, Curran C, McCaffrey N, Shields CJ, McEntee GP. Adductor tenotomy in the management of groin pain in athletes. *Intern J Sports Med.* 2011;32(1):45-48.
5. Falvey EC, Franklyn-Miller A, McCrory PR. The groin triangle: a patho-anatomical approach to the diagnosis of chronic groin pain in athletes. *Br J Sports Med.* 2009;43(3):213-220.
6. Hölmich P, Uhrskou P, Ulnits L, et al. Effectiveness of active physical training as treatment for long-standing adductor-related groin pain in athletes: randomised trial. *Lancet.* 1999;353(9151):439-443.
7. Meyers WC, McKechnie A, Philippon MJ, Horner MA, Zoga AC, Devon ON. Experience with «sports hernia» spanning two decades. *Ann Surg.* 2008;248(4):656-665.
8. Fricker P. Management of groin pain in athletes. *Br J Sports Med.* 1997;31:97-101.
9. Anderson K, Strickland SM, Warren R. Hip and groin injuries in athletes. *American Orthopaedic Society for Sports Medicine.* 2001;29(4):521-533.
10. Palisch A, Zoga AC, Meyers WC. Imaging of athletic pubalgia and core muscle injuries: clinical and therapeutic correlations. *Clin Sports Med.* 2013;32(3):427-447.
11. Hegedus EJ, Stern B, Reiman MP, Tarara D, Wright AA. A suggested model for physical examination and conservative treatment of athletic pubalgia. *Phys Ther Sport.* 2013;14(1):3-16.

12. Blanch P, Gabbett TJ. Has the athlete trained enough to return-to-play safely? The acute:chronic workload ratio permits clinicians to quantify a player's risk of subsequent injury. *Br J Sports Med.* 2016;50(8):471-475.
13. Beck BR. Muscle forces or gravity—what predominates mechanical loading on bone? Introduction. *Med Sci Sports Exerc.* 2009;41(11):2033-2036.
14. Cook JL, Purdam C. Is compressive load a factor in the development of tendinopathy? *Br J Sports Med.* 2012;46(3):163-168.
15. Kaeding C, Best TM. Tendinosis: pathophysiology and nonoperative treatment. *Sports Health.* 2009;1(4):284-292.
16. Khan KM, Scott A. Mechanotherapy: how physical therapists' prescription of exercise promotes tissue repair. *Br J Sports Med.* 2009;43(4):247-252.
17. Frost HM. Wolff's law and bone's structural adaptations to mechanical usage: an overview for clinicians. *The Angle Orthodontist.* 1994;64(3):175-188.
18. Almekinders LC, Weinhold PS, Maffulli N. Compression etiology in tendinopathy. *Clin Sports Med.* 2003;22(4):703-710.
19. Cook JL, Purdam CR. Is tendon pathology a continuum? A pathology model to explain the clinical presentation of load-induced tendinopathy. *Br J Sports Med.* 2009;43(6):409-416.
20. Cook JL, Purdam C. Is compressive load a factor in the development of tendinopathy? *Br J Sports Med.* 2012;46(3):163-168.
21. Kaeding C, Best TM. Tendinosis: pathophysiology and nonoperative treatment. *Sports Health.* 2009;1(4):284-292.
22. Orchard J, Cook J, Halpin N. Stress shielding as a cause of insertional tendinopathy: the operative technique of limited adductor tenotomy supports this theory. *J Sci Med Sport.* 2004;7(4):424-428.
23. Khan KM, Scott A. Mechanotherapy: how physical therapists' prescription of exercise promotes tissue repair. *Br J Sports Med.* 2009;43(4):247-252.
24. Giles K, Penfold L, Giorgi A. *A Guide to Developing Physical Qualities in Young Athletes—An Instructional Handbook.* Queensland, Australia: Movement Dynamics; 2005.
25. Verrall G, Hamilton I, Slavotinek J, et al. Hip joint range of motion reduction in sports-related chronic groin injury diagnosed as pubic bone stress injury. *J Sci Med Sport.* 2005;8(1):77-84.
26. Hogan A, Lovell G. Pubic symphysis stress tests and rehabilitation of osteitis pubis. In: Spinks W, Reilly T, Murphy A, eds. *Science and Football IV.* London, United Kingdom: Routledge; 2002.
27. Walheim G, Selvik G. Mobility of the pubic symphysis. In vivo measurements with an electromechanic method and a roentgen stereophotogrammetric method. *Clin Ortho Relat Res.* 1984;191:129-135.
28. Hanna CM, Fulcher ML, Elley CR, Moyes SA. Normative values of hip strength in adult male association football players assessed by handheld dynamometry. *J Sci Med Sport.* 2010;13(3):299-303.
29. Thorborg K, Petersen J, Magnusson SP, Hölmich P. Clinical assessment of hip strength using a hand-held dynamometer is reliable. *Scand J Med Sci Sports.* 2010;20(3):493-501.
30. Thorborg K, Serner A, Petersen J, Madsen TM, Magnusson P, Hölmich P. Hip adduction and abduction strength profiles in elite soccer players: implications for clinical evaluation of hip adductor muscle recovery after injury. *Am J Sports Med.* 2011;39(1):121-126.
31. Fulcher ML, Hanna CM, Raina Elley C. Reliability of handheld dynamometry in assessment of hip strength in adult male football players. *J Sci Med Sport.* 2010;13(1):80-84.
32. Crow JF, Pearce AJ, Veale JP, VanderWesthuizen D, Coburn PT, Pizzari T. Hip adductor muscle strength is reduced preceding and during the onset of groin pain in elite junior Australian football players. *J Sci Med Sport.* 2010;13(2):202-204.
33. Hrysomallis C. Hip adductors' strength, flexibility, and injury risk. *J Strength Cond Res.* 2009;23(5):1514-1517.
34. Robinson P, Bhat V, English B. Imaging in the assessment and management of athletic pubalgia. *Semin Musculoskelet Radiol.* 2011;15(1):14-26.
35. Verrall G, Hamilton I, Slavotinek J, et al. Hip joint range of motion reduction in sports-related chronic groin injury diagnosed as pubic bone stress injury. *J Sci Med Sport.* 2005;8(1):77-84.
36. Wollin M, Lovell G. Osteitis pubis in four young football players: a case series demonstrating successful rehabilitation. *Phys Ther Sport.* 2006;7(3):153-160.
37. Johnson D, Smith R. Outcome measurement in the ACL deficient knee—what's the score? *The Knee.* 2001;8:51-57.
38. Plisky P, Rauh M, Kaminski T, Underwood F. Star excursion balance test as a predictor of lower extremity injury in high school basketball players. *J Orthop Sports Phys Ther.* 2006;36(12):911-919.
39. Padua DA, Marshall SW, Boling MC, et al. The Landing Error Scoring System (LESS) is a valid and reliable clinical assessment tool of jump-landing biomechanics: the JUMP-ACL study. *Am J Sports Med.* 2009;37(10):1996-2002.
40. Gustavsson A, Neeter C, Thomeé P, et al. A test battery for evaluating hop performance in patients with an ACL injury and patients who have undergone ACL reconstruction. *Knee Surg Sports Traum Arthrosc.* 2006;14(8):778-788.

34

don't forget the
thorax

Tracey Vincel, PT, MPhty, CBBA
Andrew Barr, DPT, MSc Spt Sci, BSc (Hons) Physio, CSCS

Editors Note: *I asked one of my favorite physical therapists and her colleague to write this chapter. Tracey represents just what I want in therapists with whom we work—(1) a keen understanding of the core principles, (2) judicial creativity within the framework of the concepts, plus (3) a flexibility to work with the injury-specific approaches.*

Our rehabilitation principles break many old tenets of physical therapy while getting most patients/players speedily back to full performance. For example, most postoperative core muscle repair patients begin with pretty vigorous muscular activity on Day 0 or 1 postoperatively. The amount and type of activities depend on the specific injury. Activity differs drastically for a de-stabilizing injury vs a non-destabilizing one. Scar is usually our enemy, yet sometimes becomes a friend. Rest is almost always bad. One gigantic factor in the rehabilitation formulae is the relative proportions of hip vs core muscle involvement. Tracey's emphasis on the thorax blends with the important core principles. Read carefully how Tracey includes the back as part of "the thorax." Then look back at Chapters 5 and 6, and see that her definition fits so well with the rest of our characterization of the core. Tracey uses her own lingo and defines her terms well, which makes the chapter practical to follow. Okay, it is time to keep on our physical therapy hats and roll up our work sleeves. Let's try practicing physical therapy the way Tracey and Andy do it.

Variety is the spice of lithe.

—The chapter authors.

No matter how you understand the terms *athleticism, agility,* or *beautiful movement*, each requires the body to assume postures and move freely in and out of them without pain or stress on the joints or soft tissues. To perform a specific posture or movement, the mind and body have endless possibilities. An optimally functioning central nervous system chooses the best movement strategy and moment for that specific task. Life—and lithe—can be beautiful. If only life were always perfect…

It's time to burst that bubble. Whenever pain or dysfunction is present, movement choices shrink. Variability lessens. Loss of variety causes muscle imbalances and strain on joints, perpetuating pain and pathology.

In other words, pain limits our agility—our "litheness" (our dreadful play-on-words again). Bad habits and/or injury exaggerate the defects and reduce the movement options further, forcing us into suboptimal movement choices, a process we call *compensation*. Then compensation leads to injury and more injury.

In sports and everyday life, we rely on specific movements to accomplish our tasks. Naturally, we would love to accomplish those tasks in as strong and easy a way as possible. The movements that we seek vary from one person to another. The important movements vary, depending on the specific tasks we want to accomplish, the sport or position we play, plus our own physical or mental limitations and advantages.

Let's start with a simple story to illustrate how dysfunctional movement can easily be restored to optimal movement when you take the time to do a detailed evaluation. We then introduce some of our physical therapy terminology to help you understand how we communicate this.

JEAN-MICHEL THE ICE HOCKEY WARRIOR

Consider Jean-Michel, the archetypal 2-nights-a-week recreational hockey player: "My life's passion is hockey. Unfortunately, I've always had groin injuries. My first was in high school, I had one every season after that, one side then the other. I keep my groin muscles strong and stretch religiously…as soon as I get back to full play, my groin gets me again. We are talking 8 or 9 times just in high school and college. I took a couple of years off after college and just joined a hockey league at Chelsea Piers. Argh, I pulled my right groin again last night!" So JM comes to us, expecting a cure.

As physical therapists, with a specialty in analyzing movement, we did our thing. We looked at his whole body and how it moved, with a keen eye for dysfunction, a driver for his recurring groin issues. We looked at the kinetic chain, compensatory patterns, load analysis, specifically looking at what happened as he transferred his weight to his right leg. Of course, we concentrated on movements that mimic hockey, although we were limited by the non-ice, wood surface of our physical therapy clinic.

He did something consistently as he went through certain routines, postures, and steps. As JM transferred his weight onto his right leg, there was an obvious translation of his rib cage to the left, affecting the position of his center of mass over his feet.

He was on the hard surface inside our studio, and we wondered if this rib cage shift would also occur while on skates. We decided to observe him the next day on the ice.

Sure enough, on skates he not only displayed the same rib cage movement, but also with each stride, that movement became exaggerated. Did this rib cage shift have anything to do with his groin pain? The next week, we had JM go through some more weight transfer drills in our studio. There became no doubt that the transfer of weight to his right triggered his pain and that this shifting movement had something to do with it.

Then came the "eureka" moment. We saw that with each weight transfer, he was, in our lingo, "translating his fourth thoracic ring." He basically was losing his center—his core balance. He was shifting his center of mass from the midline to the left, trying to recruit additional muscles to power his right side as he shifted direction. This was affecting his entire kinetic chain, causing nonsequential muscle activation and altering loading patterns down the chain. Specifically, Jean-Michel's left thoracic translation was keeping him from firing his right gluteus medius and maximus muscles. The compensatory pelvic rotation created a false axis for his right hip. The natural protectors of his hip—the pectineus, adductor longus, and adductor brevis—were overfiring in order to brace the hip. The result was a no-brainer—right groin pain! In our minds, his thorax was the culprit. It was driving his groin pain.

The rest of the story: We addressed the thoracic movement disorder and returned Jean-Michel to hockey. He has been pain-free for over 2 years…another cure.

So, what the heck are we talking about? What are these things: the center, core balance, thoracic ring, kinetic chain alteration, etc?

First, let's first look at the way things have been (and to a large extent still are). And then, let's look at the way we think they should be.

The greatest obstacle to discovery is not ignorance—it is the illusion of knowledge.
—Daniel Boorstin, former US Congress Librarian.

THE WAY THINGS CONTINUE (TO A LARGE DEGREE)

Frank, a 44-year-old lawyer from Charlottesville, Virginia, comes into the office with 9 months of pain in the left groin, abdomen, chest, and buttock that has now spread to the other side. Frank played lacrosse at the University of Virginia and by his admission "let myself go" for years after college. He occasionally jogged and played golf and paddle tennis. Work and family had higher priorities than staying in shape. "So I tried P90X."

Now take a step back from Frank. Think of what the 21st century advertising culture has added to our 2 AM television watching: Cross-fit, Insanity, spin, boot camps, Ab Rail, Bowflex, Chair Fitness, Total Gym, iGallop, Zumba, the 20-Minute Work-out, and, of course, Suzanne Somers's Thighmaster, and Shake Weight. Wee-hour TV watching has added a whole new level of total confusion to the core. Some of these "training" techniques are hilarious. Add all these new training techniques to the yoga, Pilates, and P90X revolutions and what do you get? Well, if it is not total madness, consider the following.

Through subliminal thought, these late-night ads might (hopefully not) bring the following **wrong** "core training principles" to our minds*:

- Ab training is paramount.
- It's all about pulling the belly button to the spine.
- Don't be bothered to get out of the chair to exercise.

In the past few years, the health and fitness industry, armed with our ever-expanding advertising culture, has also attempted to influence our understanding of the "core," packaging and branding equipment to deliver the aesthetic and perceived performance improvements that the public "need." There is a lack in clarity in the concepts and the communication between professionals and athletes, and a disconnection between sports medicine and health and performance circles regarding the best methods of delivering core stability programs.

Okay, let's get back to Frank. All Frank did was what most of us are prone to do. A former athlete, Frank decided he needed to get back into shape. He chose one of the more popular programs, which really does have some excellent aspects to it. Only it turned out that Frank wasn't ready for the immediate vigor of the program. Within days of joining the program, Frank ripped off his rectus abdominis, pectineus, and a portion of his iliopsoas. He was compensating like mad through, among other structures, his thoracic rings. He ended up requiring surgery to correct the core instability and then several months of core rehabilitation with special attention to the thorax. Believe it or not, he is now using a routine similar to P90X, only after a 2-month ramp-up.

Let's use a fitness analogy and take a step back. Our main point is not to knock all the fitness programs on late-night television. Our issue is with the misleading information that the programs might convey, which is potentially dangerous. In this chapter we want to emphasize that the development of core stability and strength should form part of any rehabilitative or preventative training program, but this goes beyond simple abdominal crunches and requires consideration of the transfer of load through the entire body in 3 planes of motion and in low- and high-load conditions.

Two Old Medical/Physical Therapy Myths That Just Won't Go Away*

Myth 1: Core Bracing Is Good for Low Back Pain

It is commonplace for "abdominal bracing" exercises to be prescribed for low back, pelvic, and hip pain. Unfortunately, many of these people do not feel better, and sometimes get worse with these general "core bracing" type exercises. Is it possible that this training is making people stiffer? Has the body adapted to pain by tensing superficial muscle as a protection strategy for low-load activity? Is it possible that we are only feeding into this poor motor control strategy when we prescribe planks and other similar high-load "core stabilization" exercises when the underlying issues have not been addressed?

---

*Keep in mind these principles are the wrong ones.

Truth

When rigid bracing strategies are adapted, movement options are lost, and the remaining options do not allow adaption for the loads or the tasks at hand. Bracing is not the right strategy. With that strategy, injured patients cannot utilize the deeper stabilizing and other muscles. Timing and activation get worse. Overall core function is less efficient. In the next sections, we shall talk more about bracing and rigidity and the superficial and deep muscles.

Myth 2: The Thoracic Spine Is Stable and Stiff

For years, we have regarded the thorax mainly as the stiff component of the overall spine[1-4]; therefore, not of too much use in rehabilitation and performance training.

Truth

The above could not be further from the truth. The thoracic spine is a part of an enormous, 3-dimensional unit integrated with the ribs and abdomen via huge and hopefully strong attachments. This unit is not "stiff" as generally regarded. Instead, it is dynamic, integrating, and shock-absorbing.[4]

One should think of this whole unit like a giant Original Slinky, capable of important changes in shape and character that we may use to implement core movement strategies. With this concept, we physical therapists have a lot to work with. The thorax is not a stiff box; it is a lively Slinky with 10 or so rings. It can create (drive) or correct proximal or distal problems.[5-7] We should not be addressing the thoracic spine in isolation; instead, we should be considering its influence on the body above (the neck) and the body below (pelvis, lumbar spine, and hip; Figure 34-1).

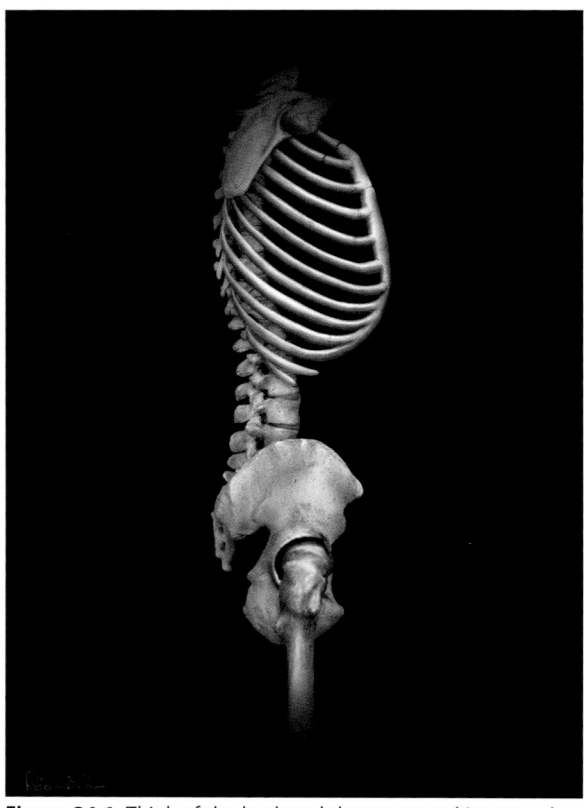

Figure 34-1. Think of the back and thorax as working together, and also connected to the pelvis.

If you always do what you have always done, you will always get what you always got.

—Henry Ford, the first automaker.

THE WAY THINGS SHOULD BE

We shall now teach you new lingo. As you read this new nomenclature with the associated assessment and treatment modalities, keep Jean-Michel the Ice Hockey Warrior in mind. A detailed assessment permitted us to identify a dysfunctional movement pattern plus a thoracic "driver." With that, we restored optimal neuromuscular control and took away his groin pain.

We provide some detail here to show therapists how we did this, and, hopefully, to use these concepts on their own clients.

New Nomenclature

- **Kinetic chain:** Movement that is created through an assembly of body segments connected by joints. This system efficiently distributes forces created during motion through the entire body. For example, movement at the ankle is linked to movement at the knee, which is linked to movement at the hip, through the pelvis and spine, thorax, and so on. Joints should not be viewed in isolation as dysfunction in one joint may be causing pain in another through poor mechanical function of the kinetic chain.
- **Failed load transfer:** Occurs when the body transfers load (ie, center of mass over the base of support) and there is (1) nonoptimal alignment, (2) nonoptimal biomechanics, or (3) nonoptimal control.[5,6]
- **Compensatory patterns:** Movement within the kinetic chain that is nonoptimal. For example, if one joint in the kinetic chain is restricted, then another joint may show a compensatory pattern by moving excessively.
- **Driver:** The area of failed load transfer in the body that happens first in time and space and, when corrected (with optimal alignment and/or control), corrects all other areas of failed load transfer occurring in the body for that functional movement.[8]
- **Nonsequential muscle activation:** A delay in the timing of the deeper stabilizing muscle activation in anticipation to joint motion. This delay increases the shearing forces through the joint and produces suboptimal alignment by an overpull from the more superficial mobilizing muscles.
- **False axis:** A joint that creates motion in suboptimal alignment, due to the overpull from a superficial mobilizing muscle.
- **Core balance:** The optimal function of the 3-layer muscular system of the core. This includes sequential activation of the local stabilizer muscles and ideal recruitment patterns of the global stabilizer and global mover muscles.
- **An Integrated Approach to the Thorax:** An assessment and treatment approach developed by LJ Lee and Diane Lee[4,5,8] that incorporates current research on the thorax and considers the thorax as a series of stacked rings and how they interact and function as a complete circle relative to the neck, shoulder girdle, and pelvis. It proposes multiple mechanisms for how the thorax can drive pain and dysfunction in other regions of the body.[9,10]
- **Thoracic ring:** Refers to the true functional unit of the thorax, the "ring" (Figures 34-2 amd 34-3).[4,5-8] The ring can be defined as 2 ribs of the same number plus the 2 vertebrae to which the ribs attach and all the joints that connect them (eg, ring = vertebra [T4 and T5] + disc + 2 ribs [right and left fifth rib] + other small joints). There are 13 joints per typical ring, totalling 136 joints in the thorax.[10]

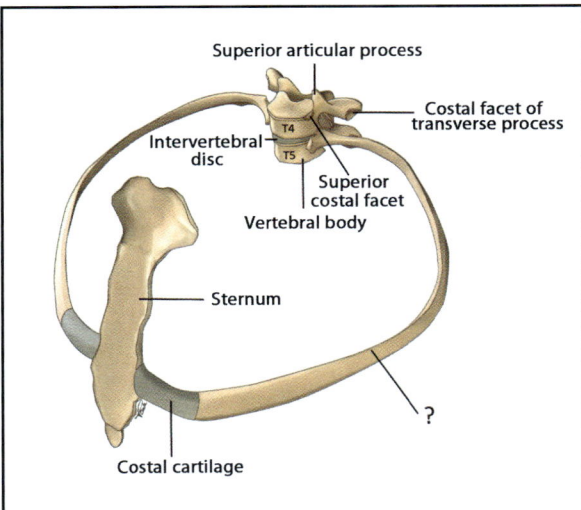

Figure 34-2. The concept of the thoracic ring. The vertebrae plus the ribs act as individual units. (© LJ Lee Physiotherapist Corp. Used with permission from Dr. Linda-Joy Lee.)

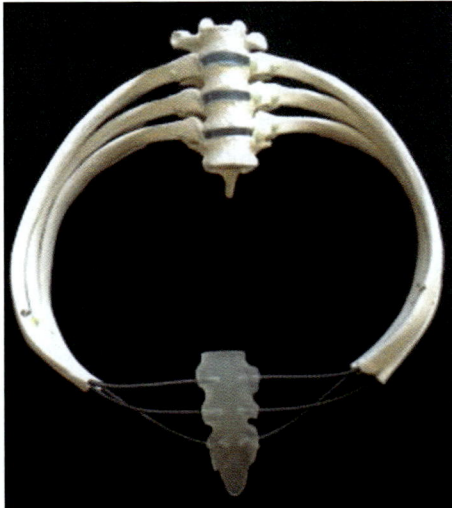

Figure 34-3. Model of a thoracic ring that we use in the clinic.

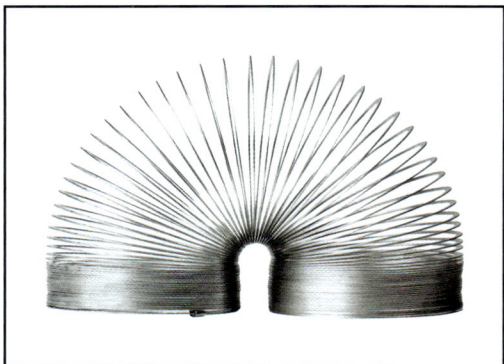

Figure 34-4. A Slinky toy.

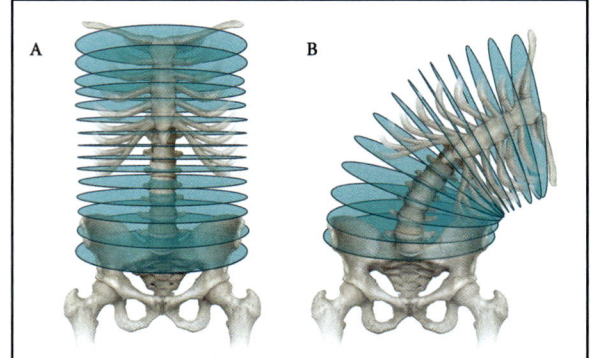

Figure 34-5. Putting the Slinky concept inside the body. (A) Straight-on view. The spine with its "rib planes" acting as separate units. The concept extends inferiorly into the pelvis. (B) The "Slinky" bends in many dimensions. "Bendability" diminishes as you go lower and lower.

- **Thoracic Slinky** (Figures 34-4 and 34-5): An analogy for the series of stacked rings or ribs that make up the thorax.
- **Optimum load transfer strategies for the trunk**[5,8]: Refers to several maneuvers that:
  ◊ Balance stability and joint mobility of all joints for each task; joint motion is controlled without rigidity and in order to maintain sufficient intra-abdominal pressure, balanced between intrathoracic and intracranial pressure
  ◊ Allow the rib cage to expand for optimal respiration
  ◊ Allow sufficient mobility (ie, the "give" in the system that dampens and reacts to perturbation)
  ◊ Create qualitative and quantitative features for functional and performance goals
  ◊ Affect a lot of systems when there is no optimal strategy
  ◊ Have choice (ie, different neuromuscular options for developing optimal strategies)
- **Optimum load transfer of the thorax**[5,8]: Refers to:
  ◊ Optimal lumbopelvic function
  ◊ The ability to attain neutral spinal alignment with the thorax and in relationship to the cervical and lumbosacral curves
  ◊ The ability to consciously recruit and maintain a tonic, isolated contraction of the local stabilizers of the thorax to ensure segmental control of neutral zone
  ◊ The ability to maintain and control neutral spinal alignment during increased loading from the upper and lower extremities
  ◊ The ability to move in and out of neutral spinal alignment (flex, extend, rotate, and side bend) without segmental or rotational collapse
  ◊ The ability to maintain all the above plus perform functional, sport-specific movements

New Eyes on Thoracic and Back Anatomy

Except for respecting the vital organs it encloses, we often overlook the thorax. Consider its obvious importance with respect to the musculoskeletal core. Representing over half the vertebral column and 20% of the body's length, the thorax takes the brunt of transferring loads between the upper extremities and head and the lower body. Think of the stable base it provides for the shoulder and all its rotational movement and transmission of power and torque from the lower back and pelvis. It also is the attachment for the diaphragm—the center of our breath and a muscle that plays a critical role, along with the transversus abdominis, multifidus, and pelvic floor, in stabilizing our deepest core. Let's look at the thorax and back in a different way. Let's think of it as the same thing, or at least functionally as the same overall unit (Figure 34-6).

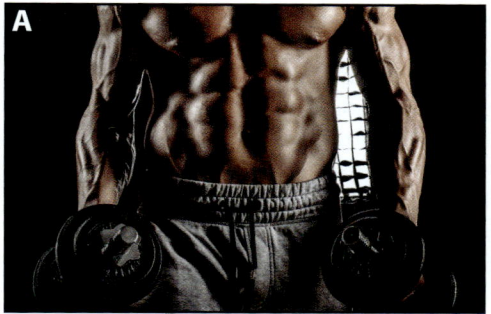 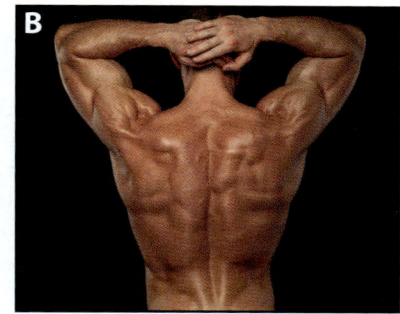

Figure 34-6. Think of the thorax in a much more inclusive way. Think about all the skeletal muscle in this region of the ribs and spine, both (A) "front" and (B) "back," as belonging to both the thorax and lumbosacral spine at the same time. From a functional standpoint, think of this region as performing like one unit.

Conceptually, regard the thorax as both a passive and an active system.

The passive thoracic system comprises the vertebral bodies, pelvic and hip bones, thorax, and connecting restraints. We divide this passive system into 4 regional segments[5,8]:

1. The vertebro-manubrium or upper thorax (T1-T2, 1st and 2nd ribs plus the manubrium)
2. The vertebro-sternum or middle thorax (T3-T7, 3rd through 7th rib plus the sternum)
3. The vertebro-chondrum or mid-lower thorax (T8-T10, 8th through 10th ribs)
4. The thoracolumbar region or low thorax (T11-T12, 11th, 12th, and, if present, 13th ribs)

The active thoracic system comprises smaller contractile muscle and noncontractile tissue enveloping the spine plus the bigger muscles. We divide the bigger thoracic core muscles into 3 groups[5,8,11,12]:

1. **Deep stabilizers:** The deep muscles closest to the spine; these provide a "stiffness" to the posture, as well as considerable sensory input to the spine. Examples—segmental thoracolumbar multifidi, superficial longissimi, diaphragm, pelvic floor muscles, and psoas.
2. **Global stabilizers:** The next deepest muscles; most of these can be thought to be involved with single vertebral body or regional segments and most important in the transverse plane. These create many interconnected slings complexly involved in trunk rotation and other movement. Physical therapists, yoga instructors, and other trainers utilize these muscles the most for optimizing posture and vertebral body alignment. Examples—internal and external obliques, superficial multifidi, medial quadratus lumborum, gluteus medius, and proximal adductors.
3. **Global movers:** The most superficial large muscles. These cross multiple vertebral levels are the most important in the longitudinal plane. These muscles "move" the vertebral joints or regions. Generation of joint motion, of course, occurs mainly in the sagittal plane. Examples—rectus abdominis, erector spinae, quadratus lumborum, latissimus dorsi, superficial lateral gluteus maximus, adductor longus, adductor magnus, and tensor fascia lata.

This is what happens when an unstoppable force meets an immovable object.

—The Joker, talking about Batman in *The Dark Knight*.

New Eyes on Thoracic Biomechanics

When unstoppable smart people see things in new light, concepts emerge that move the previously immovable. For years, the thorax was a spoiled rich kid, stiff and minimally controllable. Therapists regarded the thorax as just the thoracic spine or just the ribs, important in its proximity to important structures but fixed in their intrinsic positions. The new concept of the musculoskeletal core has changed all that. Think about the professional soccer goalie making a save on a penalty kick to his/her right, the sleek, coordinated movement (Figure 34-7).

Not only does the goalie push off on his/her right, the goalie lifts his/her thoracic spine to the left with strength and grace. Think of the ease of the Slinky walking down the stairs. Yoga masters have had some sense of this rather uniform, smooth movement for years (eg, the crescent moon posture). Think of the converse that can also happen, the disjointed movements when you frantically remember you must run back to the house to get your keys, the sudden reaction of an American football defensive back who impulsively adjusts to being out of position. Good or bad, the thorax comes into great play every day. It literally plays a pivotal role in much of what we do…hence, the concept of the thoracic ring.

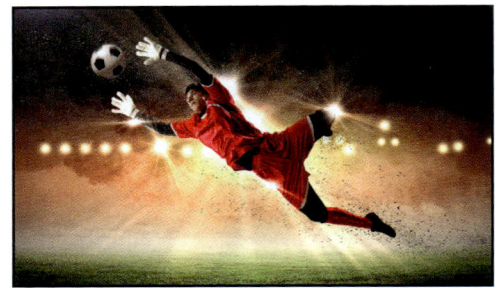

Figure 34-7.

The concept is simple. The thorax is not just the spine, it is a series of parallel rings connected by a variety of attachments that allows it to do amazing things. Transverse planes connecting the vertebral bodies to the ribs and sternum and connecting soft tissue comprise each ring. It is as simple as that. One can then make the concept as complicated as one may seek. Therefore, the true functional unit of the thorax is the ring. Each ring may be expressed mathematically as:

ring = 2 vertebral bodies + disc + 2 ribs

One can get a lot more complicated: 13 articulations per ring equaling 136 joints in the thorax. The articulations make the rings mobile.

The concept is pretty useful though, if you keep it simple.

Each vertebra joins the vertebra above or below via articular facets and strong radiate ligaments, creating leverage that move the vertebral pairs. Most of the time there are 12 ribs and corresponding bodies, so since the top and bottom vertebrae have to join to something, there are just 10 rings.

No doubt, the overall system is complex, reminding us to remember that the utility of a concept depends on its simplicity. Consider one of Dr. Lee's original descriptions: "The capacity for movement within and between the segments of the thorax, along with the requirements for control of upright posture and respiration, requires complex coordination of muscle activity by the central nervous system to meet the demands of stability and movement."[8,9] No doubt, the overall system reaches into fourth and fifth dimensions.

In other words, we can get a lot deeper into this point, but won't. Here are a few examples of how discussions of this thoracic ring concept get complex:
- With thoracic perturbations in the sagittal (flexion/extension) plane, the rings recruit the deep multifidus and superficial longissimus to control challenges to stability.[13,14]
- When challenges to stability occur in the transverse plane, the central nervous system controls the deep multifidus and superficial longissimus differentially.[13,14]
- Differential control of these 2 layers of thoracic paraspinal muscles becomes apparent only in the ring with the greatest movement.[15]

We shall keep things relatively simple. Loss of optimal neuromuscular control between the thoracic rings may have consequences throughout the body. Consequent nonoptimal loading may derive from conditions as diverse as hip impingement, arthritis and groin pain, pelvic and back pain, incontinence, Achilles tendinopathy, patellofemoral pain, or shoulder impingement. Radical believers in the thoracic ring approach get very specific with their assessment.[4,9,16,17] At this point, let's keep the concept cookbook simple because the thorax does link the upper body to the rest of the core in a clear and simple way.

Practical Know-How

The following represents some of our assessment methods. The tests themselves convert easily into therapy.

Breathing

One of the central roles of the thorax is, of course, breathing. Breathing truly plays an important role in core stability.

The diaphragm is the most efficient respiratory muscle. During inspiration, the diaphragm descends and pulls the central tendon inferiorly through a fixed set of the twelfth ribs and the L1-L3 verterbrae. These "lower ribs" rotate backward, creating an outward and backward expansion of the rib cage. Further inspiration rotates the "upper ribs" backward, further increasing the front to back dimension of the thorax. Exhalation should occur passively as the diaphragm relaxes.[5]

When motion of the lower ribs is limited by overactivation of the global system (obliques abdominals and erector spinae), outward expansion of the thorax becomes restricted, and 2 nonoptimal breathing patterns are common:

1. Abdominal bulging (belly breathing)
2. Apical upper rib breathing

Poor breathing patterns lead to inefficient core stabilization strategies. Research indicates that spinal stiffness changes through the respiratory cycle.[18,19] Stiffness increases during both inspiratory and exhalation efforts, more so with exhalation. This is consistent with the natural behavior to expire when performing demanding tasks such as lifting. This research also argues that stiffness is greater with the glottis open and trunk muscle contraction maintained; therefore, it might be beneficial to recommend this action when attempting procedures requiring greater spinal stability.[5,18,19]

Spine Core Stability

Neutral Zone Test[20,21]

Everybody has what we call "neutral zones" for various parts of the body. These correspond to what anatomists call the *normal anatomic position*. Normal anatomic positions are species-specific and account for why we walk on 2, rather than 4, legs. Of course, the human derives its set of neutral zones from cavepersons. We can find neutral zones for each part of our trunk, and the most important neutral zones apply to the lumbar, thoracic, and cervical spine curvature. For example, the neutral zone for the lumbar spine is defined by the range between maximal and minimal lordosis. One first arches the back as much as possible, and then flattens it. The resultant range is called the *lumbar neutral zone*. The same maneuvers repeat themselves to define the *thoracic neutral zone*.

The neutral zone test is the ability to maintain the spine's neutral zone when challenged by varying loads. Everyone has his/her limits. The limits may be used as a measure of the athlete's level of core stability. If the core cannot be somewhat kept in the neutral zone when challenged, the cause is a lack of either awareness or core muscle strength. For example, core control of the thoracic spine can be challenged by trying to maintain thoracic neutral zone when the arms are extended. Uncontrolled flexion of the spine with minimal perturbation reflects poor core stability. Therefore, positive tests indicate passive structures must be under continual strain in order for the person to have to bend over from minimal perturbation (Figure 34-8).

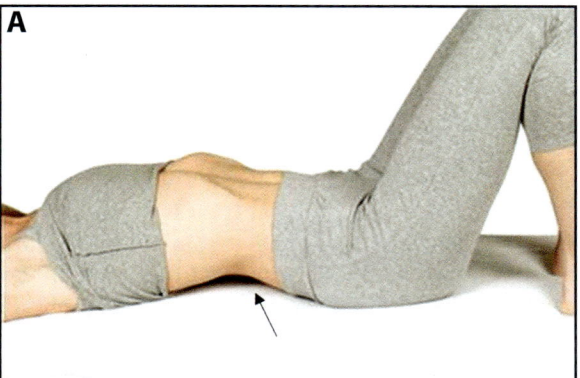 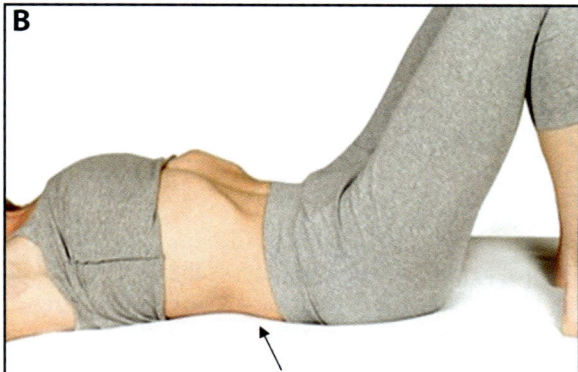

Figure 34-8. Abdominal and paraspinal (A) contraction and (B) relaxation change the spinal angle (arrows).

Dissociative Neutral Zone Test[11,12]

This describes testing the neutral zones by passively or actively moving upper or lower extremity joints. Abnormalities are called *dissociative movements*. One may train core stability by repeated introductions of movements aimed to dissociate. We used both types of neutral zone tests as therapy for Jean-Michel, our recreational "Ice Hockey Warrior." We increased the intensity of the attempted perturbations systematically.

Active Straight Leg Raise Test[22]

A supine patient lifts his/her straight leg a few inches off the table, then repeats the maneuver on the other side, while the therapist observes his/her strategy used to stabilize at the thorax, low back, and pelvis. The patient then states the leg that feels heavier, or harder to lift, particularly on initiation of the movement. Once one figures out which leg feels heavier (the "positive" leg), then various passive pelvic compressions or decompressions are added as the patient repeats the tests. The aim is to force the thorax into new positions that counter the defect.

Compressions and Decompressions With the Straight Leg Raise Test[8,22]

Compressions are just what you might guess they are—manual applications of gentle force that externally simulate muscular actions. They are used to either stabilize or destabilize different parts of the core. We apply them routinely to the following:

- Anterior pelvis (anterior to posterior ischial spines, ie, ASIS to ASIS): Working with the lower fibers of the transversus abdominis alongside other structures
- Anterior pelvis at the level of the pubic symphysis: Aiming to reinforce the anterior pelvic floor
- Posterior pelvis (ie, PSIS to PSIS): Simulating the sacral multifidus
- Posterior pelvis (one ischial tuberosity to another): Forced simulating of the posterior pelvic floor muscles
- Alternate pelvis (or hemipelves): Simulating the anterior pelvic floor on one side and the posterior floor on the other

The pattern of compression that makes the leg easier to lift directs the therapist to prescribe exercises to train the muscles capable of producing the same compressive forces. It is also useful to cue on individual core muscles and identify whether contraction of one particular muscle makes the leg easier to lift.

If **none** of the compressive patterns improve the active straight leg raise or, alternately, make it heavier, the whole system may already be undergoing too much compression. It is not indicated at this time to do exercises that increase stability. The active straight leg raise should then be retested using thoracic decompressions.

Decompressions are aimed to decrease hyperactivity of the thoracic erector spinae muscles. The therapist tester places one hand under the back of the thorax to capture the hypertonic fascicle of longissimus, iliocostalis, or spinalis, and, at the same time, the other hand on the front of the thorax at the same level. The active straight leg raise is performed while the traction force is applied.[8]

If the active straight leg raise with decompression improves the ease of leg lift, then techniques of decompression are applied first, then again with compressions. This process helps us decide when core stability training should begin.

Thoracospinal Stability

Rib Cage Wiggle Test[8]

This maneuver tests what we call *thoracic rigidity*, a loss of separation of thoracic and abdominal muscular action. The therapist applies force on the lateral chest while the patient is supine (low-load test) or sitting (medium-load test). The therapist repeats the test systematically at different rings. The amount of lateral movement during small applications of force should be relatively equal. Loss of equality represents a "positive rib cage wiggle" and high rigidity, presumptively due to excessive superficial muscle activity. We then focus on techniques to reduce hypercompression by the superficial mobilizer muscles. We want to facilitate the deep stabilizers.

Seated Trunk Rotational Range of Motion Test[8]

Seated trunk rotational testing, as well as other tests of posture, helps the clinician to identify excessive compression from the myofascial system. We usually want to correct abnormalities of this sort, before initiating core stability programs. Again, we look for rigidity (ie, the loss of separation of muscular actions). With rigidity, the normal relaxation of the contralateral longissimus muscle is lost, preventing full rotational range of motion. The test is performed with the patient seated on a table and feet on the floor.

Deep Core Muscles

To test the deep core muscles, we attempt to isolate the contractions of individual muscles. Often, we place the patient in a side-lying, unloaded position with the spine in the neutral zone. We examine the client's cognitive capability to activate and sustain contraction of individually isolated muscles. Real-time ultrasonography may improve the accuracy of all of the below techniques.[8] Some examples are below.

Transversus Abdominis Test

- **Step 1:** Find the lumbar lordosis neutral zone.
- **Step 2:** Attempt to isolate activation of the transversus abdominis (ie, palpate the muscle directly while assessing maintenance of the neutral position).
- **Step 3:** Assess opposite side.
- **Negative test:** Easily assessed activation without pain or abnormal respiration 3 times in succession (with 15 seconds of activation followed by 15 seconds of relaxation), or what we call *easy activation*.
- **Positive test:** Any breath holding, bracing, or rigidity in any core muscle group, or even a perception of high contractile effort or bulge.

Segmental Deep Multifidus Test

- **Step 1:** Position the patient prone or side-lying with lumbar spine in the neutral zone.
- **Step 2:** Attempt an isolated activation of the multifidus muscle while the examiner palpates it in a relatively deep location just lateral to the spinous processes. Repeat at each level of the lumbar spine, creating a perception of bringing the vertebrae closer to each other. Keep the low back neutral throughout the test. Muscle activation in this location actually feels like "swelling" (ie, slight muscular enlargement). Assess each side independently, noting the side of recent pain.
- **Step 3:** Assess opposite side.
- **Negative test:** Easy activation as described for the transversus abdominis.
- **Positive test:** Any breath holding, bracing, or rigidity of the superficial multifidus, quadratus lumborum, or erector spinae, or even a perception of high effort.

Load Transfer Assessment

We look at how the body moves between postures (ie, how it transfers weight, or load), taking into account both the movement and ground reaction forces if applicable. We look for what area(s) fails first and the influence of corrections. We may be trying to turn patients into rockets, but this is not rocket science. The patient tells us his/her meaningful tasks (ie, movements that are most important to him/her), as well as what feels "off." We identify where control is poor. Remember Jean-Michel. He had trouble transferring weight to his right lower extremity. Standing on one leg was his meaningful task, and the fourth thoracic ring was where he failed first, his load transfer failure. When the fourth thoracic ring was corrected, right hip alignment was restored, his glutes fired optimally, and his adductors relaxed.

After identifying the failure, we make judgments about spinal alignment and other alterations of biomechanics. We identify a specific site and direction of failed load transfer such as the pelvis, hip, lumbar segment, knee, or foot. With respect to the thorax, we look for nonoptimal ring biomechanics as well as relationships with both the lumbar and cervical spine. Maintenance of stability and control should be maintained while performing specific sport or functional movements.

All of this helps us become more specific in our therapy. We design therapy either to (1) strengthen certain muscle group alone or in tandem with complementary muscles, (2) eliminate sources of resistance or pain, or both (1) and (2). We make sure the patient is aware of our goals and agrees with them. We gradually introduce progressive loads, multiplane tasks, and carefully planned exercises to reduce fatigue or to work through fatigue.

In addition, we design various load strategies. The athlete needs to be efficient with trunk movements, and even this does not provide protection from seemingly innocuous sudden movement or posture changes. We teach the athletes to be "light on their feet." For example, the athlete does not need high-load strategies (eg, large muscle bracing) for low-load tasks. That creates unnecessary wear and tear and fatigue. Consequently, repetitive high performance suffers, low-load tasks get more difficult, and optimal power is lost for high-load tasks. One example is putting vs driving in golf. Why use bracing strategies for low-load putting? Another is uncontested dribbling in soccer vs making the long, cross-field pass. Efficiency leads to fewer abrupt changes in posture or movement and less error and injury. We believe that this sort of teaching not only preserves the global mover muscles, but also heightens central nervous system performance. Some examples are below.

Low-Load Test

We are looking at the control of the lower back and weightbearing hip during thoracic and opposite hip dissociative movements.

- **Step 1:** Find the lumbar neutral zone and stand on one leg.
- **Step 2:** Slowly flex the hip of the nonstanding leg up to 90 degrees. Hold the position, then flex and extend the upper back 15 degrees each way, then rotate the upper back 20 degrees each way.
- **Step 3:** Abduct the hip 30 degrees and then adduct to center.
- **Step 4:** Next, keeping the knee bent to 90 degrees, lower the leg so the thighs are parallel. Then extend the hip 5 degrees, and rotate the hip 20 degrees in each direction.
- **Step 5:** Repeat Steps 1 through 4 with the opposite leg.
- **Negative test:** Patient maintains the lumbar neutral zone and weightbearing hip control without any notable flexion, extension, or rotation.
- **Positive test:** Inability to maintain the lumbar neutral zone or prevent motion or other loss of alignment in the weightbearing hip.

High-Load Test (or Plank Transition Test; Figure 34-9)

- **Step 1:** Position the patient in a side plank with both the outside border of the bottom foot and the inside border of the top foot touching the floor.
- **Step 2:** Hold for 30 seconds (times may vary).
- **Step 3:** Transition into a front plank pivoting onto the toes and hold again for 30 seconds.
- **Step 4:** Transition into the opposite side and repeat. The upper and lower back must stay as one block.
- **Negative test:** The thoracolumbar region remains still (maintains its neutral zones). No flexion/extension, rotation, side bending, or other alignment loss during holds or transitions.
- **Positive test:** Undo movement or inability to maintain the neutral zone(s).

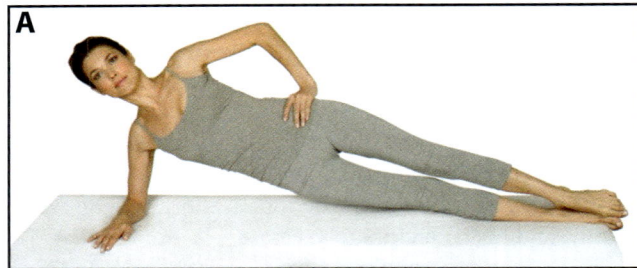 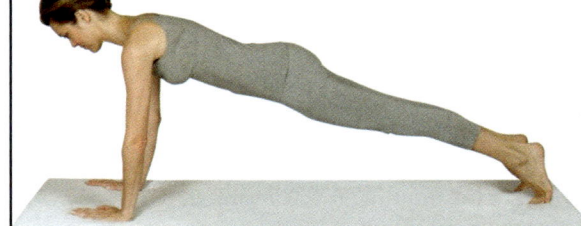

Figure 34-9. (A) Side plank and (B) front plank.

Jean-Michel's Core Assessment and Treatment Plan

JM's report illustrates how we summarized his core stability findings and planned therapy (Table 34-1). We have found this approach instructive and useful for communicating findings and progress.

Table 34-1
Jean-Michel's Report Card

Test Type	Test Detail	Result	Findings	Implication	Correction
Load transfer	Right foot standing	Positive	Fourth ring left translation, involves right sacroiliac joint and right anterior hip	Thoracic driver	Prioritize thoracic neuromuscular vector release
Core mobility-compression release	Seated trunk rotation	Positive	30% left rotation 75% right rotation	Excessive global muscle tone in thoracic erector spinae, external oblique, etc, causing rotation loss	Prioritize thoracic neuromuscular vector release
	Thoracic wiggle	Positive	Pathology involves rings 3/4 and 7/8	Intercostals causing compression by "gluing" rings	Prioritize thoracic neuromuscular vector release
Deep core	Transversus abdominis	Positive	Poor transversus abdominis isolation; 100% improvement by ring 7/8 correction	Thoracic "twist" causing neutrally mediated (T7–L1/2) abdominal wall dysfunction	Optimize ring 7/8 biomechanics before training transversus abdominis
Low-load transfer	Active straight leg raise and one leg bridge	Positive	Right active straight leg raise caused pelvic rotational control loss; ring 3/4 correction profoundly improved biomechanics and ease that maneuver	Poor rotational control with low threshold tasks	Optimize ring 3/4 biomechanics Paramount importance for retraining
	One leg standing/rotation	Positive	Rotational dissociation between hip and thorax	Poor rotational control at the hip with low threshold tasks	Retraining paramount—Test becomes the exercise
High-load strength-endurance movement	Ice hockey—square hop and hold test	Positive	Bilateral poor rotation left to right leg	Poor rotational control with high loads	Retraining paramount—Test becomes the exercise
Strength	Gmed/Gmax	Positive	Weakness throughout range	Consequent results	Improve strength after biomechanical correction

Summary

Okay, you made it through the fresh new concept, new lingo, and the many applicable tests.

Let us finish by saying simply that the thorax plays an integral, often overlooked core function in conjunction with the back. Understanding this requires new eyes, and throwing away the old concept of the thorax as just a block of immovable concrete. The musculoskeletal thoracic core is not just the ribs or the spine.

The new concept analogous to a huge Slinky brings into play the vertebral column, ribs, and sternum acting as a unit with multiple parallel rings. Muscles interlink the rings in fascinating ways that endow way more precision to the Slinky. The science is just developing. Nevertheless, the new concept proves helpful for diagnosis and treatment.

Selected Readings

Lee DG. *The Thorax—An Integrated Approach*. White Rock, British Columbia, Canada: Diane G. Lee Physiotherapist Corp; 2003.
  This is a "classic" physical therapy textbook on the thorax and its integration into the rest of the body.

Lee D. The thorax—an integrated approach. Learn With Diane Lee. https://learn.dianelee.ca/thorax-integrated-approach/. Accessed September 26, 2016.
  We now recognize the thorax as a primary contributor to multiple sites of pain in many conditions. Diane Lee's website has information about online and live classes on this subject.

Lee LB. Thoracic ring approach. Dr. Linda-Joy Lee International. https://ljlee.ca/teaching-models/the-thoracic-ring-approach/. Accessed September 26, 2016.
  The Thoracic Ring Approach challenges long-held beliefs with regard to function of the thoracic spine and rib cage. Linda-Joy Lee's website includes innovative assessment and treatment frameworks based on a broader understanding of how these areas are designed to function optimally in the context of whole body movement.

Lee LJ. Thoracic ring control: a missing link? *MPA In Touch Magazine*. 2013;4:13-16.
  If you want one article to sum up the concepts we just presented on the thorax, this is it.

References

1. Geelhoed MA, McGaugh J, Brewer PA, Murphy D. A new model to facilitate palpation of the level of the transverse processes of the thoracic spine. *J Orthop Sports Phys Ther*. 2006;36(11):876-881.
2. Lee DG. The thorax—an integrated approach. Learn With Diane Lee. https://learn.dianelee.ca/thorax-integrated-approach/. Accessed September 26, 2016.
3. Takeuchi T, Abumi K, Shono Y, Oda I, Kaneda K. Biomechanical role of the intervertebral disc and costovertebral joint in stability of the thoracic spine. A canine model study. *Spine (Phila Pa 1976)*. 1999;24(14):1414-1420.
4. Lee LJ. The essential role of the thorax in whole body function and the thoracic ring approach. Assessment and treatment videos. White Rock, British Columbia, Canada: Linda-Joy Lee Physiotherapist Corp; 2012.
5. Lee LJ. Restoring force closure/motor control of the thorax. In: Lee DG, ed. *The Thorax—An Integrated Approach*. White Rock, British Columbia: Diane G. Lee Physiotherapist Corp; 2003.
6. Lee LJ. A clinical test for failed load transfer in the upper quadrant: how to direct treatment decisions for the thoracic spine, cervical spine, and shoulder complex. Proceedings of the 2005 Orthopaedic Symposium of the Canadian Physiotherapy Association; London, Ontario, Canada; 2005.
7. Lee LJ, Chang AT, Coppieters MW, Hodges PW. Changes in sitting posture induce multiplanar changes in chest wall shape and motion with breathing. *Respir Physiol Neurobiol*. 2010;170(3):236-245.
8. Lee LJ. Discover Physio Series NYC. 2012 course notes.
9. Lee LJ. Thoracic ring control: a missing link? *MPA In Touch Magazine*. 2013;4:13-16.
10. Standring S. *Gray's Anatomy: The Anatomical Basis of Clinical Practice*. 40th ed. Edinburgh, Scotland: Churchill Livingstone; 2008.
11. Comerford MJ, Mottram SL. Functional stability retraining: principles and strategies for managing mechanical dysfunction. *Man Ther*. 2001;6(1):33-14.
12. Comerford MJ, Mottram SL. Movement and stability dysfunction: contemporary developments. *Man Ther*. 2001;6(1):15-26.
13. Lee LJ, Coppieters MW, Hodges PW. Differential activation of the thoracic multifidus and longissimus thoracis during trunk rotation. *Spine*. 2005;30:870-876.
14. Lee, LJ, Coppieters MW, Hodges PW. En bloc control of deep and superficial thoracic muscles in sagittal loading and unloading of the trunk. *Gait & Posture*. 2011;33(4):588-593.

15. Lee LJ, Coppieters MW, Hodges PW. Anticipatory postural adjustments to arm movement reveal complex control of paraspinal muscles in the thorax. *J Electromyogr Kinesiol.* 2009;19(1):46-54.
16. Lee LJ. Motor control and kinematics of the thorax in pain-free function. PhD thesis, University of Queensland, Australia, 2013.
17. Lee LJ, Lee DG. An integrated multimodal approach to the thoracic spine and ribs. In: Magee DJ, Zachazewski JE, Quillen WS, eds. *Pathology and Intervention in Musculoskeletal Intervention.* St. Louis, MO: Elsevier; 2008.
18. Richardson CA, Jull GA, Hodges PW, Hides JA. *Therapeutic Exercise for Spinal Segmental Stabilization in Low Back Pain—Scientific Basis and Clinical Approach.* Edinburgh, Scotland: Churchill Livingstone; 1999.
19. Shirley D, Hodges P, Erikson AEM, Gandevia SC. Spinal stiffness changes throughout the respiratory cycle. *J Appl Physiol.* 2003;95:1467-1475.
20. Lee DG, Vleeming A. Management of pelvic joint pain and dysfunction. In: Boyling JD, Jull GA, eds. *Grieve's Modern Manual Therapy.* 3rd ed. Edinburgh, Scotland: Elsevier.
21. Panjabi MM. The stabilizing system of the spine. I: function, dysfunction, adaptation and enhancement. Part 11. Neutral zone and instability hypothesis. *J Spinal Disord.* 1992;5(4):383.
22. Lee D. *The Pelvic Girdle: An Integration of Clinical Expertise and Research.* 4th ed. Edinburgh, Scotland: Churchill Livingstone; 2011.

35

the yin and yang of yoga

Biz Magarity, MBA, C-IAYT, 500 E-RYT

Editor's Note: *At the Vincera Institute, we incorporate yoga into many core rehabilitation programs. After hip or core muscle surgery, we often begin a judiciously designed set of yoga postures into the overall rehabilitation on Day 1 postoperatively. We intend for the postures to continue well past the final rehabilitation phase.*

The problem with promoting our approach comes from the wise statement associated with Bikram Yoga, synthesized from traditional hatha yoga *techniques: "There is yoga, and, then, there is yoga."*

The statement is so true. On researching the subject, we found way over 100 different popular disciplines. Common to all the disciplines that we researched were postures that seemed dangerous to many people's hips. Therefore, the athletic trainers, physical therapists, and yogini at Vincera collaborated and removed the universally dangerous postures from the routines. In point of fact, certain postures are safe for certain hip morphologies and dangerous for others. So, the best-fit postures, in fact, vary from one person to another.

The bottom line is that yoga can create great benefit. On the other hand, it can also, often subtly, cause substantial harm.

I asked our super-smart, lead yoga instructor, Biz Magarity, to provide comments on yoga and the core, for both the short and long terms.

Modern Yoga—A Contrast From the Early Days (Figure 35-1)

Modern yoga looks dramatically different from its origins. It has become a booming industry since it journeyed into the West in the mid-19th century. According to the *2016 Yoga in America Study*, the present-day count of 36 million US yoga practitioners represents a doubling in the past 4 years. The perception that modern yoga is primarily for young women is changing. More women (72%) continue to practice yoga, but the male proportion of practitioners is also nearly doubling. Plus, many older people are getting into it. The over-50 demographic is now only 5 percentage points behind the 30-to-49-year-old participation rate. The new segments of practitioners are contributing to the thriving niche economy, with about $16 billion dollars spent on yoga clothing, equipment, classes, and accessories just last year (Figure 35-2).[1]

Contrast this with the way yoga used to look. Yoga has been around since the 5th or 6th century BC (Figure 35-3). It started in pre-Vedic India and has roots in all Indian antiquity, Buddhism, Macedonia, and even China. The earliest yoga practices were mentioned in the Rigveda, which dates back to the 4th millennium BC. "Classical" yoga dates from 200 BC to the 5th century AD and Patanjali's writings called the *Yoga Sutras*.[2] Post-classical yoga brought a variety of different schools of yoga and a stronger focus on "unlocking" the body's hidden potential. Early yoga was male-dominated. Since the post-classical era began, pelvic core muscles and hips have been integral parts of yoga. Physical postures developed that allowed practitioners to sit comfortably for long periods of meditation or pranayama (breath and energetic practices). Yogi (male masters) were sustained by a quest to "transcend" the physical world and enter a higher level of consciousness. Yogini (female masters) came along a lot later.

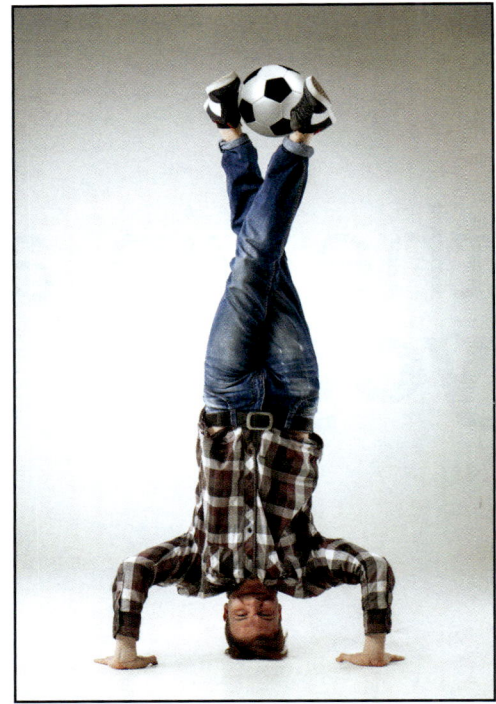

Figure 35-1.

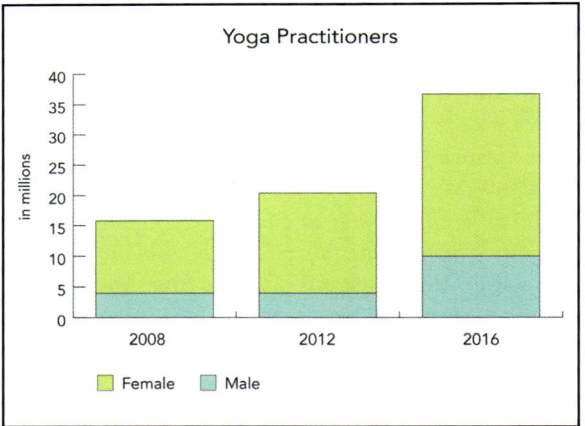

Figure 35-2. US yoga practitioner growth 2008-2016. (Data from the 2016 Yoga in America study.[1])

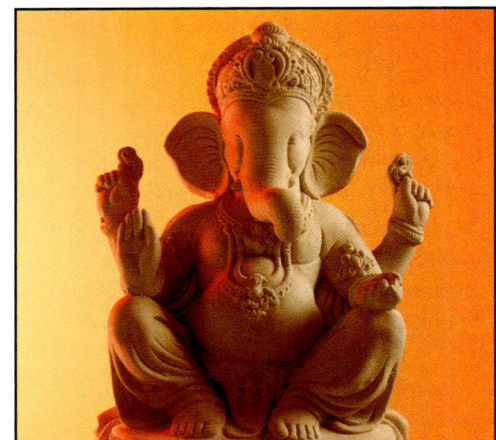

Figure 35-3. The elephant doing yoga in the statue represents the 5th century Hindu deity Ganesha, known as the "remover" of obstacles.

Now, we have designer yoga wear, self-proclaimed gurus on social media outlets, and gravity-defying, body-bending poses. We have "power" and "fitness" yoga. We have "hot" yoga, which usually refers to doing yoga in 100°F or so temperatures, but can apply also to hot, naked yoga. It may be easier now to find beer-tasting yoga than "enlightenment" yoga. A quick internet search shall easily reveal hundreds of different styles of yoga. One probably does not need to state that believers in ancient disciplines of yoga find themselves at odds with these American trends. Defenders of ancient ways say that yoga is now "all movement" and no "stillness." They go on with their critique and say that modern yoga has become more of a "distraction" than an "enlightener."

The conversations weighing the good and the bad of the modern movement have become more and more passionate within the yoga community. Blogs trigger disagreement and competition among the different schools and styles, which seems ironic considering that early yoga was all about peace and harmony. There is a yin and a yang to all this.

At least one good thing comes from all this controversy. So many varieties of yoga exist that no one discipline dominates the industry. The governing bodies of yoga cannot take sides. Therefore, would-be regulators remain loose and lenient. This leniency means that all new yoga disciplines or other new developments within the yoga world must remain "on the table"—to be accepted or rejected by anyone with access. This leniency strikes a sharp contrast with the medical world, where all new procedures, devices, or drugs must meet certain standards and pass Food and Drug Administration and/or other regulatory approvals. True regulatory agencies for yoga do not exist. Therefore, no bureaucracy can block someone from doing something new. Yoga approval remains purely a matter of popularity.

Of course, a bad side to that lack of regulation also exists.

A Blurring Definition

Defining *Yoga* has become super-complicated within the modern context and "noise" generated by the unregulated yoga market. "Yoga" comes from Sanskrit. Its root *yuj* or *yoke* means to unite or join, such as the harnessing of oxen. Many compound words in Sanskrit contain yoga, such as the medical term *chakrayoga*, which means applying a splint. In just about all modern traditions, the term yoga has come to mean "connecting" your inner self with a higher universal consciousness or spirit. Most everyone agrees that yoga involves more than just physical exercise: it has both meditative and spiritual parts.

The most recognizable component of yoga is the physical postures and practices, designed to "purify the body" and to create awareness and some level of control over the inner state. Other components of yoga include meditation, mantra, selfless service, devotion, and spiritual liberation. Less palatable in modern society, these latter pieces remain essential for a conscience-driven definition of yoga. They remain the hope to link modern yoga with science.

We still believe that advances in the physical sciences eventually unlock the profound mysteries of the obscure ancient practices. The common drive of all of those practices was, and still should be, to reverse our natural tendency to live primarily with an outward focus. By drawing our whole being inward, we will become more established within our "self," and more able to manage our own health and well-being.

The Benefits Include New Eyes

Yoga provides the tools and practices to develop a new set of eyes. A key principle is *svadyhaya*, meaning self-study. You first learn the whole subject of yoga: the postures, the breathing, and the meditation exercises. Then you study yourself within that framework. How did the posture affect your performance or mood? How did the breathing affect your sleep or ability to concentrate? How did the meditation affect your energy or ability to practice new postures? Did that heightened sense of awareness during the yoga practice translate to faster reaction times on the field?

Yoga should be empowering, and allow the practitioner to heighten his/her own intuition. Then the practitioner becomes the clinician. This can be a powerful set of tools for athletes or all who consider fitness an important parameter in their lives. Athletes are, in general, a group of people likely to become what we call "disembodied" at some point in their lives, on account of lifestyle or injuries. If someone has spent his/her entire life creating a physical specimen of a body and that has become the means to success and identity, then what happens when the perfect body no longer works properly? One can play through the pain by mentally detaching oneself from that injured part of the body. How many athletes do not recognize when they are really hurt, when pain is no longer just soreness? And then someone says, "You should have addressed this earlier." Yoga trains the awareness and intuition. The awareness and intuition muscles are the ones that tell the yoga practitioner/athlete to tell the coach, "I cannot play with this any longer."

As has been said before in this book, the urologist, gynecologist, gastroenterologist, and orthopedist all see the pelvis as particular parts or systems. Yoga also provides a more holistic or universal set of eyes. Yoga means "union" and encompasses all those systems, particularly the musculoskeletal, hormonal, circulatory, and respiratory ones. Yoga defines a "being" in terms of multiple layers, or koshas (Figure 35-4). Three layers are the physical, mental, and energetic bodies. Within the framework of yoga we look at the physical parts, as well as the thoughts, feelings, and energy and how all those things affect the body. A woman sees the integration of these different aspects at childbirth. And childbirth happens in the pelvis, the center of the core. Medicine and yoga practitioners need study this more scientifically. We see this as a huge argument for why the core should be considered a distinct and separate specialty.

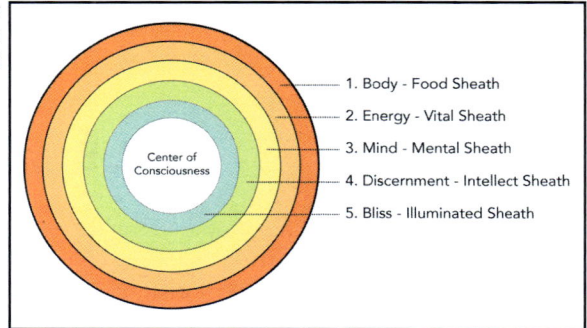

Figure 35-4. The kosha model represents a long-established yoga philosophy and a holistic approach to wellness. Postures, breathing, and meditation are the primary means of travel from the outer layers (1 to 3) into the inner layers (4 and 5), and, eventually, the inner consciousness.

CLINICAL PRACTICE EXAMPLES

"Deep" in Touch With the Universal Consciousness

A *Kriya* is a specific set of actions designed to get closer to a specific outcome. The intent is to cleanse or to remove something blocking the practitioner from "higher consciousness." Most Kriyas involve the core. Jala Basti, or JB, is an example of one such Kriya. In JB, a master practitioner squats in the river (nowadays, a tub of water) and inserts a bamboo shoot through the anus. The practitioner engages his/her pelvic floor muscles and lower abdominal muscles, and rhythmically tightens and loosens the sphincters; then sucks water up to the rectum and sigmoid colon, all the way up into the descending colon. An abdominal movement called *Nauli* swishes around the water. Finally, the practitioner expels the noxious mixture that had been keeping him/her grounded on the physical world. Then, Sh'bam…a new, higher consciousness! The practitioner becomes clean as a whistle, and this obstacle to higher consciousness has vanished.

Talk about an icebreaker for doing pelvic floor exercises.

The serious point is that we are just now coming to appreciate the value of various long-practiced postures and internal pelvic strength. As mentioned in earlier chapters, correct postures and Kegel maneuvers play important parts in core rehabilitation, performance, and everyday life. The right yoga disciplines enhance all this.

Yoga in Professional Baseball

Pat, a young Minor League Baseball player, incorporated yoga into his postoperative rehabilitation beginning the day after he had core muscle surgery. His team planned to add yoga to their training regimen, so he was eager to learn. Pat struggled through the first session, partly because of the recent surgery and partly because he had never done this before. The program included proprioception exercises, specific breath and physical movement combinations, and physical alignment cues. Pat got better throughout the week. More importantly, he began to feel confident in integrating his body, mind, and breathing rhythm into the practice. At the week's end, he commented that his body never felt so awake. The player would end up modifying his team's program, based on what he learned. His team won the triple-A championship, and Pat was brought up to the Majors at the end of the season. We yogini, of course, take full credit for Pat's and his team's successes.

With wide-open eyes and heightened awareness, the body wakes up. Yoga increases the connection and understanding of the individual for his/her own body. A radiologist may pinpoint details of an injury, the surgeon then may repair it, and afterward, the physical therapist rebuilds strength and coordination. Yoga provides the owner of that body with insight and confidence that modulates the body as he/she needs from that time forth. Yoga offers clues to "unlocking" habitual movement patterns that place the individual at risk for injury. The practice identifies and modulates those risky movement patterns to increase the chance to boost performance and avoid injury (Figure 35-5).

Yoga and World Championships

The 2014 Super Bowl champion Seattle Seahawks developed and integrated a yoga and meditation program in 2011.[3] The discipline emphasized core postures, breathing, and daily meditation. Some in the organization say this was a game-changer. According to the yoga instructors' explanation, they "replaced hard-ass apps with happiness apps and guided meditation." Yoga, plus, perhaps, a few other things, led the team to the world championship. The players were encouraged to focus inward, visualize success, and then quiet their minds through conscious breathing. The team's ethos became promotion of positivity and a "mature" mind. Several players taken in the draft prior to their Super Bowl year say they were selected on the combination of emotional maturity and physical promise. One player says that the world championship would not have happened without the yoga program. "We all felt less 'earth-bound' and 'soared' with more 'fluidity' and balance."

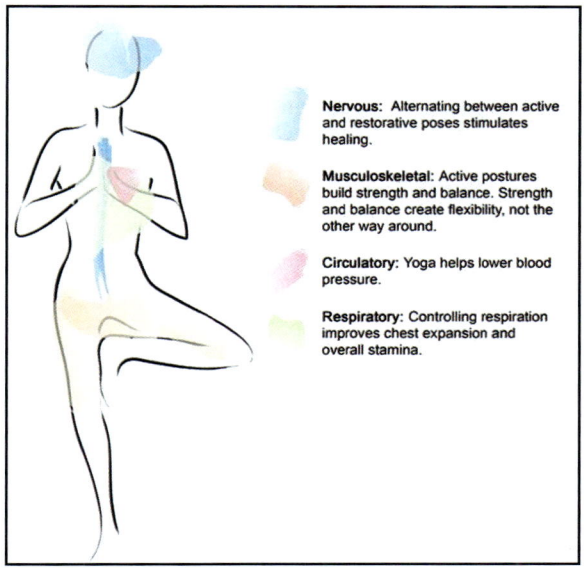

Figure 35-5. Yoga effects on 4 biological systems.

A Super Bowl ring isn't exactly "enlightenment," but it sure beats an unenlightened second place. We core yoga people, of course, again take full credit for all the successes.

That's one small step for man, one giant leap for mankind.

—Neil Armstrong, the first man on the moon.

Bandhas—Part of the Yoga Yang

A traditional yoga practice involves the use of *bandhas*, or body locks, that bridge the physical body and the energetic body. The first 2 bandhas, of course, are located at the pelvic floor and the lower abdomen. They are associated with Kegel exercises. The practitioner engages the pubococcygeal muscles, as if to lift the perineum up. Simultaneously, the transversus abdominals engage and draw the navel toward the spine. This posture tones the involved muscles and brings awareness and intuition to an otherwise oft-ignored part of the body. When practitioners appreciate the new awareness, they report increased stability and feeling "lighter" even in the more complicated poses (Figure 35-6).

Here's a more concrete example of the above mind-body-energy connection. If you are intentionally activating that musculature, you are bringing both your mind and body to one point of focus. Sustained engagement of the physical "locks" during breath retention brings a feeling of tremendous energy release, and delivers a deliberate aftershock to the nervous system that may be cleansing, calming, or energizing. The first lock associated with the pelvic floor is called *muladhara*, meaning root. It serves as a metaphor for the practitioner's intention to create unity between thought and action. The root of all action is thought. By binding the mind and body physically and energetically toward one focal point, the practitioner can act under heightened circumstances and perform more and more challenging tasks with decreasing effort. In other words, contracting your perineum is one small step toward breaking a bad habit, and toward exceeding expectations. It allows a giant leap forward and a Jedi-like focus and resilience against adversity.

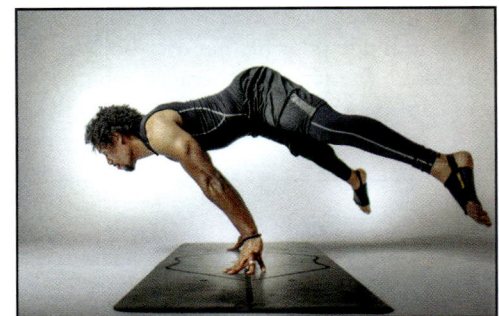

Figure 35-6. An arm balance posture. Total engagement of core musculature can make you feel "light" and as though you defy gravity. This is called "walking on the moon." The practitioner is yoga teacher Khalief Walker. (Reprinted with permission from Elliot Polinsky.)

An Anxious NFL Star Turns Core Muscle Yoga Advocate

A star NFL defensive end, let's call him Peter, expressed surprise that he was beginning yoga so soon after combined hip and core muscle surgery. In actuality, his NFL team was way ahead of the curve and had already begun incorporating yoga as part of routine training. Peter's previous experience with yoga permitted the creation of postures building on ones that he already knew. From the yoga, he quickly grew confidence, which allowed him to push safely through the normally tough rehab required by the complex surgery. This plan was all about increasing strength, mobility, and balance. Peter would have to break a sweat and test his strength before he got to the recovery and restorative postures. The team's yoga instructor was quite pleased that his strength was already so good when he returned. The transition from rehabilitation to performance yoga became easy. It was all about the vigorous rehabilitation yoga practice framework.

That's putting it mildly. Peter freaked out. This whole concept was new to him. The adrenaline rush was probably worth it. He recovered from combined surgery in record time and had 2 great NFL seasons to show for it. In retrospect, Peter commented: "I continue with the routine. Being a professional athlete recovering from such a severe core injury, yoga seemed essential. It brought back balance, core muscle strength, and elongation of the area. It played a huge role in my feeling comfortable on the field, as well as the confidence to perform the difficult task and demands of being an NFL professional athlete."

THE YIN OF YOGA

According to Chinese philosophy, yin and yang describe how opposite or contrary forces actually complement, interconnect, or "interdepend" within the natural world. *Yin* usually refers to the shady side and *yang* to the bright side. Consistent with that and as described in our introduction, yoga has both bright and shady sides.

The word ignorance, or *avidya*, comes up repeatedly in the yoga sutras of Patanjali. Ignorance may lead to all kinds of pain and suffering. Yogi believe that most physical pain and injury are unavoidable. Certain styles of yoga are inherently more risky than others, and some are not appropriate for every aspirant. A yoga teacher must be qualified enough to modify postures and exercises safely and effectively. Without any sort of regulation, no one can ensure that. Here are several specific things to mitigate chances of injury:

- **Avoid jumping right back into things.** As with other physical activities, injury happens too frequently after a sustained absence from an activity and then jumping back in too quickly. Even if you once were a great runner in high school, running a marathon after a 20-year hiatus poses a huge risk of injury. We recently saw a very fit man who had torn his rectus abdominis muscle while attempting an advanced backward bend in a yoga class that he had attended religiously for many years before he took a "sabbatical." He says he "knew" this might happen before he attempted the pose. The awareness muscles were asleep or he didn't listen to his intuition. That happens after a long hiatus.
- **Balance effort and appropriate movement.** This avoids overuse or repetitive motion injuries. Always ask if the yoga practice is deepening existing patterns of imbalance or misalignment? These injuries do not come from a single occurrence, but, instead, from a pattern of repeated small injuries. Consider the Warrior 3 posture, a standing balance pose. A very common error among instructors is to overemphasize the balance component of the posture. By so doing, one misses the opportunity to work the abdominals, adductors, and abductors muscles together, as a unit. A false alignment results that causes back, knee, or hip problems over time.

- **Avoid following en masse instructions.** The rise in yoga makes it available to anyone. Problems arise when classes are crowded or a teacher insists that everyone follow the exact same set of directions and attempt all the poses. A recent article[4] in *The New York Times* compared yoga-related hip injuries between men and women. In men, injuries, reportedly, occurred mostly by forcing relatively inflexible bodies into complicated poses. Injuries in women came from being too flexible and not having enough "compatible" strength to protect the joints. We recommend you seek out trusted yoga teachers for private instruction. Some of the recommendations in Chapter 32 for how to find the right physical therapist might also apply for the purpose of finding the right yoga instructor. The buzzword wizardry will be more ethereal, but the same 8 tips still hold. In the early days, yoga instruction was always one on one. We recommend that you don't deny yourself that "luxury" today. A private lesson from the right instructor is safer, and may be crucial for long-term yoga benefits.

Physical Injuries

A range of injuries occurs in yoga. These include thoracic outlet syndrome, aggravation of arthritis, acute disc rupture, retinal tears, and yoga foot drop.[5] The list is long. With the absence of regulation, it is impossible for yoga instructors to be aware of the many risks.

A Common and Scary Example of Yoga Yin

A high-level yoga practitioner does 2 passive hip maneuver poses—the wind-removing pose and then janushirasana. While doing the first pose, the instructor sits on his/her feet. Then, during the second pose, the instructor leans on her, "back-to-back." During the second "instructive" maneuver, the practitioner suddenly feels a subtle, deep, and slightly painful sensation. At first, she minimizes the new sensation. It seemed fleeting. When she gets up, it hurts a little to walk. The next day, she can hardly walk.

The worry here is that the instructor has been too active in her instruction, and forced the ball (femoral head) of the practitioner's hip to rub against the socket (acetabulum) and tore the practitioner's cartilage (labrum).

ONE CORE MUSCLE YOGA PRACTICE EXAMPLE

Below is an example of an exercise from our core muscle protocol. This is an active yoga posture that we use in the early stages of postsurgical recovery. Enough information is provided for you to attempt the posture on your own, as a teaser. We recommend you not try unless accompanied by a health professional or yoga instructor who has screened you for pre-existing medical conditions that might precipitate injury. This example represents one part of a total program. Do not expect a significant response from these exercises alone. Each exercise should be accompanied by feedback and dialogue between the practitioner and instructor. Each practice should stimulate an "awakening moment." (See Figure 35-7 and Video 1.)

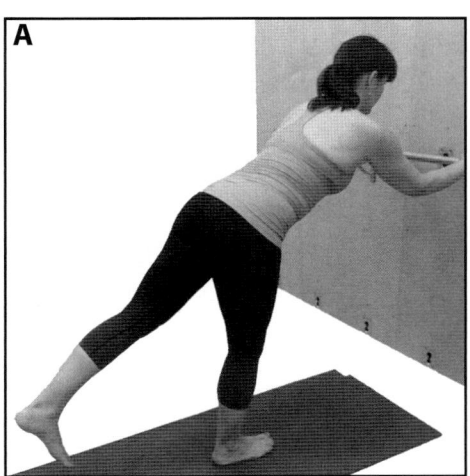
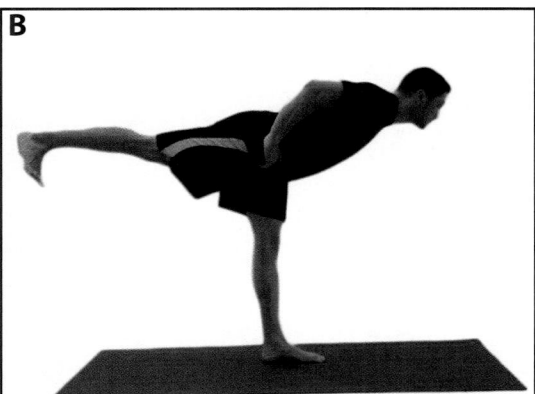

Figure 35-7. Warrior 3 posture for strengthening and postural awareness. (A) Postoperative day 1 after adductor repair. Note: (1) limitation of extension and (2) the athlete's hands on the wall. (B) Postoperative day 3. Note near full extension and hands near hips.

SAVASANA AND ONWARD TO A HIGHER CONSCIOUSNESS

Injury prevention is not the only reason to add a yoga practice to an athlete's rehabilitation or performance program. A generally accepted goal of yoga is relief from suffering and an opportunity to move to a higher state of consciousness. Marrying ancient concepts with modern science will get us there. Modern yoga classes should embrace the ancient tradition of saying "Namaste" as an acknowledgment of the higher state and divine light within each of us. If divine light is our aim, then the benefit, of course, goes way beyond the musculoskeletal system. A more aware and intuitive core permits a greater appreciation of Namaste.

SELECTED READINGS

Iyengar BKS. *Light on Yoga.* New York, NY: Shocken Books; 1979.
   This book has become a bible of Modern Yoga. A modern master provides a thorough overview of yoga theories and practices.
National Center for Complementary and Integrative Health. NCCIH 2016 strategic plan. https://nccih.nih.gov/about/strategic-plans/2016. Accessed September 17, 2016.
   This NIH-endorsed plan highlights and reviews the increased scientific understanding of yoga and other complementary arts, and the integration of these arts into more and more therapeutic settings.
International Association of Yoga Therapists. http://www.IAYT.org. Accessed September 17, 2016.
   This website, maintained by a self-governing body of yoga professionals, presents a great deal of information about the therapeutic applications of yoga

REFERENCES

1. 2016 yoga in America study conducted by Yoga Journal and Yoga Alliance. https://www.yogaalliance.org/Portals/0/2016%20Yoga%20in%20America%20Study%20RESULTS.pdf. Accessed June 3, 2016.
2. https://www.yogajournal.com/yoga-101/philosophy/yoga-sutras. Yoga Journal. Accessed September 14, 2018.
3. Roenick A. Lotus pose on two. ESPN. http://www.espn.com/nfl/story/_/id/9581925/seattle-seahawks-use-unusual-techniques-practice-espn-magazine. Published August 21, 2013. Accessed May 27, 2014.
4. Broad WJ. Women's flexibility is a liability (in yoga). *The New York Times.* http://www.nytimes.com/2013/11/03/sunday-review/womens-flexibility-is-a-liability-in-yoga.html?_r=0. Published November 2, 2013. Accessed May 27, 2014.
5. Broad WJ. How yoga can wreck your body. *The New York Times Magazine.* http://www.nytimes.com/2012/01/08/magazine/how-yoga-can-wreck-your-body.html?_r=0. Published January 5, 2012. Accessed May 27, 2014.

VIDEO

1. https://youtu.be/ClKHNfUmFQg

36

perspectives of **nonoperative** sports medicine physicians
(A) nonoperative interventions for the management of "**hip**" pain

Eugene Hong, MD, CAQSM, FAAFP
Sarah C. Hoffman, DO, FAAP, CAQSM

Editor's Note: *I asked my close colleague Gene Hong to write on the core from the perspective of a nonoperative physician, yet someone who actively participates in sports medicine. Gene is the head of sports medicine at Drexel and team physician for a number of the college and high school teams in the Philadelphia area. Gene knows his stuff. He is an excellent diagnostician and carries an ultrasound probe in his hand much of the day. I was guessing he would talk about noninterventional topics. Instead, he chose to talk intervention, with needles and small knives. I should have predicted that. Indeed, a huge part of the perspective of "nonoperative" sports physicians nowadays is operative. Dr. Hong asked his sports medicine colleague Sarah Hoffman to join in the writing.*

Determining the etiology of "hip" pain can be difficult, since pain from the same pathology can be referred to multiple anatomical regions. Therefore, it is a mistake to think in terms of a location being specific for one particular condition. For example, pain from the ball-and-socket hip joint may occur in the buttock, lateral thigh, inguinal crease, or adductor region.

Once one makes a definitive diagnosis, a variety of treatment options materialize. Our goal in this chapter is to describe a number of the "nonoperative" interventional options for "hip" pain, as well as to expound on their effectiveness when evidence permits. We will consider both intra- and extra-articular causes of pain. These include osteoarthritis or degenerative joint disease, femoral acetabular impingement, core muscle injuries, acute or chronic tendinopathy, and other conditions.

While physical and manual therapy options have been shown to be effective for some of these conditions, those treatment modalities will not be discussed. We also shall not discuss in this chapter the generally accepted initial steps in the treatment of many conditions (ie, oral nonsteroidal anti-inflammatory drugs [NSAIDs] or catabolic steroid, corticosteroid injections, ice, rest, or activity modification). Specific pathologies we shall not discuss include stress fractures; pediatric conditions such as slipped capital femoral epiphysis (SCFE) or Legg-Calvé-Perthes disease (LCPD), avulsion fractures, apophysitis, lumbar radiculopathy, and nonmusculoskeletal etiologies such as rheumatoid arthritis or infection.

PLATELET-RICH PLASMA

The autologous blood product derives from spinning whole blood and separating out a concentration of platelets.

Various preparations of platelet-rich plasma (PRP) have been used for a variety of pathologies, although definitive evidence of short- or long-term benefit remains skimpy. In vitro studies have shown increased synthesis of proteoglycans and collagen when PRP stimulates chondrocytes.[1] Several animal studies have shown that PRP improves healing.[2] Basic science studies suggest the treatment will be beneficial in patients, but clinical studies have not provided the evidence yet to prove that statistically due to a lack of power.[3]

Few studies focus on the intra-articular hip joint itself, making it necessary to postulate from the data for treatment of other pathologies, such as patellar tendinopathy or knee osteoarthritis.[3-5] Several authors have found statistical improvement in patient outcome scores compared to hyaluronic acid injections for large joint arthritis. The benefit lasted just 6 to 12 months. The majority are case studies (ie, low level of evidence). In general, the small sample sizes and wide variability in treatment makes it difficult to draw conclusions.[6,7] Only one of the above studies involved injection into the hip, and that study was inconclusive.[6]

The authors acknowledge the circular sent out to professional teams (see Chapter 10) concerning a potential danger of heterotopic ossification in the adductor region. Nevertheless, so far the published data support PRP to be safe in patients with tendinopathy. A 2011 case series by Finnoff et al[5] demonstrated that the combination of tenotomy and PRP was safe in patients with chronic tendinopathy. PRP injections did not seem to carry the risk of tendon degeneration or other systemic effects that injections of corticosteroid injections seem to have, nor, of course, the risks of surgery.[3]

A systematic review in 2014 found that a variety of studies that looked at PRP for articular cartilage pathology. There was limited evidence of short-term benefit in symptomatic knee arthritis patients. On the other hand, definitive conclusions have been impossible due to bias and generally poor quality of those studies.[7]

PLATELET-RICH PLAMSA AND PERCUTANEOUS TENOTOMY

One interesting study compared PRP to extracorporeal shock wave therapy (ESWT).[8] Forty-six athletes with jumper's knee were randomized to receive either therapy. PRP treatment came out better than ESWT. However, there was no control group; plus, it was not clear if the benefit was due to the tenotomy performed at the same time as the PRP injection. Also, the authors did not comment on whether or not the patients had failed eccentric exercises, currently the gold standard for treatment of patellar tendinopathy.

Percutaneous tenotomy means functionally aggressive "needling." This can be performed with a needle or a tiny scalpel blade. Variable amounts of cutting of fascia, epimysium, true tendon, or muscle fibers may occur. The procedure may be performed with or without PRP. Some examples of possible locations for tenotomy include but are not limited to proximal hamstrings or adductors, gluteus medius and minimus, distal rectus abdominis, and piriformis.

Percutaneous tenotomy is a step up in invasiveness and has been studied in the lateral elbow, patella tendon, and Achilles tendon. Results on those parts of the body have shown some promise. Data remain lacking for the role of tenotomy in "hip" tendinopathies and core muscle injuries.

HYDRODISSECTION

Hydrodissection is a method for separating nerves from adjacent tissue using injection of fluid, usually saline with anesthetic and/or steroid, and ultrasound guidance. It has been used for suspected peripheral nerve entrapment. Results are mixed. This has been used primarily in the abdominal wall, lateral thigh, and proximal adductor regions. One author describes an ultrasound-guided percutaneous neuroplasty of the lateral femoral cutaneous nerve for meralgia paresthetica. That resulted in immediate and long-term relief.[9] A 2015 retrospective case series reported relief of medial knee pain after total knee arthroplasty after hydrodissection of the infrapatellar branch of the saphenous nerve with anesthetic and corticosteroid.[10]

ANESTHETIC INJECTION

Anesthetic alone has improved pain and function in the long term for "hip pointers."[11,12] Seventy-five percent of rugby players in the latter study felt the injection was very helpful, while the remaining 25% called it somewhat helpful. The roundness of the numbers and vagueness of the measurements suggest a low-powered study with bias. Probably, pure anesthetic has been tried in other core anatomic regions for long-term relief, but we could not find publications on this.

TOPICAL NITROGLYCERIN

Nitroglycerin also has had variable success in reducing pain with tendinopathy, but elsewhere in the body. The hip/groin region, so far, seems unstudied. In a randomized controlled trial for chronic lateral epicondylosis, topical nitroglycerin reduced pain.[13] Similar results appeared in the literature for Achilles tendinopathy. The latter randomized controlled trial involved a glyceryl trinitrate patch plus physical therapy vs physical therapy alone. Another similar randomized controlled trial, which included placebo topical patches plus eccentric exercises, did not demonstrate significant changes.[14]

PROLOTHERAPY

Prolotherapy involves injection of irritant solutions, such as concentrated sugar, into the soft tissues. In theory, pain relief comes from either growth factors or ischemia triggered by the resultant inflammatory response.[15] There is some evidence of improved outcomes for tendinopathy and osteoarthritis.[16] In one study of elite male kicking-sport athletes with chronic groin pain, 20 of 24 patients had no pain and 22 of 24 remained "unrestricted" at 32 months after treatment. They had monthly injections of dextrose and lidocaine.[17]

ACUPUNCTURE

Limited studies exist about the effectiveness of acupuncture for hip and other joint pain. In 2007, Moe et al[18] found no "moderate quality" evidence that acupuncture affected pain or function in patients with osteoarthritis. In one case report, the pain from a calcifying tendinitis of the gluteus medius completely resolved in a 68-year-old man after 3 months of treatment. He still had no pain and the calcifications had disappeared at 6 months.[19] Crespin et al showed significant short-term pain relief with acupuncture after hip replacement. In that study, acupuncture was given at the same time as pharmacologic management.[20]

Extracorporeal Shock Wave Therapy

Theoretically, ESWT works for tendinopathy via some sort of mechano-biological mechanism. Reportedly, the ultrasonographic technique has analgesic and healing effects. Supposedly, ESWT promotes angiogenesis and bone remodeling. It does release substance P in rabbit femurs.[21] In the knee, ESWT reduced "patients' perceptions" of the clinical severity of their osteoarthritis compared to placebo.[22] Moderate evidence suggests the technique may be effective for greater trochanteric pain syndrome when compared to home training and corticosteroid injection in short and long terms.[23]

Other Modalities

We could find no good studies in the sports medicine literature on the use of botulinum toxin, cryotherapy, or radiofrequency ablation in this region of the body. Logically, the use of each of those modalities makes sense for particular conditions, but, to our knowledge, we do not yet have good clinical scientific trials in the use of these interventions for core muscle injuries.

Summary

The athlete's core remains a largely unstudied area of the body with respect to the use of many of the therapeutic interventions described above. A number of these nonoperative interventions show potential promise in the lab as well as in the limited studies thus far. And while we have described a number of nonoperative therapies that are currently being used in clinical practice, there may be other interventions that are being employed and for which there are even less data. There is certainly a need for further research into the optimal nonoperative interventions to treat "hip" pain. At this point in time with our current understanding of the literature, the authors recommend that each clinical case, each athlete, be evaluated for the appropriate use of nonoperative therapies, and that treatment be tailored to the specific individual based on the diagnosis and contributing factors, including the expectations of the provider and the athlete.

Selected Readings

Fortier LA, Hackett CH, Cole BJ. The effects of platelet rich plasma on cartilage: basic science and clinical application. *Oper Tech Sports Med*. 2011;19(3):154-159.
  An interesting article on the basic science potential of PRP for cartilage injury.
Fitzpatrick J, Bulsara M, Zheng MH, et al. The effectiveness of patelet rich plasma in the treatment of tendonopathy: a meta-analysis of randomized controlled clinical trials. *Am J Sports Med*. 2016;44(6):1379-1381.
  Current meta-analysis of the limited number of randomized controlled trials using PRP to treat tendonopathy—the good, the bad, and the better.
Van Leeuwen MT, Zwerver J, Van den Akker-Scheek. Extracorporeal shockwave therapy for patellar tendinopathy: a review of the literature. *Br J Sports Med*. 2009;43:163-168.
  Good review article on the use of ESWT for patellar tendon injury.
Gambito ED, Gonzalez CB, Oquiñena TI, Agbayani RB. Evidence on the effectiveness of topical nitroglycerin in the treatment of tendinopathies: a systematic review and meta-analysis. *Arch Phys Med Rehabil*. 2010;91(8):1291-1305.
  If you are interested in a better understanding of topical nitroglycerin in the treatment of tendon injury, start with this article.

REFERENCES

1. Akeda K, An H, Okuma M, et al. Osteoarthritis and cartilage. *Osteoarthritis and Cartilage.* 2006;14(12):1272-1280.
2. Taylor D, Petrera M, Hendry M, et al. A systematic review of the use of platelet-rich plasma in sports medicine as a new treatment for tendon and ligament injuries. *Clin J Sport Med.* 2011;21(4):344-352.
3. Mautner K, Kneer L. Treatment of tendinopathies with platelet-rich plasma. *Phys Med Rehabil Clin N Am.* 2014;25:865-880.
4. Mishra AK, Skrepnik NV, Edwards SG, et al. Efficacy of platelet-rich plasma for chronic tennis elbow. *Am J Sports Med.* 2014;42(2):463-471.
5. Finnoff J, Fowler S, Lai J, et al. Treatment of chronic tendinopathy with ultrasound-guided needle tenotomy and platelet-rich plasma injection. *PM&R.* 2011;3:900-911.
6. Tietze D, Geissler K, Borchers J. The effects of platelet-rich plasma in the treatment of large-joint osteoarthritis: a systematic review. *Phys Sportsmed.* 2014;42(2):27-37.
7. Dold A, Zywiel M, Taylor D, et al. Platelet-rich plasma in the management of articular cartilage pathology: a systematic review. *Clin J Sports Med.* 2014;24(1):31-43.
8. Vetrano M, Castorina A, Vulpiani M, et al. Platelet-rich plasma versus focused shock waves in treatment of jumper's knee in athletes. *Am J Sports Med.* 2013;41:795-803.
9. Mulvaney S. Ultrasound-guided percutaneous neuroplasty of the lateral femoral cutaneous nerve for the treatment of meralgia paresthetica: a case report and description of a new ultrasound-guided technique. *Curr Sports Med Rep.* 2011;2:99-104.
10. Clendenen S, Greengrass R, Whalen J, et al. Infrapatellar saphenous neuralgia after TKA can be improved with ultrasound-guided local treatments. *Clin Orthop Relat Res.* 2015;473:119-125.
11. Hall M, Anderson J. Hip pointers. *Clin Sports Med.* 2013;32:325-330.
12. Orchard J, Steet E, Massey A, et al. Long-term safety of using local anesthetic injections in professional rugby league. *Am J Sports Med.* 2010;38:2259-2266.
13. Ozden R, Uruc V, Dogramaci Y, et al. Management of tennis elbow with topical glyceryl trinitrate. *Acta Orthop Traumatol Turc.* 2014;48(2):175-180.
14. Steunebrink M, Zwerver J, Brandsema R, et al. Topical glyceryl trinitrate treatment of chronic patellar tendinopathy: a randomized, double-blind, placebo-controlled clinical trial. *Br J Sports Med.* 2013;47:34-39.
15. Alfredson H, Ohberg L. Sclerosing injections to areas of neo-vascularisation reduce pain in chronic Achilles tendinopathy: a double-blind randomised controlled trial. *Knee Surg Sports Traumatol Arthrosc.* 2005;13(4):338-344.
16. Distel L, Best T. Prolotherapy: a clinical review of its role in treating chronic musculoskeletal pain. *PM&R.* 2011;3(6S):78-81.
17. Topol G, Reeves D, Hassanein, K. Efficacy of dextrose prolotherapy in elite male kicking-sport athletes with chronic groin pain. *Arch Phys Med Rehabil.* 2005;86:697-702.
18. Moe RH1, Haavardsholm EA, Christie A, Jamtvedt G, Dahm KT, Hagen KB. Effectiveness of nonpharmacological and nonsurgical interventions for hip osteoarthritis: an umbrella review of high-quality systematic reviews. *Phys Ther.* 2007;87(12):1716-1727.
19. Lin W, Liu C, Tang C, et al. Acupuncture and small needle scalpel therapy in the treatment of calcifying tendonitis of the gluteus medius: a case report. *Acupuncture Medicine.* 2012;30(2):142-143.
20. Crespin DJ, Griffin KH, Johnson JR, et al. Acupuncture provides short-term pain relief for patients in a total joint replacement program. *Pain Med.* 2015;16:1195-1203.
21. Gerdesmeyer L, Wagenpfeil S, Haake M, et al. Extracorporeal shock wave therapy for the treatment of chronic calcifying tendonitis of the rotator cuff. *JAMA.* 2003;290(19):2573-2581.
22. Zhao Z, Jing R, Shi Z, et al. Efficacy of extracorporeal shockwave therapy for knee osteoarthritis: a randomized controlled trial. *J Surg Res.* 2013;185:661-666.
23. Mani-Babu S, Morrissey D, Waugh C, et al. The effectiveness of extracorporeal shock wave therapy in lower limb tendinopathy: a systematic review. *Am J Sports Med.* 2015;43:752-761.

(B) we need more **studies**

DAVID STONE, MD

Editor's Note: *I also asked one of the great sports medicine physicians in the country to provide his viewpoint on the core—how he thinks about the whole concept, etc. The University of Pittsburgh's David Stone provides some insightful comments.*

"THE CORE"

In sports medicine, we generally view the core of the body as a muscular box that begins at the diaphragm and ends at the bottom of the pelvis. The abdominal muscles make up the front of the box, and the paraspinals and gluteal muscles, etc, the back of the box.[1] Some authors include the anatomy as low as the thighs or as high as the deltoids.[2] The core concept serves as a model for training athletes and enhancing performance.

The underlying assumption of the model is: Controlling the position of the trunk allows for optimal production, transfer, and control of force and motion.[3] The same concept also applies to prevention of injuries to the knee, ankle, and upper extremities.

I'm all about that bass.
—This Meghan Trainor/Kevin Kadish song was the third best-selling single of 2014 and now a top seller of all time. The "bass" refers to the back and booty, etc. According to Trainor, the song and accompanying video promote "body confidence." Some consider the lyrics controversial.

THE LITERATURE SUGGESTS THE CORE IS ALL ABOUT THE BACK

A perusal of the literature provides an impression that the core concept applies mostly to the back and back pain. The core concept, of course, applies to much more of the body, but this generally is what you will read. The literature focuses on rehabilitation.[4] The rehabilitation approaches vary radically, yet 2 general observations persevere:
1. Endurance, or one might say the opposite (ie, wear and tear), of muscles relate to symptoms[5]
2. Motor control and spinal stability go together[4]

The chief concerns translate to worry about the consequences of incorrect spinal loading or poor posture.

The following is my quick and dirty synopsis of some of the back rehabilitation techniques in this literature. Spinal exercises are performed with consideration of the neutral spine posture, abdominal co-contraction, and functional bracing.[4] Authors emphasize unisegmental multifidi, the quadratus lumborum, iliocostalis and longissimus muscles, and the abdominal wall. They underscore the importance of the transversus abdominus in particular. Isometrics, and not weights, are the primary rehabilitation instruments. Correlating with this theme is the fact that isometric exercises produce about 45% of the maximum voluntary contraction of the lumbar paraspinals muscles. The overall goal is to restrict spinal range of motion. Experts encourage conscious simultaneous contraction of the abdominal muscles at the same time as abdominal hollowing (drawing the navel toward the spine in a dynamic fashion). The exercises progress to various flexion positions and such isometrics as a rowing exercise for one hand while the other hand supports the trunk.[6]

The efficacy of these exercises has been conclusively demonstrated in patients with chronic back pain and radiographic evidence of spondylolysis or spondylolisthesis.[6] When performed under strict guidance, those exercises reduced pain significantly at 30 months. The control group consisted of a variety of different regimens left to the original treating practitioners. The fact that effectiveness was demonstrated for only this select group of patients does not seem to matter, considering that these type exercises get applied to back pain patients in general.

WHAT ABOUT ATHLETES?

Interestingly, while back pain is extremely common in athletes,[7] those spinal stabilization exercises are not well studied in this population.[8] The focus on the core in sports has been with the global muscle system (ie, the large torque-producing muscles that act on the spine but do not directly attach to it).[9] The "global" muscles include the rectus abdominus, external oblique, and iliocostalis lumborum pars thoracis. In contrast to the local muscles that attach directly, these muscles do not exert a direct effect on the spine. For asymmetric tasks, Danneels[9] demonstrated that the external oblique, gluteus maximus, iliocostalis lumborum pars thoracis, and latissimus dorsi, as a group, created significant differences in recruitment compared to the rectus femoris, multifidus, and internal oblique muscles. The latter muscles, however, became the main global stabilizers and prime movers when the spine goes into extension. The gluteus maximus and gluteus medius also provided stability to the pelvis. In general, the latissimus dorsi counterbalanced the torso forces.

Maarten et al conclusively demonstrated the importance of the core muscles in athletic tasks.[10] The authors studied force development during vertical jumping, and found that hip extensors helped generate forward and upward movement rather than an upward and backward movement when subjects went from a squat into their vertical jumps. "Jump height" very sensitively followed small variations in the timing of muscle firing patterns. The force generation of the knee and ankle appeared dependent on the hip. Jump height correlated strongly with the firing of the gluteus maximus.

As might be expected, lack of core stability also correlated with injury.[10,11] Those studies were performed in college track and basketball players. Leetun et al analyzed hip abduction, external rotation, and core flexor, lateral trunk, and extension strength.[11] The physiotherapists used side planks, a straight leg lowering test, the Biering-Sorensen test, and flexor endurance tests. Significant increases in injury occurred in 2 situations: when the hip abductors and external rotators were weak or when the abdominal muscles were weak. Male athletes generated greater core stability scores than female athletes. Together, those studies demonstrated the importance of the hip in transferring forces from the lower extremity in terms of both performance and the risk of injury. For both sexes, hip external rotation seemed a useful predictor of injury.

Intriguingly, studies exist that suggest that core strengthening does not reduce pain. For example, Nadler et al introduced Division 1 college athletes to a core strengthening that highlighted abdominal, paraspinals, and hip extensor strengthening.[12] The program may have helped in some body regions but not in the incidence of back pain. On the other hand, hip abductor weakness definitely predicted injury, so the authors, of course, speculated that more abductor strengthening might have been better.

The ultimate measure of a man is not where he stands in moments of comfort and convenience, but where he stands at times of challenge and controversy.

—Dr. Martin Luther King Jr.

DIFFICULTIES CORRELATING GOOD CORES WITH PERFORMANCE

Probably the most concrete interpretation of this MLK Jr quote you ever heard applies to the scientific study of the importance of core strength with respect to athletic performance. The studies must be done with the body under some stress and a slant toward measuring endurance. Clearly, the body needs to be challenged in order to see the importance of the core. Most of the studies on this subject have, thus far, simply not done that.

Common sense would say that since the core is the body's engine room, good core conditioning would enhance athletic performance. However, that has been hard to prove definitively. An example of that difficulty is the well-known Stanton study.[13] Stanton utilized the Sahrmann core stability test and the Swiss ball prone stabilization core stability test to measure core stability and its effect on running economy. The authors evaluated maximal aerobic power as the highest oxygen volume (VO_{2max}) during the last minute of exercise, and running economy as the volume of oxygen consumption at 60% to 90% velocity/maximal oxygen uptake. They also analyzed trunk angle utilizing treadmill videos. The core training program lasted 6 weeks. It turned out that the Swiss ball training improved core strength, but not running economy or VO_{2max} or running posture. Back-treading because the results seemed to defy logic, the authors concluded that perhaps the subjects were only moderately well-trained. Instead of calling this a negative study, they questioned whether their Swiss ball regimen, in reality, produced an adequate training response.

Similarly negative findings have been found by others. Scibek et al[14] scrutinized swimming performance, Nesser et al[15] studied college football players, and Thompson et al[16] found similar results in golfers. The football study was exhaustive, computing countermovement vertical jumps, shuttle runs, 20- and 40-yard sprints, bench presses, squats, and power cleans. The variables also included trunk flexion, extension, and side-lying bridge positions. Remarkably, hip strength was not one of the variables. Weak to moderate correlations between performance and core strength were not consistent. The authors side-barred that one-time explosive movement tests may not truly measure core stability, which involves more isometrics and endurance than bursts of activity. The authors concluded that the core muscles work as a unit and should not be evaluated with single exercises of sports performance.

Enter the Functional Movement Screen (FMS). The FMS was developed, in part, to address this question whether conditioning can be studied in a dynamic fashion over time with respect to both performance and injury. One can consider that the incidence of injury measures an extreme of performance or lack of performance. The FMS consists of 7 movements, evaluating ranges of joint motion and stabilizations, balance, and symmetry. The 7 movements involve:

1. Deep squats
2. In-line lunges
3. Hurdle steps
4. Shoulder mobility
5. Active straight leg raises
6. Rotary stability
7. Trunk-stability push-ups

The tests place the athlete in extreme positions designed to detect weakness or muscle imbalance by either the appearance of compensatory movements or just plain poor performance. Each person creates a baseline and gets measured over time.

Kiesel et al demonstrated significant injury correlations with low FMS scores in footballers.[17] FMS scores and injury prevention also improved with a certain core training programs.[18] Likewise, Tee et al showed the FMS to predict severe injuries in rugby players.[19] In-line lunges and active straight leg raising seemed so sport specific that the authors' recommended tests and results be interpreted taking into account both demands of the sport as well as the specific participants. Hodges and Richardson demonstrated that trunk activity precedes motor activity of the lower extremity, consistent with the concept of the core creating the stable platform for lower extremity movement.[20]

One must note that the FMS does not address strength, power, endurance, or agility. Therefore, it should be considered somewhat unidimensional and incomplete.[21,22] The FMS does certainly set the stage for measuring performance over time, even though it is not perfect.

The Core, the Central Nervous System, and the Knees

Proprioception involves the back and central nervous system. Deficits in proprioception have been shown to increase the risk of knee injury. In female college athletes, Zazulak[23] easily demonstrated that deficits in active lumbar spine repositioning increased ligamental and meniscal injury. In contrast, passive proprioceptive repositioning did not make a difference. Active motion requires feedback from muscle spindles, and passive motion does not, probably explaining the change as well as highlighting the importance of core strength. A follow-up study[24] found that truncal displacement was much greater in the injured female athletes. Forward and lateral flexion, extension, and a history of back pain all predicted injury. Lateral truncal displacement was the strongest predictor of anterior cruciate and other ligament injury. In a study that correlates with Zazulak's, Myer et al found that plyometric exercise, dynamic stabilization, and balance training improved both drop vertical jump and medial drop landing movements (ie, markers for risk of knee injury in female athletes).[25]

We are all in the gutter, but some of us are looking at the stars.

—Oscar Wilde, from *Lady Windermere's Fan.*

It's Not About the Naysayers

Even though the concept of the core may now seems obvious to some of us, that visualization requires new eyesight and new thinking. As Oscar Wilde insinuates, we all can live with what we got, but why not take the risk to look up and see what else is out there?

Almost unbelievably, the concept of the core of the body is not universally accepted. Lederman has noted that the distinction between global vs core muscles is "purely anatomic" and "has no functional meaning."[26] Grenier and McGill saw increased spinal stability with co-contraction of the abdominal muscles and without any contribution from the transversus abdominis, seemingly refuting one of our key concepts of core stability.[27] Wirth et al questioned whether the altered muscle firing patterns seen on electromyography of core muscles might actually be the result and not the cause of problems.[28] The latter authors also question the entire notion of training on uneven surfaces, citing a gross lack of evidence to support one of our key concepts of core strengthening.

That said, we must challenge those and other "experts" in our field to flee their notions and come up with alternative hypotheses for how the core works. Like it or not, those experts shall be forced to recognize that this region of our body is here to stay.

Selected Readings

Leetun DT, Ireland ML, Willson JD, et al. Core stability measures as risk factors for lower extremity injury in athletes. *Med Sci Sports Exerc.* 2004;36:926-934.
   This fun, although somewhat controversial, article exposes a positive correlation between the core and injury. The data may be underpowered; nevertheless, they provoke, from my viewpoint, the right thoughts.

Wirth K, Hartmann H, Mickel C, Szilvas E, Kelner M, Sander A. Core stability in athletes: a critical analysis of current guidelines. *Sports Med.* 2007;47(3):401-414.

The article provides good criticisms of some previous articles and addresses some important aspects of core training.

Kibler WB, Press J, Sciascia A. The role of core stability in athletic function. *Sports Med.* 2006;36(3):189-198.

Although some may consider this article "ancient," it addresses important core concepts that I use in the office with my throwers.

REFERENCES

1. Akuthota V, Ferreiro A, Moore T, Fredericson M. Core stability exercise principles. *Curr Sports Med Rep.* 2008;7(1):39-44.
2. Hibbs AE, Thompson KG, French D, Wrigley A, Spears I. Optimizing performance by improving core stability and core strength. *Sports Med.* 2008;38(12):995-1008.
3. Kibler WB, Press J, Sciascia A. The role of core stability in athletic function. *Sports Med.* 2006;6(3):189-198.
4. McGill SM. Low back stability: from formal description to issues for performance and rehabilitation. *Exerc Sports Sci Rev.* 2001;29(1):26-31.
5. Biering-Sorenson F. Physical measurements as risk indicators for low back trouble over a one year seriod. *Spine.* 1984;9:106-119.
6. O'Sullivan PB, Phyty GDP, Twomey LT, et al. Evaluation of specific stabilizing exercise in the treatment of chronic low back pain with radiologic diagnosis of spondylolysis or spondylolisthes. *Spine.* 1997;22:2959-2967.
7. Jonassan P, Halidin K, Karlsson J, et al. Prevalence of joint related pain in the extremities and spine in five groups of top athletes. *Knee Surg Sports Traumatol Arthrosc.* 2011;19:1540-1546.
8. Stuber KJ, Bruno P, Sajko S, et al. Core stability exercises for low back pain in athletes. A systematic review of the literature. *Clin J Sports Med.* 2014;24:448-456.
9. Danneels LA, Vanderstraeten GG, Cabier DC, Witvrouw EE, De Cuyper HJ. A functional subdivision of hip, abdominal and back muscles during asymmetric lifting. *Spine.* 2001;26(6):E114-E121.
10. Maarten B, Zandwijk V, Peter J. Dynamics of force and muscle stimulation in human vertical jumping. *Med Sci Sports Exerc.* 1999;31:303-310.
11. Leetun DT, Ireland ML, Willson JD, et al. Core stability measures as risk factors for lower extremity injury in athletes. *Med Sci Sports Exerc.* 2004;36:926-934.
12. Nadler SF, Malnga GA, Bartoli LA, et al. Hip muscle imbalance and low back pain in athletes: influence of core strengtening. *Med Sci Sports Exerc.* 2002;34(1):9-16.
13. Stanton R, Reaburn PR, Humphries B. The effect of short term Swiss ball training on core stability and running economy. *J Strength Cond Res.* 2004;18(3):522-528.
14. Scibek JS, Guskiewicz KM, Prentice W, et al. *The effect of core stabilization training on functional performance in swimming.* Master's thesis. University of North Carolina, Chapel Hill, NC; 2001.
15. Nesser TW, Huxel KC, Tincher JL, et al. The relationship between core stability and performance in division 1 football players. *J Strength Cond Res.* 2008;22(6):1750-1754.
16. Thompson CJ, Myers Cobb K, Blackwell J. Functional training improves club head speed and functional fitness in older golfers. *J Strength Cond Res.* 2007;21(2):131-137.
17. Kiesel K, Plisky P, Voight M. Can serious injury in professional football be predicted by a preseason functional movement screen? *N Am J Sports Phys Ther.* 2007;(2):147-158.
18. Kiesel K, Plisky P, Butler R. Functional movement test scores improve following a standardized off-season intervention program in professional football players. *Scan J Med Sci Sports.* 2011;21:287-293.
19. Tee JC, Klingbiel FG, Collins R, Lambert MI, Coopoo Y. Preseason functional movement screen component tests predict severe contact injuries in professional rugby union players. *J Strength Cond Res.* 2016;30(11):3194-3203.
20. Hodges PW, Richardson CA. Feed forward contraction of transversus abdominus is not influenced by the direction of arm movement. *Exp Brain Res.* 1997;114:362-370.
21. Cook G, Burton L, Hoogenboom BJ, Voight M. Functional movement screening: the use of fundamental movements as an assessment of function, part 1. *Int J Sports Phys Ther.* 2014;9:396-409.
22. Cook G, Burton L, Hoogenboom BJ, Voight M. Functional movement screening: the use of fundamental movements as an assessment of function, part 2. *Int J Sport Phys Ther.* 2014;9:549-562.
23. Zazulak BT, Hewett TE, Reeves NP, Goldberg B, Cholewicki J. The effects of core proprioception on knee injury. *Am J Sports Med.* 2007;35(3):368-373.
24. Zazulak BT, Hewett TE, Reeves NP, Goldberg B, Cholewicki J. Deficits in neuromuscular control of the trunk predict knee injury risk. *Am J Sports Med.* 35(7):1123-1130.
25. Myer GD, Ford KR, McLean SG, Hewett TE. The effects of plyometric versus dynamic stabilization and balance training on lower extremity biomechanics. *Am J Sports Med.* 2006;34(3):445-455.
26. Lederman E. The myth of core stability. *J Bodyw Mov Ther.* 2010;14(1):84-98.
27. Grenier SG, McGill SM. Quantification of lumbar stability by using 2 different abdominal activation strategies. *Arch Phys Med Rehab.* 2007;88(1):1254-1265.
28. Wirth K, Hartmann H, Mickel C, Szilvas E, Kelner M, Sander A. Core stability in athletes: a critical analysis of current guidelines. *Sports Med.* 2017;47(3):401-414.

37

an **osteopath's** view of the core universe
manipulative therapies
a **functional** approach

JASON HARTMAN, DO
PHILIP J. KOEHLER III, DO, MS
VERONICA WILLIAMS, DO, ILLUSTRATOR

Editor's Note: *My osteopathic colleague Jason Hartman pens his perspective on the core. It is very different from mine. Yet, Jason's profound understanding of the anatomy and integrative approach encompasses what the core is all about. Jason is transforming me into a believer. Jason invited one of his gifted students, Philip, to join in the writing of this chapter. Another of Jason's talented students, Veronica Williams, illustrates this chapter.*

It is much more important to know what sort of a patient has a disease than what sort of a disease a patient has.
—Sir William Osler, considered the ultimate diagnostic physician ever.

This whole chapter constitutes a plea for all health professionals who participate in the care of athletes, and everyone else who desires to stay fit, to think out of the box and in terms of manipulative therapy. Manipulative medicine is where it is at. (See Figure 37-1.)

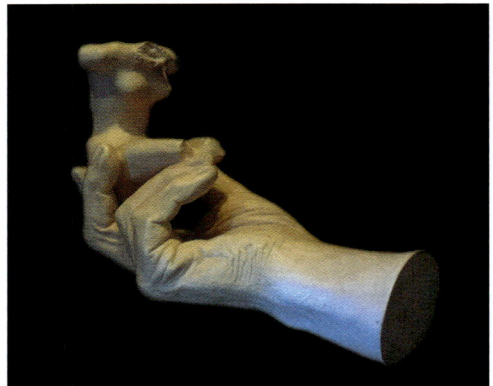

Figure 37-1. *Hand of Rodin Holding a Torso.* Shortly before the death of artist Auguste Rodin (1840-1917), his assistant casted Rodin's hand and fit this plaster fragment of a previous Rodin work into it. The sculpture resides in the Rodin Museum in Philadelphia, Pennsylvania.

	Bone/Joint	Muscle/Tendon	Fascia	Ligament	Nerve	Viscera
OMM	*	*	*	*	*	*
Acupuncture		*	*	*	*	
Chiropractic	*			*		
Massage		*	*			
ART		*	*			
Graston/Astym		*	*			
Rolfing		*	*			
Dry Needling		*	*			
Shiatsu		*	*			
Strain Counterstrain		*	*			
MFR		*	*			
LAS/BLT	*			*		
Craniosacral	*				*	
Visceral Tech						*

Figure 37-2.

Osteopathic manipulative medicine sanctions more than 30 categories of manual manipulation that incorporates thousands of distinct techniques. Osteopathic physicians commonly employ just 4 broad categories of techniques: soft tissue, high-velocity-low-amplitude (HVLA), myofascial release, and counterstrain[1] (Figure 37-2). A recent meta-analysis and systematic review revealed that manual modalities and multimodal treatments shorten the return to play time for many high-level athletes with core injuries.[2,3] Ask yourselves the following question: If this is true for athletes, why should manipulative therapy not work for all of us?

A Straightforward Sentinel Case

Mary, a 60-year-old athletic female with osteoarthritis of the left hip, gets referred to my office for manipulative therapy after many years of left-sided pubic area pain that had taken her away from recreational running and most other physical activities that she enjoyed. After initial assessment, I sent her for rectus abdominis core muscle repair. Thereafter, she faithfully employed manipulative therapy, and she has done extremely well for the past number of years.

For a long time before Mary came to us, her caring physicians identified her as another aging patient experiencing a "typical" progression of hip arthritis. Mary was being viewed through the old lens of structural reductionism. That was unfortunate. We had to ask the question: "What if her new physicians had seen her 20 years earlier? Would that have altered her outcome?"

We were the ones who asked the question. Of course, the answer is yes.

Structural Reductionism

Reductionism is the philosophy that molecules constitute all systems, and the interactions of molecules establish all hierarchies of chemical, biological, and physical properties. The earliest reductionist was Thales (born circa 636 BC in Asia Minor), who hypothesized that the fundamental substance of the universe was water; water composed all things. Descartes, the mapper, became the most famous promoter of this philosophy.[4]

We propose the term *structural reductionism* as a narrow condensation of reductionism to just the musculoskeletal system. Basically, this philosophy means restoration of the proper structure to the body restores function. Traditional medicine abides by this approach, but in an even narrower way. Their approach assumes a paradox that different structures within the musculoskeletal system can function independently from each other; yet, if you fix just one thing, you can fix it all.

In short, traditional medicine goes by the philosophy that pathophysiology can be reduced to a simple defect in a muscle, ligament, bone, or other relevant structure and does not have to take into account the complexity and interdependency of the whole organization (ie, the overall form and function). Of course, we are exaggerating somewhat its philosophy. Hopefully you get the point.

Osteopathy breaks this mold. It looks at the body as totally connected components. In this chapter, we want you to become Descartes. View the universe as water. That way, you will broaden your scope and see how to manage the entire body.

Structural reductionism occurs at all levels of health care. Health care professionals at the front line of musculoskeletal complaints—massage therapists, athletic trainers, physiotherapist, and physicians, to name a few—usually perceive pain through the lens of structural reductionism. The result is that they will achieve success in a certain percentage of patients, but will not in others because they cannot access the full spectrum of problems.

PUBIC PAIN—THE WAY IT WAS

Just like in our sentinel case, the physical exam is the only place "it" is at. The site of pain determines most everything. The diagnosis is a rectus abdominis issue. Treatment begins with rest, ice, nonsteroidal anti-inflammatory drugs, and then corticosteroid injections; when that ceases to work, surgery comes to the rescue. This is diagnosis and treatment by mode of structural reductionism. Six months later, adductor pain begins, and then anterior thigh pain. Then other things happen.

CORE PAIN—THE WAY IT SHOULD BE

Manual therapies help us understand the body from a wider perspective. The roots of manual therapies involve "holism," effectively the opposite of reductionism. Holism traces back to Aristotle: "The whole is more than the sum of its parts."[5] Likewise, each medical disorder is more than the sum of enzymatic or cellular dysfunctions.[6]

We are applying Aristotle to the musculoskeletal system. Think of the musculoskeletal system as complex yet interdependent anatomy.

This system functions as a whole and has units beyond regular Newtonian dynamics. The functional units—call them *biokinetic chains*—influence each other. When one chain falters, the entire system falters. One simple dysfunction affects posture, gait, movement, and the homeostasis of the entire musculoskeletal system. We need everybody to believe it is naive to think that dysfunction can be solved only by the simple reapproximation of a defective attachment. Human movement and posture are determined by complex interactions between bones, joints, muscles, ligaments, nerves, blood vessels, lymphatics, and hollow and solid viscera.

Mary

Let's turn back to Mary. In other hands, Mary might have been treated in a more "holistic" manner. From the initial assessment, she would have undergone analyses of movement, gait, and posture. She would have been observed to have a functionally short left leg, pelvic torsion, and an internally rotated hip. She would have undergone complete evaluation of the hip, and that would have revealed laxity of her hip capsule. Mary also would have multiple myofascial trigger points (MTrPs) involving her hip flexors and adductors. She also would exhibit extensive functional weakness of her glutes, which would have contributed to her generally weak core.

Various conceptual frameworks have been applied to explain what manipulative therapies address. Among these is osteopathy. We shall also discuss other therapies, to some extent, in this chapter.

The key to being a great goalkeeper lies in the strength of the core.
—Gordon Banks, the best soccer goalkeeper of all time, and not just because he said this.

Diagnosis

Osteopathic philosophy emphasizes looking at patients in the entire context of their lives, and not just their chief complaints. When we talk to and examine a patient, we keep 4 doctrines in mind:
1. The person is a unit, all organ systems connect.
2. The body self-regulates, self-maintains, and self-heals.
3. Structure and function interrelate complementarily.
4. Rational treatment comes from understanding the above 3 doctrines.

The History

Patients with pelvic pain often have a myriad of somatic and visceral complaints. For example, patients with interstitial cystitis see 5 to 7 physicians before the diagnosis is made. Like patients with Crohn's disease or angina, they have multiple co-morbidities. They are 2 to 3 times more likely to suffer from low back pain or tension headaches, and 10 to 20 times more likely to have fibromyalgia or vulvodynia.[7]

There is no doubt that these patients have neurologically mediated reflexes that go in 2 directions, from the organs to the musculoskeleton (viscerosomatic) and vice versa (somatovisceral). The reflexes lead to a heightened neurologic state and easy excitability of both the central and autonomic nervous systems, so much so that it becomes impossible to distinguish between the chicken and the egg. Successful treatment of the patient has to break that vicious cycle. It must somehow shrink the ease with which the central and autonomic nervous systems bolt into the picture. Success requires multidisciplinary approaches targeted at both somatic and visceral pathologies. (See Figures 37-3 and 37-4.)

We must ask about the problem's chronicity, exacerbating and alleviating factors, previous medical or manual treatments, lifestyle, and psychosocial and other factors that might help design optimal ergonomics (eg, typical day at work, leisure, and exercise). We must do a complete review of systems and complete sexual and surgical histories. All organ systems and past treatments apply. This knowledge base helps design optimal manual therapies.

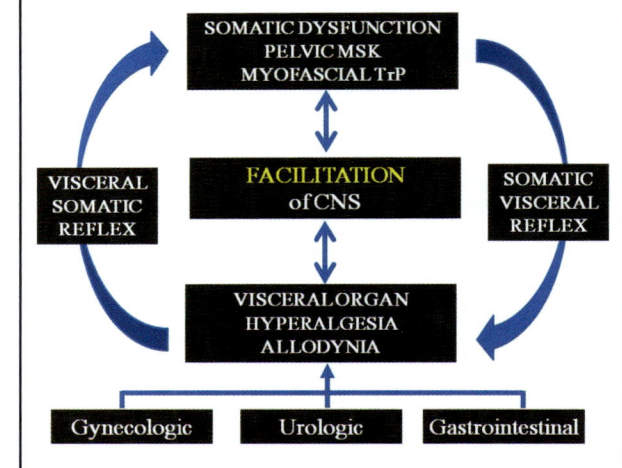

Figure 37-3.

The Structural Exam

The purpose here is to identify physical problems (ie, somatic dysfunction). Somatic dysfunction, in essence, indicates the need for osteopathic manipulative therapy. The diagnosis of somatic dysfunction requires at least 1 of 4 criteria: tenderness, tissue texture change, restricted range of motion, and asymmetry. There are 3 parts to the structural examination: observation, palpation, and functional assessment.

Observation begins when the patient walks into the office and continues throughout the visit. Look for motion abnormalities of the pelvis or postural or functional compensations that might be secondary to pain or structural discrepancies. Spot antalgic gaits, asymmetries of normal anatomic landmarks, and posture and possible pelvic tilt imbalances. Here is when we might pick up upper/lower cross syndrome, iliopsoas syndrome, short-leg syndrome, an anteriorly rotated pelvis as a result of hip flexor and erector spinae hypertonicity,[8] or a posteriorly rotated pelvis due to hamstring hypertonicity.[9]

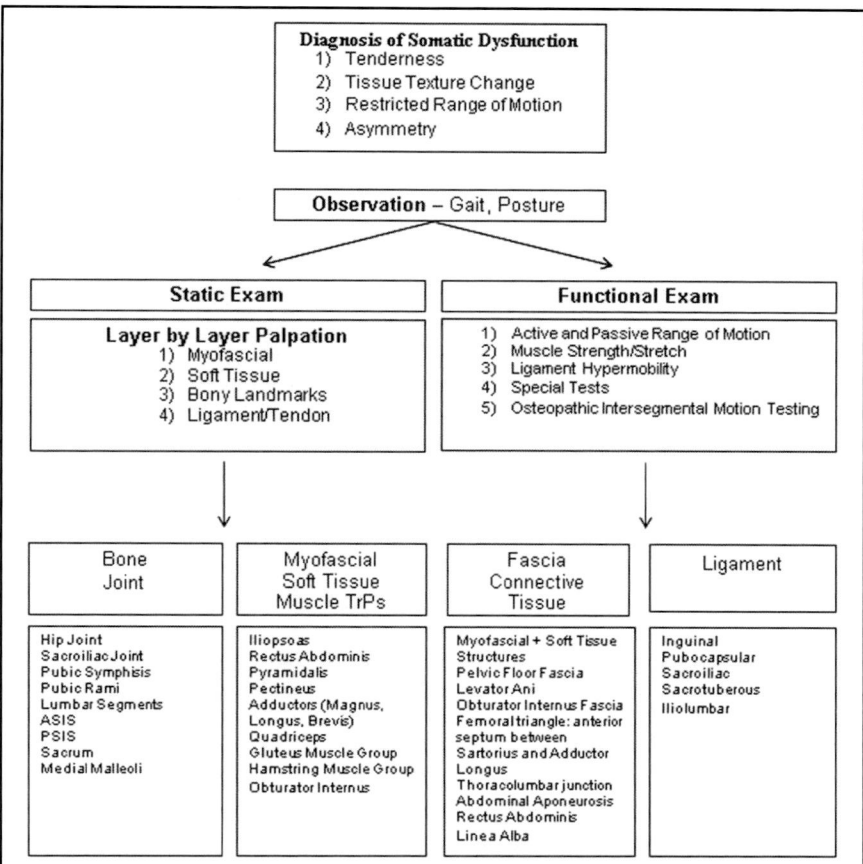

Figure 37-4.

Palpation begins with a static exam. Palpation might find acute or chronic changes of hypersympathetic tone with chronic texture changes. The tissue may feel cool, while looking pale and mottled, or boggy with a fibrotic ropy muscular texture.

We might start with the pubic bodies and/or rami and look for tenderness, then the various muscles, ASIS, PSIS, and back. We check for alignment. For example, we may palpate a posteriorly rotated innominate bone on the left, and confirm this with a cephalad left medial malleolus. Then we know we are working with a short leg on the left. From the static palpation exam, patterns arise, from acute or chronic trauma, poorly healed injury, or various postural forces. The more chronic the patterns, the more compensatory layers appear.

We examine all the core muscle groups detailed in Section One of this book. We identify "trigger points," areas when touched or otherwise stimulated set off cascades of pain. Trigger points travel along predictable "Travellian" lines or with spasmodic or chronically contracted muscle. Leg shortening signals the possibility of an ongoing protective mechanism and atrophy resulting from fatigue and weakness.

Next, we examine the ligaments of the core (eg, inguinal, pubocapsular, sacrotuberous, sacroiliac, iliolumbar). Pelvic or hip instability may manifest itself along ligaments. We look for the same patterns of tenderness and texture. Instability often creates alterations in the location of trigger points. That, by itself, can be a clue. For example, hip instability often manifests at the pubic symphysis or one of the bodies, owing to massive compensatory shifts.

The final level of static palpation is the fascia and other connective tissue. The book *Anatomy Trains: Myofascial Meridians for Manual and Movement Therapists* by Thomas Myers[10] dedicates itself to understanding the continuity of connective tissue throughout the musculoskeletal system. An important fascial level is the obturator internus fascia, which becomes continuous with the adductor fascia. Fascial lines connect the adductors to the contralateral rectus abdominis on top of the pubic plate and contribute to the physical therapy concept of slings. Manual techniques sometimes aim to normalize the forces across those planes and balance core. A small fascial disruption may disrupt a delicate balance and create major dysfunction. Resultant alterations in posture and movement create an instability and susceptibility to injury.

Functional assessment becomes the primary assessment tool after completion of the history and the first 2 parts of the structural exam. At Vincera, we developed resistance tests for each of the core muscles attaching to or crossing the pubic symphysis or joint (Figure 37-5). Interpretation of each test involves 3 considerations:
1. Does the test cause pain?
2. Does the resultant pain correlate to the muscle being tested?
3. Does the resultant pain recreate the pain causing the athlete's disability?

For the hip, functional assessment means primarily range of motion without interference from contracting muscles. These include the standard flexion-abduction-external rotation (FABER) and flexion-adduction-internal rotation (FADIR) tests, plus other rotational or hyperflexion/hyperextension tests aimed to isolate anterior, posterior, or lateral impingements or other pathology. Nearby tenderness sometimes helps solidify diagnoses, but pain may also come from more remote inflammation and cause confusion.

There are several standard functional tests for the sacroiliac joint[11,12]:
- Gaenslen
- FABER/Patrick's test
- Thigh thrust/femoral shear test
- ASIS distraction/compression (supine)
- Sacral compression (lateral recumbent)
- Standing and seated flexion tests

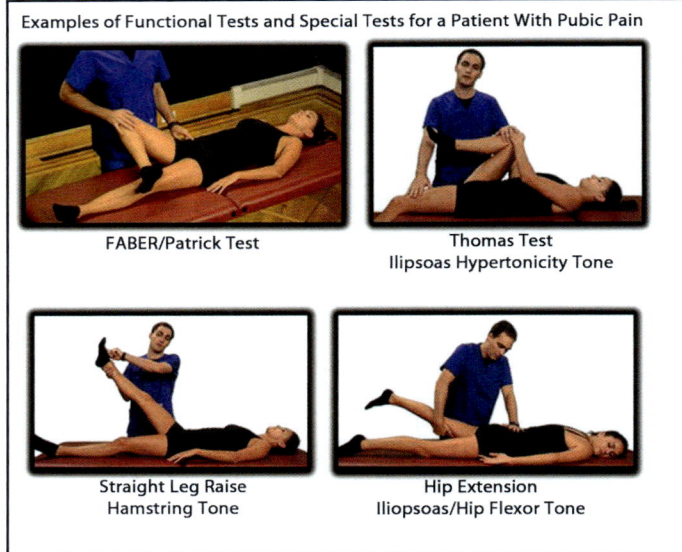

Figure 37-5. (Reprinted with permission from MedQuest Educational Services.)

Do not ignore the lumbar spine when using manual therapy. This is the longitudinal axis that manages axial weight and posture. First, assess the lumbar curvature and designate whether it is normal, hyper-, or hypolordotic. The degree of lumbar lordosis greatly affects pelvic tilt, and then sequentially the hip, core muscles, and fascial and ligamentous balance. Chronic low back pain may directly relate to weak gluteus muscle groups or hamstrings or tight iliopsoas. What happens to the deconditioned weekend warrior, who promises to play in that adult men's hockey league? Bad things, of course. A compromised core creates secondary low back pain and different varieties of core injury.[8]

Common Sources of Dysfunction

The Dirty Half Dozen

Greenman identified 6 common patterns of somatic dysfunction in patients with back, buttock, and thigh pain. Fifty percent of 183 patients exhibited 3 or more of these patterns at the same time.[13] Three of these dysfunctions are described in this section.

Iliopsoas Syndrome

Janda lower cross syndrome is an example of postural compensation predisposing to injury. One iliopsoas muscle becomes hypertonic and shortened, and this creates a kinetic chain of compensatory events. The components of the chain are: (1) an anteriorly rotated innominate and externally rotated limb on the side of the psoas dysfunction, (2) a contralateral pelvic shift, (3) a hypertonic contralateral piriformis and quadratus lumborum, and (4) consequent sciatica. Abnormalities have also been see in vertebral mechanics, particularly at the origins of the psoas major (T12-L3). (See Table 37-1.)

Correspondingly, when the hip flexes past 90 degrees, it externally rotates.[14] We infer that this shortens the other external rotators. Prolonged shortening leads to hypertonicity and trigger points. That's what happens with prolonged sitting. By that mechanism, the obturator internus may also become a primary pain generator. Pelvic floor dysfunction may result related to common attachment with the pelvic diaphragm. Resultant diaphragm flattening distorts the normal pelvic bowl, thus shortening the levator ani and coccygeus and creating additional trigger points. So, postural (ie, "lower cross") injury, iliopsoas syndrome, and lifestyle (eg, prolonged sitting) all can disrupt the kinetic change and create back, pubic, and pelvic pain. (See Figures 37-6 and 37-7.)

An Osteopath's View of the Core Universe—Manipulative Therapies—A Functional Approach

Table 37-1
Iliopsoas Syndrome (Right)

Structure	Somatic Dysfunction
Right innominate	Anterior
L1/L2	F SRRR (non-neutral)
Sacrum	Posterior dysfunction (left on right)
Left leg	Externally rotated
Pelvis	Left side shift
Left piriformis, quadratus lumborum	Hypertonic

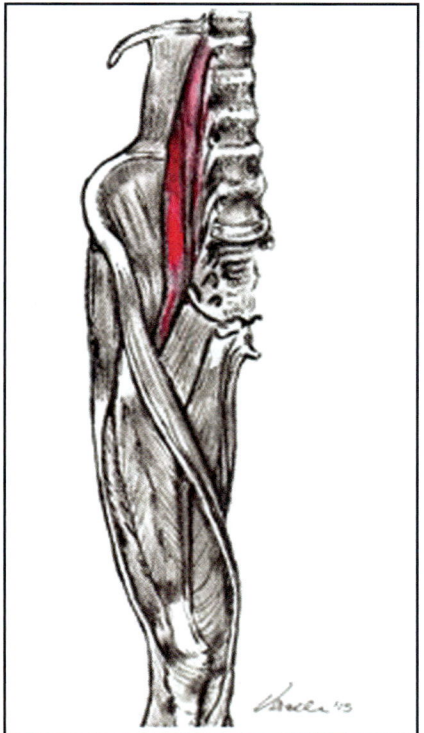

Figure 37-6.

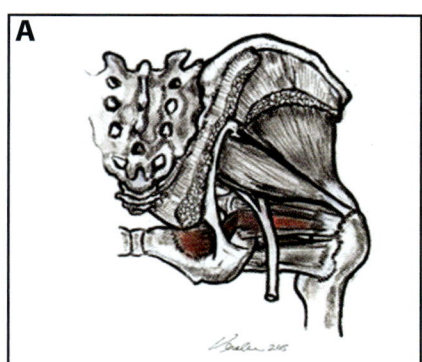

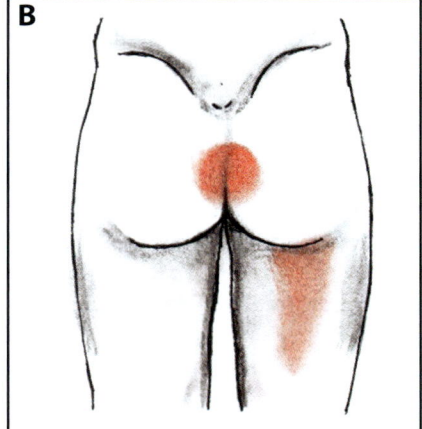

Figure 37-7.

Short Leg Syndrome

Short leg syndrome is implicated in about every type of core pain: low back, lower abdomen, pubis, and pelvis.[15] For example, in a patient with a structural short leg, a specific change of specific kinetic compensatory patterns emerge (Figure 37-8).

For example, the changes 5 through 8 in Figure 37-8 produce the hypertonic hamstring short leg shown in Figure 37-7. Thoracolumbar musculature eventually fatigues, which leads to compromise of fascial integrity. Ligaments press to maintain postural balance. The iliolumbar ligament is often the first site of pain. Therefore, it should be tested by palpation when the syndrome is suspected.[15] According to Wolf's law, areas of repetitive mechanical stress or force cause a reflexive deposition of bone to reinforce areas of mechanical weakness.[16] It is not hard to conceptualize any of these things—iliolumbar calcification, contractures, and scoliosis—turning structural. These are all arguments for early intervention.

Pubic Shear

Pubic shear is pain commonly believed to come from osseous misalignment secondary to muscular imbalance. Diagnosis requires a positive lateralization test (eg, ASIS compression, standing flexion or prone sacroiliac motion tests) demonstrating both dysfunction and a restricted sacroiliac joint. Shear may occur at any of the sites of muscular attachment or at the symphysis and are so named: superior, inferior, cephalad, caudad, and symphyseal. It so happens that our osteopathic understanding of what is going on here fits precisely with what Meyers described as a likely cause of "athletic pubalgia."[17] Perhaps we should tell Meyers to look for osseous misalignment in his patients! (See Figure 37-9.)

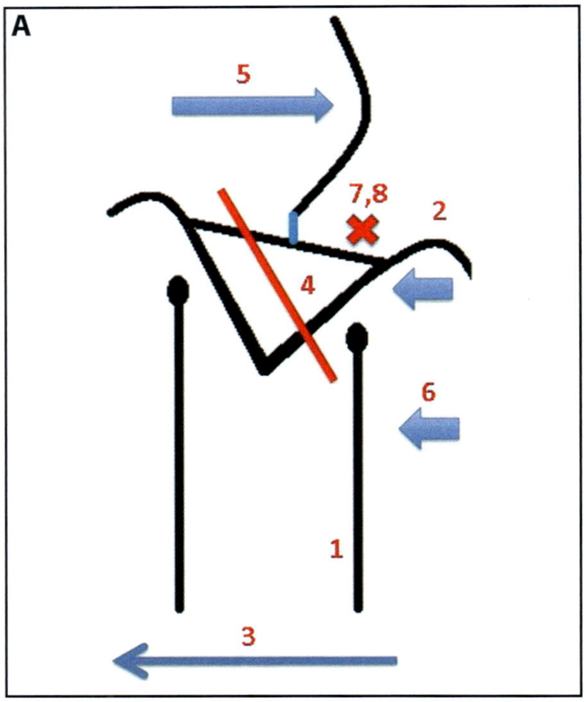

Treatment

As much as it may seem that we poo-pooed, in the introduction, medicine's traditional goal of structural reductionism, that is also the goal of osteopathic manual manipulation. But, we want restoration of proper structure and function at all levels of the somatic framework. We are talking about a dynamic, sequential treatment process, involving multiple levels—biomechanical, neural, metabolic, respiratory-circulatory, and psychosocial.

The cynic will say that all manual medicine is doing is "making tight things loose." This is actually not so far from the truth. We do correct structures that are tight. We then peel back the somatic layers and often find things that are "loose" or unstable. To correct these dysfunctions, we choose weapons that affect multiple levels. We employ exercise, acupuncture, prolotherapy, and, yes, even surgery.

In fact, we love combinations of therapies. A Cochrane review of 5 high-quality randomized controlled trials showed prolotherapy to be effective for back pain with other treatment modalities such as osteopathic manipulative medicine and exercise.[18] We also love to change or combine techniques of osteopathic manipulative medicine during a given treatment course. We always pay most attention to what we call the *key lesion*, the one with the greatest restriction or tenderness. We continually reassess and redirect, to achieve the key goal of correcting at multiple levels. Homeostasis can only come from this sort of multidirectional attack. A great example is how correcting a costal dysfunction affects respiration. Yes, our goal is structural reductionism, but at all levels.

Effective treatment of pubic pain illustrates, in spades, what we are talking about. Mary is the case in point. Think of all that we have had to treat: functional short leg, postural imbalance, Janda lower cross syndrome, altered gait, hip osteoarthritis, and visceral problems.

Figure 37-10 represents a Venn diagram for the specific techniques used for Mary, our sentinel patient.

Compensation Patterns Common to an Anatomic Short Leg (Posterior View)

1) Anatomical right short leg
2) Sacral base unleveling with a caudad sacral base on ipsilateral side
3) Pelvic side shift to contralateral side
4) Sacral torsion
5) Functional convex scoliosis
   - Sidebending to contralateral side and rotation to ipsilateral side
6) Anterior innominate with hypertonic and shortened quadriceps on ipsilateral side creating a functionally longer leg
7) Postural compensation of thoracolumbar musculature
8) Ligamentous stress of iliolumbar and sacroiliac ligaments on ipsilateral side

Figure 37-8. (Reprinted with permission from MedQuest Educational Services.)

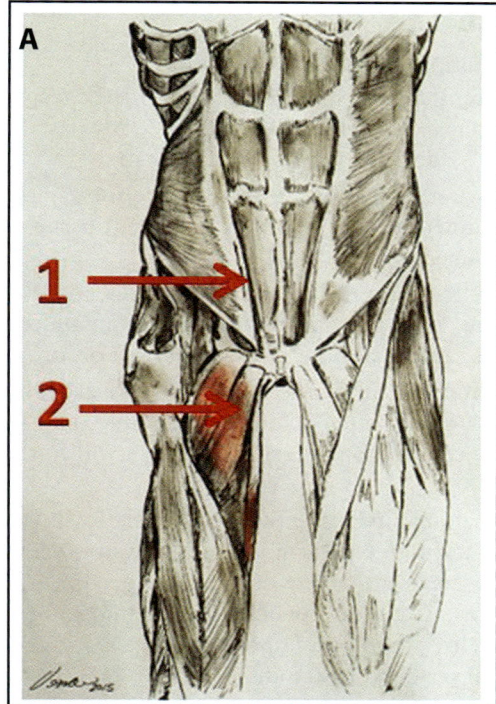

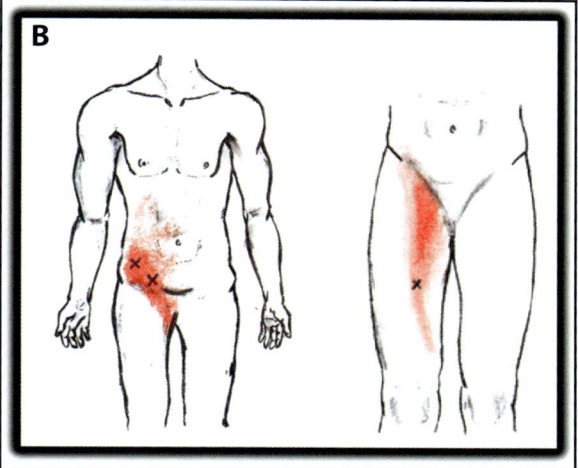

Figure 37-9.

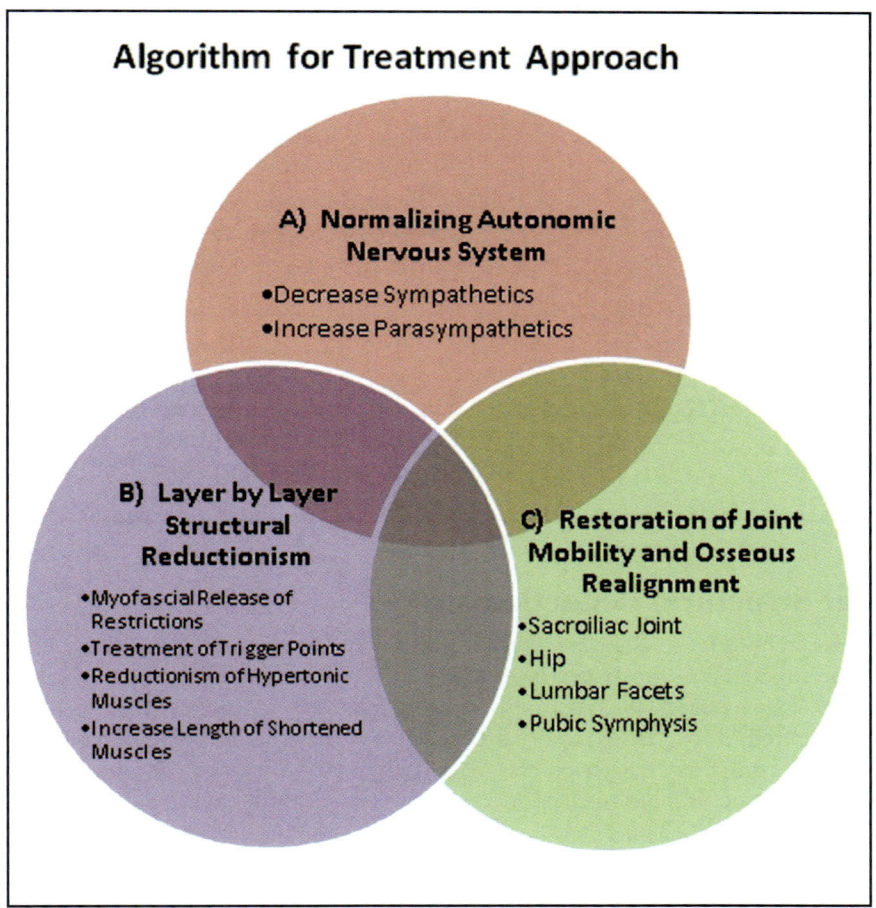

Figure 37-10.

Normalization of Autonomic Nervous System

To break her vicious cycle of autonomic facilitation our goal, multiple modalities were used:

1. Myofascial release of the linea alba and other anterior abdominal wall structures, including the respiratory and pelvic diaphragms. This aim was to decrease sympathetic tone to tissues supplied by T5-L2. Myofascial release in that region targets 3 sympathetic collateral ganglia. Table 37-2 details some of that information.

2. Suboccipital and sacral treatments were aimed to increase parasympathetic influences via the vagus nerve and sacral nerve plexus. Fortunately, these tissues respond to numerous techniques including soft tissue or ischemic compression, acupuncture, dry needling, and trigger point injections.

    The vagus nerve exits the cranium at the jugular foramen. Relaxing the muscles in the area possibly increases cranial-sacral movement and increased vagal neural outflow. The spinal accessory nerve (cranial nerve XI) also exits in that region. Perhaps relaxation of the trapezius musculature and sternocleidomastoid occurs and helps.

3. HVLA was also likely effective in the same occipito-atlantal and atlanto-axial upper cervical segments. This modality is designed for restricted vertebral segments. A "thrust" often achieves an audible "pop," indicating movement of the joint through a barrier.[16] The pop likely results from release of bubbles within the synovial joint.[19]

    The terms *mobilization* and *manipulation* apply to spinal manipulative therapy, which HVLA represents. HVLA is a manipulation, which refers to a lower velocity technique than mobilization. It also uses repetitive, short-amplitude burst thrusts (ie, just like mobilization). A Cochrane review of 26 randomized controlled trials with over 6000 patients identified high-quality evidence for effectiveness of this type technique for short-term improvement. Functional status measured by several disability scales also improved.[20] In theory, HVLA works by affecting mechanics of restricted (ie, relatively immobile) vertebral facet joints.

Table 37-2
Facilitation of the Central Nervous System

Anatomic Nerve	Spinal Levels	Sympathetic Autonomic Level	Visceral Organ	Collateral Sympathetic Ganglion
Greater splanchnic	T5-T9	T5-T9	Upper GI: stomach, liver, spleen, pancreas, duodenum	Celiac
Lesser splanchnic	T10-T11	T10-T11	Middle GI: duodenum to promixal two-thirds of transverse colon, kidneys, gonads, adrenals, upper ureters	Superior mesenteric
Least splanchnic	T12			
Lumbar splanchnic	L1-L2	T12-L2	Lower GI/GU: distal one-third of transverse colon to rectum, lower ureters, bladder, penis/clitoris, prostate	Inferior mesenteric

Layer by Layer Structural Reductionism

While we apply these techniques to all layers, the fascial layer evokes a special sweet spot in the mind of osteopaths. Kuchera summarizes the functions of the fascial layer of the somatic framework by "the 4 P's": packaging, protection, posture, and passageways.[21] It envelopes all structures including muscles, visceral organs, and ligamentous and articular structures. In this layer, we find MTrPs as well as other trigger points in general. Three popular books[22-24] describe how to treat somatic dysfunction using these trigger points. Again, combination therapy (ie, osteopathic manipulative therapy with wet or dry needling, acupuncture) has the best success.

Ischemic compression/soft tissue/massage may be the overall most popular form of manual therapy. This involves compressing soft tissue directly over MTrPs. Pain production guides the amount of compression and reduction of pain is one of the aims of therapy. Pain reduction supposedly coincides with disappearance of a taut band.[25] Some believe that the beneficial effect comes from mechanical disruption of muscle architecture. A potential physiological explanation is the activation of noiciceptive c-fibers and release of neuroinflammatory factors. The main point is that it works but nobody knows why.

TABLE 37-3
COMPARISON OF TRIGGER POINTS AND TENDER POINTS

Trigger Point (Travell)	Tender Point (Jones)	Both
Muscle tissue	Muscle, tendon, ligament, fascia	Locally tender—pea-sized tissue texture change
Radiating pain pattern	No radiation of pain	Located in muscle
Taut band of tissue	Not taut band	"Jump sign" when palpated
Elicits twitch response	No twitch response	

Counterstrain (or Strain-CounterStrain [SCS]) therapy is a gentler, "indirect" osteopathic manipulative therapy technique, also known as *positional release therapy*. As you can tell, we manual therapists have a lot of names that describe essentially the same things. Lawrence Jones, an osteopath, brought this technique to life in 1955, and his "tender point" therapy has become popular among all brands of manual therapists, not just osteopaths.[26] The locations of his tender points are similar to the locations of trigger points described by Travell and Simons.[22] (See Table 37-3.)

The proposed mechanisms for the beneficial effects of counterstrain are fascinating. They involve "inappropriate proprioceptive reflexes,"[26] "gamma efferent activity" in the muscle spindle, and reflex lengthening of antagonist muscles and fascia.[17] "Gamma gain" is thought to be the chief player of a vicious "pain-spasm-pain cycle." Electromyography studies support the latter concept.[27]

Basically, SCS consists of the practitioner palpating definite tender points in a targeted region of the body. Then the patient assumes a position, and then, with the practitioner's help, holds that position for 90 seconds.[28]

Counterstrain deserves recognition as a first-line treatment for iliopsoas problems. Figure 37-11 shows the tender points and a summary of the technique. Jones's tender points correlate with classic trigger points described for pubic, pelvic, and low back pain.[26]

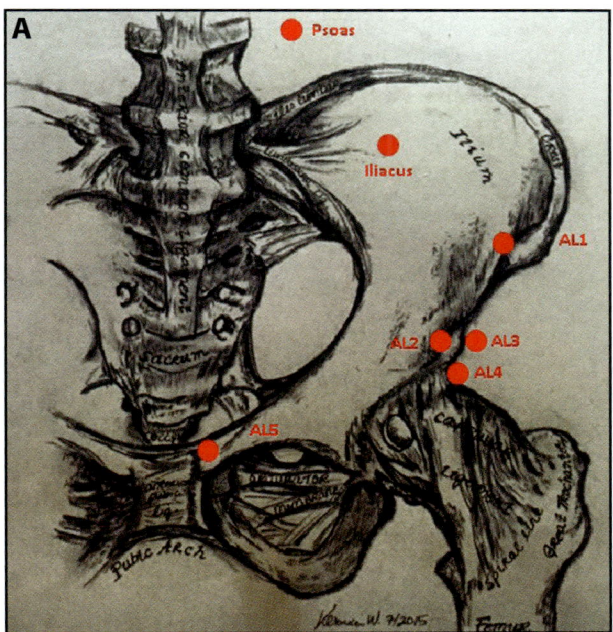
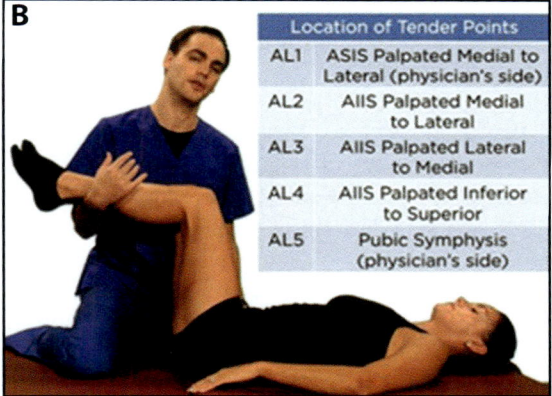
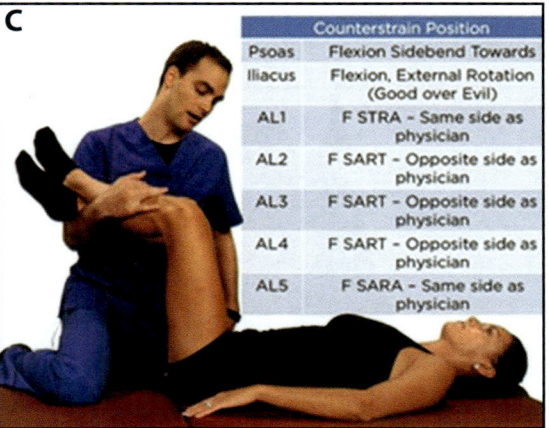

Figure 37-11. ([B, C] Reprinted with permission from MedQuest Educational Services.)

Wet needling describes injecting medications into trigger points. Local anesthetics work by reversibly blocking sodium channels and inhibiting ion flux and nerve transmission. Thereby, anesthetics decrease nociceptive pain at the same time as mechanical disruption of MTrPs by the increase in blood flow due to the needle itself. Increasing blood supply increases ATP production, which unlinks actin and myosin bridges and allows for muscular relaxation. This technique applies to the pelvic floor and has become popular for myofascial plane syndromes.[29,30] Botulinum toxin with or without local anesthetic adds a particular flair to the treatments.[31]

Dry needling commonly describes a solid filiform, approximately 30-gauge or acupuncture needle inserted perpendicularly into an MTrP. Deeper depths can elicit a twitch response. The success rates may be similar to wet needling, which suggests mechanical disruption to be the effective mechanism. A recent article notes that ischemic compression combined with dry needling decreased soreness.[31] A Cochrane review of 35 randomized controlled trials showed dry needling to be effective for chronic low back pain and myofascial pain syndromes. In that study, acupuncture was also effective. For multiple reasons, we believe combinations of the 2 modalities make particular sense.[32]

Restoration of Joint Mobility and Osseous Realignment Using Muscle Energy

Muscle energy is an osteopathic technique developed by Mitchell in 1979.[33] We use it to lengthen shortened muscles, to mobilize restricted articulations, and to reduce muscle tone or myofascial restriction.

The most well-known form is post isometric relaxation and repositioning muscle energy. The patient voluntarily contracts the affected muscle mildly against an externally applied counterforce by the practitioner. After 3 to 5 seconds of isometric contraction, the patient relaxes as the practitioner passively moves the muscle or joint through the restricted barrier.[28]

The physiologic mechanism of muscle energy therapy remains unclear. Nevertheless, a Cochrane review of muscle energy techniques of 12 randomized controlled trials and 14 comparisons showed the technique to be commonly used and safe across multiple manual modalities.[34]

This technique helps restore joint mobility and osseous realignment. It helps break the action of hypertonic muscles surrounding a joint, thereby restricting the range of motion. By the same mechanism, it helps release compression of articular surfaces and friction coefficients. The technique even helps joints that have become fixed over time due to fibrosis and contracture. The mechanism then involves extra-articular mobilization of muscles and nearby ligaments with beneficial compensation capabilities. Cerebral palsy or upper motor neuron lesions serve as dramatic examples of the fixed contracture situation.

Three examples show how this technique may be employed. Super pubic shear involves a hypertonic rectus abdominis pulling the pubic bodies cephalad (Figure 37-12). The physician using muscle energy recruits the adductor muscles to contract, pulling the bodies and rami inferiorly and helping to achieve osseous realignment. In theory, osseous realignment loosens muscles and reduces spasm, as it restores tone.[35] The second example is anterior innominate dysfunction, when the innominate bone rotates anteriorly due to a hypertonic quadriceps (Figure 37-13). The third example is the so-called innominate out-flare, which involves an overactive external rotator group (Figure 37-14).

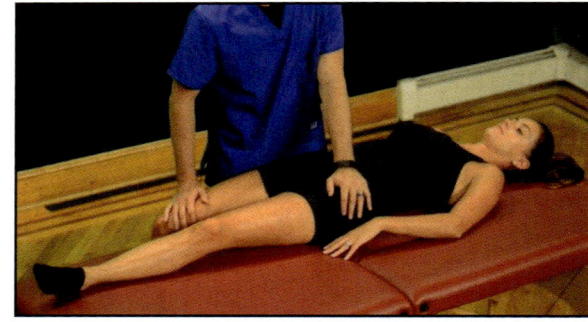

Figure 37-12. Super pubic shear. (Reprinted with permission from MedQuest Educational Services.)

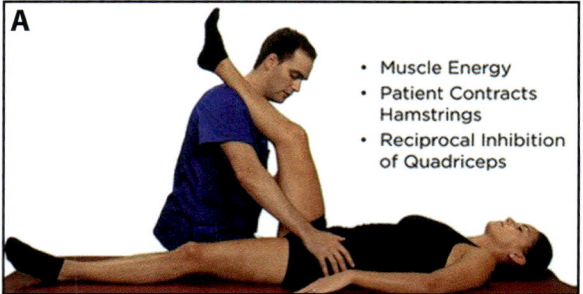
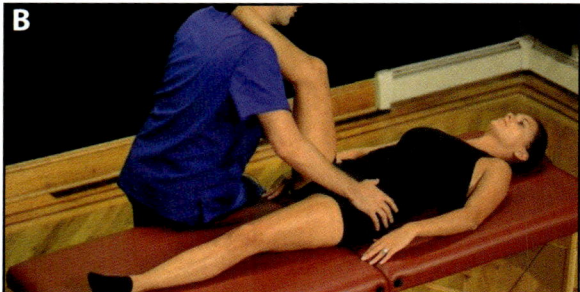

Figure 37-13. Anterior innominate dysfunction. (Reprinted with permission from MedQuest Educational Services.)

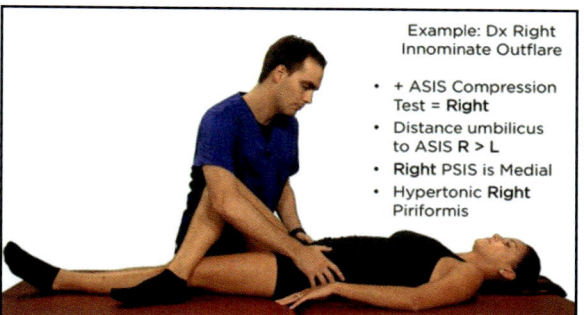

Figure 37-14. Innominate out-flare. (Reprinted with permission from MedQuest Educational Services.)

The way a team plays as a whole determines its success. You may have the greatest bunch of individual stars in the world, but if they don't play together, the club won't be worth a dime.

—Babe Ruth, the greatest baseball player of all time.

OUR VIEWPOINT

We osteopaths see things from a holistic perspective. Manual modalities offer preventative, primary, and adjunctive angles to patients with core problems. The body's capability to heal depends on restoring normal structure at all layers of the somatic and visceral frameworks.

No specific manual modality is a gold standard. Optimal treatment involves a multilayered approach using combinations of therapy and the incorporation of detailed anatomic knowledge after comprehensive examinations.

We employ multiple manual modalities as adjunctive treatment for patients after core muscle and hip repairs. Particularly promising are protocols that target new scar tissue formation. A central theme of our treatments encompasses restoration of balance of muscle and fascial components. Manual modalities help the body recover, and also correct potential future dysfunctions that are created during the body's attempts to achieve homeostasis. Let's face it, injury and surgery change everything. From our holistic perspective, it is vital that the body get all the way back.

By no means is postsurgical recovery our only collaboration within the health care paradigm. We believe that manual modalities help prevent muscle imbalances that predispose people to somatic trauma that requires surgical repair. The modalities also offer adjunctive and primary treatment.

In essence, our holistic thought process is the new approach to musculoskeletal dysfunction. By its very nature, the core is central to our theme. As Babe Ruth said in the above quote, the whole is what determines overall success.

We are learning much more combining our knowledge about responses to manual treatment with the various pathologic entities that we continue to identify. The future of the new field of "core medicine" is bright.

SELECTED READINGS

Still AT. *Philosophy and Mechanical Principles of Osteopathy.* Kansas City, MO: Hudson-Kimberly Publishers Company; 1902.
   In this book, the founder of osteopathy, Andrew Taylor Still, describes his then novel-philosophy. He explains his landmark observations about interdependence of structure and function, and connections to health and disease.

Nicholas AS, Nicholas EA. *Atlas of Osteopathic Techniques.* 3rd ed. Philadelphia, PA: Lippincott Williams & Wilkins; 2016.
   This very complete atlas of osteopathic techniques takes the prospective osteopath through the different steps of manipulation techniques ranging from high-velocity mobilization to myofascial release.

Myers TW. *Anatomy Trains: Myofascial Meridians for Manual and Movement Therapists.* 3rd ed. New York, NY: Elsevier; 2014.
   This textbook brings a functional view of anatomy to the health care professional from the perspective of the continuity of fascia throughout the body. This continuity offers an understanding of how a change in mechanical function in one part of the body may affect function at a remote site.

Chila AG, American Osteopathic Association. *Foundations for Osteopathic Medicine.* 3rd ed. Philadelphia, PA: Lippincott Williams & Wilkins; 2011.
   This popular textbook of osteopathic manipulative medicine provides the osteopathic student with an overview of the history, science, and range of techniques.

Travell JG, Simons DG. *Myofascial Pain and Dysfunction: The Trigger Point Manual*. Vol 2. Baltimore, MD: Williams & Wilkins; 1992.
This very thorough investigative book describes all the muscles, trigger points, and radiation patterns within the musculoskeletal system. It is a must-have for musculoskeletal medicine practitioners.

REFERENCES

1. Johnson SM, Kurtz ME. Osteopathic manipulative treatment techniques preferred by contemporary osteopathic physicians. *Journal of the American Osteopathic Association*. 2003;103(5):219-224.
2. King E, Ward J, Small L, Falvev E, Franklyn-Miller A. Athletic groin pain: a systematic review and meta-analysis of surgical versus physical therapy rehabilitation outcomes. *Br J Sports Med*. 2015;49(22):1-7.
3. Serner A, Hölmich P, Weir A, van Eijck C, Beumer B, deVos, R. Study quality on groin injury management remains low: a systematic review on treatment of groin pain in athletes. *Br J Sports Med*. 2015;49(12):813.
4. Descartes R, Cottingham J, Stoothoff R, Kenny A, Murdoch D. *The Philosophical Writings of Descartes in 3 Volumes* and *The Philosophical Writings of Descartes, Volume 3: The Correspondence*. Cambridge, United Kingdom: Cambridge University Press; 1988.
5. Aristotle's *Metaphysics* translated with an introduction by H. Lawson-Tancred. London, United Kingdom: Penguin; 1998.
6. Beresford MJ. Medical reductionism: lessons from the great philosophers. *QJM: An International Journal of Medicine*. 2010;103(9):721-724.
7. Nickel JC, Tripp DA, Pontari M, et al. Interstitial cystitis/painful bladder syndrome and associated medical conditions with an emphasis on irritable bowel syndrome, fibromyalgia and chronic fatigue syndrome. *J Urol*. 2010;184:1358-1363.
8. Janda C. Evaluation of muscular imbalance. In: Liebenson C, ed. *Rehabilitation of the Spine*. Baltimore, MD: Williams & Wilkins; 1996.
9. Kendal FP, McCreary EK. *Muscle Testing and Function*. 3rd ed. Baltimore, MD: Williams & Wilkins; 1983.
10. Myers TW. *Anatomy Trains: Myofascial Meridians for Manual and Movement Therapists*. 3rd ed. New York, NY: Elsevier; 2014.
11. van der Wurff PL, Buijs EJ, Groen GJ. A multitest regimen of pain provocation tests as an aid to reduce unnecessary minimally invasive sacroiliac joint procedures. *Arch Phys Med Rehabil*. 2006;87(1):10-14.
12. Laslett M, Aprill CN, McDonald B. Provocation sacroiliac joint tests have validity in the diagnosis of sacroiliac joint pain. *Arch Phys Med Rehabil*. 2006;87(6):874; author reply 874-875.
13. Greenman PE. Syndromes of the lumbar spine, pelvis, and sacrum. *Phys Med Rehabil Clin North Am*. 1996;7:773-785.
14. Hammoud S, Bedi A, Voos JE, et al. The recognition and evaluation of patterns of compensatory injury in patients with mechanical hip pain. *Sports Health: A Multidisciplinary Approach*. 2014;6:108-118.
15. Kuchera WA, Kuchera ML. *Osteopathic Considerations in Systemic Dysfunction*. 2nd ed rev. Dayton, OH: Greyden Press; 1994:129-158.
16. American Osteopathic Association. *Foundations for Osteopathic Medicine*. Philadelphia, PA: Lippincott Williams & Wilkins; 2011.
17. Meyers WC, Yoo E, Devon ON, et al. Understanding "sports hernia" (athletic pubalgia): the anatomic and pathophysiologic basis for abdominal and groin pain in athletes. *Oper Tech Sports Med*. 2012;20:33-45.
18. Staal JB, de Bie R, de Vet HCW, Hildebrandt J, Nelemans P. Injection therapy for subacute and chronic low-back pain. *Cochrane Database of Systematic Reviews*. 2008;3.
19. Evans DW. Mechanisms and effects of spinal high-velocity, low amplitude thrust manipulation: previous theories. *J Manipulative Physiol Ther*. 2002;25:251-262.
20. Rubinstein SM, van Middelkoop M, Assendelft WJ, de Boer MR, van Tulder MW. Spinal manipulative therapy for chronic low-back pain: an update of a Cochrane review. *Spine (Phila Pa 1976)*. 2011;36(13):E825.
21. DiGiovanna EL, Schiowitz S, Dowling DJ. *An Osteopathic Approach to Diagnosis and Treatment*. 3rd ed. Philadelphia, PA: Lippincott Williams & Wilkins; 2005.
22. Travell JG, Simons DG. *Myofascial Pain and Dysfunction: The Trigger Point Manual: The Lower Extremities*. Vol 2. Baltimore, MD: Williams & Wilkins; 1992.
23. Gunn CC. *The Gunn Approach to the Treatment of Chronic Pain*. 2nd ed. New York, NY: Churchill Livingstone; 1997.
24. Baldry PE. *Myofascial Pain and Fibromyalgia Syndromes*. Edinburgh, Scotland: Churchill Livingstone; 2001.
25. Martín-Pintado-Zugasti A, Pecos-Martin D, Rodríguez-Fernández ÁL, et al. Ischemic compression after dry needling of a latent myofascial trigger point reduces postneedling soreness intensity and duration. *PM R*. 2015;7(10):1026-1034.
26. Jones LH, Kusunose R, Goering E. *Jones Strain-Counterstrain*. Boise, ID: Jones Strain-Counterstrain, Inc, 1995.
27. Wynne MM, Burns JM, Eland DC, Conatser RR, Howell JN. Effect of counterstrain on stretch reflexes, hoffmann reflexes, and clinical outcomes in subjects with plantar fasciitis. *J Am Osteopath Assoc*. 2006;106(9):547-556.
28. Nicholas AS, Nicholas EA. *Atlas of Osteopathic Techniques*. 2nd ed. Philadelphia, PA: Lippincott Williams & Wilkins; 2011.
29. Weiss JM. Pelvic floor myofascial trigger points: manual therapy for interstitial cystitis and the urgency frequency syndrome. *J Urol*. 2001;166(6):2226-2231.
30. Moldwin RM, Fariello JY. Myofascial trigger points of the pelvic floor: associations with urological pain syndromes and treatment strategies including injection therapy. *Curr Urol Rep*. 2013;14(5):409-417.
31. Jeynes LC, Gauci CA. Evidence for the use of botulinum toxin in the chronic pain setting—a review of the literature. *Pain Pract*. 2008;8:269-276.
32. Furlan AD, van Tulder MW, Cherkin D, et al. Acupuncture and dry-needling for low back pain. *Cochrane Database of Systematic Reviews*. 2005;1. Art No: CD001351. doi: 10.1002/14651858.CD001351.pub2.
33. Mitchell FL. *The Muscle Energy Manual*. Vol 1. East Lansing, MI: MET Press; 1995.
34. Franke H, Fryer G, Ostelo RW, Kamper SJ. Muscle energy technique for non-specific low-back pain. *Cochrane Database Syst Rev*. 2015;27(2):CD009852.
35. Still AT. *Philosophy and Mechanical Principles of Osteopathy*. Kansas City, MO: Hudson-Kimberly Publishers Company; 1902.

38

a **chiropractor's** perspective
the knee bone's **connected** to the thigh bone...

Marc Legere, DC, BS, BA

Editor's Note: *I asked my friend Marc Legere while he was the Phillies' chiropractor to offer his viewpoint on the core. As you will see, Marc makes complex things simple and fun.*

As a physician who specializes in physical pain, I often have patients describe pain throughout different parts of their body. What is often surprising to them is that, more times than not, the pain that they feel in one part of their body is due to a problem or dysfunction coming from another, "unrelated" area.

One thing that you have to keep in mind as we discuss injuries in this section is that your musculature is the true key to proper functional movement. If a muscle is injured, shortened, or doesn't function properly, you can develop issues in your joints, ligaments, tendons, discs, and nerves locally or at another location in the body. With that said...

The knee bone's connected to the thigh bone...
—Well-known American spiritual song. The melody was composed by author and songwriter James Weldon Johnson (1871–1938). The lyrics were inspired by Ezekiel 37:1–14.

THINK OF THE SONG AND THE KINEMATIC CHAIN

Remember that song "Dem Bones"?[VID 1] That's the song that says "The knee bone's connected to the thigh bone, the thigh bone's connected to the hip bone, the hip bone's connected to the back bone...". As funny as it may sound, that song is more true than you know. This "bone connected to another bone" lyric describes what in medical terms is referred to as the *kinematic chain*. The word to focus on in the word kinematic is "kine." Kine is short for kinesiology, which according to the *Merriam-Webster Dictionary* is "the study of the principles of mechanics and anatomy in relation to human movement." Now look at what, according to www.thesciencedictionary.com, is the definition of the word kinematic chain. That definition is: "A number of links connected to one another to allow motion to take place in combination. It becomes a mechanism when so constructed as to allow constrained relative motion between its links." What both of these are saying is that a muscle or bone in one location can affect another muscle or bone at another location because of a chain of related movements.

PROPER EVALUATION

Keeping this in mind, in order for a physician to properly evaluate a patient for the first time, he/she should possess an in-depth knowledge and understanding of how the body works as a unit to properly diagnose what the actual problem is. Most of our clinical knowledge comes from information that isn't found in many textbooks. While anatomy and injuries are taught in school, the clinical connections that are seen in practice are not. With that said, we need to consider both core and non-core muscles in order to properly fix a core muscle injury. If we simply focus on fixing a painful muscle, we may be setting the patient up for future problems. We need to expand our scope to consider the damaged and causative muscles at the same time.

OK, so you may be saying to yourself, now that I know that I can't just focus on the core, where else should I look?

During an examination, I always like to focus on all of the non-core muscles first, and then work my way back to the core muscles, ensuring that I don't miss anything. With that said, let's take a look at a motion below the pelvis and then one above the pelvis to see how they can affect our core muscles.

THE FOOT, THE BRAIN, AND THE NECK

An improperly functioning foot can wreak havoc on our core muscles. Let's reference our "Dem Bones" song to help us trace our way up to the pelvis. "The foot bone's connected to the shin bone, the shin bone's connected to the knee bone, the knee bone's connected to the thigh bone, the thigh bone's connected to the hip bone." You can see how the domino effect that occurs in the foot can connect to the hip due to these connections.

When the foot collapses inward, "losing your arch," a stress occurs on the inside portion of the knee. This creates an opening of the inside portion of your knee joint. This opening causes the inner portion of the thigh to move even farther inward. That movement can either pinch the inner muscles of the thigh or cause the muscles that prevent the inner motion of the thigh to have to work harder and therefore become painful or damaged. If we look at a foot that rotates in the opposite direction of the arch, a stress occurs on the outside ankle joint. That stress puts additional pressure on the outside portion of the knee. This leads to either an opening between the pelvis and thigh or an outward rotation of the leg, which causes a shortening of the muscles in the posterior pelvis and hip. In either case, these far away areas create problems in the pelvis.

Now you may be asking yourself, if I have foot problems, why doesn't it feel like they are working improperly? Well, it's a pretty simple answer...the brain! Our brains are amazing machines that can adapt to different stimuli or challenges very quickly. The ability to learn a new pattern or motion is called *neuroplasticity*.[1] Exactly how fast does the brain adapt? Within 24 hours.

What I mean is that your brain has already started making changes to muscular firing patterns as soon as it experiences pain or restricted motion. After approximately 48 hours, the body has made global changes to movement that begin to feel normal. It is the concept of practice makes perfect or learning a new golf swing. If you start to learn a new swing, at first it feels very awkward, but, over time, your body has made the necessary changes to its firing patterns and movements.

With that in mind, we can see how an ankle sprain 2 to 3 years ago set the stage for a core muscle injury today. That improperly moving, normal-feeling ankle has begun the domino effect all the way into the pelvis.

To examine another muscle group far from the core, that still affects the core, let's look at the neck. Our "Dem Bones" connection here is: "The neck bone's connected to the back bone, the back bone's connected to the hip bone." If you have bad posture, you usually hold your head forward of where it should be. This is common for people who work at desk jobs because their monitor is too low or because their chair is too high in relationship to their keyboard. When the head moves forward, the mid-back arches forward to compensate. Because the mid-back arches forward, the low back increases its arch, which in turn pulls on the core muscles in both the front and back of the pelvis, similar to pelvic tilt discussed in Chapter 28. In the front side of the body, the abdominal muscles are stretched and the thigh muscles are shortened. In the posterior portion of the body, the joints in the back are compressed, and the hamstrings are stretched out.

Let's Talk Specifics

So now that we are on the same page about how our core muscles are truly global muscles, let's talk specifics. Once we can diagnose the true cause of our pain, we then need to look at all of the methods of treatment that can be utilized to either prevent injuries or to recover from injuries in the fastest way possible. If we look at all of the medical specialists that can help prevent or recover from core muscle injury, the list can be long. In my interactions with professional athletes, they use one or all of the following specialties to help with an injury:

- Surgeon
- Chiropractor (modern)
- Physical therapist
- Yoga instructor
- Primary care physician
- Sports medicine physician
- Pain management physician
- Massage therapist
- Athletic trainer
- Nutritionist
- Strength and conditioning specialist

The list of specialists is quite long and can be overwhelming if you do not know where to start. This is where an integrated institute comes into play. The Vincera Institute has developed a truly unique team of specialists who look at a patient's injury from a global point of view. By working as a team, they can all focus on what we do best with one goal in mind, patient injury prevention and recovery.

For this chapter, I am focusing on how a modern-day chiropractor should address your physical injuries. I am not sure what first pops (Get it? "...pops"?) into your head when you think of chiropractors, but the first thoughts can be negative and rightfully so. Chiropractic has needed to evolve, and has finally begun to evolve in recent years. A much better term for what a chiropractor is should be *manual* (meaning hands on, nonsurgical) *physician*. Having said that, let's stick with the title of chiropractor or chiropractic for the chapter just to keep things simple.

Adjustments

Before I get going, I want to address 2 topics: (1) what an adjustment or manipulation actually is and (2) what happens during one? First, to me and the rest of the medical world, an adjustment is, in its most simple sense, a stretch. Yup, that's it...just a stretch. Now, there is nothing wrong with that, and as we all see or feel it throughout our lives, a stretch can be really beneficial. But to claim that it does anything more than restore motion in a fixed or improperly moving joint is difficult; unless you can prove it, don't claim it. There is research on adjustments/manipulations that show that an adjustment can help with nonmuscular conditions, but where we can make our biggest impact on our patients is when there is physical pain.

Second, let's address the infamous "pop" that happens during an adjustment. The popping that occurs during an adjustment is one of two things:

416   Chapter 38

1. The sound of a pop is air escaping a restricted or stuck joint (Figure 38-1). The bone is never out of place and a manipulation does not put a bone back into place. We know through our study of the kinematic chain that muscles are the movers of joints and if a muscle is restricted in its motion, the joint is restricted in its motion as well.

   Muscles on one side of a joint need to move well enough so that muscles on the opposite side of a joint can pull the bone through a specific range of motion. If the antagonistic, opposite muscle of a pulling muscle is tight, the joint cannot easily move through its normal range. Imagine a tug of war between 2 teams pulling on a rope or in our case a bone. The stronger one side pulls, the harder the other side has to pull in order to get movement.

   During normal movement of a joint, air moves in and is released out of a joint. In an improperly functioning joint, the air moves into a joint but does not have enough movement to leave the joint. This creates an accumulation of air in a joint until an adjustment/manipulation or stretch comes along. By creating a movement that opens up the joint, the air finally has enough space to release and then the infamous "pop" is heard. Think of opening a bottle of soda. When you give the air inside the bottle a place or way to escape, it makes a popping sound.

2. The second time that you hear a pop is when you have created enough movement in a joint where a tight or shortened muscle that is caught or stuck behind a bony growth or bump finally gets stretched enough to pass over the bump and slaps down onto the bone (Figure 38-2).

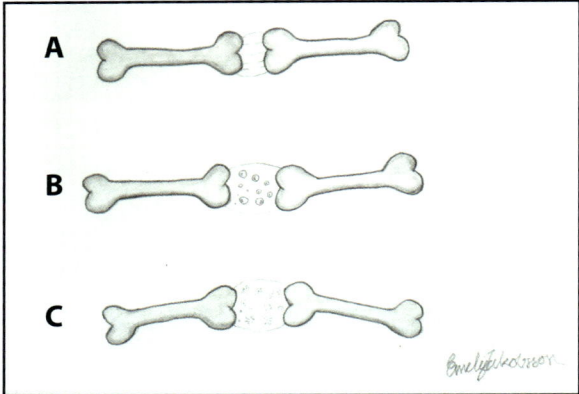

Figure 38-1. What happens when you hear a joint "pop" just once, and then it does not pop again for minutes or hours? The obvious example is your knuckles. This same reason applies to the spine or other joints during adjustment. This happens, usually, within a tight joint or one that does not have normal movement. (A) The joint space between the 2 bones starts to open. (B) Air bubbles appear. (C) When the joint finally opens enough, the air suddenly escapes and you hear a blunt pop. Think of what happens when you open a can of soda "pop." Trapped air suddenly escapes. (Illustrated by Emelie Jakobson.)

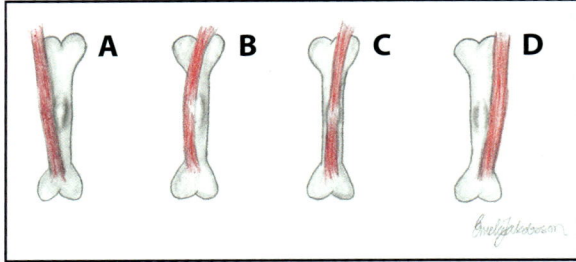

Figure 38-2. Here is the second type of "pop," the one you get when you move muscle, ligament, or other soft tissue over any sort of ridge. For example, when a muscle gets "tight" from being over- or underused, it gets "caught" on one side of a bump. This type of adjustment pop comes from the muscle traversing from one side of the bump to another. This pop happens outside of a joint, and, unlike the pop in Figure 38-1, you can reproduce this pop repeatedly. (A) Muscle on one side of a bony ridge. (B) Muscle starts to bend around the bony bump, building up pressure at this point, and possibly causing mild discomfort. (C) The muscle finally passes over the bump. (D) The muscle has now "slapped down" on the other side, often producing some relief. (Illustrated by Emelie Jakobson.)

BACK TO THE FOOT

Now that we have cleared up what happens during an adjustment, let's take a look at "Dem Bones" again to see how the most common non-core injuries can cause core muscle injuries, and how core muscles can cause non-core injuries. Once we know this, we know what needs to be done to fix these injuries utilizing our nonsurgical methods.

Let's start with a common foot injury, and then work our way to the core. Every year, more than 2 million people are treated for plantar fasciitis. This common injury is caused when the muscles of the foot fail to support your arch and the foot falls inward. This collapse causes the fascia tissue on the bottom of the foot to pull at its attachment sites on the foot. This pulling causes irritation of the foot and eventually creates a change in the way that a person will walk to avoid the pain.

Guess what happens next? The body starts to compensate for this new movement and that pesky kinematic chain kicks into high gear. People who experience plantar fasciitis often avoid walking on the inside of their foot so they hobble along the outside portion of their foot. Since the foot is not used in the way that it was intended, the body compensates by walking gingerly, and loads the core muscles to swing the leg in a shortened range of motion instead of bending at the hip.

One of the main muscles that gets affected by this change is the iliopsoas or, as they are better known, the hip flexors. These muscles are the main lifters of the leg. Remember the saying: If you don't use it, you lose it? Well, if you don't use the range of motion of the hip, you lose the motion of the hip. Since the hip flexors lift the leg at the hip, their range of motion is crucial for normal function. If they are tight or short and then stretched out through movement, they pull on their attachment sites, which are at the low back and the thigh. When a physician looks to fix hip flexor pain, he/she needs to not only fix the hip flexor itself, but also correct the problem that initially caused the injury, which, in this example, is the foot. Without proper care, the patient will have temporary relief of symptoms in the hip flexors, but will remain more prone to future injuries in that same area because the actual cause of the pain was never addressed.

If we stay focused on the same area of core muscle and foot injuries, we can look at the same condition chain, but work in reverse. In the case of a damaged or injured core muscle, a patient can develop plantar fasciitis. When a patient has tight or restricted muscles in the glutes, his/her foot is rotated to the side. This rotation doesn't just affect the foot. It also affects the groin muscles, the knee, and the foot.

Some of the more common injuries that occur because of this rotation are groin pulls or tears, knee arthritis, and plantar fasciitis, to name a few. The reason why you can develop plantar fasciitis with restricted muscles in the glutes is pretty simple when you look at the mechanics of the foot and ankle.

The foot is intended to move in an up-and-down motion like you are pressing the gas pedal in a car. When you move your foot in this motion, the muscles on the bottom of the foot are contracted and nicely developed. When you stop using your foot in this manner, your muscles weaken and fail to hold the arch of your foot. (Just a brief side note, another big contributor of plantar fasciitis is footwear, because it changes the way you activate the muscles of the foot.) Now back to our injury, the position of having a nice arch creates slack in the plantar fascia. When your arch collapses, the foot actually gets longer, which, in turn, pulls onto the attachment sites of the plantar fascia.

Now to the Elbow

As you saw in both of these examples, the core muscles and foot are intimately tied together, yet you may be asking yourself: But what about muscles of the elbow? This joint cannot develop an injury because of the muscles of the core... right?

Well, guess again. Of course it can, and because we can use the kinematic chain, again it will make sense.

Let's take a look at the motion of a pitcher in baseball and see how a core muscle can create elbow problems. One of the more common injuries of professional or collegiate baseball pitchers is a tear of the ligament in the inside of their elbow joint (the ulnar collateral ligament). A tear of this tendon often leads to a procedure called *Tommy John surgery*. So how do our core muscles cause a tear in the elbow?

Well, before I address that, I need to teach you about a baseball term called a *slot angle*. The slot angle is the position of the shoulder joint during the motion of a pitch. Most pitchers have different slot angles, but the lower the slot angle the more likely the pitcher is to tear this ligament.

Now is about the time where you begin asking yourself, so how do my core muscles change a slot angle? Well, one of the main reasons that a pitcher's slot angle changes is because the hips have decreased their ability to rotate. When the muscles of the gluteal area become tight, they rotate the foot outward, just as they do for people who develop plantar fasciitis. This increase in outward rotation reduces the ability for the hips to rotate inward.

A pitcher gains most of his/her pitch speed and momentum from his/her core muscles. Rotation of the core starts the motion of a pitch, and for the most part, the arm follows through like a whip. If the core muscles don't function as well as they should, the pitcher has to compensate in one way or another. More times than not, the compensation that occurs is that the slot angle lowers, and an increase in stress develops on the inside of the elbow joint. Over time, this stress loads the ligament more and more, and then so much that it eventually tears or rips right off of the bone.

When it comes time to preventing elbow problems, it is crucial to focus on the core so that the same bad habits or restrictions don't develop again.

An ounce of prevention is worth a pound of cure.
—Philadelphian Benjamin Franklin wrote this under an assumed name about fire safety—
not health care, as commonly believed.

THE MODERN CHIROPRACTOR

Now that we have seen 3 different core/non-core muscular injuries, let's spend some time on how a modern chiropractor (manual physician) can help with prevention and recovery. It's important to remember that old saying displayed above. Those 10 little words are some of the most true and understated words in medicine today. In the world of physical medicine, what that means is, if you are willing to do a little work up front to prevent an injury, you will save yourself a lot of work recovering from one.

Patients are often surprised with how much work it takes to recover from a surgery. I try to stress the importance of preventative medicine because, as most people learn, surgery is just the beginning of the recovery process. Some surgeries take weeks to recover from, whereas others take upward of a year. Don't you think that, in general, trying a course of 1 to 2 weeks of nonoperative treatments is worth a shot, before you go down the surgical path that could take months? I do!

WAYS TO PREVENT INJURY

Now, let's take a look at some of the best ways to prevent core muscle injuries. When we take a look at the 3 examples that I mentioned earlier in the chapter, there are 2 primary things that would have helped prevent the injuries: (1) proper muscular use and (2) proper muscle health.

Remember how I referenced the first 24 hours of having an injury? Well, this is where the body has begun to learn a new firing pattern to avoid the pain or to compensate for a weak muscle. These changes over time feel normal but they start to create problems in joints as well as in the muscles that move the joints.

Unfortunately, this compensation creates stresses in new tissues and joints, which ultimately develop scar tissue. Scar tissue both reduces ranges of motion and increases pain. Since these 2 areas of dysfunction cause the highest amount of injuries, let's try to fix them. When we try to fix an improperly functioning core muscle, pelvic muscle, leg, or even toe, we **must** remember "Dem Bones" and the kinematic chain. In order to fix the imbalance, we need to change the way that the tissue is functioning. We do this by increasing a person's proprioception. "Proprio what?" you may be saying? You read me right…proprioception.

Let's calm down and let me explain what proprioception is.

It's the ability to control movement in an area of your body. For example, someone who has bad proprioception has difficulty touching his/her finger to his/her nose or standing on one leg. Someone with good proprioception can hop on one leg while juggling chainsaws. The reason that bad proprioception can cause a core muscle injury is that you aren't or can't control the body in the way that it should, or is intended to, work.

The body is very much a machine with respect to how it uses bones, muscles, and joints to accomplish a very specific motion. If the angle of a motion for a joint is off by only a few degrees and you repeat that motion over and over and over, then you will develop an uneven wearing of that joint, and eventually develop arthritis or a muscular tear.

With regard to scar tissue, the cycle works a little different. To help understand how scar tissue develops, let's use another example. Try making a fist, and now imagine that your fist is actually a muscle. Do you think that blood can penetrate deeper into a loose fist or a tightly clinched one? A loose one, right?

Well, your muscles aren't too different from this. When a muscle is tight because of overuse or improper use, it gets tighter and tighter. Sometimes, they feel knots or "trigger points." These knots do not allow blood to penetrate easily into them, so a condition of decreased oxygen delivery occurs. (Don't forget that blood is what carries oxygen to a muscle.) When a muscle senses that it is not getting enough blood, probably because it is being overused, it calls to the body for help and the body responds by sending scar tissue to that area of the body.

The scar tissue starts to work overtime and grabs onto anything and everything that it can to hold that muscle in place. Since they body thinks that the scar tissue is needed and because scar tissue is a naturally occurring event, the body never removes it once it is there. That means, that unless you do something like PATCH technique (we will get to PATCH in the next paragraph) to remove the scarring, it is there to stay, and like I mentioned earlier, scar tissue doesn't move well and causes a lot of pain. Some great methods of managing healthy proprioception are physical therapy, yoga, or Pilates. The Vincera Institute is lucky to have highly skilled therapists and instructors who know how to greatly increase the body's movement and function.

Addressing the scar tissue is where I come in. In order to be able to properly move in physical therapy or yoga, a patient needs to be able to get into the proper positions. Unless scarring is removed prior to movement, the patient will only get flexible in his/her healthy tissue instead of in his/her damaged or scarred tissue. I utilize a proprietary technique called the *PATCH technique*. The PATCH technique is a nonsurgical, hands-on method of breaking up scar tissue by utilizing specific movements and hand contacts.

This method quickly, and thoroughly, breaks up scar tissue to restore proper blood flow and body function. The other great thing about the PATCH technique is its ability to not only fix damaged tissue but its ability to prevent scarring as well. Remember, as the body gets overused or improperly used, it tries to help with the use of scar tissue. With the PATCH technique, I can continually ensure proper blood supply and muscular movement. By addressing these factors in a proactive manner, I can keep the professional or amateur athlete out of pain for an extended period of time.

SUMMARY

When the proper chiropractic and hands-on methods are used in conjunction with other surgical or nonsurgical procedures, patients should recover from injuries in a significantly expedited time frame. Just remember "Dem Bones" when you start to feel any aches and pains around your body. And ask yourself, "Is this painful because I injured it, or is it sore because of something else going on in my body?"

SELECTED READINGS

Myers TW. *Anatomy Trains: Myofascial Meridians for Manual and Movement Therapists.* 3rd ed. New York, NY: Elsevier; 2014.
   This book does a great job showing how so many of our muscles or body parts connect through movement. If you want to check out how a foot injury contributes to future pelvic injuries, this book is a great read.

Perry J, Burnfield J. *Gait Analysis: Normal and Pathological Function.* 2nd ed. Thorofare, NJ: SLACK Incorporated; 2010.
   I really like this book because of how well it breaks down movement. Injuries often come about because of dysfunction in one part of the body triggering compensation or pain in another. Gait analysis helps you see how the body should move and, therefore, what to correct when there are discrepancies.

REFERENCE

1. Hallett M. Neuroplasticity and rehabilitation. *J Rehabil Res Dev.* 2005;42(4):xvii-xxii.

VIDEO

1. https://www.youtube.com/watch?v=pYb8Wm6-QfA

section **five**

life is a **journey***

*from "Life is a journey and not a destination," attributed to Transcendentalist poet
Ralph Waldo Emerson and revisited by AM O'Shea, a very smart CEO

39

putting it **all** together
a **patient's perspective** on the core

Esra Roan, PhD

Editor's Note: *Totally unsolicited, one of my patients, a biomedical engineer, requested to contribute to this book. She wrote me this note:*

"Dr. Meyers, during one of our many conversations, I heard that you were writing a book on the core. As you know, I am an associate professor in biomedical engineering, and I came to your practice through extensive scientific search and a healthy dose of serendipity. I think patients deserve better, and perhaps an easier route to a diagnosis! I would love to put this all together from a patient's perspective. I have come across so many women that complain about similar problems. I strongly believe that this may affect many people who travel in circles trying to get a diagnosis on their lower abdominal pains. Even though I personally am very vocal about my experience, having this written may help patients, physicians, and physical therapists in how they approach a patient like me."

I did not refuse the request.

The greatest evil is physical pain.

—Saint Augustine (354-430 AD).

It seems that I had been dealing with this pelvic injury for nearly 15 years!

Recently, I heard Dr. Meyers was writing this book, so I asked him if I could contribute a chapter. Over the years, when I shared my experiences with other women, I heard many of them say that they knew someone with a similar experience. People need to know about this new evolving field. It bridges medicine and health.

In this chapter, I will present my personal experience of what I shall now call *core pain* from its early onset to postsurgical recovery. The road was very long. At times, there was no hope!

Please bear with me. I want to tell this story. I think it is important and you may know someone who is experiencing it.

MY STORY

Over the past few years, much press has surfaced about famous quarterbacks, elite hockey players, and world-class pitchers with some sort of hip, "sports hernia," athletic pubalgia, or other problem, and they all somehow seem to get fixed. That publicity is probably what kept my ears open to the possibility that I might have a fixable problem.

I now have to ask: What happens to those who are not elite athletes, but may be suffering from core muscle injuries?

This is my story. After you read it, I want you all to ask that same question.

Tennis Days

I was a high-performing tennis player. I played for the national team of my home country Turkey and in some professional tournaments as well. I decided to pursue a collegiate career and played for a small college—Tennessee Technological University (Cookeville, Tennessee). We played hard, and our seasons were long. I was able to get a top 50 NCAA Division I ranking once. In other words, I played a lot of tennis when I was young and got injured a lot as well. During my teenage years, I complained of back pain, while during college years more injuries piled on. But, my desire to maintain rankings and scholarship never allowed me really to take proper care of my body.

Sometime during my senior year in college, I began to have lower abdominal pain and complained of this to the team physician. Being a female athlete, I was immediately referred to an OB/GYN and was placed on hormonal drugs with the thought that I had endometriosis. Then, the first laparoscopy came, which did not alleviate the pain, so the physician suggested removal of my left ovary: I was 22!

I walked out hastily, went to a second physician, and had another laparoscopic surgery within a year of the first one.

In both circumstances, the physicians found low levels of endometriosis not commensurate with the level of symptoms I experienced. I went through my senior year of tennis with the same lower abdominal pain, but also experienced a serious shoulder injury, so I sat out a few months, and complained less of the abdominal pain. Afterward, I stopped playing for a while.

Pregnancies…Endometriosis

The next phase of lower abdominal pain (which never went away in the first place) began to creep into my life postpregnancy in 2004. This time, I met an endocrinologist who did another laparoscopic surgery (my third!) before pregnancy and again confirmed that I had minimal levels of endometriosis. Once I was pregnant, I stopped chasing answers to my abdominal pain problems. However, my son Ben was born after a nearly 36-hour labor that ended with an emergency cesarean section. I remember, once I recovered from the procedure, my abdominal pain immediately flared up and I was at my doctor's office.

At this time, she was convinced it was something other than endometriosis, and she sent me to a specialist acupuncturist and also a pelvic floor physical therapist. Both of these people were instrumental for me to understand that my problems were not necessarily related to OB/GYN or gastroenterology fields. It was unfortunate that I moved to Memphis, Tennessee, at about the time that we were probably approaching a diagnosis. Also, I was expecting my second child.

Once I gave birth to my second son, I decided it was time now to become active again. It was 2007. I began running, swimming, and playing mild levels of tennis. Immediately, my left hip got inflamed, and I showed up at the local orthopedic physician's office. I was diagnosed with bursitis. A nurse walked in with a big needle, and I walked out refusing this treatment. I knew somehow that everything was tied together, but did not know how. I decided to rest.

A few years ago, again I decided that it was time to become active again. I started playing tennis, swimming, and running. Needless to say, 3 to 6 months into it, I was again in pain and could not continue with any exercise.

It is important to note that each time I started over with exercise, I did it at a reduced level, and despite that the pain worsened. In the last trial, I was unable to build up enough strength or courage even to jog. At this time, I was extremely frustrated and depressed. The pain was present not only during limited exercise, but my daily life also was being impacted. I did not know where to go, but I knew I had a serious chronic pain problem that was making life difficult for both my family and me.

More Doctor Specialists

When the pain was so bad that I actually made a visit to the ER, I decided to begin the same process that I went through in Cincinnati, Ohio, with OB/GYN, gastroenterology, etc. Late in 2012, I was put on hormonal therapy to see if it would help, thinking again that it was endometriosis. This was not helping and I refused to take the sixth month dose, since I was knowledgeable of the side effects of these drugs. During this time, I was sent to a GI specialist and also to a urologist. I underwent a colonoscopy and endured every test in the world that one can have done, and no definitive diagnosis emerged. In the end, all physicians looked at me and I felt as though they wanted me to go away. I was left with a lot of pain and no help. The only person who was again providing some help in the form of pain relief with myofascial release treatments was the pelvic floor therapist. She was also the one to say for the first time that I had a "defect" for sure in the abdomen and potentially pelvic floor.

The Lightbulb

During the latest cycle of treatments, I became even more frustrated, and partially from the statements being made by my physical therapist, I began reading voraciously. I ran across research papers talking about chronic pelvic floor pain, "athletic pubalgia," pelvic floor muscle issues, etc.[1,2] My therapist and I would share the articles and talk about them during my sessions. During this time, I remember a lightbulb going off in my head and thinking these articles describe my symptoms. Could I have this? I contacted a hip surgeon whom I know from work and inquired about the plausibility of my conclusion. I asked him for a referral to the orthopedic surgeon in town who treats the most athletes. Five minutes into that appointment, the physician was convinced that I probably had this condition and he referred me to a hernia specialist to rule out actual hernia. Then came more diagnostic imaging!

But, finally, I was in the hands of 2 savvy surgeons who knew something about the abdomen and pelvis. Dr. Guy Voeller knew that these were not hernia issues and also knew that most general surgeons tried to treat them that way. I am not sure he knew what the problem was exactly, but he knew where to send me. He and my other physicians in Memphis referred me to Dr. Meyers in Philadelphia, Pennsylvania.

My Symptoms

So, what were my symptoms that made it so difficult to diagnose?

My symptoms went from mild in 1998 to severe in the fall of 2013. They began with mild abdominal pain. I cannot recall whether it impacted my tennis performance, but I remember having pain. After my first pregnancy, I knew muscles were involved, because every time I sneezed or laughed, I began experiencing abdominal cramps. Another symptom for me was related to the joint laxity in the pelvic region, which represented itself when I began to play tennis at very low intensity in 2005. When I would run-stop-return (ie, change directions on the court), I began to feel laxity in my pubic area and also spasms in the pelvic floor muscles (Figure 39-1).

Transitioning from pain during exercise to pain during daily life occurred after 2007 (ie, after the birth of my second son). Until then, I experienced a low level of abdominal pain (2 to 4 out of 10) depending on the time of day. Sometime during 2008 and on, as I attempted to get more active, the pain levels during off times increased. I began to struggle sitting down for prolonged periods of time, and as my abdominal muscles began to spasm, I began to take more over-the-counter pain medication during this period, and it helped.

During the final stages, which began with an episode of trochanteric (hip) bursitis, I was unable to focus on my work and get any relief from over-the-counter pain medication. I experienced a high level of pain (9 out of 10) on the lateral side of the left hip, and I even felt feverish. Once the bursitis subsided, I struggled on a regular basis with lateral hip pain on the left in addition to abdominal spasms. Another symptom that began creeping in at this stage was a feeling of a bruised pubic symphysis. The levels of chronic pain did increase to the point where over-the-counter medications did not relieve pain.

Sleep has always been difficult with this condition. However, it was not until the latter phases that, even with pain medications, I could find a comfortable position to sleep. During the final stages, I would wake up in the middle of the night with abdominal spasms as I changed directions. These were always very painful episodes.

In the end stage, between the core injury diagnosis in May 2013 and the surgery in December 2013, my symptoms worsened drastically. The symptoms became more hip-related than abdominal or core muscle-related. In less than 5 minutes of walking, I would begin to feel a very sharp pain deep and lateral in my thigh that I was supposing was my hip. That would result in my eyes tearing up. About the time of surgery, I could not complete my lectures, which were 90 minutes in length, standing up. At the end of the day, the location where the left hamstring attached to the hip would be in so much pain that, again, I struggled with sleep and virtually every other activity relating to daily life.

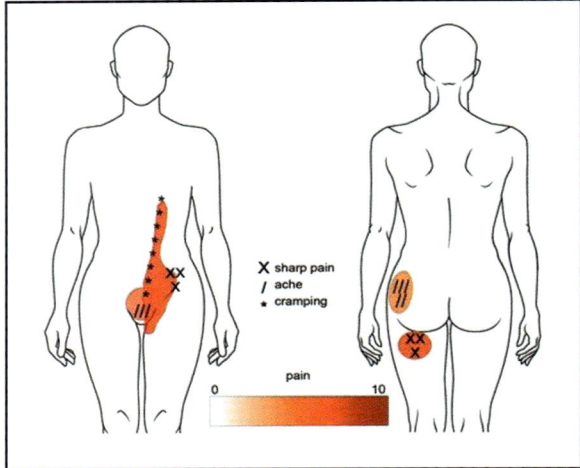

Figure 39-1. My symptoms progressed from being vague and almost tolerable to severe and continuous cramps aggravated by coughing and sneezing.

The Diagnosis

I first had a consultation and in-office examination with Dr. Meyers in May 2013. I presented him my history, and I remember very clearly that he listened for about 15 minutes. This was a first for me, as I always struggled to get physicians to listen to my story. After examination, he said that I probably had a core muscle injury, but I would need diagnostic imaging to fully confirm this. He suspected the hip was also involved. Moreover, he also pointed out that hip pathology was often encountered in this situation and that I should consider a hip arthrogram and MRI. So, I scheduled another trip from Memphis to Philadelphia in June 2013 to get the hip and lower abdominal imaging done. The diagnostic imaging revealed that I had core muscle injuries and hip impingement with labral tears. I was diagnosed at last!

Surgeries

Once I was diagnosed with core muscle and hip pathologies, I was offered multiple avenues to repair these conditions. One alternative was to have 2 surgeries—repair the core muscles and hip separately.

Another option was to wait until the Vincera Institute opened its doors and have the 2 surgeries done together—what they call a *combination surgery*, during which 2 surgeons operate to repair the core muscles and hip at once. Based on my condition in June, I opted for the latter. However, the December 5th date of surgery could not have come sooner, because my symptoms worsened dramatically.

First Surgery

I underwent a combination surgery on December 5, 2013, at the Vincera Institute. Dr. Struan Coleman was the hip surgeon, while Dr. Meyers repaired the core muscles. The surgery went uneventfully, though the 2 surgeons found a substantial amount of damage in soft tissue surrounding the hip and in core muscles. During the surgery, the rectus abdominis, psoas tendon, round ligament in the hip, and hip labrum were all repaired. The bruised feeling of the pubic symphysis was related to the muscles tearing the fibrocartilage cover off the pubic bone (what most people call "osteitis pubis"). Dr. Meyers did inject some steroid between the bone and the cover so that the fluid would decrease and allow the cover to seal back quicker. Multiple muscle groups, including adductors and psoas, were repaired, loosened, or lengthened. Both cam and pincer lesions were taken down. In addition, a small, totally coincidental inguinal hernia was also found and repaired. The silver lining in all of this was that there was no damage to the cartilage in the joint.

Opposite Side Symptoms

As I went through physical therapy, my physical therapist asked me to do lunges about 3 to 4 months out. I remember going down and not being able to get up with a pain in my right (the opposite) hip. So, I utilized the check-up for the left surgery, and talked to both physicians about the right side. Because of the facilities, I was able to undergo an arthrogram on the spot before my flight to Memphis at 5pm! It was clear that I had the same type of issues on the right side, but with symptoms that were not as intrusive of my daily life. I remember asking Dr. Coleman, "How long do I have before I need surgery?" He answered: "Come back in 3 months."

This is where it got very complex for me. I knew if I waited long, I risked getting to the end stage of excessive pain, but more importantly, I was concerned about cartilage damage. So, I began to make plans for the surgery. Here is the main caveat: Not expecting that I would need another surgery, my husband and I chose an insurance plan that was not as good as the previous year. Considering the travel, cost of surgery, cost of rehabilitation, and in- and out-of network benefits, I began to worry very much about the cost of the second surgery. My husband and I researched the cost-effectiveness of the second surgery and tried to navigate the insurance world. I knew I wanted to have this surgery done as soon as I could and prevent further damage, so we moved ahead.

On July 17, 2014, I underwent the second combination surgery involving the right hip. The findings were very similar to the left, but definitely less severe. Again, I had hip labral repair and core muscle repairs, as well as repairs and compartmental releases (like a fasciotomy) of the adductors and psoas muscles as well as the pubic bone surgery. Again, there was no damage to the hip cartilage, which again made the whole experience worthwhile.

Cycling the Day After Surgery

At the end of both surgeries I went to my hotel room and began ice treatments immediately. I remember thinking before the surgery, "How will I be able to apply ice in this spot?" The new high-end icing equipment makes it very easy. Following both surgeries, I spent the first 24 hours in the sleeves of the icing systems, in which the machine activated every 30 minutes.

The doctors and the therapists ask you to get on a stationary bike the day after the surgery. After the first one this was difficult, as I was feeling weak and sick, due to lack of appetite. I was already a pro at that after the second one, and getting on the bike for 10 minutes was no problem. Both surgeries took place on a Thursday. I returned to Memphis on Tuesday and Sunday after the first and second surgeries, respectively. Although I attempted to get direct flights both times, during the first surgery, a major snowstorm caused us to have a difficult trip back through Atlanta, Georgia.

Before I had the first surgery, I searched for a physical therapist in Memphis who would be willing to work with me and made an appointment in advance. When I got back from Philadelphia to Memphis, I went to see the local physical therapist and began therapy immediately. Although the Vincera Institute provides guidance and answers any questions that arise, having a very good and creative physical therapist made the recovery a lot better. For example, he suggested that I begin with water therapy the first week, and this really helped. Later, he found additional exercises and his weekly check-ups led me to change my routines according to guidelines. My local physical therapist also suggested numerous resources for me to read and listen to as I rehabilitated. We also read some interesting articles together.[3,4]

After the first surgery, I was on 2 crutches for 3 weeks and a single one until the sixth week postoperation. In contrast, after the second one, I was down to a single crutch within 10 days and soon after no crutches. I think that the level of pain and damage was lower on the right side, and that led to a faster short-term recovery.

The series of exercises that are prescribed are focused greatly on the core muscles and the muscles that surround the hip. Many exercises are challenging, and I went through routines at least 3 times a week. My visits to physical therapy that were spaced 2 weeks apart after 3 months served as check-ups and provided time to discuss the assignments of new exercises. Even though I felt the progress every week, the check-ups helped with finding the muscle groups that need to be worked on and that I may have omitted.

SOME PARTING THOUGHTS

I still consider myself to be very lucky.

I was able to get to the bottom of this unexplained lower left quadrant pain that was chronic and worsening over the years (Figure 39-2). Moreover, I had the means to go to Philadelphia and undergo the surgeries. It is really important to note that insurance companies do not cover the core muscle injury repair. It is ironic that they covered every diagnostic test and treatment that I was prescribed in the prior 12 years of searching for diagnosis! Imagine that they still call these surgeries "experimental"!

Even as I do a literature survey today while I am writing, I see mostly "elite athletes" and "high-performing athletes" in the titles of scientific publications relating to this topic. What about people like me? Was I an elite athlete? No. Was I a good tennis player? Yes. Did I practice a lot? Yes. When I was seeking diagnosis, was I an athlete? NO! It becomes my, the patient's responsibility almost to self-diagnose by pulling all the information together. This is why maybe there are books on hip impingement, for example, *The Entrepreneurial Patient* (http://theentrepreneurialpatient.com). I always think that I got lucky, since my research is in the field of biomechanics of soft tissue, and I regularly read scientific publications. But then, how can a patient who is not a researcher get diagnosed?

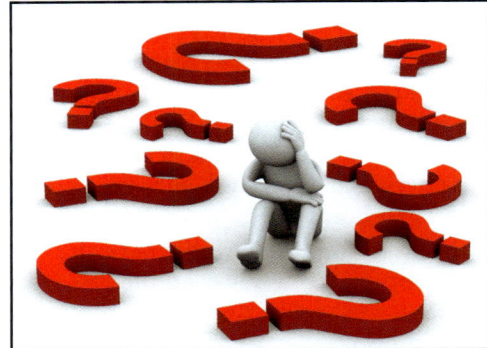

Figure 39-2. I felt so alone and had so many unanswered questions.

The source of lower left quadrant pain was difficult to diagnose for multiple reasons.

There is also a big picture issue here relating to health care of collegiate athletes. A recent study by Simon and Docherty looked at the health-related quality of life in former Division I athletes and showed that they have worse eventual outcomes than the rest of the population when it comes to physical function, depression, fatigue, etc.[5] The authors suggest that the price that many athletes pay is high for the short athletic careers in college.

The broader conversation relating to this will be ongoing, but I would like also to speculate whether this is partly because some of our lingering musculoskeletal issues go undiagnosed for so long?

If you find yourself midlife in similar pain, choose wisely and research extensively! There are not many physicians in the world who know how to repair core muscle injuries. Find a center or a surgeon who does many of these on an ongoing basis. Do not underestimate your chronic pain, it wears you down. At first sight, the quote "The greatest evil is physical pain" seems a bit extreme, but once you have a chronic pain situation, then you realize how true this is! So, take care of yourself.

Those who know me personally are aware of my long history of this issue and also know that I am usually very open about my experience. I suspect that there are a lot of women, and men, who are out there with unexplained abdominal pain. I hope that what I am presenting here may trigger some people to think about the possibility of having a core muscle problem—or a subtle hip problem or both—especially if there is athletic history.

SELECTED READINGS

Lester D. *da Vinci's Ghost: The Untold Story of Vitruvian Man.* London, United Kingdom: Profile Books; 2011.
  Vitruvian man is da Vinci's most famous drawing, and the sketch depicts the pubic bone or an area just above it as the center of our body. Appreciating this fact leads to an understanding of the core and the problems I suffered. The author examines the forces that converged in 1940 to turn an idea that had been around for centuries into this iconic image.

REFERENCES

1. Chaitow L. Chronic pelvic pain: pelvic floor problems, sacro-iliac dysfunction and the trigger point connection. *Journal of Bodywork and Movement Therapies.* 2007;11:327-339.
2. Meyers WC, Kahan DM, Joseph T, et al. Current analysis of women athletes with pelvic pain. *Med Sci Sports Exerc.* 2011;43(8):1387-1393.
3. Pope D. Physio Edge Podcast 11. Hamstring tendinopathy with Dr. Alison Grimaldi. 2012. Accessed September 26, 2016.
4. Pope D. Physio Edge Podcast 9. Lateral hip pain with Dr. Alison Grimaldi. 2012. Accessed September 26, 2016.
5. Simon JE, Docherty CL. Current health-related quality of life in former National Collegiate Athletic Association Division I collision athletes compared with contact and limited-contact athletes. *J Athl Train.* 2016;51(3):205-212. doi:10.4085/1062-6050-51.4.05.

final chapter
seeing things a **whole new way**

Somewhere over the rainbow, bluebirds fly...if happy little bluebirds fly beyond the rainbow, then why oh why can't I?

—From the 1939 musical comedy-drama fantasy film produced by Metro-Goldwyn-Mayer, *The Wizard of Oz*. Based on a book by Frank Baum, this icon of American popular culture is commonly acclaimed the most watched movie of all time.[VID 1]

DOROTHY

It's one of the most famous moments in movie history.

After viewing Dorothy Gale's dreary Kansas world only in stark black and white and surviving with her the horrible twister that lifted her house off its moorings, we get the reward, the big reveal. The house crashes to the ground, on top of that nasty, stripe-socked Wicked Witch of the East. And Dorothy, having been knocked unconscious by a loose window, awakens to stillness. Gone is the howling terror of the tornado; in its place, a surreal calm.

Dorothy gets out of bed. With her dog, Toto, securely under her arm, she grabs her basket and walks, wide-eyed, to the back door, and throws it open. What she sees changed Hollywood forever: Technicolor (Figure 40-1).

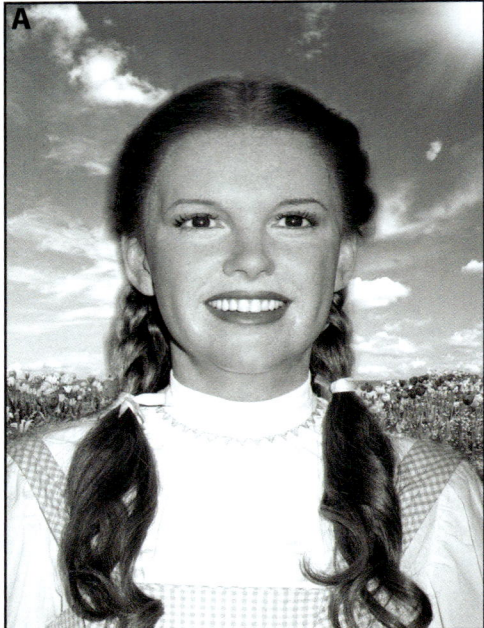 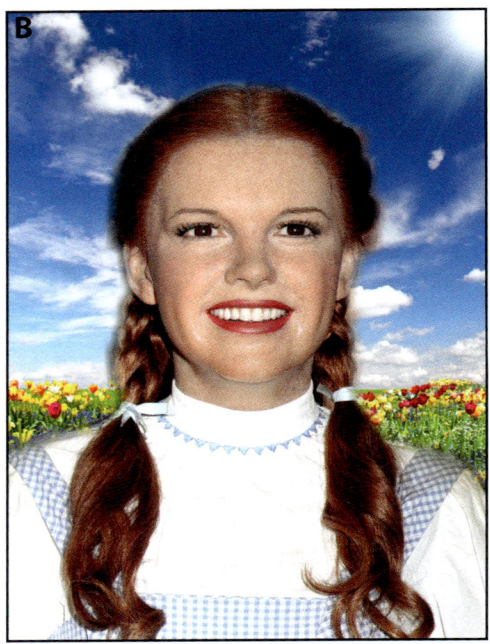

Figure 40-1.

Not just color, but the vivid Technicolor of a wild imagination that creates an impossibly vibrant world. As she enters Oz, Dorothy experiences a world beyond her imagination, so much more than the grim landscape of her home, no matter how much she later yearns to return there. Dorothy has been changed forever, thanks to the sights that she will never forget.[VID 2]

Toto, I've a feeling we're not in Kansas anymore.

—Dorothy, addressing her dog after the tornado as she enters Oz, in the new world of Technicolor.

SURVIVING THE TORNADO

So, too, has the medical world been altered by the ideas and images that precede this final chapter. Old ways have been left behind in a heap, the way we discarded previous thoughts about the sun's orbiting the earth and New Coke. No more shall the medical community even think to call a core injury a "sports hernia," just as no one should ever talk about personal organizers, dial-up modems, or *Caddyshack II*.

Gone are the "old eyes," which had us looking at the body's core in olden ways and treating injuries with methods practically akin to medieval barbers' using leeches to bleed impurities from unfortunate villagers. It's no longer enough to lump all core muscle injuries into one steaming pile or to ignore the impact of a weakened engine room on the rest of the body. Those days are gone. Long gone. (See Figures 40-2 and 40-3.)

Final Chapter—Seeing Things a Whole New Way 431

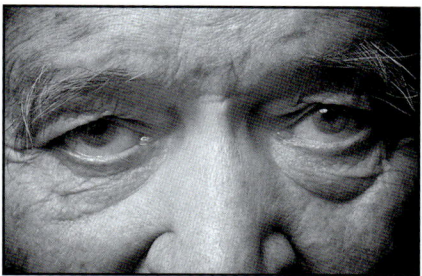

Figure 40-2.

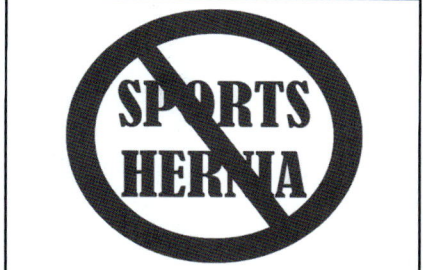

Figure 40-3.

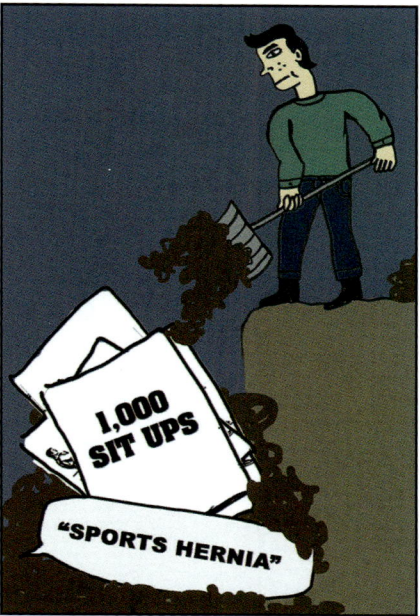

Figure 40-4.

Ding Dong! The Wicked Witch is dead!
—Sung by the Winkies after a Wicked Witch melts away.

That doesn't mean there still aren't troglodytes hiding in caves and refusing to look at the new world. They still use terms like sports hernia to describe core injuries, sounding about as intelligent as 70-somethings talking about the "Internet machine" or that "newfangled rap music." We can try to bury them. But if we can't, let them stay in the dark, although their continued use of old eyes has sometimes-catastrophic impacts on their patients (Figure 40-4).

The real voyage of discovery consists not in seeing new sights, but in looking with new eyes.
—A slightly different translation of the same Marcel Proust quote used to lead off Chapter 2.

THE JOURNEY IN TECHNICOLOR

You, on the other hand, have left the darkness. As did the great trailblazers of mankind, like da Vinci, Einstein, and Elvis, you have joined the vanguard. You also have joined forces with Cinderella, Eminem, and Rodney Dangerfield, at least with respect to the core muscles named after them. The new universe of core understanding and medicine has brought you clear descriptions of the anatomy in a way that allows you to see how it is all interrelated and therefore different than the previous views of the body's most crucial area—brain excluded. (That's pretty vital, too.) (See Figures 40-5 and 40-6.)

What was once thought to be as mysterious as the Bermuda Triangle has been simplified. It all fits together neatly and makes sense now. Imagine that. No more working as if the lights had been turned out.

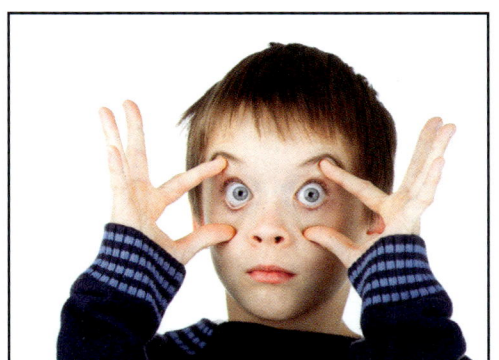

Figure 40-5.

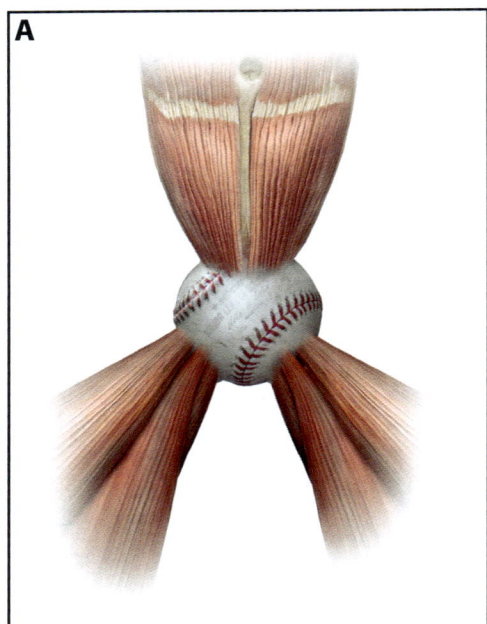
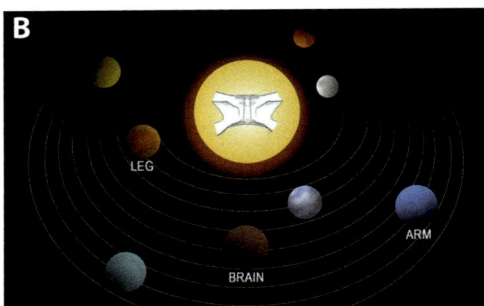

Figure 40-6.

And how about that hip? Until now, nobody knew that it was quite so important to the rest of the body. It has so much to do with the core that it deserves a lot more attention than ever before. Thanks to what's been presented in this book, you'll be certain to provide that consideration. In their chapters, both Byrd and co-editor Philippon give credit for their innovations to Ganz, from Bern, the same town, interestingly, where Albert Einstein linked acceleration and gravity and created his theory of relativity. Perhaps, that's the secret; perhaps, we should all move to Bern.

Pardon us for this, but, wherever you are, you may now officially consider yourself hip to the hip. Feeling good?[VID 3]

There's no place like home. There's no place like home. There's no place like home...
—Dorothy, returning home to Kansas having learned so much from her vibrant journey.

THE PROMISE OF A NEW DAWN

It should feel great. You have learned how to diagnose, treat, repair, rehabilitate, and prevent. It's a continuum on which the entire medical community should travel. Perhaps, you had your own Eureka moment. No doubt, it came after reading one of the chapters of this book. Possibly, it came in a dream*, like it did with Dorothy or Paul McCartney**.

Guaranteeing good core health is a group effort, and those who refuse to collaborate will be operating in a vacuum— and mistreating patients. This is no longer a case of the physicians being the only one who could possibly know what to do. First, do no harm. Then call the yoga studio and make sure your patient can get in for some classes to make sure that psoas muscle injury doesn't recur.

---

*In a cute article advertising the FORTH innovation methodology by Gijs van Wulfen, the polling of 348 managers and professionals revealed dreaming to be the number 2 situation where Aha! moments occur. Interestingly, showering, true to Archimedes, took the number one spot.
**Apparently, McCartney awakened one morning with the tune of the most-recorded song in history, *Yesterday*, in his head. The working title became *Scrambled Eggs*. Fortunately, McCartney had a second Aha! moment later which brought better lyrics.[VID 4]

Three of Dorothy's life lessons—the value of the journey, self-sufficiency, and appreciating home—apply in spades to our journey with the core. Dorothy's route back to Kansas was not simple, even though a simple solution—the red, sparkly shoes—was there from the beginning. She profited from her new eyes, the danger, the Wizard's duplicity, and then his reveal as an ordinary man. She saw right and wrong play out through the witches. She learned to trust herself and what she saw and experienced. With new confidence, she had her Aha! moment and found new eyes and the solution to get back to Kansas. The new sights gave her much more insight, and taught her how to navigate the oft-times treacherous and confusing adult topography.

Likewise, Dorothy learns about self-sufficiency. The Scarecrow, who considers himself brainless, possesses brains. Compassion fills the Tin Man's heart, which, he thinks, is lacking. And the Lion by no means needs courage or nobility. In the same vein, Dorothy already possesses the right shoes to get her back to Kansas. The moral of inner strength prevails.

With her new eyes and sense of self-sufficiency, Dorothy returns home and appreciates that everything, in fact, fits together. The movie began with Dorothy's and Auntie Em's frustrations about whether everyone could live and work together. Em admonishes Dorothy to go "find yourself a place where you won't get into any trouble." Dorothy does that and finds the answer "over the rainbow." It turns out she really doesn't have to look any further than her back yard. The solution lies in the strength, the intricate framework, and the amicable harmony that exists right there.

It just so happens that the same thing holds for the core. With our new eyes open and a more confident appreciation of Bill Belichick's admonition, "It is what it is," we find out it is all about our home, our back and front yards, and everything in the middle. The 4 parts to the core—the back, the hips, the core muscles, and everything else—all live and work together. Our job is to appreciate this more and more, to find out how things work, and to make everything even more harmonious. The core belongs to all of us (Figure 40-7).

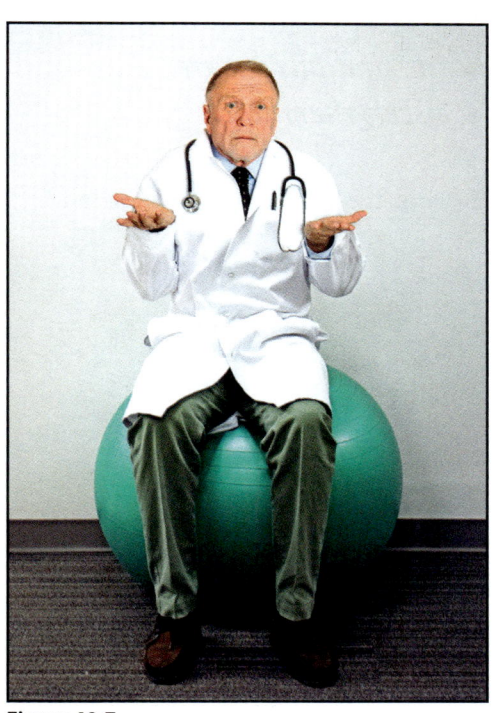

Figure 40-7.

When the whole community works together to ensure good health, society wins. When egos, small minds, and old eyes prevail, it's impossible to complete the job. The goal is performance, whether we're talking about an elite athlete's returning to competition from an injury or a mom's ability to lift her crying 3-year-old and comfort him/her. Those who try to do it alone don't get it. Just as the core is an interrelated collection, so, too, is its treatment a collaborative concern. Continued attention to the body's most important area will minimize future trouble.

Let's not forget the most important part of all this: the patient. Those who choose to adhere blindly to old ways will often be more interested in their own perspective than that of the person whom they are supposed to be treating. It's not about ego. It's not about arguing over whose methods are more successful. The evidence is clear, and you are holding it in your hands. The goal now is to apply it in a way that does the most good for the most people. In other words: make sure your heads never get so far into your gluteus maximi that you stop caring about the patient.

The patient should be the focus. There is no question about that. You have read the case histories about the physical pain and emotional angst people with undiagnosed and mistreated core injuries have endured. They search. They yearn for relief. And that comes only when physicians take the time to address the problem in a thorough and holistic way.

And with new eyes.

It's time for the medical community to open the door and to use those eyes to see what is outside. You can bet that the world looks brilliant, just as Oz did to Dorothy. But while she was discovering a new world and marveling at its wonders, you have been educated fully on the core and its vital role. Step boldly ahead and be among those who are ready to spread the gospel.

It's a new dawn (Figures 40-8 and 40-9). And you're feeling good.^{VID 5}

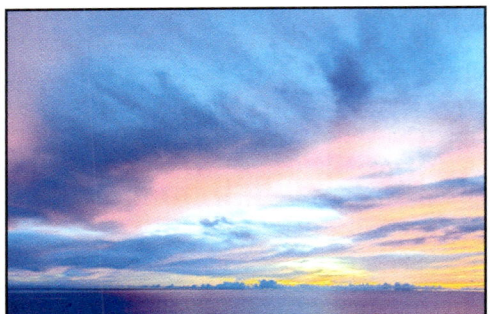

Figure 40-8.

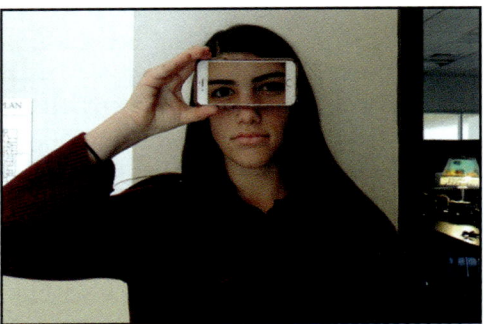

Figure 40-9. Put on your new eyes.

We live in a wonderful world that is full of beauty, charm, and adventure. There is no end to the adventures we can have if only we seek them with new eyes wide open.

—Slight modification of a famous quote from Jawaharlal Nehru, the first Prime Minister of India.

VIDEOS

1. https://www.youtube.com/watch?v=PSZxmZmBfnU
2. https://www.youtube.com/watch?v=x6D8PAGelN8
3. https://www.youtube.com/watch?v=Edwsf-8F3sI
4. https://www.youtube.com/watch?v=btC2_t8HZP4]
5. https://www.youtube.com/watch?v=D5Y11hwjMNs

quiz **answers**

- **Figure 5-24.** Can't tell. Sure he's got a great-looking 6-pack but, as you know, that is just one small piece of the core.
- **Figure 5-25.** Good. Maintaining a seemingly effortless side plank with excellent form takes excellent core strength. This probably means she has a good core.
- **Figure 5-26.** Can't tell. You may have your suspicions, based on age and sagginess, and they may be correct, but... We cannot draw definitive conclusions from the information in this photo.
- **Figure 5-27.** Can't tell. The same logic applies as in the previous answer. Just because you bench-press does not mean you have a good core.

financial disclosures

Dr. James Rheuben Andrews has no financial or proprietary interest in the materials presented herein.

Dr. Enrique Aradillas has no financial or proprietary interest in the materials presented herein.

Dr. Andrew Barr has no financial or proprietary interest in the materials presented herein.

Mr. Michael J. Bradley has no financial or proprietary interest in the materials presented herein.

Dr. Jacqueline M. Brady has no financial or proprietary interest in the materials presented herein.

Ms. Karen K. Briggs has no financial or proprietary interest in the materials presented herein.

Dr. J. W. Thomas Byrd has no financial or proprietary interest in the materials presented herein.

Dr. Struan H. Coleman has no financial or proprietary interest in the materials presented herein.

Dr. Christopher C. Dodson has no financial or proprietary interest in the materials presented herein.

Mr. Rob Gordon has no financial or proprietary interest in the materials presented herein.

Dr. Fares S. Haddad has no financial or proprietary interest in the materials presented herein.

Dr. Jason Hartman has no financial or proprietary interest in the materials presented herein.

Dr. Sarah C. Hoffman has no financial or proprietary interest in the materials presented herein.

Dr. Eugene Hong has no financial or proprietary interest in the materials presented herein.

Dr. Bryan Talmadge Kelly has no financial or proprietary interest in the materials presented herein.

Dr. Philip J. Koehler III has no financial or proprietary interest in the materials presented herein.

Dr. Eric J. Kropf has no financial or proprietary interest in the materials presented herein.

Mr. Michael William Krzyzewski has no financial or proprietary interest in the materials presented herein.

Dr. Marc Legere has no financial or proprietary interest in the materials presented herein.

Ms. Biz Magarity has no financial or proprietary interest in the materials presented herein.

Dr. Hal David Martin has no financial or proprietary interest in the materials presented herein.

Mr. Jim McCrossin has no financial or proprietary interest in the materials presented herein.

Mr. Alex McKechnie has no financial or proprietary interest in the materials presented herein.

Dr. William C. Meyers has no financial or proprietary interest in the materials presented herein.

Dr. William R. Mook has no financial or proprietary interest in the materials presented herein.

Dr. Kevin O'Donnell has no financial or proprietary interest in the materials presented herein.

Dr. Marc J. Philippon has no financial or proprietary interest in the materials presented herein.

Dr. Alexander E. Poor has no financial or proprietary interest in the materials presented herein.

Dr. Anil S. Ranawat has no financial or proprietary interest in the materials presented herein.

Dr. Brian J. Rebolledo has no financial or proprietary interest in the materials presented herein.

Dr. Esra Roan has no financial or proprietary interest in the materials presented herein.

Dr. Johannes B. Roedl has no financial or proprietary interest in the materials presented herein.

Dr. Marc R. Safran has no financial or proprietary interest in the materials presented herein.

Dr. John P. Salvo Jr has no financial or proprietary interest in the materials presented herein.

Dr. Joshua Sampson has no financial or proprietary interest in the materials presented herein.

Mr. Andrew Small has no financial or proprietary interest in the materials presented herein.

Dr. David Stone has no financial or proprietary interest in the materials presented herein.

Dr. Konstantinos Tsitskaris has no financial or proprietary interest in the materials presented herein.

Ms. Tracey Vincel has no financial or proprietary interest in the materials presented herein.

Dr. Veronica Williams has no financial or proprietary interest in the materials presented herein.

Dr. Daniel P. Woods has no financial or proprietary interest in the materials presented herein.

Dr. Feras Ya'ish has no financial or proprietary interest in the materials presented herein.

Dr. Adam C. Zoga has no financial or proprietary interest in the materials presented herein.

index

abdominal bracing exercises, 367-368
abdominal hernias, 9
abdominal muscles, overfocus on, 43-44
abdominal obliques, full-thickness avulsion of, 164
abdominal organs, as pain source, 195
abdominal pain. *See also* pelvic floor pain
    after vomiting, 199-200
    of lower left quadrant, 424-427
acetabular osteotomy, 255
acetabulum
    development of, 210
    early efforts at reshaping, 231
    morphologic variations of, 287
    undercoverage of, 210
    version of, 300-301
ACL injuries, core muscle injuries and, 60-61
acupuncture, 391
adductor brevis, 25, 106
adductor complex, 74
    avulsed, 32

adductor harness avulsion, treatment of, 222-223
adductor longus, 25, 106
    torn and retracted, 115
adductor magnus, 106
    injury of, 115
    muscle belly injuries of, 115
adductor magnus origin avulsions, 315
adductor-plate disruption, natural history of, 113-114
adductor/pubic symphysis disruption, 112
adductor/quadriceps tumor, 159
adductor releases, 107
    anatomy of, 107
adductors, 52-53, 149
    anatomic realities of, 108
    attachments of, 106, 107
    avulsions of, 112-113
    belly strain of, 109
    disorders of, 109-116
    functions of, 105-106
    heterotopic ossification of, 110-111

important facts about, 106-107
injuries to, 106
    repairs of, 106
    strictures of, 108
    tears in, 105
    varieties of, 107
most important, 106
old beliefs about, 107-108
adjustments, 415-416
adolescent athletes, 253-254
adolescents
    hip conditions in, 253-266
    hip dysplasia of, 259
    hip pathologies to consider in, 262
    hip surgery subspecialty for, 255
    history and physical examination of, 256-257
    radiologic assessment of, 257
afferent pathways, 62
agility, pain limiting, 366
aging process, 217-218
anesthetic injection, 391
antalgic gait, 257
anterior impingement test, 288
anterior innominate dysfunction, 410
anterior pelvic tilt, 297
    excessive, 299
apical upper rib breathing, 373
apophyseal avulsions, 259-260
apophysitis
    ASIS, 167
    ischial tuberosity, 167
arm balance posture, 386
arthritis
    of hip, 276
    under- or overestimating effect of in hip arthroscopy, 249
arthro-endoscopic procedures, 272
arthroscopic techniques
    for hip, evolution of, 232-234
    for hip impingement with vulvodynia, 240
    in interest in sports hip disorders, 230
    minimally invasive, 284-285
    for vulvodynia, 241-243
arthroscopic tenotomy, 272
articular cartilage defects, 289
ascites, 158
ASIS apophysitis, 167
athletic pubalgia, 287, 425
    current literature on, 34-35
    landmark article on, 230

athletic trainers
    importance of, 345-346
    right principles of, 349-354
athletic wisdom, 224-225
athleticism, xxiv, 8, 48, 52, 60, 82, 88
autologous chondrocyte implantation, 273
autonomic nervous system, normalization of, 408
avascular necrosis, 174, 284
avidya, 386
avulsions. *See also specific muscles*
    of abdominal obliques, 164
    central, fixing, 222
    partial hamstring, 166
    rectus femoris, 166

back, 45-47
    anatomy of, 370-371
    conceptualizing, 50-51
    definition of, 46
    injuries to, 64
    in literature on core, 395
    muscles of
        spasmodic contractions of, 64
        in stability, 153-154
    in pelvic pain, 171-172
    posterior and, 312
back pain, 195
    in barrel racer, 197-198
    diagnosing, 197-198
back rehabilitation techniques, 395
balance, xxv, 52, 88, 95, 180, 351
balance training, 354, 386, 397, 406
bandhas, 385-386
Baryshnikov, Mikhail, 60
baseball pitcher hockey goalie syndrome, 109-110
    treatment of, 222
Bassett, Frank, 25
Beckenbauer, Franz, injury of, 59-60
belly breathing, 373
biomechanical axis alignment, 317
biomechanics, 296-301
    altered with core muscle injuries, 303-307
    lack of knowledge about, 131-132
    thoracic, 371-372
blood vessels, 205
body transmission, 59-60
bone tumor, pubic, 160
botulinum toxin, 392
brachial plexus, 192
bracing strategies, 367-368

Bradley, James, 7
brain
    connected to core muscles, 414-415
    connecting to harness, 87-88
    core interaction with, 62-63
    in harnessing core power, 53
breathing, 373
    poor patterns of, 373
bridle muscles, 51-52
Brown, Sheldon, core injury of, 6
buttock claudication, 315
buzzwords, 348
Byrd, Jairus, core injury of, 63

cam
    deformity of, 283
    enhancement of, 211
    femoroacetabular impingement with injuries to, 304-305
    impingement of, 210
        arthroscopy for, 289
cam-associated asphericity, 274
cam resections, computerized navigation and robotics for, 270-271
capsular adhesions, after arthroscopy, 289
central core muscle injuries, requiring surgery, 221
central nervous system (CNS)
    facilitation of, 408
    proprioception and, 397
central sensitization, 194
cervical plexus, 192
chakrayoga, 383
charlatans/scammers, in fitness world, 331, 346, 348, 374
cheilectomy, 230
chiropractors
    modern, 418
    perspective of, 415-419
chronic pain syndromes, 205
Clemens, Roger, injury of, 110
"clincher" tests, 189
cognitive function
    diminished with core injuries, 62-63, 363
    harness injuries triggering deficits in, 87
compartment syndrome, rectus femoris, 125
compartmental releases, 106
compensation, 366
    creating new injuries, 418
    for foot injury, 416-417
compensatory injuries, 222
compensatory patterns, 369

complex regional pain syndrome (CRPS), 173, 194, 205
    as mimicker of core injury, 222
compressions, with straight leg raise test, 374
computed tomography (CT), 187
computerized navigation, for cam resections, 270-271
consciousness, higher, 384, 388
Copenhagen Hip and Groin Outcome Score (HAGOS), 353
core
    acting as unit, 8-9, 26-27
    anatomy of, 44-48
    brain in harnessing, 53
    brain interaction with, 12, 62-63
    complexity of, 7, 17
    definition of, 14, 16, 46
    as engine and transmission, 4-5
    as epicenter of body, 11-12
    in everyday life, xxv, 4
    fourth part of, 17, 48
    gender distinctions of, 48-50
    instability of, 150, 395
    need for more studies of, 394-397
    nerves of, 191-200
    organs and systems of, 6, 17
    in power and athleticism, xxiv, 8, 48, 52, 60, 82
    public interest in and commercialization of, 15
    serious problems of, 65
    sports medicine view of, 394
    stability of, 135, 147-155, 367, 373-376, 396-397
    universe of, 204-206
core balance, 366, 369
core bracing myth, 367-368
core development, 207-214
core forces, in women vs men, 50
core injuries, 7. *See also specific injuries*
    assessing outcomes of, 353
    characteristics of, 221
    definition of, 46
    diminished cognition with, 62-63, 87, 363
    fixing, 220
        case examples of, 222-224
        decision-making factors in, 220-221
        guidelines for, 221-222
        when, why, and how, 218
    frequency of, 65-66
    harness, 115
    perfect storm for, 220
    prevention of, 213, 418-419
    serious conditions mimicking, 65
    tricky, diagnosing and managing, 349-350
    when, why, and how to fix, 218

core medicine, 72
core mobility-compression release test, 377
core muscle yoga
    advocate of, 386
    practice example of, 387
core muscles, 45, 47
    anatomy of, ignorance of, 171
    attached to pubic bone, 73
    avulsions of, 3-4
        treatment of, 222-223
    in control of extremities, 60-62
    deep, 375
    definition of, 46
    development of, 211-213
    in femoroacetabular impingement, 249
    foot and knee problems connected to, 414-415
    in gait cycle, 306-307
    hip interaction with, 63
    injuries of
        current literature on, 34-35
        definition of, 46
        diagnosis of, 426
        elbow injuries in, 417
        femoroacetabular impingement and, 234-235, 304-305
        foot injuries in, 416-417
        hip involvement in, 54-55
        new way of viewing, 430-434
        plantar fasciitis with, 417
        prevention of, 418-419
        psoas bursitis with, 136
        recognition of, 230
        seen as sports hernia, 31-34
        surgery for, 219, 426-427
    power, 74
    skeletal, as pain source, 195
    steroid injections into, 222
    surrounding pubic bone, 75
    of thorax, 371
core neutral posture, 21, 354
core pain
    diagnoses to consider in, 185
    history taking for, 184-186
    imaging for, 187-189
    physical examination for, 186
core principles, 180-181
core rehab principles, 351-353
core research, focus of on back pain and rehab, 395
core stability, iliopsoas in, 135
corticosteroid injections, for proximal hamstring avulsion, 340
counterstrain, 400, 409

coxa profunda, 274
coxa recta, 211
coxa rotunda, 211
coxa saltans, classification of, 261-262
crippling injury, 84-85
Crohn's disease
    in groin pain, 174
    with thickening of terminal ileum, 157
    treatment of, 224
Crohn's disease fistula, 65
cryotherapy, 392
Curry, Steph, 61

da Vinci, Leonardo, Vitruvian man, 44, 70
decision-making, 333
decompressions, with straight leg raise test, 374
deep core muscles, tests for, 375
deep core test, 375, 377
deep derrière, 309-311, 324
    anatomic considerations in, 312
    anatomical landmarks of, 311-314
    back and, 312
    pain in
        clinical and imaging features of, 321-322
        diagnostic traps of, 320
        imaging and ancillary tests for, 320
        locating, 314-320
        main disorders of and anatomic associations, 315
        nonoperative treatment of, 320
        patient history of, 314-315
        physical examination for, 317-319
        surgical treatment of, 323-324
        tests for, 316-317
deep gluteal syndrome (DGS), 311, 314-315
    clinical and imaging features of, 321
    vs ischiofemoral impingement, 317-319
deep posterior pelvic muscles, 152-154
deep stabilizers, 371
degeneration, defined, 217
degenerative disc disease, 205
degenerative disease, 234, 249, 254, 258-261
degenerative joint disease, 272, 275-277
degloving quadratus femoris fascial injury, 162
development
    of core, 208-214
    definition of, 208
    embryonic, 208-209
    questions to consider regarding, 213
developmental dysplasia of the hip (DDH)
    definition of, 255
    hip arthroscopy for, 272

diagnosis
    lack of experience in, 171
    universe of, 204-206
diastasis syndromes, 100-101
differential infections, 189
disc extrusion, 163
dissociative movements, 374
dissociative neutral zone test, 374
doctor-parent-child triad, 256
driver, 369
dry needling, 410
dynamic stabilization, 397
dysfunction, common sources of, 404-406
dysplasia, advantages and disadvantages of, 210-211

early activation, 351
efferent pathway, 62
elbow injuries, core muscle problems in, 417
electromyography (EMG), for deep derrière pain, 320
embryonic development, 208-209
    of core muscles, 211-213
    of femur and other pelvic bones, 209-210
    similarities of to evolutionary process, 211
empiricism, 8, 10, 170
    pros and cons of, 247
endometriosis, 65, 174, 424-425
endoscopic techniques
    for ischiofemoral impingement, 323
    for posterior pain issues, 323-324
epigastric artery pseudoaneurysm, 174
epigastric artery syndrome, 101
Erector Set model, 54-55
Eureka moments, 22-25
evaluation
    clinical knowledge needed in, 414
    diagnoses to consider in, 185
    general surgeon's approach, 184
    history taking in, 184-186
    imaging in, 187-189
    orthopedic surgeon's approach, 184
    physical contact in, 186
    physical examination in, 186
    practice problems of, 175-177
    specialists' approach, 184
evolutionary process, 70-71
    similarities to embryological processes, 211-212
exercise
    choosing proper system of, 354
    harmful, 331
    importance of, 9
experience, importance of, 331
experimental procedures, 218

external rotation, excessive, 257
extracorporeal shock wave therapy, 392
extremities, control of, 60-62

FABER test, 199, 257, 316, 404
FADIR test, 199, 404
failed load transfer, 369
false axis, 369
femoral head
    early efforts at reshaping, 231
    fractures of, 275
    ossification of, stages of, 209
femoral neck
    isthmus growth plate of, 209-210
    osteochondroplasty of cam resection of, 270
    stress fracture of, 163
    version of in ischiofemoral impingement, 312
femoroacetabular impingement (FAI), 108
    in adolescents, 261
        case study of, 265-266
        mixed-type, 265-266
    arthroscopy for, 291
    bad hip anatomy in, 281-282
    with cam lesions, 304-305
    categories of, 210
    causes and implications of, 291
    clinical presentation and exam of, 288-290
    core muscle injuries and, 234-235, 304-305
    current concepts about, 287
    effect of on gait cycle, 307
    etiology of in childhood, 275
    evolving understanding of, 231
    frequency of in athletes, 283
    history of, 284
    landmark article on, 230
    mixed-type, 265-266, 283
    morphologic challenges of, 273-275
    morphologic variations leading to, 287
    pelvic pain and, 238-243
    prevention of, 291
    surgery for, 139, 238
        psoas retraction after, 137
    types of, 283
    with vulvodynia, 238-243
    work-up for, 247
femur
    cam bump on, 211
    development of, 209-210
    morphologic variations of, 287
    pistol grip deformity of, 231
    version of, 300, 312

fibrocartilage pubic plate, 74, 76-77
fibrocartilage pubic plate separation, 83-84
fitness, integrated with medicine, 9-10
fitness industry
    advertising culture of, 367
    deception in, 347
    new training techniques of, 15, 367
fluoroscopy, for deep derrière pain, 320
foot injuries, core muscle problems and, 414-417
function, restoring, 353
functional assessment, in osteopathic practice, 402-404
Functional Movement Screen (FMS), 396-397
functional performance measures, 361

Gaenslen test, 316
Gagne, Simon, injury of, 63
gait
    analysis of in evaluating posterior pain, 317-318
    patterns of with hip pathologies, 257
gait cycle, 306-307
Ganz, Reinhold, landmark FAI article of, 230, 284-285
Garciaparra, Nomar, groin injury of, 82, 94
Garrett, William, 25
gastrointestinal system, 174, 205
Gay, Tyson, 4, 6, 142
gender differences, anatomic, 48-50
genitourinary problems, benign and malignant, 174
Glick, Dr. James, 284
global movers, 371
global stabilizers, 371
glute-mede
    anatomy and functions of, 144
    injuries of, 145
gluteal (gluteus) muscles, 142, 149, 240
    injuries of, missing in hip arthroscopy, 251
gluteus maximus, 142
    anatomy of, 143
    claudication of, 322
    features of, 143
    functions of, 143
    size of, 143
    tear in, 168
gluteus minimus, 144
gluteus region, importance of, 141
goal-setting, practical, 332
Goldner, J. Leonard, 131-132
good shape, defining, 218-219-220
gracilis muscle, 106
greater trochanteric ischial impingement, 321
greater trochanteric pelvic impingement, 312, 315
    sciatic nerve and, 313

groin injuries, 22
    current literature on, 34-35
    ignorance about, 23-24
    seen as sports hernia, 31-34
groin pain
    changing patient profiles over 2 decades, 28
    Crohn's disease in, 174
    in cyclist, diagnosing, 198-199
    prospective studies on, 28
    thoracic movement disorder in, 366
    treatment of, 224
groin pulls, foot injuries in, 417
group-think problem, 33
growth, 208
    processes of, 331
    questions to consider regarding, 213
gynecologic problems, in pelvic pain, 65, 174, 424-425

Hamilton, Josh, core muscle avulsions of, 3-4
hamstring active test, 316, 319
hamstring origin avulsion, clinical and imaging features of, 322
hamstring origin tendon avulsion, 315
hamstring syndrome, 313
hamstring tendon pathologies, 314
hamstrings
    anatomy and functions of, 336
    chronic rupture of, 341
    importance of, 335
    injuries of
        current management of, 338-342
        early management approaches to, 338
        frequency of in athletes, 337-338
        surgical procedure for, 323
    nomenclature of, 338
    partial avulsion of, 166
    in posterior impingements, 313
    ruptured proximal, 335-340, 343
        case examples of, 342
        diagnosis and treatment algorithm for, 343
        management of, 340-341
        outcomes in, 342
    workouts for
        bad, 336
        good, 337
harness
    adjacent muscles and bones of, 87
    affecting pubic bone, 88-89
    in athleticism, 52-53, 82
    brain and, 87-88
    connections of, 87-88

at control center, 88
deep structure connections to, 87
definition of, 46, 86
direction of forces on, 86
function and malfunctions of, 82-84
importance of rectus abdominis muscle in, 97
injury of, 32, 84-85
    requiring surgery, 221
muscles of, 51-53, 149
protecting, 352-353
rectus abdominis in, 102

harness adductors
    injuries of, 115
    in protection of hip, 108

harness and bridle, 46
Hasek, Dominik, injury of, 105
head tilt deformity, 284
hernia repair, 218
    commercial interests in, 38
    inappropriate, 32
    success reported for, 27

heterotopic ossification
    adductor, 110-111
    postoperative, 250-251
    of rectus femoris, leading to hip impingement, 125

high-load strength-endurance movement test, 377
high-load test, 376
high-velocity-low-amplitude (HVLA) manipulation, 400, 408
Hill, Grant, 62
hip, 47
    anatomic variations of, 210-211
    anatomy of in femoroacetabular impingement, 281-282
    arthritis of, osteopathic manipulation for, 400
    arthro-endoscopic procedures around, 272
    biomechanics of, 306
        altered with core muscle injuries, 303-307
        in gait cycle, 306-307
    with core muscle injuries, 54-55, 222
    decreased rotation of in elbow problems, 417
    definition of, 46
    degeneration of, 284
    embryology of, 209-210
    exponential recognition of disorders of, independent forces on, 230-231
    harness adductors protecting, 108
    injuries of
        affecting adolescents, 253-266
        during spring training, 282-283
    intrinsic anatomical stabilization of, 151
    not knowing anatomy of, 171
    pubic bone connection to, 26
    tilt and version dynamics of, 250
    tissue layer components of, 151-152

hip/abductor injuries/weakness, 116, 395
hip arthroscopy
    in arthritic hip, 276
    arthro-endoscopic procedures of, 272
    in complex pediatric deformities, 275-276
    computerized navigation and robotics in, 270-271
    as developing field, 246
    eligible patients for, 248
    evolution of, 232-234
    failed, management for, 291
    for femoroacetabular impingement, 273-275, 284-285, 288-289, 291
        work-up for, 247
    frontiers in, 270
    hip dysplasia after, 245-246, 249
    for hip impingement with vulvodynia, 240
    hopes for, 248
    learning curve for, 248, 276-277
    limitations of, 273
    minimally invasive nature of, 284-285
    for painful total hip evaluation, 271-272
    for symptomatic hip dysplasia, 272
    traps of, 248-251
    for vulvodynia, 241-243

hip-core muscle interaction, 63
hip deformities
    active neglect in treatment of, 254
    in adolescents
        case studies of, 263-266
        clinical experience with, 255-262
        current treatment of, 255
        nomenclature for, 255
    complex pediatric, 275-276
    gait patterns in, 257

hip dysplasia
    case study of, 265
    evaluation and treatment of, 259
    hip arthroscopy for, 245-246, 249, 272

hip impingement, 54, 55
    causing nonoptimal movement patterns, 239
    cortisone injections for, 239
    diagnosis and surgery for, 426-427
    pelvic pain and, 238-243
    physical therapy for, 240
    protection against, 108
    psoas bursitis with, 137
    with rectus femoris heterotopic ossification, 125
    referred pain from, 239

surgery for, 240
    rectus femoris compartment syndrome complicating, 125
  with vulvodynia, diagnosis management flow chart for, 239
hip instability
  after hip arthroscopy, 249
  anatomical components of, 150-152
  definition of, 149-150
  road to, 147-148
hip joint, ball-and-socket, 11, 45, 47, 54
  chronic inflammation of with pelvic pain, 238-239
  complexity of, 284
  environment of, 285
  ossification of, 210
  as pain source, 195
hip pain
  etiology and diagnosis of, 389
  hip arthroscopy for, 271-272
  nonoperative management of, 390-392
hip replacement, total
  for hip/adductor injury, 116
  iliopsoas pain after, 135
  psoas stricture after, 138
hip-spine syndrome, 315
  clinical and imaging features of, 322
hip stability
  layer concept of, 150-152
  from tension, 211
homeostasis, 406
Hooke's law, 51
hoverboards, dangers of, 15
hydrodissection, 391

ice treatment, 427
iliacus hematoma syndrome, 262
iliacus muscles, 87, 130, 132, 134
  strain of, 166
iliopsoas muscle/tendon, arthro-endoscopic procedures on, 272
iliopsoas (psoas) muscle, 52-53, 149
  affected by foot injury, 417
  anatomy of, 130-131
  bursitis of, 159
    complex, 159
    with core muscle injury, 136
    with hip impingement, 137
    mimicking tumor, 159
    straightforward, 136
  in core stability, 135
  development and growth of, 212-213
  doing too much or too little to in hip arthroscopy, 250
  function of, 134
  impingement of, arthroscopic tenotomy for, 272
  injuries to, 129, 135-138
    femoroacetabular impingement surgery for, 139
    subtlety of, 135
    treatment algorithm for, 138-139
  irritation of
    with hip impingement, 239
    with paralabral cyst, 165
  location of, 130-134
  mysteriousness of, 130-132
  primary and secondary issues of, 138
  questions about, 139
  retraction of after femoroacetabular impingement surgery, 137
  sarcoma of, 158
  strength of, 134
  stricture of after total hip replacement, 138
iliopsoas syndrome, 404-405
iliotibial band, 150-152
imaging, 187-189. *See also* computed tomography (CT); magnetic resonance imaging (MRI); plain radiography
  for deep derrière pain, 320
  for femoroacetabular impingement, 288
  of hamstring injuries, 339-340
immune system, 205
impingements. *See also specific areas of*
  advantages and disadvantages of, 210-211
  tilt and, 299-300
inflammatory pelvic mass, 65
injury prevention, 213, 418-419
innominate out-flare, 410-411
instability, 150. *See also* core, instability of; hip instability
insurance companies
  issues of in misdiagnoses, 177
  labeling procedures as experimental, 218
Integrated Approach to the Thorax, 369
intercostal sensory pain, 99
internal rotation, excessive, 257
internal snapping hip syndrome, 213
interstitial tearing, 217
intrapelvic nerve entrapment, 315
ischemic compression, 408
ischial tuberosity apophysitis, 167
ischial tunnel syndrome, 313, 315
ischiofemoral impingement (IFI), 163, 250, 311
  clinical and imaging features of, 321
  femoral neck and lesser trochanter version with, 312
  patient history in, 314-315
  surgical procedure for, 323
  vs deep gluteal syndrome, 317-319

ischiofemoral impingement test, 317
ischiofemoral ligament strain, 315

Janda lower cross syndrome, 404
janushirasana, 387
joint mobility, restoration of, 410
joint "pop," 415-416

Kegel maneuvers, 384
key lesion, 406
kinematic chain, 311, 414, 416-419
kinesiology, definition of, 414
kinetic chain, 62, 160, 235, 239, 366, 369, 401, 404
King, Rob, hamstring workout of, 337
knee joint, connecting to foot and core muscles, 414-415
kosha model, 384
Krahn, Bryan, on finding right therapist, 347-348
Kriya, 384
Krzyzewski, Mike, 71

labral deficiency, 275
labral reconstruction, arthroscopic, 289
labral tears/detachment, 289, 315
    in adolescents, 260-261
    clinical and imaging features of, 322
    in dysplastic hips, 289
Landry, Carl, 120
Lee, David, 119
left rectus abdominis-adductor plate, 90
leg roll, 257
Legg-Calvé-Perthes disease (LCPD)
    case study of, 264
    challenges of, 276
    definition of, 255
    evaluation and treatment of, 258-259
life, wear and tear of, 217-218
ligamentum teres injury, missing in hip arthroscopy, 251
limitations, knowing your, 330-331
load, concept of, 360
load monitoring, 360
load transfer test, 375-377
locker room examinations, 176
long biceps femoris, long head of, 338
long-stride walking test, 316
low back pain, with excessive anterior pelvic tilt, 299
low-load test, 376
low-load transfer test, 377
Lowry, Kyle, mysterious injury of, 349-350
lumbar facet weightbearing test, 198
lumbar nerve root, pinched, 200
lumbar neutral zone, 373

lumbosacral plexus, 192
lymphatic issues, 175
lymphocele, retroperitoneal, 175

magnetic resonance imaging (MRI), 187-188
    for deep derrière pain, 320
    of hamstring injuries, 339-340
    T2 axial obliques sequence of, 189
massage, 408
McCarthy's flexion-extension maneuvers, 257
McElhinney, Curtis, 112
McKibbin instability index, 301
McNabb, Donovan, groin injury of, 31-32, 129
medical community
    ignorance of core in, 15, 17, 218
    integrated with fitness, 9-10
    specialization of, 8-10, 24
men, core anatomy of, 48-50
mesh plug, 166
mesh syndromes, 98
Meyers, Bill, 12
    athletic pubalgia article of, 230
microtraumatic injuries, 213
midline rectus abdominis-adductor plate, 90
Miller, Heath, 7
mind-body-energy connection, 385-386
mini-open surgical approach, for posterior pain issues, 323-324
modified Harris Hip Score, 353
Montana, Joe, 64
mosaicplasty, 273
movement, 18
    active and passive, 397
    categorizing, 360
    reduced variability of with injury, 366
    3 phases of, 351
muladhara, 386
muscle energy, 410
musculoskeletal core, 82
musculoskeletal overuse injuries, 213
myofascial release, 400, 408
myofascial slings, 352

Nadal, Rafael, injury of, 64
Nauli, 384
neck, connection of to core muscles, 414-415
nerve branches, messages transmitted along, 193
nerve entrapment syndromes, 99, 315
nerve fibers, covering body, 193
nerve plexus, 192

nerve roots
    as pain source, 195
    problems of, 198-199
nerves
    core, 191-200
    impingements of, 172
    as pain source, 195
    pinching of, 198
    recognizing more than one injury, 193-194
nervous system, 205. *See also* central nervous system (CNS); nerves; *specific nerves*
neurological cheat sheet, 196
neurological syndromes
    in pelvic pain, 173
    with rectus abdominis injury, 101-102
neurologists, characterizing and diagnosing pain, 195-196
neurophysiology, crucial concepts of, 192-194
neutral zone test, 373
Nippert, Howard, 89
nitroglycerin, topical, 391
nonoperative sports medicine physicians, perspectives of, 389-392
nonsequential muscle activation, 369
nonsteroidal anti-inflammatory drugs (NSAIDs), for proximal hamstring avulsion, 340
normal anatomic position, 70

Ober's test, 257
obstetric problems, in pelvic pain, 174
obturator nerves, in pelvic pain, 172, 196
optimal core health, magic formula for, 330-333
    application of, 333-334
optimizing body, for different purposes, 219-220
optimum load transfer strategies for trunk, 370
orthopedic surgeon, patient evaluation by, 184
osseous realignment, 410
ossification
    centers of, 210
    postoperative heterotopic, 250-251
osteitis, 83
osteitis pubis, 77
    definition of, 89-90
    imaging tests for, 188
    primary, 89-90
    as reactive process vs primary, 222
    secondary, 89-90
osteoarthritis, hip, 276
osteochondral allograft transplantation, 273
osteochondral defects, 273
osteoid osteoma, 160
osteopathic manipulation, categories of, 400

osteopaths, perspective of on core, 399-411
Oswalt, Roy, injury of, 61, 110
ovarian cysts, 174
Owens, Terrell, 43-44

pain. *See also specific sites of*
    anatomy of, 192
    characteristics of, 195
        cheat sheet for, 196
    diagnosing, 195-196
    with instability, 149-150
    limiting movement and agility, 366
    sources of, 194-195
    stereo, 194, 200
paralabral cyst, with psoas irritation, 165
PATCH technique, 418-419
patient factors, 221
patient history, 184-186
    in adolescent hip deformities, 256-257
    in osteopathic practice, 402
    in treatment plan, 360-361
patient's perspective, 423-428
pectineus, 25, 106
    avulsion of, 113
pectineus squeeze test, 360-361
pediatric deformities, complex, 275-276
pelvic bones, 45, 47
    development of, 209-210
pelvic examinations, 175
pelvic floor disorders, 175
pelvic floor muscles, 154-155
    exercises for, 384
    as pain source, 195
pelvic floor pain, patient's perspective on, 423-428
pelvic hernias, 9
pelvic inflammatory disease, 174
pelvic internal rotator tear, 224
pelvic muscles, deep posterior, 152-154
pelvic organs, as pain source, 195
pelvic pain
    femoroacetabular impingement and, 238-243
    lack of knowledge about, 169-170
    missing diagnosis of, 171-175
    nerves in, 192
    poor evaluation practices for, 175-177
pelvic rotational wink, 257
pelvic tilt, 285-287, 296
    anterior, 297, 299
    bad, 299-300
    extremes of, 298
    lateral, 297

posterior, 297
ways to think about, 286
when it matters, 297-298
pelvic varicosities, 174
pelvis
anatomy of, 10
biomechanics of, 296-301
bony, 195
female vs male, 49
medical ignorance about, 24
3 orientations of, 296
weak spots in, 54
percutaneous tenotomy, platelet-rich plasma and, 390
performance
difficulty correlating good core with, 396-397
principles of, 354
performance anxiety, 12
performance level, getting athlete back to, 354
periacetabular osteotomy, 255
peripheral muscle injury, self-healing, 222
peripheral nerves, 87
in pelvic pain, 172-173, 192
physical examination, 186
in adolescent hip deformities, 256-257
in treatment plan, 360-361
physical therapists, importance of, 345-346
physical therapy
for deep derrière pain, 320
myths about, 367-368
pincer deformities, 283
pincer impingement, 210
arthroscopy for, 289
tilt and, 299-300
piriformis muscle test, 319
active, 317
passive seated, 316
piriformis stretch test, 319
piriformis syndrome, 161, 272
pistol grip deformity, 231, 284
pitchers, elbow injuries in, 417
pitcher's vertebral stress reaction, 162
plain radiography, 187
for deep derrière pain, 320
of hamstring injuries, 339
plank transition test, 376
plantar fasciitis, with core muscle injuries, 417
plate injuries, Roedl classification of, 90
platelet-rich plasma (PRP), 110, 205, 222, 390
plyometric exercise, 397
positional release therapy, 409

posterior femoroacetabular impingement, 315
clinical and imaging features of, 322
posterior impingement test, 288
posterior rim impingement test, 317
posture
in back pain, 395
default, 354
reinforcing correct, 354
of yoga, 383
power, harnessing, 352
power muscles
central harness and, 51-52
control of, 52-53
injuries of, 222
prolotherapy, 391
proprioception, 397, 418
proximal hamstring avulsion, 343
case examples of, 342
diagnosis and evaluation of, 338-339
imaging of, 339-340
management of, 340-341
outcomes for, 342
proximal hamstring tendinopathy, 342
chronic, 338
proximal hamstring tendon avulsion, 337-340
psoas muscle. *See* iliopsoas (psoas) muscle
psoas snap, 261
pubic area, taboos about, 72
pubic body, definition of, 89-90
pubic bone, 10
in athleticism, 82
balance of forces around, 78
baseball model of, 73-74
as center of core, 35, 72, 88-89, 204
reasons for not accepting, 36-39
at center of normal anatomic position, 70-71
changes in with age and soft tissue injury, 27
core muscles surrounding, 75
evolution of, 71
fibrocartilage cover of, 73-74, 86
fibrous dysplasia of, 160
functions of, 69-70
gross anatomy of, 73-76
harness and, 88-89
interactions with surrounding, 89
microscopic anatomy of, 77-78
muscular attachments to, 78
pain sites around, 25
stresses on, 89

pubic bone joint, 73
    connection to hip, 26
    stabilizing muscles of, 25
pubic bone marrow edema, 188
pubic complex, 25
pubic pain
    common sources of, 404-406
    manual therapies for, 401
    old diagnosis and treatment of, 401
    osteopathic diagnosis of, 402-406
    osteopathic treatment for, 406-410
    treatment algorithm for, 407
pubic plate
    adductor attachments onto, 107
    normal and injured, 84
    progression of injury to, 91
pubic plate separation, 83-85, 188
pubic ramus
    definition of, 89-90
    osteoid osteoma of, 160
pubic shear, 406
    super, 410
pubic symphyseal joint, 73
    disruption of, 89
pubic symphysis
    definition of, 89-90
    formation of symphyseal capsule of, 211
pubic symphysis stress test, 360-361
pudendal nerve
    entrapment of, 315
    irritation of, clinical and imaging features of, 321
    issues of, 314
    in pelvic pain, 172

Q angle, 48
quadratus femoris strain, 163
quadratus lumborum strain, 164
quadriceps mechanism, 122

radiofrequency ablation, 392
rectus abdominis/adductor muscles, development and growth of, 212-213
rectus abdominis compartment syndrome, 98
rectus abdominis diastasis, 100-101
rectus abdominis hematoma, 95
rectus abdominis muscle, 52-53, 73-74, 94, 149
    abuse of, 96
    atrophy of, 97-98
    avulsions of, 99-100
    development of, 211
    endometrioma of, 157
    hip joint and, 26
    importance of in harness, 97, 102
    injuries of, 93-94
    parts of, 95
    problems with, 97-102
    subtleties of, 96
    surgeon's knowledge of, 97
    tears of, 99
    torn at attachment, 115
    tumors of, 102
    variable anatomy of, 97
    weakened, 25
rectus femoris compartment syndrome, complicating hip impingement surgery, 125
rectus femoris muscle, 149
    acute complete avulsion of, 122-123
    anatomy of, 122
    avulsion of, 166
        complete, return to full play after, 126
        complete, without repair, with other injuries, 124
        fixing, 222
        heterotopic ossification following, 125
        indirect head, 124
        proximal, routine nonoperative treatment of, 121-122
        repairs of with good results, 123
        second complete after first untreated, 123
    heterotopic ossification of leading to hip impingement, 125
    indirect head tear of, 165
    injuries to, 119-120, 122-126
        treatment algorithm for, 126-127
    size and position of, 102-121
    surgeons' lack of respect for, 121-122
reductionism, 400-401, 408-410
referral bias, 177
reflex sympathetic dystrophy, 194
rehabilitation
    acute phase of, 361-362
    current practice in, 359-363
    final stage of, 357-363
    first part of, 357
    in literature on core, 395
    old way of, 359
    of Olympic diver, 358-359
    principles, 351-353
    subacute stage of, 361-362
return to play
    early, 353
    full
        criteria for, 361
        getting to, 354, 357-363

return-to-play therapy, 362
rib cage wiggle test, 374
right rectus abdominis-adductor plate, 90
robotics, for cam resections, 270-271
Rose, Derrick, injury of, 60-61
rower's rib syndrome, 99

sacral stress fracture, 161
sacroiliac distraction test, 316
sacroiliac joint
    pain/dysfunction of, 199, 315
        clinical and imaging features of, 322
    septic arthritis of, 161
sacroiliac joint lateral compression test, 317
sacrotuberous ligament avulsion, 315
sartorius strain, 165
scammers, 331, 348
scar tissue, 418-419
Schilders whole-mounts, 77
sciatic nerve, 313
    decompression of, 272
    entrapment of, 315
        clinical and imaging features of, 321
        patient history in, 314
    impingement of, 321
    in pelvic pain, 172
    rehabilitation exercises for, 323
seated trunk rotational range of motion test, 375
segmental deep multifidus test, 375
self-knowledge, 332
semimembranosus tendon, 338
semitendinosus tendon, 338
sequential activation, 351
set position, 71
sex, 17
    pubic bone and, 69
shock wave therapy
    extracorporeal, 392
    for proximal hamstring avulsion, 340
    vs platelet-rich plasma, 390
Shockey, Jeremy, 6
short leg syndrome, 405-406
short limb dip, 257
sitting
    in pelvic tilt problems, 299
    in posterior pain, 314
6-pack abs, focus on, 96
Slinky movement model, 50-51, 370, 372
slipped capital femoral epiphysis (SCFE), 266
    in adolescents, 253-254
    case studies of, 263
    cheilectomy for, 230
    definition of, 255
    evaluation and treatment of, 258
    treatment of, 275
slot angle, 417
Smith, Brad, 113
snake oil salesperson, 346
snapping hip syndrome, 213
    in adolescents, 261-262
soft tissue manipulation, 400, 408
specialists
    approach of to patient evaluation, 184
    in diagnosing pelvic pain, 425
    involved in core health, 330-331
    narrow knowledge of, 24
    working with sports injuries, 415
specific adaptations to imposed demands (SAIDs), 360
spermatic cord lipoma, mesh plug and, 166
spicules, 77
spigelian syndrome, 101
spinal loading, incorrect, 395
spinal manipulative therapy, 408
spinal nerve roots, as pain source, 171-172, 195
spinal stabilization exercises, 395
spine
    disorders of in posterior pain, 315
    muscles around, 51-52
    in pelvic pain, 171-172
spine core stability, 373-374
sports hernia, 7
    core muscle injuries seen as, 31-34
    misdiagnosing, 27
    rejection of term, 430-431
sports hip disorders, exponential recognition of, 230-231
sports injuries, 21
    early specialization in, 213
stability, 148-149. *See also* core, stability of; hip stability
    defining, 149-150
    before mobility, 352
    muscle groups in, 152-155
    spine core, 373-374
    thoracospinal, 374-375
stabilizers, 395
    dynamic and static, 285
    pelvic, 149, 234
    of thorax, 370, 371
standing, in pelvic tilt problems, 299
steroid injections, 222-223
    for deep derrière pain, 320
    for proximal hamstring avulsion, 340

straight leg raise test, 200
    active, 374
        compressions and decompressions with, 374
streaming, 360
strength coaches, importance of, 345-346
strength test, 377
strike zone, xxiii
structural exam, in osteopathic practice, 402-404
structural reductionism, 400-401
    layer by layer, 408-410
suboptimal consultations, 176
surgeons, patient evaluation by, 184
synovial cell sarcoma, 65
Szaro, Richie, core injury of, 11, 23

tender points, 409
tendinopathy
    extracorporeal shock wave therapy for, 392
    prolotherapy for, 391
    topical nitroglycerin for, 391
tensor fasciae latae, 150-152
terminal ileum, thickening of, 157
testing, active and passive, 186
therapies, cataloging, 332-333
therapist
    clients of, 348
    colleagues of, 348
    finding right, 347-349
    flexibility of, 348
    training of, 348
    ultra-aggressive, 348
thigh thrust test, 316
"things we cannot unsee" theory, 36-38
thoracic movement disorder, 366
thoracic neutral zone, 373
thoracic rigidity, 374
thoracic ring, 369
thoracic Slinky, 370, 372
thoracic spine, as stable and stiff, 368
thoracic system, active and passive, 371
thoracospinal stability, 374-375
thorax, 365, 378
    anatomy of, 370-371
    assessment techniques for, 373-377
    biomechanics of, 371-372
    conceptualizing, 50-51
    deep core muscles of, 375
    deep stabilizers of, 371
    global movers of, 371
    global stabilizers of, 371
    optimum load transfer of, 370
    ring structure of, 372

3-dimensional imaging, in hip arthroplasty, 270-271
tilt, 296
    bad, 299-300
    types of, 297
    when it matters, 297-298
Tommy John surgery, 417
traction, for ischiofemoral impingement, 323
training methods, dangerous, 15
transversus abdominis test, 375
Trendelenburg gait, 54, 257
Trendelenburg sign, positive, 318
trigger points, 409
    injections into, 410
trochanteric bursitis, 425-426
truncal displacement, lateral, 397
trunk, optimum load transfer strategies for, 370
tumors
    in pelvic pain, 173
    rectus abdominis, 102

ulnar collateral ligament tear, 417
ultrasound, 187
upright posture
    evolutionary and embryonic processes in, 212-213
    pelvic tilt problems and, 298-299
uterine fibroid, 161
uterine fibrosis, infarcted, 174

vascular disease, in pelvic pain, 174
Verlander, Justin, 61
version, 296, 300-301
    acetabular, 300-301
    femoral, 300
    in ischiofemoral impingement, 312
vertebral body stress reaction, 162
vertebral column, muscles around, 50-51
vertebral disc extrusion, 163
vulvodynia, 238
    arthroscopy for, 241-243
    diagnosis management flow chart for, 239
    hip impingement and, 238, 243
    pelvic floor and hip physical therapy for, 241

weightlifter's syndromes, 101
wet needling, 410
wind-removing pose, 387
Wojtys, Dr. Edward, 213
women, core anatomy of, 48-50
workout regimes, overly aggressive, 220

X-ray, 187

yoga
- benefits of, 383-384
- in clinical practice, 384-386
- core muscle example of, 387
- definition of, 383
- history of, 382
- holistic philosophy of, 384
- injury prevention in, 388
- modern, 382-383
- NFL advocate of, 386
- physical injuries occurring in, 387
- potentially dangerous, 381
- preventing injury in, 386-387
- in professional baseball, 384-385
- world championships and, 385
- yang of, 385-386
- yin of, 386-387

young adult hip surgery subspecialty, 255

Zimmerman, Ryan, rectus abdominis injury of, 93-94